ANNALS OF THE NEW YORK ACADEMY OF SCIENCES

Volume 637
December 12, 1991

THE MALE GERM CELL: SPERMATOGONIUM TO FERTILIZATION[a]

Editor
BERNARD ROBAIRE

AF851160

Scientific Organizing Committee
ANDRZEJ BARTKE, KEVIN J. CATT, YVES CLERMONT, CLAUDE DESJARDINS, MARIA DUFAU, E. MITCH EDDY, LARRY L. EWING (deceased), NORMAN HECHT, DOLORES J. PATANELLI, BERNARD ROBAIRE (Chairman), RICHARD SHERINS, and ELIZABETH WILSON

CONTENTS

[a] This volume is the result of The XIth North American Testis Workshop, which was entitled **The Male Germ Cell: Spermatogonium to Fertilization** and held by McGill University in Montréal, Québec on April 24–27, 1991. The workshop was dedicated to the memory of Larry L. Ewing.

Part III. Hormonal Control of Testicular Function

Part IV. Structure and Function of Germ Cell Organelles

ANNALS OF THE NEW YORK ACADEMY OF SCIENCES

THE MALE GERM CELL: SPERMATOGONIUM TO FERTILIZATION

♾ *The paper used in this publication meets the minimum requirements of American National Standard for Information Sciences—Permanence of Paper for Printed Library Materials, ANSI Z39.48-1984.*

The drawing on the softcover version of this volume was made by Margo Orltzschner from a design by Yves Clermont. It represents the life span of a spermatozoon, from its initiation in a seminiferous tubule, to its maturation in the epididymis and finally to its interaction with the zona pellucida of the egg and fertilization.

Library of Congress Cataloging-in-Publication Data

The Male germ cell : spermatogonium to fertilization / edited by Bernard Robaire.
p. cm.—(Annals of the New York Academy of Sciences, ISSN 0077-8923 ; v. 637)
Result of the XIth North American Testis Workshop held by McGill University in Montréal, Québec on April 24–27, 1991.
Includes bibliographical references and index.
ISBN 0-89766-709-3 (cloth : alk. paper). — ISBN 0-89766-710-7 (paper : alk. paper)
1. Spermatogenesis—Congresses. I. Robaire, Bernard. II. McGill University. III. North American Testis Workshop (11th : 1991 : Montréal, Québec) IV. Series.
[DNLM: 1. Spermatogenesis—physiology—congresses. 2. Spermatogonia—physiology—congresses. 3. Testis—physiology—congresses. W1 AN626YL v. 637 / WJ 834 M245 1991]
Q11.N5 vol. 637
[QL966] 500 s—dc20 [599'.0166]
DNLM/DLC
for Library of Congress 91-38987
CIP

46

CCP
Printed in the United States of America
ISBN 0-89766-709-3 (cloth)
ISBN 0-89766-710-7 (paper)
ISSN 0077-8923

Part V. Specific Gene Expression During Spermatogenesis

Part VI. Cell-Cell Interactions in Seminiferous Tubules

Part VII. The Epididymis: Site for Sperm Maturation

Part VIII. Post-Epididymal Changes in Spermatozoa

This workshop was supported by grants from:

- Fonds de la Recherche en Santé du Québec
- Medical Research Council of Canada
- National Institute of Child Health and Human Development

Other financial assistance was received from:

- Genetics and IVF Institute
- Hoffmann-La Roche Inc.
- Merck Frosst Canada
- Pharmascience Inc.
- The R.W. Johnson Pharmaceutical Research Institute
- Serono Canada
- Sterling Drug Inc.

Dedicated to

LARRY L. EWING

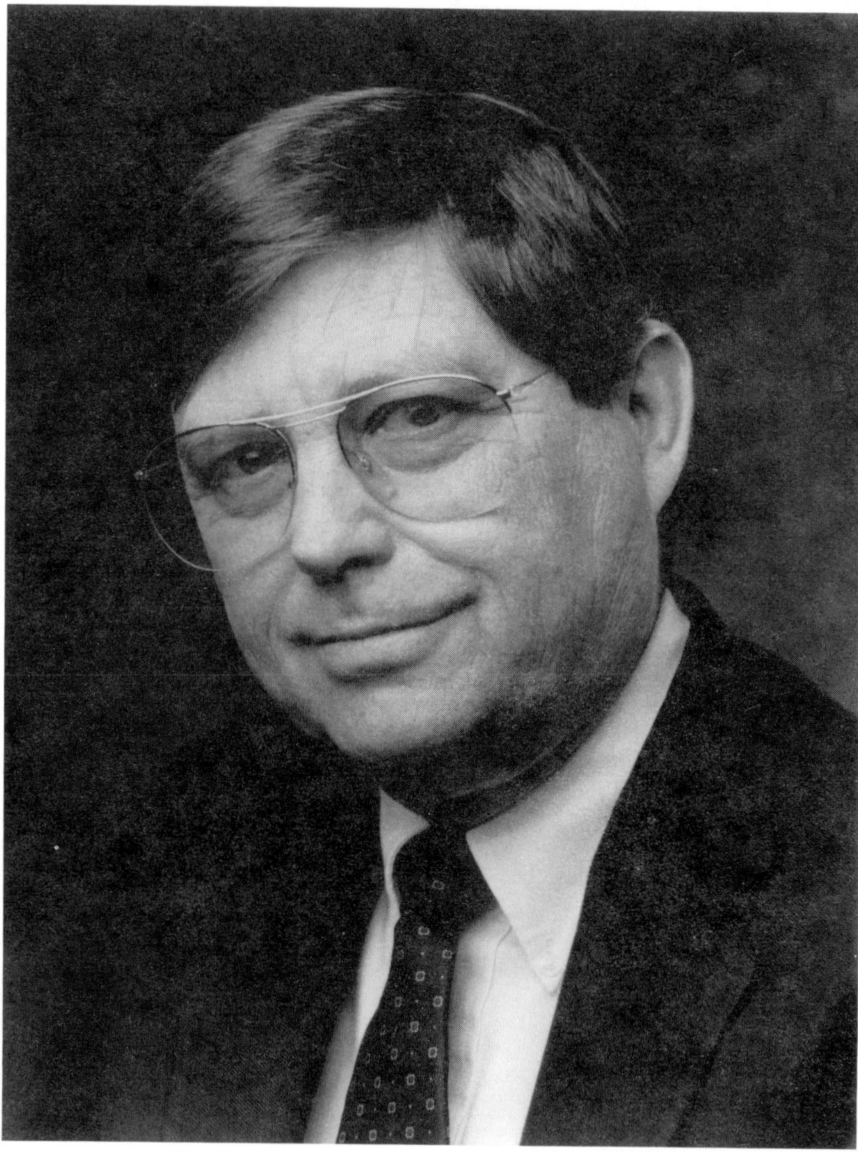

Dedication

On August 13, 1990, Larry L. Ewing died suddenly. His untimely death has created a void in the hearts of the many scientists who knew him well and respected him for his honesty, his breadth and depth of knowledge about male reproduction, and his sincere concern for his students, colleagues and friends.

At the time of his death, Larry was Professor, Division of Reproductive Biology, The Johns Hopkins School of Hygiene and Public Health. Larry's contributions to the scientific community went well beyond the major scientific accomplishments outlined in the first chapter of this volume. They included his service and commitment to several scientific societies, participation in numerous government task forces, and active involvement on many peer review panels. Most notably, he was a Founding Member of the Society for the Study of Reproduction, and became its President and Editor of its journal (*Biology of Reproduction*). He was also President of the American Society of Andrology. Since 1981, Larry served on the organizing committee of the Testis Workshop. He planned and hosted the Tenth Workshop in Baltimore in December 1988. His contributions were pivotal to making the present workshop a success.

Larry's absence was deeply felt during the Workshop by all the participants. This volume is dedicated to his memory.

Preface

The conference represented by this volume was the Eleventh North American Testis Workshop. It was held April 24–27, 1991 and was hosted by McGill University in Montréal, Québec, Canada.

The meeting opened with a talk delivered by Barry Zirkin celebrating the scientific contributions of Larry Ewing. A personalized view of the major developments, over the last four decades, in the field of research on the testis was then presented by Yves Clermont—a prime mover in our present-day understanding of the process of spermatogenesis. The last component of the plenary session focused on the major breakthroughs recently made in the mechanism of steroid hormone action.

Several major concepts were presented during the meeting. First, the complex regulation of spermatogenesis was made apparent. The genetic factors determining when the testis will and will not develop are being elucidated. A clear understanding of the nature of the species differences with respect to the role played by specific hormones in allowing spermatogenesis to take place is developing. Second, the intimate relationships between structure and function in the formation of the intricate organelles that constitute spermatozoa became strikingly apparent in the elegant presentations on the nuclear matrix and annulus, cytoskeletal elements and the acrosome. Third, the extent to which spermatozoa possess specific genes that are expressed in a highly controlled manner was underscored by studies on protamine and homeobox genes. Fourth, the intricate, site specific changes that take place in the epididymis and the potential ways these changes allow for the maturation of spermatozoa was highlighted. Finally, assessment of the value of computer aided semen analysis, the molecular events underlying the acrosome reaction and sperm-egg interaction, provided valuable insights in the significance of new technologies and newly discovered molecules.

This Workshop would not have been possible without the major financial support of the NICHD, MRC (Canada), FRSQ (Québec), Serono (Canada) as well as several other corporate sponsors. There are many individuals who provided major support and encouragement in the preparation of the meeting and this volume. In addition to the members of the local arrangements committee, I should like to express my special appreciation to Larry L. Ewing (deceased), D. J. Patanelli, R. Sherins, K. J. Catt and B. Hales, as well as to those who so skillfully helped assemble and bring to press this volume: Bill Boland, Sheila Kane, and Joyce Hitchcock.

BERNARD ROBAIRE

A Thirst for Science: An Overview of the Scientific Contributions of Larry L. Ewing (1936–1990)

BARRY R. ZIRKIN

Division of Reproductive Biology
The Johns Hopkins University
School of Hygiene and Public Health
Baltimore, Maryland 21205

BERNARD ROBAIRE

Department of Pharmacology and Therapeutics
Centre for the Study of Reproduction
McGill University
Montréal, Québec, Canada H3G 1Y6

INTRODUCTION

The scientific contributions of Larry L. Ewing spanned many areas of the male reproductive system. His excitement about research, his own as well as that of others, and his drive to pursue an objective, whether it was testing a novel concept, a technically complex study, or the resolution of a scientific question, were the hallmarks of his approach to science. Our objective in this chapter is to highlight the remarkable scientific contributions that Larry made, throughout his career, to our knowledge of the male reproductive system with particular emphasis on testicular function and structure.

Larry was born in Valley, Nebraska in 1936. With his wife, Aggie, he left Valley in 1954 to begin undergraduate work at the University of Nebraska, graduating in 1958 with a B.Sc. from the University of Nebraska School of Agriculture. He then entered a graduate program in reproductive physiology in the Department of Dairy Science at the University of Illinois, where he studied with Noland VanDemark. When Larry joined the VanDemark laboratory, he was asked what he wished to study. Having just read an article on organ perfusion, he immediately responded that he wanted to develop methods for maintaining the normal function of the testis by *in vitro* perfusion. In 1962, four years after he began graduate work, he had met the first of his many scientific goals and received the Ph.D. degree.

The first of the three publications that resulted from Larry's thesis[1] was entitled "Factors affecting testicular metabolism and function. 1. A simplified perfusion technique for short-term maintenance of rabbit testis." This paper was the beginning of Larry's life-long contribution to the understanding of testicular function. In it, he first described the development of "a simple and inexpensive apparatus for perfusing the mammalian testis" (FIG. 1). To examine the regulation of Leydig cells, Larry was to use testicular perfusion (along with numerous other methods) throughout his scientific

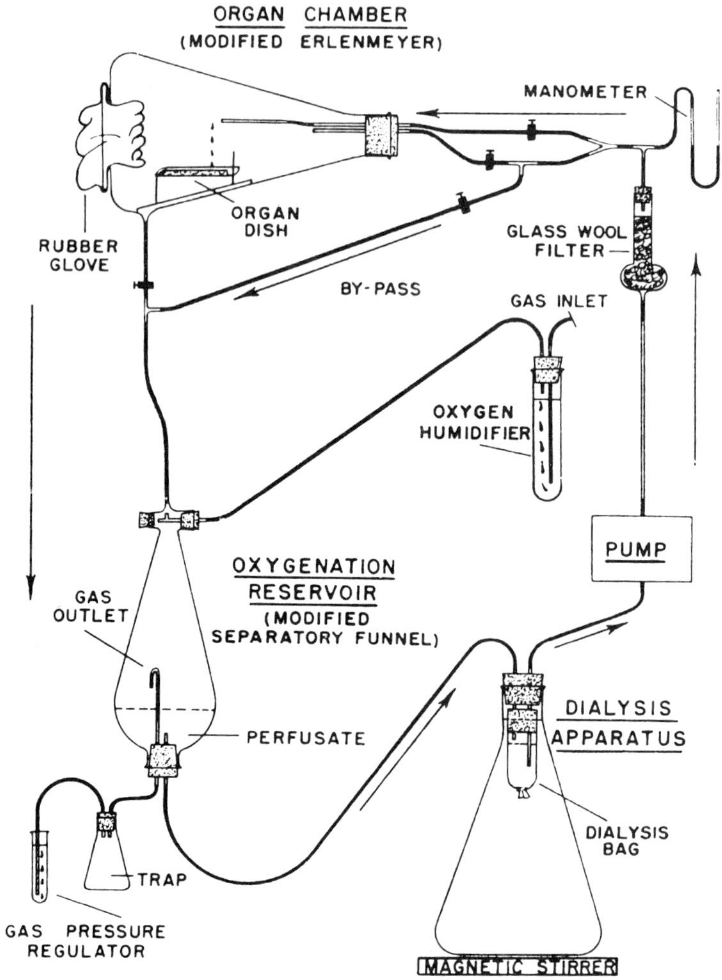

FIGURE 1. Apparatus used in perfusing isolated rabbit testes. (From ref. 1, reprinted with permission.)

career. He recognized that the power of the perfusion method was that it allowed an investigator to examine testicular function apart from extratesticular influence, but without compromising the three-dimensional architecture of the testis.

In 1962, immediately after completing his Ph.D., Larry accepted the position of Assistant Professor at Oklahoma State University. He was then 26 years old.The first of what would be his numerous successful NIH grant applications, entitled "The effect of stress and aging on testicular metabolism," was funded shortly thereafter. Contributions to the topic of aging of the male reproductive system spanned Larry's entire career from his first grant and first single-authored manuscript[2] to his most recent

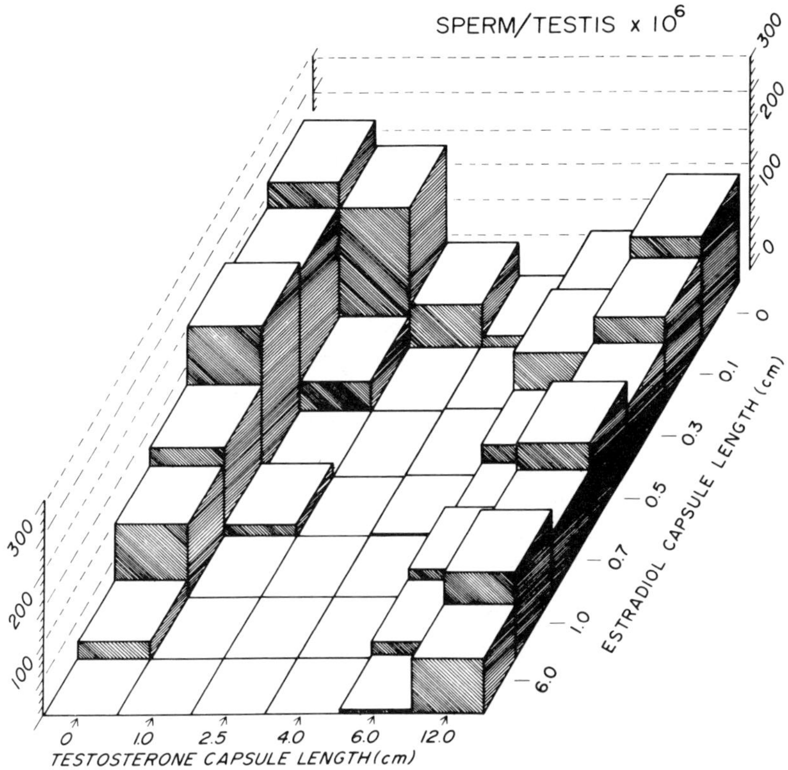

FIGURE 2. Effect of testosterone alone, estradiol alone or combinations of testosterone and estradiol on the number of sperm (condensed spermatids/spermatozoa) in adult rat testes. Animals were treated for three months with subcutaneous polydimethylsiloxane implants of various lengths filled with either testosterone or estradiol as indicated in the figure. Each bar represents the mean of values obtained from six different animals.

program grant from the National Institute on Aging entitled "Aging and male reproductive tract structure and function."

Having accepted his first academic appointment without the benefit of postdoctoral training, Larry took a leave from Oklahoma State University in 1965 to become a postdoctoral trainee with Eik-Nes at the University of Utah. The work he conducted with Eik-Nes[3] demonstrated that testosterone could be synthesized from steroid precursors by the perfused rabbit testis. Furthermore, testosterone production was found to be responsive to gonadotropins and could be maintained for several hours *in vitro*.

In 1968, Larry again took a leave from Oklahoma State University to become a Special Research Fellow at The Johns Hopkins School of Medicine in the Department of Pharmacology and Experimental Therapeutics. There he worked with Guy Williams-Ashman. One paper,[4] entitled "Protein phosphokinase reactions in mammalian testis. Stimulatory effects of adenosine 3′:5′-cyclic monophosphate on the phosphorylation of basic proteins" resulted from this leave. Far more importantly, Larry became excited

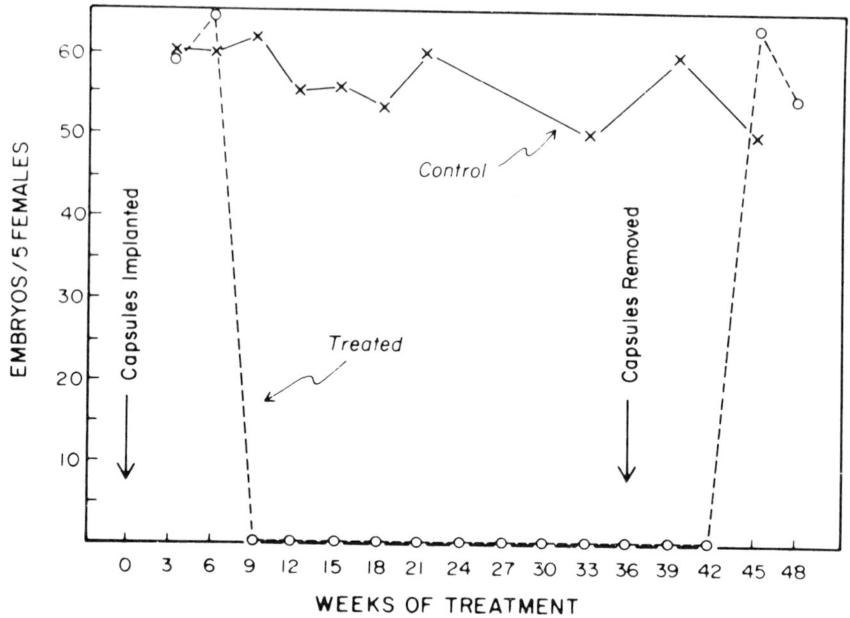

FIGURE 3. The temporal effect of 2.5 cm testosterone-0.1 cm estradiol implants on fertility of male rats. X---X equals 1 control male rat. O----O equals 1 treated rat. Each male was cohabited with 5 females for 20 days. Five different females were provided for each male every 3 weeks. (From ref. 9, reprinted with permission.)

by the environment at Hopkins, an environment that he would later join. He also first met Donald Coffey, then an Assistant Professor, who was to have a great deal to do with attracting Larry to Hopkins, and with whom Larry would interact extensively throughout his scientific career.

When Larry returned to Oklahoma, he began a long, extremely fruitful collaboration with Claude Desjardins on the regulation of Leydig cell function and of spermatogenesis. In 1973, they demonstrated, for the first time, that the administration of appropriate doses of testosterone to rabbits, via sustained release Silastic capsules, could cause azoospermia.[5] Subsequently, however, this complete suppression of spermatogenesis by the appropriate sustained release dose of testosterone was found not to occur in other species; rather, a partial suppression was obtained in both rats and monkeys.[6-9]

To obtain greater suppression of spermatogenesis, Larry, along with Claude Desjardins and Bernard Robaire, decided to enhance the inhibitory action of testosterone on luteinizing hormone (LH) secretion by the hypothalamo-pituitary axis by adding a small dose of the most potent biologically active suppressor of LH secretion then known, estradiol. A dramatic synergistic interaction on the suppression of spermatogenesis and LH was found (FIG. 2).[7,8] This synergistic combination of testosterone and estradiol made rats reversibly infertile (FIG. 3) without changing their sexual or aggressive behavior.[9] These observations on the rat were extended to the monkey[10,11] and have been used as a model to study the consequences of selectively shutting off

Leydig cells. Ultimately, the work resulted in a patent for the administration of testosterone and estradiol via sustained release devices to cause azoospermia, and thus male contraception. Larry's interest in contraception persisted to the end of his career. At the time of his death, he was testing, in collaboration with Richard Sherins,[12] the use of injectable slow release testosterone microspheres as a method for contraception in human males. Hopefully, this work will continue and be brought to fruition.

After 10 years at Oklahoma State University, Larry was attracted, in 1972, to Johns Hopkins University as Professor in the Department of Population Dynamics at the School of Hygiene and Public Health. He became the first Head of a newly created Division of Reproductive Biology within the Department. Among the first papers that Larry published from Hopkins[13] was one entitled "Formation and secretion of 5α-androstan-17β-ol-3-one, 5α-androstan-3α,17β-diol and 5α-androstan-3β,17β-diol by the perfused rabbit testis epididymis." In this paper, tritiated testosterone was infused into the artery of the isolated testis-epididymis, and the testosterone metabolites 5α-androstan-17β-ol-3-one (DHT), 5α-androstan-3α,17β-diol (3α-diol) and 5α-androstan-3β,17β-diol (3β-diol) were measured. The results showed that substantial quantities of testosterone, biosynthesized within the testis-epididymis, are converted to metabolites that are secreted into the venous effluent.

Larry's interests in the formation of 5α-reduced metabolites extended beyond the testis. With Bernard Robaire and Barry Zirkin, he demonstrated that the enzyme responsible for the formation of 5α-reduced androgens, 4-ene steroid 5α-reductase, was regulated, in the epididymis, not only by circulating androgens but also in a paracrine manner, *i.e.*, by factor(s) secreted directly into the epididymis from the testis via the efferent ducts.[14]

Larry's contributions to our understanding of the androgen microenvironment of the epididymis, as well as that of the testis, was extended in a series of papers with Terry Turner and his colleagues.[15–17] Using a combination of methods, including micropuncture, they established that there is a rapid fall in the intraluminal concentration of testosterone and a rise in dihydrotestosterone as one moves from the testis to the epididymis.

The biological significance of the presence of 5α-reduced androgens in some androgen-dependent tissues but not others fascinated Larry. He developed a close collaboration with Donald Coffey and Steve Berry to study the androgen dependence of prostatic growth and development of benign prostatic hyperplasia in the dog. They carefully sorted out the differential effects of age and of various androgens on the development of benign prostatic hyperplasia in the beagle, the best-defined model of this disease.[18–20] With Patrick Walsh, Larry tackled the issue of whether dihydrotestosterone is in fact elevated in human prostatic hyperplasia. In what has become a classical paper, they presented convincing evidence that the content of this steroid was not any higher in hyperplastic than in control tissue.[21]

With his interest in testosterone production and secretion, Larry's attention next turned to the mechanism by which testosterone escapes from the Leydig cell. With Curtis Chubb and Bernard Robaire, evidence was obtained (FIG. 4) that the diffusion of steroids from the Leydig cell was enhanced by the presence of steroid-binding macromolecules in the blood.[22] Furthermore, since the non-secreted steroid was not accumulated in the tissue, they concluded that testosterone had to feedback inhibit its own synthesis (FIG. 5). This important paper provided the first experimental evidence that the passage of steroids from the Leydig cells was facilitated by extracellular steroid-binding proteins and that the biosynthesis of testosterone was autoregulatory.

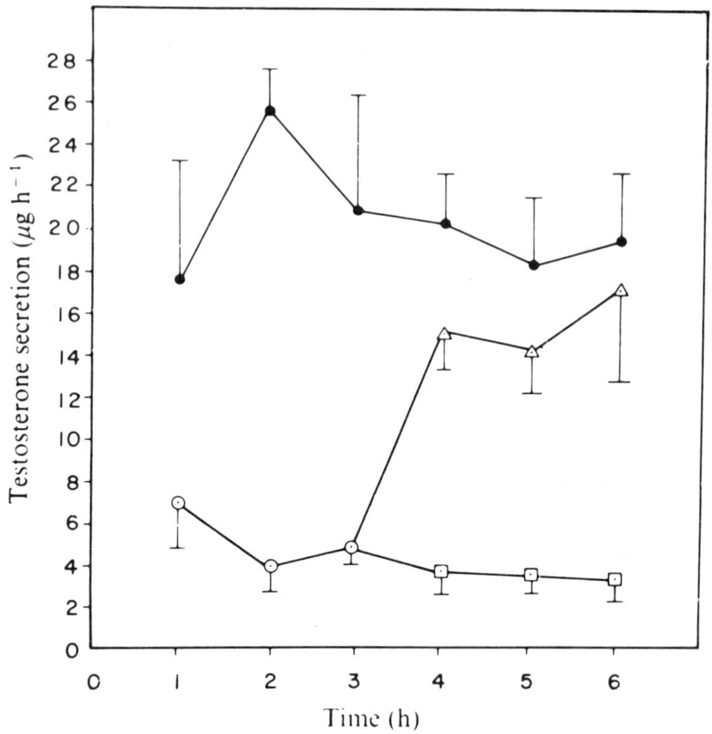

FIGURE 4. Testosterone secretion by rabbit testes minus epididymides perfused *in vitro* with medium containing either 3% (w/v) fraction V BSA or 3% (w/v) Dextran. ●, 10 testes perfused with medium containing fraction V BSA for 6 h; ○, 20 testes perfused with the medium containing Dextran for the first, second and third hours of a 6-h perfusion experiment; △, 10 testes switched to medium containing fraction V BSA during the fourth, fifth and sixth hours of perfusion. The latter 10 testes were from the same rabbits that furnished the contralateral testes simultaneously perfused with medium containing fraction V BSA for 6 h. □, 10 testes not switched but perfused with medium containing Dextran for 6 h. The line above or below each point represents the standard error of the mean. (From ref. 22, reprinted with permission.)

Larry's contributions to knowledge about the regulation of the Leydig cell continued unabated through the 1970s and 1980s. In 1979 and 1980, he and Curtis Chubb published a series of classical papers that dealt with alternative metabolic pathways, in different species, for the biosynthesis of testosterone from pregnenolone.[23-26] In one study,[25] they examined the preferred testosterone biosynthetic pathways in rat and rabbit testes; these studies were based on the concept that the activity of steroidogenic reactions could be determined by measuring the secretion products of testes perfused *in vitro* while the testes were infused with steroidogenic reaction inhibitors and testosterone biosynthetic intermediates. The results of their studies indicated that preferred testosterone biosynthetic pathways exist and are different in different species (FIG. 6).

Leydig cell regulation studies in Larry's laboratory set out in a new direction in

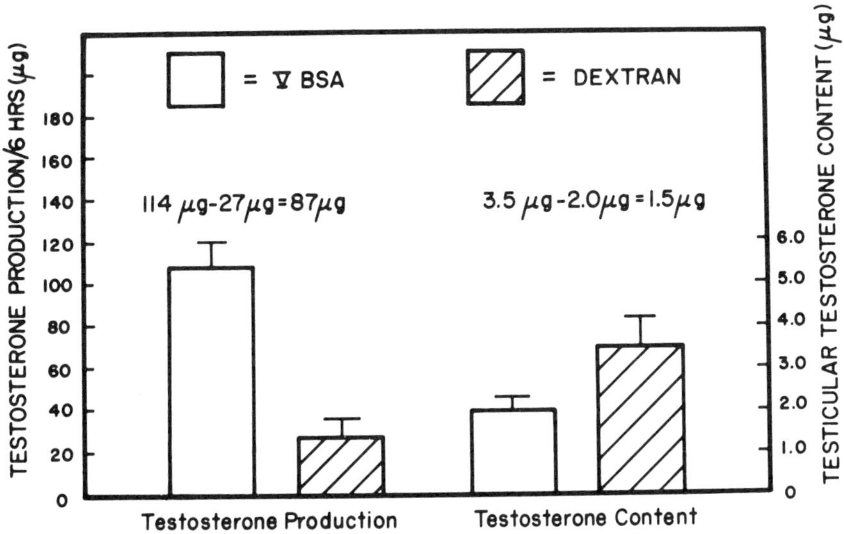

FIGURE 5. Testosterone production rate per 6 hours and testosterone content of the same testes after a 6-h perfusion period of adult rabbit testes with a solution containing either fraction V bovine serum albumin (V BSA) or Dextran. The open bars (±SEM) represent the means of values obtained from 10 adult rabbit testes perfused with the V BSA solution, while the hatched bars (±SEM) represent the means for the contralateral testes of each animal perfused with Dextran.

the later 1970s. After perfusing testes from the guinea pig, rabbit, dog, rat and hamster *in vitro* with maximally stimulating LH concentrations, Larry made the observation that there were major between-species differences in testosterone secretion which could not be explained on the basis of differences in testis weight. In collaboration with Barry Zirkin, stereological methods were used to show that differences in testosterone secretion could not be explained by species differences in Leydig cell mass, but rather by the amount of smooth endoplasmic reticulum in the Leydig cells.[27] Indeed, they established that there was a linear, positive correlation between the ability of Leydig cells in the five species studied to produce testosterone in response to LH and the amount of smooth endoplasmic reticulum of the Leydig cells (FIG. 7).[28]

With the results of this "experiment of nature," Ewing and Zirkin hypothesized that experimental inhibition of testosterone secretion would be reflected in quantitative changes in Leydig cell morphology. The recovery of steroidogenesis following removal of steroidogenic inhibition should also be coupled, then, to morphological changes in the Leydig cell. To test these hypotheses with the model developed earlier by Larry and his colleagues, rats were implanted with testosterone-estradiol capsules for the purpose of suppressing Leydig cell function and spermatogenesis. At intervals after the capsules were implanted, the testosterone secretion rate was examined in one testis from each rat, and stereological analyses of Leydig cell number and structure were done with the contralateral testes. A similar protocol was used to examine the recovery of steroidogenic capacity, *i.e.*, previously implanted capsules were removed, and testes were examined for renewed testosterone production and morphology at regular intervals thereafter. The results of these studies[29] showed clearly that significant, linear

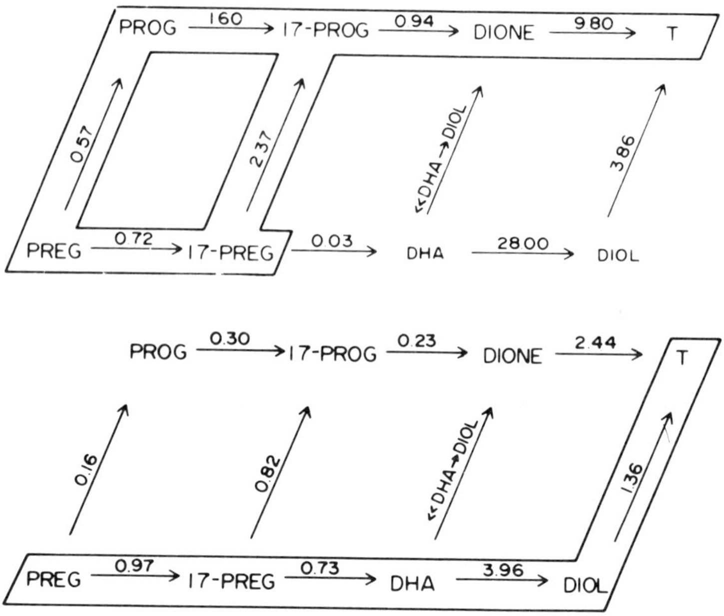

FIGURE 6. Preferred testosterone biosynthetic pathway in rat (*upper panel*) and rabbit (*lower panel*) testes perfused *in vitro*. Numbers represent fraction-of-control value of reactions. Each number multiplied by 100 equals the percentage of testosterone that could be produced by this reaction. Enclosed reactions are components of the preferred pathway. (From ref. 25, reprinted with permission.)

relationships existed between the capacity of testes to secrete testosterone and the quantity of smooth endoplasmic reticulum per Leydig cell and/or per testis (FIG. 8). These results suggested that LH regulates not only Leydig cell steroidogenesis but also smooth endoplasmic reticulum membrane biogenesis and/or turnover.

These studies of Leydig cell structure and steroidogenic function accelerated with the arrival of Tung-Yang Wing to Larry's laboratory. Ewing and Wing showed that the treatment of rats, at the time of hypophysectomy or of testosterone-estradiol implantation, with LH, but not with follicle-stimulating hormone (FSH), prolactin, thyroid-stimulating hormone (TSH) or growth hormone (GH), could maintain both Leydig cell smooth endoplasmic reticulum and the capacity of the testes to produce testosterone.[30] These results demonstrated that a trophic effect of LH on the Leydig cell is to maintain the integrity of the smooth endoplasmic reticulum, and presumably, of some or all of the enzymes responsible for testosterone production.

The next logical question Ewing and Wing asked was what would be the effect of LH withdrawal on the surface area of smooth endoplasmic reticulum and the capacity of *in vitro* perfused rat testes to carry out specific steroidogenic reactions.[31] They found that the conversion of pregnenolone to progesterone was not affected by LH withdrawal, but that the conversions of progesterone to 17α-hydroxyprogesterone, 17α-hydroxyprogesterone to androstenedione, and androstenedione to testosterone were each significantly reduced upon LH withdrawal. The decrease in the activities of these enzymes was well correlated with the dramatic decrease in the amount of smooth

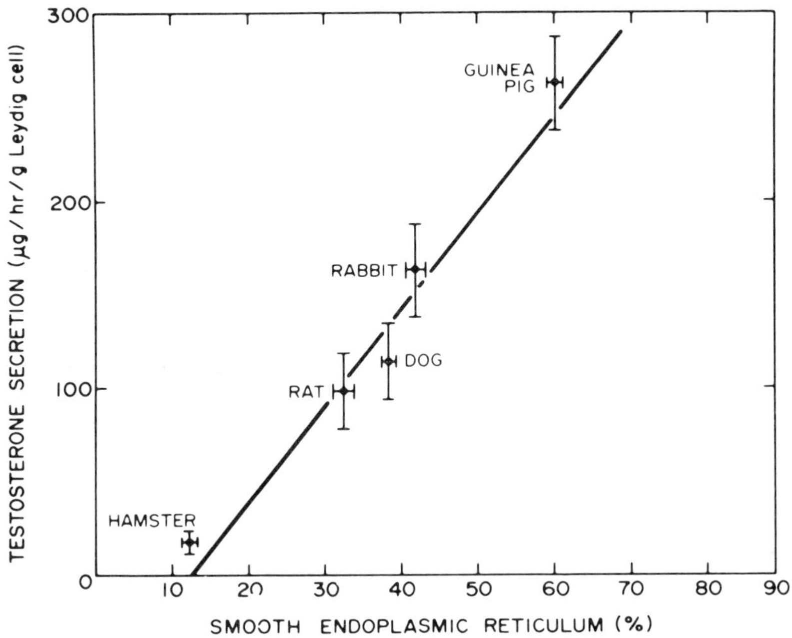

FIGURE 7. Plot of mean testosterone secretion by maximally stimulated *in vitro* perfused testes of the hamster, rat, dog, rabbit, and guinea pig (n = 5 for each species) against the mean volume density of smooth endoplasmic reticulum (SER) in Leydig cell cytoplasm of the contralateral testes. A linear positive correlation (r = 0.99) is seen. (From ref. 28, reprinted with permission.)

endoplasmic reticulum found in the Leydig cells (FIG. 9). These unexpected results suggested that the reaction responsible for the conversion of pregnenolone to progesterone in the rat testis is less dependent on LH than the reactions responsible for converting progesterone to testosterone, and that the enzyme responsible for the pregnenolone to progesterone conversion may not be associated with the classically defined smooth endoplasmic reticulum. The results of these studies culminated in a paper published in *Recent Progress in Hormone Research.*[29]

By the mid-1980s, these structure/function studies had become central to Larry's laboratory. With Diane Keeney and Chamindrani Mendis-Handagama, new stereological methods were introduced that could be used to estimate cell numbers without the bias resulting from assumptions about nuclear shape. Ewing and Keeney used these methods to examine the effects of LH deprivation on Leydig cell number.[32] Unexpectedly, they found that although Leydig cells lose volume as a consequence of LH withdrawal, cell numbers do not decrease even after 16 weeks of LH deprivation via implantation of testosterone-estradiol capsules. These results indicated that though LH is required to maintain Leydig cell structure, it is not required to maintain Leydig cell number.

Previous observations made in Larry's laboratory raised the possibility that there might be correlations between testosterone secretion rates and Leydig cell organelles other than the well-established correlation between testosterone production and smooth endoplasmic reticulum. To explore this possibility, Mendis-Handagama and Ewing

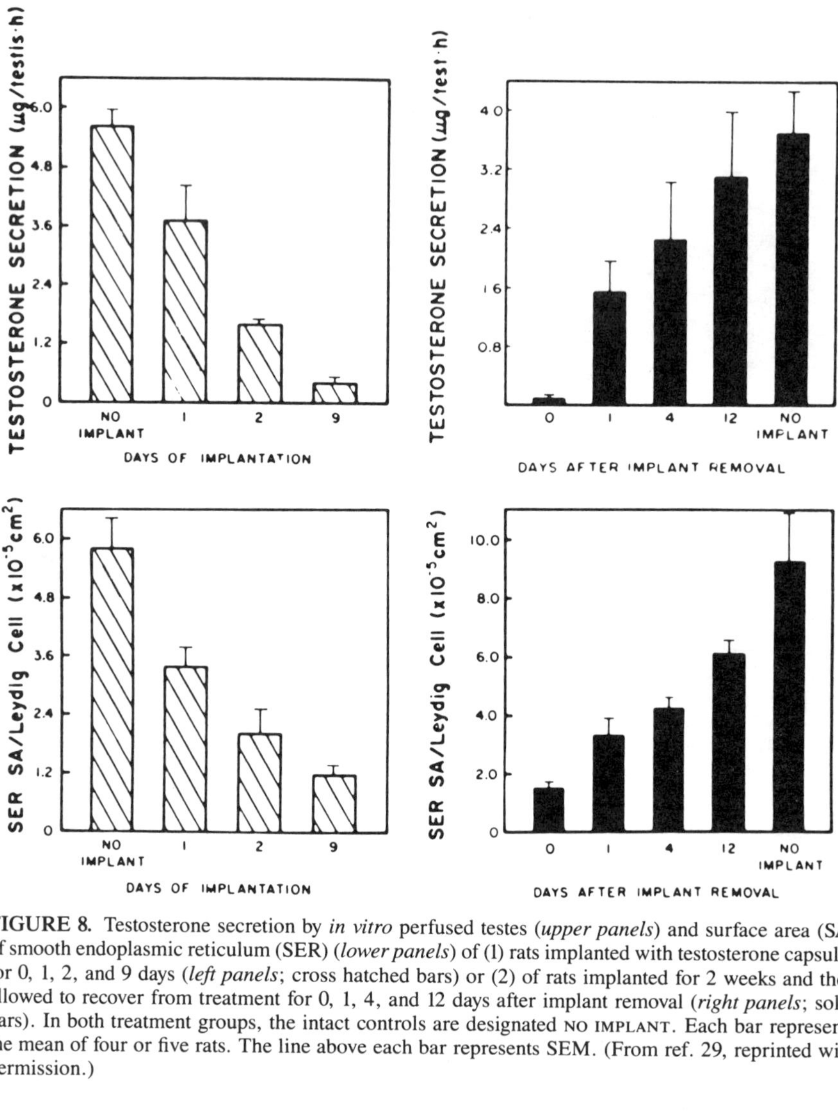

FIGURE 8. Testosterone secretion by *in vitro* perfused testes (*upper panels*) and surface area (SA) of smooth endoplasmic reticulum (SER) (*lower panels*) of (1) rats implanted with testosterone capsules for 0, 1, 2, and 9 days (*left panels*; cross hatched bars) or (2) of rats implanted for 2 weeks and then allowed to recover from treatment for 0, 1, 4, and 12 days after implant removal (*right panels*; solid bars). In both treatment groups, the intact controls are designated NO IMPLANT. Each bar represents the mean of four or five rats. The line above each bar represents SEM. (From ref. 29, reprinted with permission.)

examined the possible correlations among over 100 factors associated with Leydig cell structure and function in hamster, rat and guinea pig testes.[33] They found that the differences in testosterone production among the three species were highly correlated with only two of the factors examined: the volume and surface area of smooth endoplasmic reticulum, and peroxisome surface area. In both cases, highly significant, positive linear correlations were found. Later, using electron microscopic immunolocalization methods, they[34] demonstrated further that Leydig cell peroxisomes contain sterol carrier protein-2 (SCP-2) which is known to participate both in microsomal

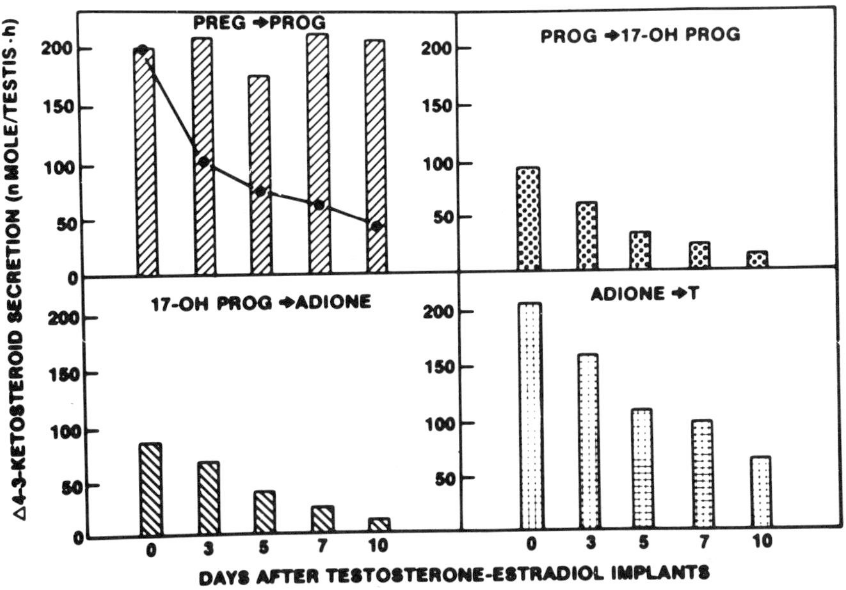

FIGURE 9. Correlation of the capacity of perfused testes to convert pregnenolone (PREG) to progesterone (PROG) (*upper left panel*), PROG to 17-hydroxyprogesterone (17OHPROG) (*upper right panel*), 17OHPROG to androstenedione (ADIONE) (*lower left panel*), and ADIONE to testosterone (T) (*lower right panel*) with the Leydig cell smooth endoplasmic reticulum (SER) surface area per testis (●; *upper left panel*) in the intact control (0-day) and 3-, 5,-, 7-, and 10-day T-E-implanted rats. The capacities to convert PROG to 17OHPROG, 17OHPROG to ADIONE, ADIONE to T were highly correlated ($p < 0.05$) with the days of treatment and the surface area of the Leydig cell SER. The capacity to convert PREG to PROG (*upper left panel*) was not affected by the treatment and was not correlated with the Leydig cell SER surface area. The surface area of the Leydig cell SER for each time point was derived from three testes, each from a single rat. The steroidogenic capacities represented by each column were derived from the mean of four testes, each from a single rat. The SEM, not shown here, was about 10% or less of the mean in most cases. (From ref. 31, reprinted with permission.)

conversion of lanosterol to cholesterol and in the intracellular transport of cholesterol into mitochondria. These results, taken together, suggested that peroxisomes may play a role in testosterone production by the Leydig cell.

Finally, with Matthew Hardy, Larry turned his attention to how the mature population of Leydig cells arises during puberty. Indirect evidence had suggested that Leydig cells arise by differentiation from mesenchymal precursor cells during puberty; however, there was no conclusive evidence that this was so. Additionally, there was evidence for division of Leydig cells, but there were no data as to the extent to which cell division (and/or differentiation of mesenchymal cells) contributed to the adult Leydig cell population of approximately 25×10^6 cells per testis. Hardy and Ewing[35] used stereological methods to show convincingly that mesenchymal cells do indeed contribute to increases in Leydig cell number 14–28 days postpartum (FIG. 10), and they used autoradiography to show that the newly differentiated Leydig cells then undergo 1–2 rounds of division to complete the final growth phase. This remark-

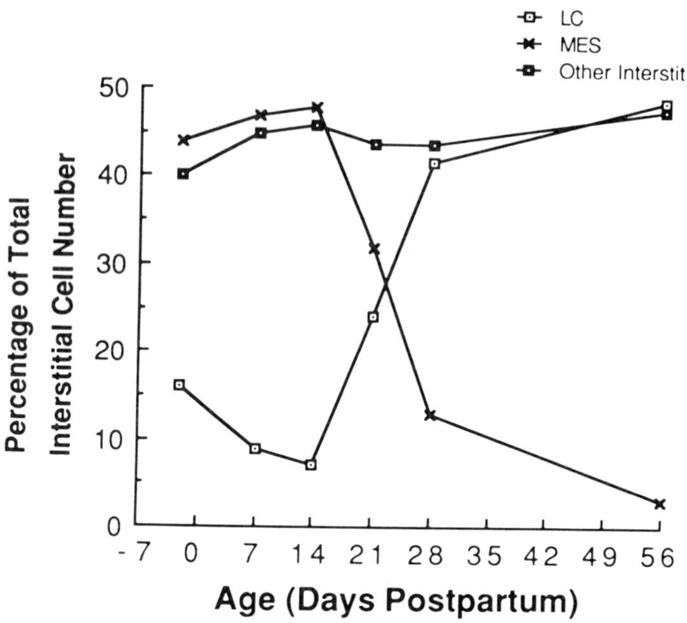

FIGURE 10. The numbers of mesenchymal (MES) and Leydig cells (LC) and combined numbers of macrophages, pericytes, and endothelial and myoid cells (other interstit), expressed as a percentage of the total number of all interstitial cells of rat testes, at six developmental times. (From ref. 35, reprinted with permission.)

able study thus showed the extent to which mesenchymal precursors and Leydig cell division contribute to the growth of Leydig cell number, and the timing of this growth.

All the while these studies of Leydig cell regulation were being conducted with the whole testis, Larry recognized the need for *in vitro* studies. But, typically, he refused to work on cells whose differentiated function (testosterone production) was significantly compromised or lost. He believed that there were no satisfactory methods available to isolate Leydig cells that were able to produce testosterone in amounts comparable to the amounts produced normally by the testis. Larry had begun the effort to isolate Leydig cells of this quality in the early 1980s.[36] He was not satisfied with the results until Gary Klinefelter[37] developed a procedure involving vascular perfusion, enzymatic dissociation, centrifugal elutriation and Percoll gradient centrifugation (FIG. 11) that achieved >95% pure Leydig cells that were well preserved, stained for 3β-hydroxysteroid dehydrogenase, and had the ultrastructural characteristics of Leydig cells. Most importantly, these cells responded to maximally stimulating LH concentrations with a 10-fold increase in testosterone production over 3 hours. The quantity of testosterone produced by these cells was many-fold higher than others had achieved, and approached the standard of the perfused testis.

Soon thereafter, Klinefelter and Ewing[38] developed methods to maintain testosterone production by these cells for 24 hours in culture. In part, this was achieved by allowing the isolated Leydig cells to attach to Cytodex beads. These cells synthe-

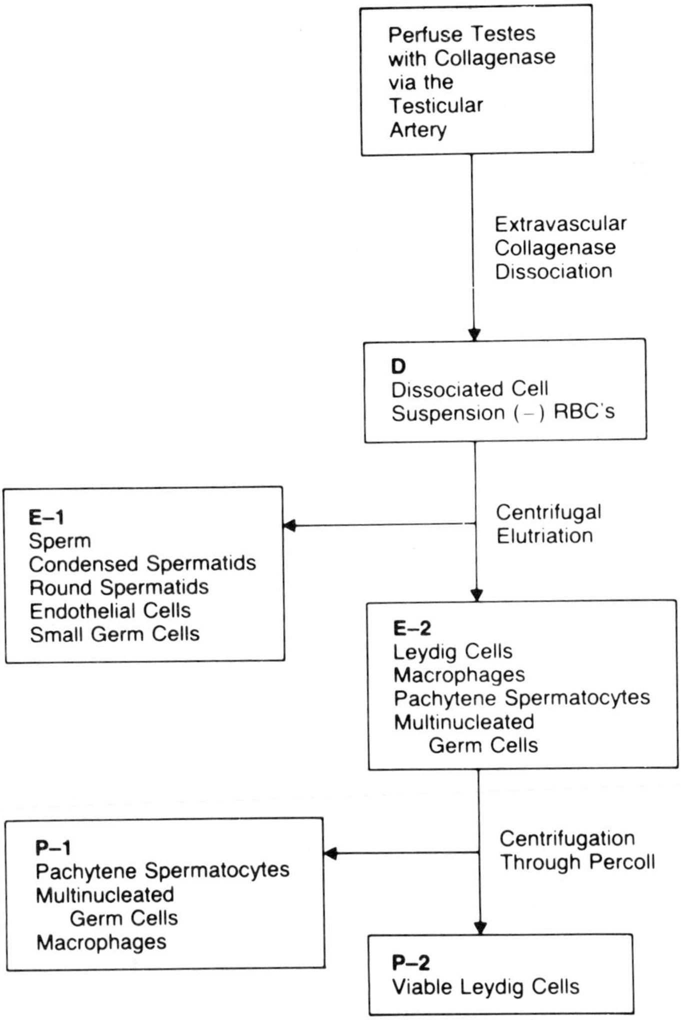

FIGURE 11. A schematic flow diagram of the sequence of steps used to purify rat Leydig cells. D = cell suspension following collagenase dissociation; E-1 = a 300-ml fraction of cells collected with an elutriator rotor speed of 2000 rpm and a 16 or 20 ml/min countercurrent buffer flow; E-2 = a 100-ml fraction of cells collected from the elutriation chamber after decreasing the rotor speed to 0; P-1 = a lighter-than-1.068 g/ml fraction of E-2 cells recovered from a continuous, linear Percoll gradient formed from 60% Percoll during centrifugation for 1 h at 20,000 gav; and P-2 = a 1.068 g/ml-and-heavier-fraction of E-2 cells recovered after Percoll gradient centrifugation. (From ref. 37, reprinted with permission.)

sized and secreted 40% of the amount of testosterone produced by equivalent numbers of Leydig cells in the perfused testis, and indeed, more testosterone than the equivalent number of Leydig cells produced *in vivo* under physiological LH stimulation. But, still not satisfied, Klinefelter and Ewing[39] modified their methods once again, reducing

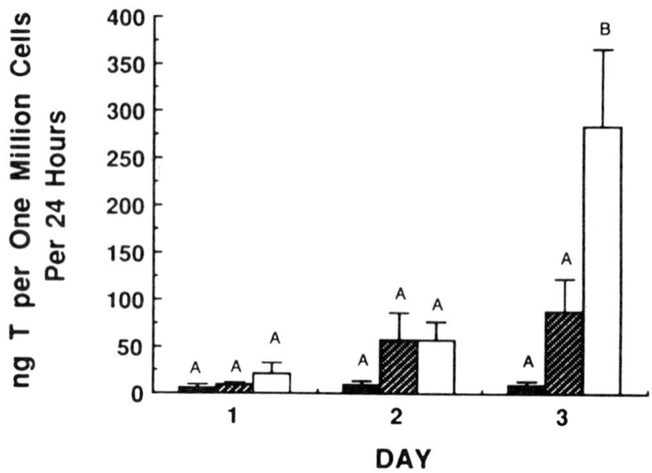

FIGURE 12. Daily testosterone secretion rate measured during *in vitro* culture of precursor cells. Solid black bars = LH; cross-hatched bars = DHT; solid white bars = LH + DHT. Groups sharing the same alphabet letter were not significantly different. (From ref. 40, reprinted with permission.)

oxygen tension so as to extend the ability of these cells to synthesize and secrete testosterone to 3 days.

The development of these important methods allowed Hardy, Kelce, Klinefelter and Ewing to conduct a remarkable experiment in which they examined the differentiation of mesenchymal to Leydig cells *in vitro.*[40] Using a modification of the techniques that had been developed for adult Leydig cells, they isolated an enriched population of mesenchymal cells from the testes of 21-day-old rats. Culture of these cells with a combination of LH and dihydrotestosterone (DHT) led to a significant (10-fold) increase in the ability of the cultured cells to secrete testosterone (FIG. 12). Remarkably, neither LH nor DHT alone had this effect. These studies suggested that androgens themselves may regulate both the morphogenic and steroidogenic processes that accompany the differentiation of Leydig cells from precursor mesenchymal cells.

In sum, the contributions that Larry made to our knowledge of Leydig cell structure, function and regulation are remarkable. The trademarks of his science were his unwillingness to accept less than excellence and his ability to provide support and assistance to anyone who was serious about his or her work. Larry's publications will continue to have influence for years to come. Those of us who were fortunate enough to have interacted with Larry personally profited greatly for having done so. The 11th North American Testis Workshop could not have been dedicated to a finer scientist, teacher, and person than Larry L. Ewing.

REFERENCES

1. VANDEMARK, N. L. & L. L. EWING. 1963. Factors affecting testicular metabolism and function. I. A simplified perfusion technique for short-term maintenance of rabbit testis. J. Reprod. Fertil. **6:** 1–6.

2. EWING, L. L. 1967. Effect of aging on testicular metabolism in the rabbit. Am. J. Physiol. **22:** 1261–1267.
3. EWING, L. L. & K. B. EIK-NES. 1966. On the formation of testosterone by the perfused rabbit testis. Can. J. Biochem. **44:** 1327–1344.
4. REDDI, A. H., L. L. EWING & H. G. WILLIAMS-ASHMAN. 1971. Protein phosphokinase reactions in mammalian testis. Stimulatory effects of adenosine 3':5'-cyclic monophosphate on the phosphorylation of basic proteins. Biochem. J. **122:** 333–345.
5. EWING, L. L., L. G. STRATTON & C. DESJARDINS. 1973. Effect of testosterone polydimethylsiloxane implants upon sperm production, libido and accessory sex organ function in rabbits. J. Reprod. Fertil. **35:** 245–253.
6. EWING, L. L., B. SCHANBACHER, C. DESJARDINS & V. CHAFFEE. 1976. The effect of subdermal testosterone filled polydimethylsiloxane implants on spermatogenesis in Rhesus monkeys (*Macaca mulata*). Contraception **13:** 583–596.
7. EWING, L. L., C. DESJARDINS, D. C. IRBY & B. ROBAIRE. 1977. Synergistic interaction of testosterone and oestradiol inhibits spermatogenesis in rats. Nature 269: 409–411.
8. ROBAIRE, B., L. L. EWING, D. C. IRBY & C. DESJARDINS. 1979. Interactions of testosterone and estradiol-17β on the reproductive tract of the male rat. Biol. Reprod. **21:** 455–463.
9. EWING, L. L., R. A. GORSKI, R. J. SBORDONE, J. V. TYLER, C. DESJARDINS & B. ROBAIRE. 1979. Testosterone-estradiol filled polydimethylsiloxane subdermal implants: Effect on fertility and masculine sexual and aggressive behavior of male rats. Biol. Reprod. **21:** 765–772.
10. EWING, L. L., R. C. COCHRAN, R. J. ADAMS, K. J. DARNEY, JR., S. J. BERRY, M. J. BORDY & C. DESJARDINS. 1983. Testis function in Rhesus monkeys treated with a contraceptive steroid formulation. Contraception **27:** 347–362.
11. LOBL, T. J., K. T. KIRTON, A. D. FORBES, L. L. EWING, P. L. KEMP & C. DESJARDINS. 1983. Contraceptive efficacy of testosterone-estradiol implants in mâle Rhesus monkeys. Contraception **27:** 383–389.
12. BURRIS, A. S., L. L. EWING & R. J. SHERINS. 1988. Initial trial of slow-release testosterone microspheres in hypogonadal men. Fertil. Steril. **50:** 493–497.
13. EWING, L. L. & B. BROWN. 1975. Formation and secretion of 5α-androstan-17β-ol-3-one, 5α-androstan-3α, 17β-diol and 5α-androstan-3β,17β-diol by the perfused rabbit testis epididymis. Endocrinology **96:** 479–485.
14. ROBAIRE, B., L. L. EWING, B. R. ZIRKIN & D. C. IRBY. 1979. Steroid Δ4 5α-reductase and 3α-hydroxysteroid dehydrogenase in the rat epididymis. Endocrinology **101:** 1379–1390.
15. TURNER, T. T., C. E. JONES, S. S. HOWARDS, L. L. EWING, B. ZEGEYE & G. L. GUNSALUS. 1984. On the androgen microenvironment of maturing spermatozoa. Endocrinology **115:** 1925–1932.
16. TURNER, T. T., L. L. EWING, C. E. JONES, S. S. HOWARDS & B. ZEGEYE. 1985. Androgens in male rat reproductive fluids: Hypophysectomy and steroid replacement. Am. J. Physiol. **248:** E274-E280.
17. TURNER, T. T., L. L. EWING, C. E. JONES, S. S. HOWARDS & B. ZEGEYE. 1985. Androgens in various fluid compartments of the rat testis and epididymis after hypophysectomy and gonadotropin supplementation. J. Androl. **6:** 353–358.
18. EWING, L. L., S. J. BERRY & E. G. HIGGINBOTTOM. 1983. Dihydrotestosterone concentration of beagle prostatic tissue: Effect of age and hyperplasia. Endocrinology **113:** 2004–2009.
19. BERRY, S. J., D. S. COFFEY & L. L. EWING. 1986. Effects of aging on prostate growth in beagles. Am. J. Physiol. **250:** R1039–R1046.
20. BERRY, S. J., D. S. COFFEY, J. D. STRANDBERG & L. L. EWING. 1986. Effect of age, castration and testosterone replacement on the development and restoration of canine benign prostatic hyperplasia. The Prostate **9:** 295–302.
21. WALSH, P. C., G. M. HUTCHINS & L. L. EWING. 1983. Tissue content of dihydrotestosterone in human prostatic hyperplasia is not supranormal. J. Clin. Invest. **72:** 1772–1777.
22. EWING, L. L., C. E. CHUBB & B. ROBAIRE. 1976. Macromolecules, steroid binding and testosterone secretion by rabbit testes. Nature **264:** 84–86.
23. CHUBB, C. & L. L. EWING. 1979. Steroid secretion by in vitro perfused testes: Secretion by rabbit and rat testes. Am. J. Physiol. **237:** E231–E238.
24. CHUBB, C. & L. L. EWING. 1979. Steroid secretion by in vitro perfused testes: Inhibitors of testosterone biosynthesis. Am. J. Physiol. **237:** E239–E246.

25. Chubb, C. & L. L. Ewing. 1979. Steroid secretion by in vitro perfused testes: Testosterone biosynthetic pathways. Am. J. Physiol. **237:** E247–E254.
26. Becker, S., C. Chubb & L. L. Ewing. 1980. Mathematical model of steroidogenesis in rat and rabbit testes. Am. J. Physiol. **239:** R184–R195.
27. Ewing, L. L., B. R. Zirkin, R. C. Cochran, N. Kromann, C. Peters & N. Ruiz-Bravo. 1979. Testosterone secretion by rat, rabbit, guinea pig, dog, and hamster testes perfused *in vitro*: Correlation with Leydig cell mass. Endocrinology **105:** 1135–1142.
28. Zirkin, B. R., L. L. Ewing, N. Kromann & R. C. Cochran. 1980. Testosterone secretion by rat, rabbit, guinea pig, dog, and hamster testes perfused *in vitro*: Correlation with Leydig cell ultrastructure. Endocrinology **107:** 1867–1874.
29. Ewing, L. L. & B. Zirkin. 1983. Leydig cell structure and steroidogenic function. Rec. Prog. Horm. Res. **39:** 599–635.
30. Ewing, L. L., T.-Y. Wing, R. C. Cochran, N. Kromann & B. R. Zirkin. 1983. Effect of luteinizing hormone on Leydig cell structure and testosterone secretion. Endocrinology **112:** 1763–1769.
31. Wing, T.-Y., L. L. Ewing & B. R. Zirkin. 1984. Effect of luteinizing hormone withdrawal on Leydig cell smooth endoplasmic reticulum and steroidogenic reactions which convert pregnenolone to testosterone. Endocrinology **115:** 2290–2296.
32. Keeney, D. S., S. M. L. C. Mendis-Handagama, B. R. Zirkin & L. L. Ewing. 1988. Effect of long term deprivation of luteinizing hormone on Leydig cell volume, Leydig cell number, and steroidogenic capacity of the rat testis. Endocrinology **123:** 2906–2915.
33. Mendis-Handagama, S. M. L. C., B. R. Zirkin & L. L. Ewing. 1988. Comparison of components of the testis interstitium with testosterone secretion in hamster, rat, and guinea pig testes perfused *in vitro.* Am. J. Anat. **181:** 12–22.
34. Mendis-Handagama, S. M. L. C., B. R. Zirkin, T. J. Scallen & L. L. Ewing. 1990. Studies on peroxisomes of the adult rat Leydig cell. J. Androl. **11:** 270–278.
35. Hardy, M. P., B. R. Zirkin & L. L. Ewing. 1989. Kinetic studies on the development of the adult population of Leydig cells in testes of the pubertal rat. Endocrinology **124:** 762–770.
36. Bordy, M. J., J. H. Shaper & L. L. Ewing. 1984. Trophic influences of luteinizing hormone on steroidogenesis by Percoll-separated rat Leydig cells in culture. Ann. N.Y. Acad. Sci. **438:** 329–345.
37. Klinefelter, G. R., P. F. Hall & L. L. Ewing. 1987. Effect of luteinizing hormone deprivation *in situ* on steroidogenesis of rat Leydig cells purified by a multistep procedure. Biol. Reprod. **36:** 769–783.
38. Klinefelter, G. R. & L. L. Ewing. 1988. Optimizing testosterone production by purified adult rat Leydig cells *in vitro.* In Vitro Cell. Devel. Biol. **24:** 545–549.
39. Klinefelter, G. R. & L. L. Ewing. 1989. Maintenance of testosterone production by purified adult rat Leydig cells for 3 days *in vitro.* In Vitro Cell. Devel. Biol. **25:** 283–288.
40. Hardy, M. P., W. R. Kelce, G. R. Klinefelter & L. L. Ewing. 1990. Differentiation of Leydig cell precursors *in vitro*: A role for androgen. Endocrinology **127:** 488–490.

Four Decades of Research on the Biology of the Male Reproductive System: A Few Landmarks

YVES CLERMONT

Department of Anatomy
McGill University
Montréal, Québec, Canada H3A 2B2

It is with great pleasure that I open the proceedings of the XIth Testis Workshop and take this opportunity to welcome to Montreal colleagues and experts from around the world. Needless to say, I find it most interesting to witness the rapid accumulation of information on the biology of the male reproductive system in general and, in particular, on the formation and maturation of spermatozoa which culminates with the fertilization of the oocyte. The present workshop, as you will see, will be an impressive demonstration of this intense research productivity.

Being among the few in this assembly who has had the chance of observing the rapid development of our field of investigation since the early fifties, I would like to take the next few minutes to do two things: Firstly I would like to describe to you briefly the status of research on the testis when I arrived here at McGill in 1949 to undertake my graduate training under the supervision of Dr. C. P. Leblond. Secondly, I would like to tell you what I consider, from my own limited point of view, as the main phases and landmarks in the history of our discipline.

STATUS OF RESEARCH IN 1949–1950

In 1949–1950 research on the histology of the testis and associated ducts, on the seminiferous tubules and spermatogenesis in particular, was, peacefully quiescent. And this "sleeping beauty" had been dormant since the beginning of the century, that is from the time when European cytologists and histologists had described spermiogenesis and the seminiferous epithelium of a number of animal species. I think in particular of the remarkable studies of the French histologist Claude Regaud (1901) who produced at the end of the last century, his remarkable descriptions on the cycle and the wave of the seminiferous epithelium of the rat.[1,2]

However, during the first half of the century, the endocrinological aspects of the testis, that is, the role of Leydig cells, the nature, biosynthesis and sites of action of steroids, as well as the control of the androgenic function by the anterior pituitary, had been extensively studied. I should indicate here that many anatomists were involved in these investigations and contributed with physiologists and biochemists to create a new branch of biomedical science: endocrinology.[3]

Similarly, prior to 1950, the cytologists-geneticists, working on a large variety of animal species and plants, had clarified many aspects of meiosis. Thus a major step had been made toward the understanding of a key feature in the formation of haploid male germ cells. I may add however that the molecular mechanisms responsible for the synapsis of homologous chromosomes have yet to be clarified.

However, when I recall the information available in 1949–1950 on the kinetic processes taking place within the seminiferous tubules, it was somewhat desert-like! The histological descriptions on the seminiferous tubules, in man in particular, were limited to what was available in the few textbooks. It is true that we had a few excellent and detailed light microscopic descriptions of spermiogenesis, in particular those of Duesberg (1908) on the rat,[4] of Meves (1899) on the guinea pig.[5] But owing to the lack of appropriate tracer methods we had no information on the duration of spermatogenesis or of the cycle of the seminiferous epithelium; we had little or no notion about the mode of proliferation, renewal and differentiation of spermatogonia—and I might add that the molecular mechanisms that would explain the behavior of spermatogonial stem cells remain unelucidated to this day. The descriptions of the development of sex cords in the rat or other mammals were rather superficial or incomplete and had to be re-examined closely. One of the major components of the seminiferous epithelium, the Sertoli cell, was in those days completely neglected and the description then available was not different from the one given by Sertoli himself in 1865.[6] Furthermore, in 1950 it was still generally believed that Sertoli cells formed a syncytium and as to its function it was described as being "sustentacular" as Sertoli himself indicated and phagocytic as suggested by Regaud in 1901.[1] Just think for a minute what has been learned about Sertoli cells since 1950. Several interesting presentations on this fascinating cell will be made here.

Thus, in 1950 the "spermatogenic kettle" was still quiescent and only purring. However, early signs of potential boiling were in the air as a consequence of the development of new techniques and instruments. I am thinking in particular of new histochemical techniques recently developed such as the Feulgen reaction for the demonstration of deoxyribonucleic acid, or the periodic acid-Schiff technique for the demonstration of carbohydrates and glycoproteins.[7] The technique of radioautography, developed a few years earlier by Leblond and collaborators permitted the use of radioactive isotopes to label and trace within tissue labeled cells or cellular components.[8] I remember vividly Dr. Leblond telling his students with great excitement that tritium-labeled thymidine had just been synthesized, and was available commercially. It could thus be used to label dividing cells and trace their progeny. We then soon utilized this tracer to determine the duration of the cycle of the seminiferous epithelium and spermatogenesis in the rat.[9]

There was also some information circulating concerning a new microscope which made use of an electron beam rather than a beam of light and which had a magnifying power far superior to that of the best microscopes we were using. So the electron microscope was around the corner. This was the case not only in principle, but in reality, since there was one such electron microscope, one of the first built by RCA, an EMU-1, located in a building next to our laboratory, the Eaton Electronic Building, where it was used by physicists to prepare electron diffraction patterns of various materials. We soon tried to use it to look at the head of rat's spermatozoa in gold shadowed whole mounts preparations, since appropriate fixation methods and ultramicrotomes were not yet available. The observations we made then were published a few years later.[10] So in the early 1950s, although research on the male reproductive system was sluggish, the stage was being set for action.

A FEW LANDMARKS OF RESEARCH ACTIVITIES IN THE DOMAIN OF THE MALE REPRODUCTIVE SYSTEM

I. The New York Academy of Sciences Meeting (1952)

One of the earliest scientific manifestations that research on the biology of the testis and on spermatogenesis in particular was engaged, although modestly, took place in 1952 at the meeting organized by Warren Nelson and John MacLeod and sponsored by the New York Academy of Sciences. This meeting took place in New York in the facilities of the Academy (FIG. 1).[11]

There was a total of 30 participants at that meeting and 16 papers were presented. As you can see on the cover page of the proceedings all the names of the participants could be printed easily in a short paragraph (FIG. 1). This would be more difficult to do with all the names (close to 350) of the participants in the present workshop!

There were only two presentations on spermatogenesis at that meeting. One was by Dr. Edward Roosen-Runge on the kinetics of spermatogenesis in mammals[12] and one was by Dr. C. P. Leblond and me on the cycle of the seminiferous epithelium of the rat in which we presented our observations on spermiogenesis as seen in sections stained with the periodic-acid-Schiff method.[13] This histochemical method outlined the evolution of the carbohydrate rich acrosomic system during spermiogenesis and we then used the steps of spermiogenesis as a key to a classification of the various cell associations or stages (14) that form the cycle of the seminiferous epithelium. The other presentations included a brief communication on the epididymis by Mason and Shaver[14] and papers on the histopathology and endocrinology of the human testis.

If we note that the proceedings of the last five Testis Workshops (since 1981) including this year's proceedings have been or will be published under the auspices of The Annals of the New York Academy of Sciences, then you have here (FIG. 1) the true ancestor and precursor of our proceedings.

II. The West Point Meeting on the **Mechanisms Concerned with Conception**

During the following decade the "spermatogenic kettle" started to boil pleasantly! This was due mainly to the addition of new information on the seminiferous epithelium and the structure of spermatozoa resulting from the use of the electron microscope. The contributions of Dr. Fawcett and of his students were particularly impressive and exciting at that time. The combined impact of the Russian sputnik (1957) and the interest of various agencies in the control of human fertility, resulted in a rapid increase of the funding of research in general and of research on reproduction in particular with, as a consequence, a rapid accumulation of information on the male reproductive system.

This led to the organization of a major meeting on The Mechanisms Concerned with Conception. Drs. C. Hartman and W. Nelson were the promoters of this meeting which took place at West Point, New York in 1959 (FIG. 2). The format of the

FIGURE 1.

ANNALS OF THE NEW YORK ACADEMY OF SCIENCES
VOLUME 55, ART. 4. PAGES 543–742

Editor
ROY WALDO MINER

BIOLOGY OF THE TESTES

BY

W. O. NELSON, J. MACLEOD (*Conference Chairmen*), C. W. CHARNY, Y. CLERMONT, A. S. CONSTON, E. T. ENGLE, M. EPSTEIN, D. GHOSH, R. Z. GOLD, N. J. HECKEL, C. G. HELLER, E. C. JUNCK, H. A. LARDY, C. P. LEBLOND, M. E. LONG, K. M. LYNCH, JR., W. O. MADDOCK, K. E. MASON, E. P. MCCULLAGH, J. H. MCDONALD, D. R. MERANZE, W. MONTAGNA, G. E. MORTIMORE, C. A. PAULSON, E. C. ROOSEN-RUNGE, C. A. SCHAFFENBURG, S. L. SHAVER, F. A. SIMMONS, AND R. C. SNIFFEN

Consulting Editor
JOHN MACLEOD

NEW YORK
PUBLISHED BY THE ACADEMY
November 20, 1952

1

FIGURE 2.

Mechanisms Concerned With Conception

Proceedings of a symposium
prepared under the auspices of the Population Council
and the Planned Parenthood Federation of America

Edited by

CARL G. HARTMAN

Chairman of the Biological Research Committee of the
Planned Parenthood Federation of America

SYMPOSIUM PUBLICATIONS DIVISION
PERGAMON PRESS
OXFORD · LONDON · NEW YORK · PARIS
1963

(2)

meeting which grouped some 70 participants and dealt with the male and female reproductive systems and fertilization was then innovative in that instead of formal presentations, each participant gave several short presentations followed by immediate and lengthy discussions, *i.e.*, the typical workshop format. I remember clearly the atmosphere of excitement that prevailed during these discussions. Dr. Fawcett presented his most recent EM observations on Sertoli cells and germinal cells, Dr. Leblond and I presented our radioautographic data on the duration of spermatogenesis in the rat, on the renewal of spermatogonia in rodents and primates, and our initial studies on the cycle of the seminiferous epithelium in man. Dr. Nelson and his student Dr. Steinberger presented their work on the effects of various factors, hormones, temperature, radiation and toxins, on spermatogenesis. At that meeting I met Dr. Carl Heller with whom I initiated a collaboration that led, a few years later, to our publication in *Science* (1963) on the duration of the cycle of the seminiferous epithelium and of spermatogenesis in man.[15] This symposium was elegantly summarized in an article written by Dr. Zolly Zuckerman and published in *Science* in 1959.[16] The proceedings were published as a book four years later.[17] It included a substantial chapter on spermatogenesis prepared by Drs. Leblond, Steinberger and Roosen-Runge, which gave an interesting summary of the research done on the testis during the preceding 10 years.[18]

III. The Ford Foundation–sponsored Report on Reproduction and Human Welfare: A Challenge to Research

Following the West Point meeting and for 15 years, there was a period during which there was intense research, and the field of reproductive biology developed rapidly. An expression of this development was the formation of new societies. The Society for the Study of Reproduction was founded in 1967 and The American Society of Andrology in 1975. In parallel, new specialized journals were published, innumerable books were printed, and dozens of special symposia were organized. Among these I should mention the Gordon Conferences and of course, the series of Testis Workshops that were initiated with the support of the NIH. The first one of these took place in Houston, Texas in 1974 and was organized by Drs. Maria Dufau and Anthony Means. In 1969, a number of investigators initiated a series of international symposia concentrating exclusively on the spermatozoon and grouped many comparative spermatologists. The first meeting of this group took place in Rome and Sienna in 1969 and was organized by Dr. Baccetti.[19] I might add in passing that the last one of these international gatherings of spermatologists was also organized by Dr. Baccetti in Sienna. It took place last August (1990) and was well attended. Many of us here today had the occasion of meeting in that lovely medieval city. Scientifically very interesting, this meeting was also the occasion for recognizing the contribution of Dr. D. W. Fawcett and his collaborators to the field of spermatology.

To return to the mid-1970s the research in the field of reproduction was indeed so intense and the accumulation of knowledge so rapid that the granting agencies supporting the research wanted to see where this work was going. Among these agencies, the Ford Foundation, initiated and sponsored a survey of the research done on the male and female as well as on the funding policies that existed then. This extensive survey was coordinated by Dr. R. O. Greep and resulted in two publications that appeared consecutively in 1976 and 1977.[20,21] The summary report of 1976 (FIG. 3) included an interesting chapter of more than a hundred pages prepared by Dr. Fawcett

FIGURE 3.

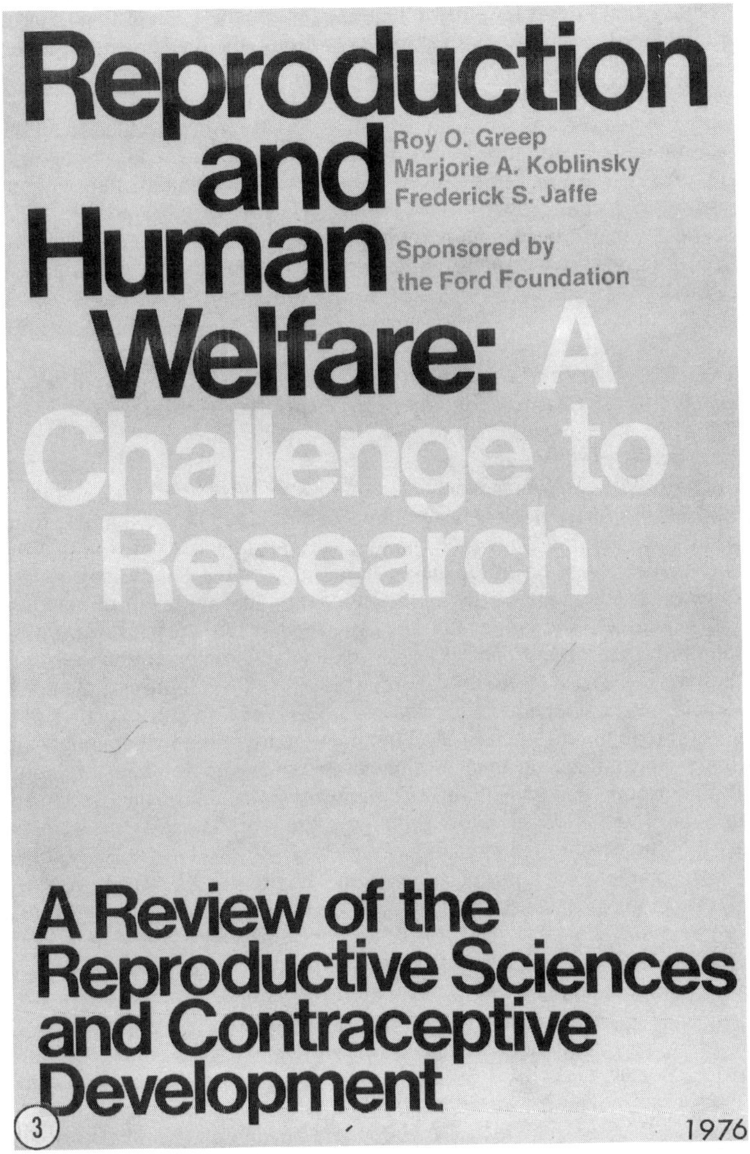
Reproduction and Human Welfare: A Challenge to Research
Roy O. Greep
Marjorie A. Koblinsky
Frederick S. Jaffe
Sponsored by the Ford Foundation
A Review of the Reproductive Sciences and Contraceptive Development
3
1976

summarizing well the work done on the male reproductive system since 1960.[21] This summation is impressive and demonstrated the remarkable and rapid progress made in our understanding of the structure and function of the seminiferous epithelium, of the interstitial tissue, and of the role of the accessory ducts system as well on the intricate process of fertilization. Many of the facts, notions or hypotheses presented in this chapter are still valid today. In fact, Dr. Fawcett was so euphoric about the progress made that he wrote in his concluding comments "There is no doubt that in the more balanced perspective of future generations, the decades from 1960 to 1980 will be considered a golden era in the progress of basic understanding of reproductive biology of the male."[21]

However, this did not mean that everything about male reproduction and fertilization had been discovered. In this regard, it is interesting to read on pages 569–584 of this report the questions in the field of reproductive sciences that the consultants and contributors to the report wanted to have clarified or answered.[21] We discover first that these queries were innumerable; second, most of these constitute the basis and object of present day research; and third, of the questions raised many have yet to be tackled.

IV. The Last 15 Years and the Present Era: Impact of Cell and Molecular Biology on Research on the Male Reproductive System

All that precedes, *i.e.*, what went on in research on the male reproductive system between 1950–1975, was, however, rather modest compared to what has taken place since the Ford Report. Of course my views here are subjective and not those of an archivist or historian, but it is evident to me, as it must be to all of you, that the "spermatogenic kettle" is not boiling peacefully any longer but is now boiling violently! This is obviously the result of the fantastically rapid development of new methodologies utilized in cell and molecular biology. Indeed, we are now riding more and more rapidly on the crest of the wave of molecular biology. Immunohistochemical methods have been used more and more efficiently at the light and electron microscopic levels; new cytochemical probes have been developed; molecular genetics is now the royal road to new ventures and more and more refined biochemical analytical methods are being utilized on an increasing number of problems related to reproduction.

With this exponential growth of information, we live dangerously so to speak but this makes our lives as investigators even more exciting. The last 3 or 4 Testis Workshops gave us an idea of the increasing complexity and diversification of the research already done on the male reproductive system; the present XIth Testis Workshop will certainly be another demonstration of the exciting research now in progress.

REFERENCES

1. Regaud, C. 1901. Étude sur la structure des tubes séminifères et sur la spermatogénèse chez les mammifères. Arch. Anat. Micr. **4:** 291–432.
2. Regaud, C. 1909. Étude sur la structure des tubes séminifères et sur la spermatogénèse chez les mammifères. Arch. Anat. Micr. **11:** 291–431.
3. Everett, J. W. & C. H. Sawyer. 1987. Endocrinology and Reproductive Biology. *In* The American Association of Anatomists 1988–1987. Essays on the History of Anatomy in America. J. E. Pauly, Ed.: 183–197. Williams and Wilkins. Baltimore, MD.

4. DUESBERG, J. 1908. La spermiogenèse chez le rat. Arch. F. Zellforschung **2:** 137–180.
5. MEVES, F. VON. 1899. Über Structure und Histogenese der Samenfäden des Meerschweinchen. Arch. Mikr. Anat. **54:** 329–402.
6. SERTOLI, E. 1965. Dell'esistenze di particolari cellule ramificate nei canalicoli seminiferi del testicolo umano. Morgagni **7:** 31–40.
7. LISON, L. 1953. Histochimie et cytochimie animales, pp. 1-607. Gauthier-Villars. Paris.
8. LEBLOND, C. P. 1987. Radioautography: The role played by anatomists in the development and application of the technique. *In* The American Association of Anatomists. 1888–1987. Essays on the History of Anatomy in America. J. E. Pauly, Ed.: 89–103. Williams & Wilkins. Baltimore, MD.
9. CLERMONT, Y., C. P. LEBLOND & B. MESSIER. 1959. Durée du cycle de l'épithélium séminal du rat. Arch. Anat. Micr. Morphol Exp. **48:** 37–56.
10. CLERMONT, Y., E. EINBERG, C. P. LEBLOND & S. WAGNER. 1955. The perforatorium—An extension of the nuclear membrane of the rat spermatozoon. Anat. Rec. **121:** 1–12.
11. MINER, R. W., Ed. 1952. Biology of the testis. Ann. N.Y. Acad. Sci. **44:** 543–742.
12. ROOSEN-RUNGE, E. C. 1952. Kinetics of spermatogenesis in mammals. Ann. N.Y. Acad. Sci. **55:** 574–584.
13. LEBLOND, C. P. & Y. CLERMONT. 1952. Definition of the stages of the cycle of the seminiferous epithelium in the rat. Ann. N.Y. Acad. Sci. **55:** 548–573.
14. MASON, K. & S. L. SHAVER. 1952. Some functions of the caput epididymis. Ann. N.Y. Acad. Sci. **44:** 585–593.
15. HELLER, C. G. & Y. CLERMONT. 1963. Spermatogenesis in man: An estimate of its duration. Science **140:** 184–186.
16. ZUCKERMAN, S. 1959. Mechanisms involved in conception. Science **130:** 1260–1264.
17. HARTMAN, C. G., Ed. 1963. Mechanisms Concerned with Conception. Pergamon Press. Oxford, London, New York, Paris.
18. LEBLOND, C. P., E. STEINBERGER & E. C. ROOSEN-RUNGE. 1963. Spermatogenesis. *In* Mechanisms Concerned with Conception. C. G. Hartman, Ed.: 1–72.
19. BACCETTI, B., Ed. 1970. Spermatologia comparata. Problemi Attuali de Scienza e di Cultura **137:** 1–575. Academia Nazionale dei Lincei, Roma.
20. GREEP, R. O. & M. A. KOBLINSKY. 1977. Frontiers in Reproduction and Fertility Control. A Review of the Reproductive Sciences and Contraceptive Development. Sponsored by the Ford Foundation. The MIT Press, Cambridge, MA, and London, England.
21. FAWCETT, D. W. 1976. The male reproductive system. *In* Reproduction and Human Welfare. R. O. Greep, M. A. Koblinsky & F. S. Jaffe, Eds.: 165–277. Sponsored by the Ford Foundation. The MIT Press, Cambridge, MA and London, England.

Updates and New Models for Steroid Hormone Action

JAMES P. LANDERS AND THOMAS C. SPELSBERG

Department of Biochemistry and Molecular Biology
Mayo Clinic and Mayo Foundation
Rochester, Minnesota 55905

INTRODUCTION

There has been exciting progress in the understanding of the mechanism of action of steroid hormones. This paper outlines the plenary lecture presented at the 1991 Testis Workshop in Montreal, presenting an update on the mechanism of action of steroids on gene expression, including receptor structure and function and a cascade model for steroid hormone action. This review is directed at those not in the field of steroid hormone action. Brief reviews of the following areas are included: 1) the model outlining the known and the speculated steps of steroid action, 2) steroid receptor structure and function, 3) the role of steroid response elements, 4) the role of transcription factors (TF) and the chromatin acceptor proteins in receptor-DNA interactions, and 5) the cascade model of steroid hormone action, including the rapid steroid regulation of the expression of the nuclear proto-oncogenes and their role as regulatory genes in this model. Owing to space limitations, the authors have cited recent comprehensive reviews with only selected specific references. We have also had to omit important discussions of various aspects of the field. For more comprehensive reviews on the steroid regulation of gene expression, the readers are referred to the following references: Rories and Spelsberg,[1] Carson-Jurica *et al.*,[2] and a recent excellent book, *Nuclear Hormone Receptors*, edited by M. G. Parker.[3]

BASIC MECHANISM OF STEROID ACTION

Since the initial discovery that ecdysone, a steroidal insect growth hormone, could induce the formation of "puffs" in polytene chromosomes, the elucidation of the mechanism by which steroid hormones exert their biological effects on target tissues has been the subject of intensive research. The model, proposed independently by both Gorski *et al.*[4] and Jensen *et al.*[5] more that 20 years ago, has provided a foundation for the proposal of ever-evolving models to explain the control of gene transcription by steroid hormones. The current model, shown in FIGURE 1, explains the mechanism of action of steroid hormones. While more detailed, this model does not differ greatly from the one originally proposed. Free steroids are thought to passively diffuse into all cells since there is no evidence for "active transport" of these molecules. Steroids are preferentially retained in target cells through the formation of stable complexes with specific intracellular receptor proteins (R) which are both steroid and tissue specific[6] and are present at a concentration of ca. 10,000–100,000 molecules per cell.

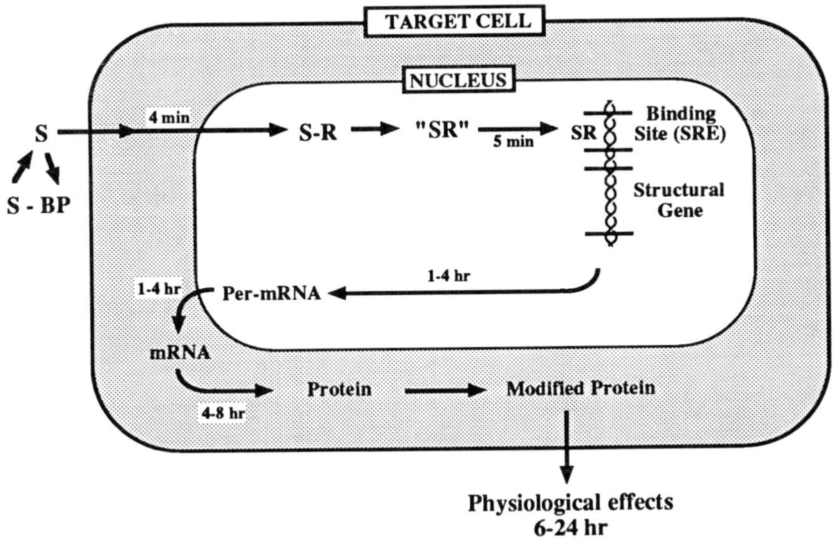

FIGURE 1. Steroid action pathway: general mechanism of action of steroid hormones. SRE = Steroid Response Element; S = Steroid; R = Receptor. The times (min) represent the interval after cell exposure to the steroid that detectable changes in the levels of the molecules are measured.

Each receptor binds its respective steroid reversibly but with high affinity; equilibrium dissociation constants (K_D) are somewhere between 10^{-10} to 10^{-8} M. Binding of the steroid induces a conformational/oligomeric "activation" of the receptor molecule which enables it to bind with high affinity to specific sites on chromatin, termed nuclear acceptor sites. Bound to the nuclear acceptor site, the activated steroid-receptor complex acts as a transcriptional regulator, altering the transcription of steroid-responsive genes and/or, in some cases, altering post-transcriptional steps causing a change in the steady-state levels of specific mRNAs and proteins.[7]

Important to both the physiological and mechanistic aspects of steroid-induced regulation of gene expression, is the chronological order with which these processes occur. In general, entrance of the steroids into the cell and the nuclear binding of the steroid receptor complex occurs within minutes after injection into an animal. Following the steroid-receptor complex (SR) formation (1–4 min post-treatment), is the binding of this complex to the nuclear acceptor sites (2–5 min), effects of this nuclear binding on RNA synthesis (minutes for "early" genes and several hours for "late" genes), and finally, changes in protein profiles due to changes in protein synthesis and protein turnover (6 hours and longer post-treatment). The major physiological effects of steroids in cells, however, are observed by 12 to 24 hours after steroid treatment. The 2 to 4 hour period between the SR binding to the nuclear acceptor sites and the late gene transcriptional response has been termed the "lag" phase or period and is still not understood. While the elucidation of SR receptor structure and the specific DNA sequences with which they interact has provided insight into their role in the elicitation of steroid-induced biologic effects, the molecular processes and

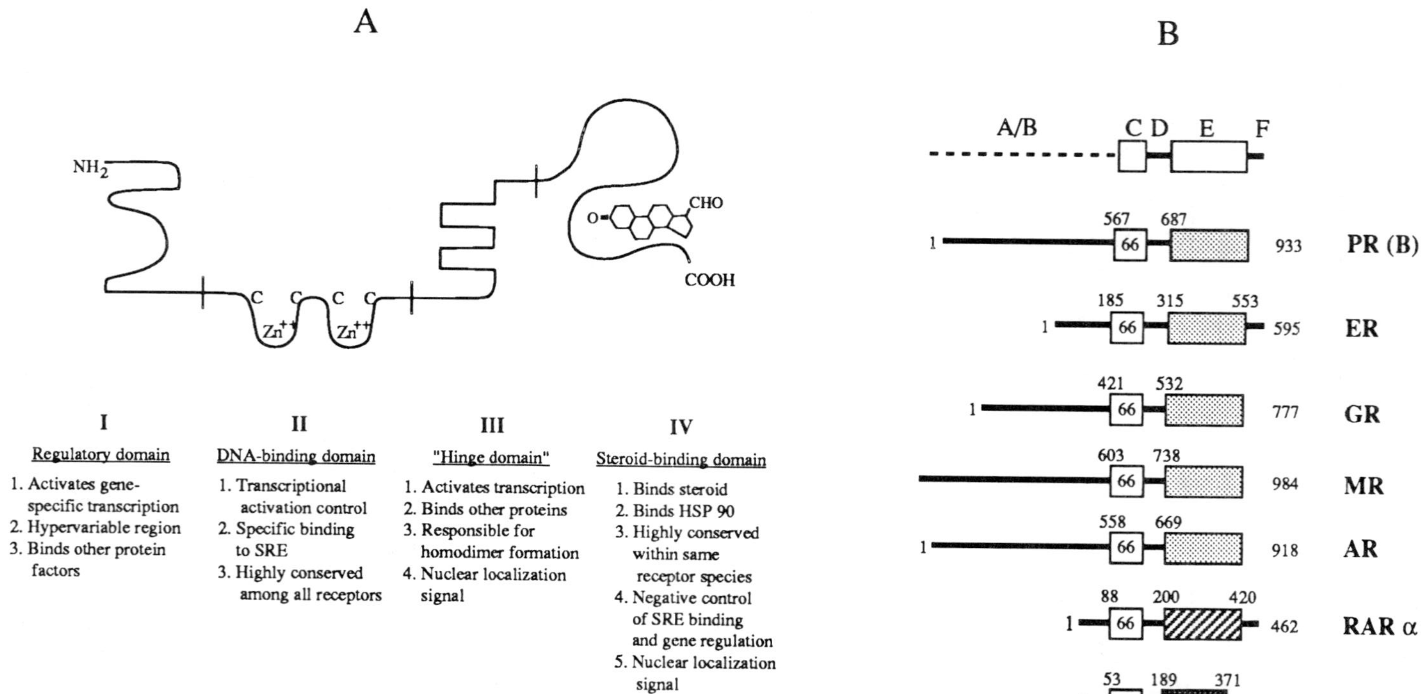

FIGURE 2. Model of the receptor domains. *Panel A* represents a model summarizing the functions of the various domains of the receptor. *Panel B* represents another type of model showing amino acid numbers at the various domain borders with a listing of each of the receptor species. PR, ER, GR, and AR are defined in the text. MR = mineralcorticoid; RARα = retinoic acid receptor; TR = thyroid receptor. (Modified with permission from Spelsberg *et al.*[156] [*Panel A*] and Jensen[155] [*Panel B*].)

specific components of the SR which govern specific gene transcription are still largely unresolved.

PRIMARY STRUCTURE OF THE RECEPTOR

General Receptor Domains

As a means to understanding how SR regulate the transcriptional activity of specific genes, extensive structure/function studies have been undertaken. Biochemical, immunological and genetic analyses of certain SR have provided strong evidence that these receptor proteins fold into three separate domains which mediate distinct functions of the receptor.[8] This has been confirmed by the cloning, sequencing, and functional analysis of cDNAs encoding the progesterone receptors (PR) from the chicken[9,10] and rabbit,[11] the glucocorticoid receptors (GR) from the mouse,[12] human,[13] and rat,[14] as well as the cDNAs encoding the estrogen receptors (ER) from human,[15] chicken,[16] mouse,[17] frog,[18] and rainbow trout.[19] FIGURE 2 illustrates the general domains of receptors which are members of the steroid receptor superfamily and outlines the functional characteristics of each domain. The receptors range in size from 427 amino acids for the vitamin D_3 receptor to 984 amino acids for the mineralocorticoid receptor. Despite this variation in size, all receptor species are extremely comparable in terms of their composition and domain functions. Reading in the N-terminal to the C-terminal direction, the receptors contain a variable (or transcriptionally regulating) domain at the N-terminal (I or A/B), a DNA binding domain (II or C) of 66–68 amino acids, a "hinge" domain (III), and a steroid binding domain (IV or E) which, in addition to steroid binding, contributes to receptor function in some, as yet, undefined manner. It should be mentioned here since it is not discussed later, that Region I, also referred to as the A/B domains, at the N-terminal end, is thought to be involved in cell type–specific regulation of gene transcription, possibly receptor-receptor homodimer formation, or receptor-receptor and receptor-transcription factor heterodimer formation. Interestingly, in comparison with other receptor species, the ER is largely deficient in Domain I, which is thought to be important in transcriptional control. The fact that many of these other domains (II, III and IV) are highly conserved in ER, PR, and GR, led to the use of the cDNAs in hybridization assays for the identification of other related genes and proteins of this family. This resulted in the discovery of a family of other receptors, such as those for mineralocorticoids,[2] retinoic acid,[20] thyroid hormone (T_3),[21] and Vitamin D,[2] were part of the steroid receptor superfamily. Still other proteins with functions that have not yet been unequivocally defined, have also been identified as part of a larger superfamily of DNA-binding proteins that regulate gene expression and include an upstream promoter transcription factor in the chicken (coup protein),[22] yeast proteins,[23] and more recently, several proteins in *Drosophila*.[24-26] Clearly the receptor superfamily represents genes that have evolved from a common ancestor.

The DNA-binding Domain (II and III)

The DNA-binding domain (II or C) of SRs is the most highly conserved region among members of the SR family (see 66–68 amino acids or Domain II in FIG. 2).

This domain contains two subregions which are encoded by two separate exons. The amino acid residues of the subregions were originally thought to fold into two adjacent protruding DNA-binding domains, termed "zinc fingers-like motifs" in recognition of their loose similarity to the zinc-stabilized DNA-binding "fingers" of *Xenopus laevis* transcription factor IIIA.[27,18] The solution structure of the DNA binding domain has only been solved for the ER,[29] and GR,[30a] and shows that the two zinc finger-like motifs actually fold to form a single structural domain unlike the independently folded units of the TFIIIA-type zinc fingers. More is discussed on the actual structure of this domain in the section on receptor binding to the DNA response elements. This DNA-binding domain in the receptors displays an enhanced binding to DNA sequences that function as enhancers of transcription of steroid regulated genes.[30b] This domain also appears to be the only portion of a receptor protein absolutely required to mediate transcription of a steroid responsive gene,[31] with the possible exception of a short piece of the flanking "hinge" region on the C-terminal side of the DNA-binding domain (Domain III in FIG. 2).[32] Part of the second zinc finger of Domain II and Domain III are speculated to interact with "other" proteins (*e.g.*, transcription factors, other molecules of the receptor complex) to form heterodimers. Domain swapping experiments show that Domain II controls which element and gene will be regulated by a receptor. Further studies with chimeric ERs have shown that three amino acids on the C-terminal side of the CI finger are critical to receptor recognition of the appropriate response element.[33]

Steroid-binding Domain (IV)

Functional analysis of GR deletion mutants[34] and protease digestion of the native receptor[35] have localized the steroid binding domain to the C-terminal one-third of the receptor protein. Similar experimental approaches have revealed that the highly conserved protein domains of the C-terminal region (roughly 250 amino acids) (see FIG. 2, Domain IV) serve analogous functions in progesterone[36] and estrogen[32,37] receptors. Studies with the GR have shown that the steroid-binding domain is key in regulating the transcriptional activity of the receptor and that this activity is relatively independent of receptor structure: repositioning the steroid-binding domain from the C-terminus to the N-terminus of the receptor molecule does not affect its control of DNA-binding activity or transcriptional regulation.[38] Interestingly, the fusion of the steroid-binding domain (IV) with an unrelated protein, the adenovirus ElA gene product, places the protein activity under hormonal control. Overall, as depicted in FIGURE 2, this domain when joined with other proteins, is known for its ability to inhibit the activities of the other proteins, *e.g.*, the inhibition of the DNA binding of transcription factors. When it is fused to these factors as a chimeric protein, it inhibits their regulatory activity and this effect is reversed when the Domain IV portion is complexed with a steroid ligand.

Specific subregions of the steroid binding domain that are specifically responsible for conferring this transcriptional activity or a "transcriptional activating function" (TAF) have been identified in certain receptor systems and, in some cases, are very similar to the "acidic activating domains" (AAD) of Gal4 and VP16.[39] TAFs in several other receptors differ structurally from the AADs of Gal4 and VP16 in that they are not acidic in nature. It is important to note that TAFs are apparently not restricted to the steroid-binding domain since they have also been identified in other receptor domains.[40]

Despite our detailed knowledge of the various domains and subdomains of the steroid receptor, there is little agreement as to the mechanistic role of the steroid in receptor function. Intrinsic in any model of steroid action is the assumption that steroid binding is essential for the "activation" of the receptor to a form that is capable of high affinity binding to DNA and the regulation of specific gene transcription. However, this simple assumption has been flawed by *in vitro* studies using purified receptors wherein receptor/DNA interactions can occur in the absence of steroid. For example, Willmann and Beato[41] showed that not only could steroid-free GR bind selectively to the mouse mammary tumor virus (MMTV) SRE, but that it did so with slightly better binding than observed in the presence of the hormone. Similar conclusions have been reached with the estrogen[42–45] and progesterone[46] receptors. Thus, the DNA binding of SR is not absolutely dependent on the presence of the hormone.

One explanation for these observations may be that in crude preparations the receptor is associated with other factors that inhibit interaction with specific DNA sequences and that hormonal treatment or purification induces the release of the inhibitory factors. Ideal candidates for these factors are the heat shock proteins (hsp90 and hsp70) which are associated with steroid receptor complexes and released upon binding hormone.[47,48] Support for this hypothesis comes from the results of *in vitro* transcription studies which demonstrate that purified ligand-bound receptors function to enhance the transcription of genes containing SRE while steroid-free receptors from crude nuclear extracts fail to activate transcriptional activity.[49] An alternative explanation has been provided by Schauer *et al.*[50] who studied the kinetics of the interaction between the receptor and DNA and showed that the steroid had a tremendous effect on the rate of receptor association/dissociation with DNA. Hormone binding dramatically increased the receptor off-rate by as much as 30-fold over the unbound counterpart, whereas the on-rate was affected to a lesser extent (~5-fold increase). Beato *et al.*[51] suggested that this effect may not be specific to the GR but may, indeed, be a general property of steroid hormone receptors since similar observations were made with the PR from the rabbit uterus. Consequently, the steroid may alter the kinetics of the receptor/DNA interaction such that the receptor scans the genomic DNA for specific binding sites, in much the same way that several proteins with DNA-binding activities are thought to function.

An alternative explanation for the apparent lack of hormone-dependence in steroid receptor–binding may simply be that other nuclear (DNA-associated) proteins are involved in the specific interactions of SR with DNA sequences. This and other laboratories have identified candidate "acceptor" proteins on chromatin that may function in this capacity. This is discussed in more detail in a later section.

QUATERNARY STRUCTURE OF STEROID RECEPTORS

There is little doubt that the cloning, sequencing, and mutational analysis of several steroid receptors has helped our understanding of the functional components of the receptor involved in both the binding of the steroid and the subsequent binding of the activated steroid-receptor complex to the DNA. However, it has become clear that the higher order structure of the receptor is important in regulating the transcriptional potency of steroid receptors. This may be accomplished through the specific interaction of the receptor with other proteins, which may ultimately regulate the receptor either prior to steroid activation (*i.e.*, stabilize the untransformed complex) or during the interaction of the transformed receptor with chromatin and the primary transcription complex.

Interaction of Steroid Receptors with Hsp90 and Other Proteins

Steroid receptors exist as part of a large multimeric complex in their unactivated state within the cell. The 8S/9S form of the receptor is typically considered the unactivated form and the 4S the activated receptor. Recent studies have shown that the 300 kDa 8S/9S form may, in fact, be derived from an even larger heteromeric complex, potentially of cytoskeletal origin.[52] The multimeric nature of steroid receptor complexes raises questions as to the identity of the other proteins which are associated with the steroid binding subunit. In this respect, the preparation of monoclonal antibodies, and particularly the advent of immunoaffinity chromatography, has revolutionized the study of steroid hormone receptor complexes, and led to the realization that steroid hormone receptors are associated with other nonsteroid-binding protein subunits. One of these nonsteroid-binding proteins, a 90 kDa heat shock protein (hsp90), has been found to be associated with most unactivated steroid hormone receptors studied thus far.[53,54] It has not yet been unequivocally determined whether any of the components of the complex other than the SR itself are required for signal transduction. However, several lines of circumstantial evidence indicate that hsp90 plays a key role in regulating receptor function. For example, studies with the GR have shown that hsp90 may be key in the maintenance of the inactive GR and the formation of a functional hormone-binding domain. When hsp90 is dissociated from the complex prior to steroid binding, the resultant receptor complex is unable to bind the steroid.[55] Further, truncated forms of the GR lacking 80 amino acids of the steroid binding domain that are key to hsp90 binding, are constitutively active (albeit at a lower level), are localized in the nucleus and display high affinity DNA binding and transcriptional regulation in the absence of steroid.[56]

The identity and number of binding sites for hsp90 within steroid receptors is controversial. The sites of interaction seem to be restricted to the steroid-binding domain since most of the N-terminal and DNA-binding regions of the receptor can be deleted without markedly affecting the hsp90 binding. Transfection studies using deletion mutants of the mouse GR (in COS cells) suggest a limited interaction of hsp90 with the steroid-binding domain.[57] A deletion of a highly conserved region of the steroid binding domain results in a receptor that is very unstable, has constitutive transcriptional activity, but very little receptor-associated hsp90. These authors propose that there are two contact sites between hsp90 and the steroid-binding domain. These data are consistent with the concept that hsp90 stabilizes the GR from proteolysis. More recent studies with PR, GR, and ER indicate that multiple contact sites may be involved in the binding of hsp90. Toft and coworkers,[58] using several deletion mutants of the steroid-binding domain (IV) of the avian oviduct PR, found that hsp90 binding was obliterated (and hsp70 binding diminished) only when the entire steroid-binding domain was deleted; three separate regions were found to be crucial for restoration of hsp90 and hsp70 binding. Cadepond *et al.*,[59] used a similar approach to study the interaction of hsp90 with deletion mutants of the human GR and concurred that multiple sites of interaction were involved. Interestingly, the ability of these specific subregions of the steroid binding domain to promote hsp90 binding was apparently sequence independent since the individual linkage of each subregion to the truncated receptor restored the formation of the 8S oligomeric complex. Similar results were found with ER where the complete deletion of the steroid-binding domain resulted in a truncated receptor that was unable to form the 9S complex.[60] In summary, several regions of the steroid binding domain (Domain IV) were found to confer hsp90 binding but no single region was particularly essential to this binding. In contrast, the N-terminal region of the receptor, including the two zinc fingers of the DNA binding domain (Domains I and II), were found not to be required for formation of the 9S complex.

The *in vivo* function(s) of heat shock proteins has not yet been defined unequivocally, although it has been speculated that they may function in the general maintenance of the cell.[61] Potential functions include the stabilization of other proteins under denaturing conditions, maintenance of unfavorable protein conformations, prevention of premature protein aggregation and, in the case of steroid receptors, the masking of DNA-binding sites. In many cases, they may function as protein "chaperones" which regulate and direct the assembly of multimeric protein complexes.[62] For the case of the PR, other non-receptor proteins, in addition to hsp90, have recently been shown to be associated with the steroid binding subunit. Avian oviduct PR isolated by immunoprecipitation was associated with hsp70,[48] hsp90 and several novel receptor-associated proteins.[63] Non-hsp proteins with apparent molecular weights of 54, 50 and 23 kDa (referred to as p54, p50 and p23) have also been shown to be part of the unactivated PR complex and have provided the basis for re-evaluation of steroid receptor transformation (see FIG. 3). These results are similar to those of Faber and colleagues who have shown the common association of a 59 kDa protein with the progesterone, estrogen, androgen and glucocorticoid receptors.[64] Interestingly, partial reconstitution of the avian PR to an oligomeric complex containing hsp90 and hsp70 could be achieved in rabbit reticulocyte lysate.[65] In a mixture containing both rabbit reticulocyte lysate and oviduct cytosol, reconstitution was markedly reduced, indicating that oviduct cytosol may contain "factors" having a negative influence on reconstitution. However, the absence of reconstitution in oviduct cytosol alone indicates that rabbit reticulocyte lysate may contain factors which promote the binding of these components to the steroid-binding subunit. Reconstitution was inhibited in the presence of hormone, consistent with the concept that hormone induces the dissociation of these proteins from the complex during "activation."

While the role of these associated proteins in steroid receptor function is still only speculative, it is likely that they do play a role in some aspect of receptor transport, stability and/or transformation. For example, it is known that receptor phosphorylation is at least one of the (many) processes involved in the transformation of the cytosolic PR to its DNA-binding counterpart. The presence of non-receptor, non-hsp proteins in the native PR complex may provide a plausible mechanistic explanation for phosphorylation concurrent with activation.[66,67] It is not unreasonable to anticipate that one of the higher molecular weight proteins (*e.g.*, p54 or p50) has kinase activity since this function is consistent with the observation that p54 was dissociable in a steroid-dependent manner. One could envisage a steroid-induced phosphorylation which would effect a conformational change in the PR with the subsequent dissociation of p54 and hsp90. These events could result in a smaller DNA-binding form which has new sites exposed on the receptor. Ideal candidates for these on the receptor sites

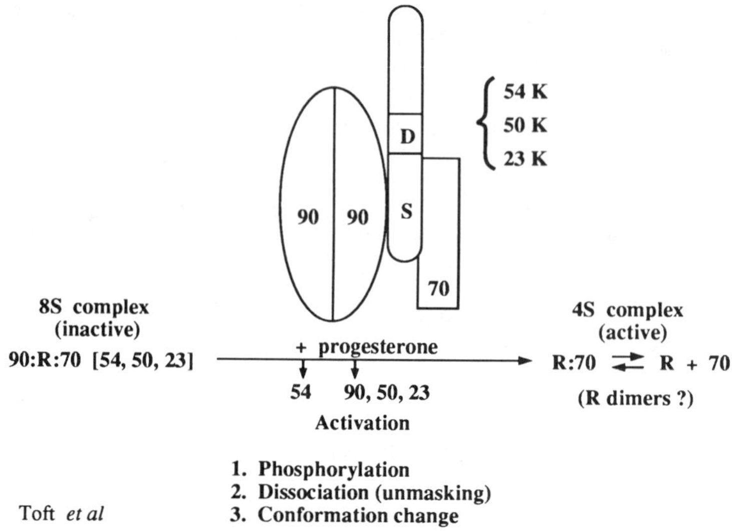

FIGURE 3. Higher order structure of PR. Hsp90 exists as a dimer and, along with hsp70, interacts with the steroid-binding domain of the progesterone receptor (R; Steroid binding (S) and DNA binding (D) domains are illustrated). The location of binding of the 54, 50, and 23 kDa nonreceptor proteins within the PR complex is not known. Their behavior in the presence of salt and molybdate is very similar to hsp90. However, it is not clear whether they interact directly with the receptor or with hsp90/70 or both. Their function in the transformation of the receptor to an active DNA-binding form is not known. Following activation *in vivo*, hsp70 appears to remain at least partially bound. Whether this is indicative of an hsp70 requirement for the specific interaction of the receptor with chromatin, DNA or other nuclear proteins is still open to question. Alternatively, hsp70, known to play a role in modulating protein folding (Rothman, 1989),[61] may be responsible for conformational or other changes in the receptor during the activation process. (Used with permission from Toft *et al.*[154])

may be other DNA-associated proteins (acceptor site proteins or docking site proteins) on chromatin proposed to play a key role in regulating early gene expression by the activated PR and GR complex (for review, see refs. 1 and 68) (FIG. 4). This idea is consistent with the studies of Edwards and coworkers[69] and Spelsberg and coworkers[1] who have identified a nuclear factor which enhances the binding of PR to specific DNA sequences. A clear potential role for non-receptor proteins in mediating the interaction of the receptor complex with specific DNA sequences and DNA-associated proteins exists, but it is not yet understood. Additional aspects of these other proteins are shown in FIGURE 4 and are discussed later.

RECEPTOR PHOSPHORYLATION

Phosphorylated forms of several steroid hormone receptors have been identified including those for the glucocorticoids, progesterone and estrogens.[53,54] Although several studies have implicated events such as phosphorylation in the regulation of steroid receptor function, the direct effect of post-translational modification is yet to be

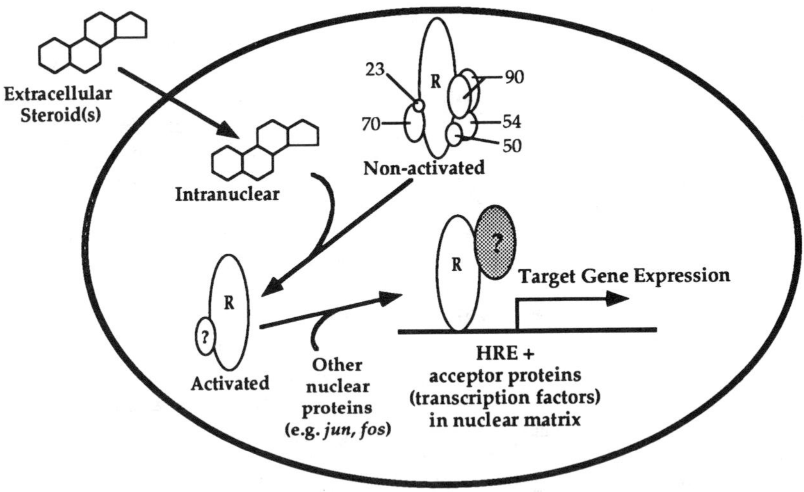

FIGURE 4. Schematic model of steroid hormone action. The steroid enters the cell where it binds to the non-activated receptor (R) in either the cytosol or the nucleus. Steroid binding brings about activation of the receptor which is thought to include the release of proteins (depicted as open circles attached to the non-activated receptor), and a change into a form able to associate with chromatin. Hsp70 or other proteins may be part of the activated receptor (depicted as hollow circle with ?). Other nuclear proteins (depicted as shaded circle with ?) may be involved when association with chromatin occurs at an appropriate hormone response element (HRE). This particular interaction with chromatin is presumably responsible for the regulation of transcription of responsive genes.

defined.[2] While earlier studies by Smith *et al.*[70] indicated that GR activation was unlikely to involve phosphorylation or other covalent charge modification, more recent studies clearly show that the GR is endogenously phosphorylated at four specific serine residues, one in the DNA-binding domain and three adjacent to this binding domain.[71] Despite the lack of evidence supporting a role for phosphorylation in the hormone regulation of receptor function, these authors proposed that the phosphorylation of a serine-rich region next to the DNA-binding domain may serve to destabilize charge interactions required for the interaction with DNA and hence play a role in receptor cycling. The importance of phosphorylation in receptor function under physiological conditions was demonstrated by Orti *et al.*,[72] who showed the hormone-dependent change in the GR phosphorylation state *in vivo.* GR agonists (*e.g.*, triamcinolone acetonide) but not antagonists (*e.g.*, RU 486) increased the number of phosphates in the GR from 3 to 5.

NUCLEAR LOCALIZATION SEQUENCES OF STEROID RECEPTORS

There are two common mechanisms by which proteins enter the nucleus: 1) a diffusion through the nuclear membrane followed by binding to some intranuclear component or 2) a nuclear signal in the amino acid sequence (nuclear localization signal) which directs the protein to the nucleus.[73] As depicted in FIGURE 2, all steroid receptors contain a sequence of basic amino acids (arginines, lysines) in the general vicinity of the second zinc finger (between the DNA- and steroid-binding domains) (*i.e.*, in the hinge region or Domain III) that, although not highly conserved, is similar to that of the SV40 large T antigen. The basic region has been implicated as the nuclear localization signal for several steroid receptors including those for the glucocorticoids,[74] mineralocorticoids,[75] estrogens,[76] androgens,[77] and progesterone.[78a] To study the GR, Picard and Yamamoto[74] attached this sequence to other proteins and showed that the resulting hybrid protein localized to the nucleus. In addition, GRs with C-terminal deletions extending into the basic region are transcriptionally inactive.[31,78b] Apparently, these sequences are also necessary for the interaction with DNA.[79,80] Studies of the PR system by Milgrom and coworkers confirm the presence of a nuclear localization signal in the vicinity of the second zinc finger.[78a] They point out that this sequence is highly conserved among PRs from other species. Moreover, if other steroid receptors are aligned through their DNA-binding domains, homologous sequences are found in all steroid receptors in exactly the same position, that is, 10 amino acids after the last conserved cysteine.

Also depicted in FIGURE 2 is the identification of additional nuclear localization signals in the hormone binding domain (Domain IV). Picard and Yamamoto[74] showed that the sequence in the hormone-binding domain of the GR was hormone-dependent. This may have some significance to the cytosolic localization of the unbound receptor. Similarly, Green and Chambon[76] report that a region important for the interaction of the ER with hsp90 may play a role in nuclear localization. The role of these localization signals is not fully understood.

STEROID-RECEPTOR BINDING TO STEROID-RESPONSE ELEMENTS (SRE)

The characteristics of the DNA-binding domain of steroid receptors has been described earlier. These conserved domains are responsible for the receptor binding to conserved DNA sequences (elements) about 13–26 basepairs in length. The regulation of gene transcription by steroid hormone receptors is now known to be mediated by specific DNA sequences located in the vicinity of the regulated gene (for a recent review, see Martinez and Wahli[81]). Such transcriptional control regions have been identified in a variety of genes, and the comparison of these sequences has allowed for the identification of a consensus sequence for steroid receptor–binding sites. The binding of steroid receptors to these consensus sequences has been confirmed by DNase I and DMS methylation protection experiments using purified hormone-bound receptor.[81,82] Synthetic oligonucleotides cloned upstream of the herpes simplex thymidine kinase (tk) promoter have been found to confer responsiveness to the receptors for glucocorticoids and progestins, estrogens, or androgens to this otherwise unresponsive transcription unit. These elements are usually found as inverted repeats (palindromes) but sometimes as direct repeats or even as single elements. Many of these elements have been identified as steroid-response elements (SREs) since many have been shown to modulate steroid regulation of gene transcription.[81] The palindromic structure of the SREs is a candidate for the binding of receptor homodimers. Evidence for the binding of receptor dimers to DNA (SREs) has been reported by several laboratories for estrogens and glucocorticoids,[83-85] as well as for thyroid hormones.[86]

The SREs of one steroid receptor often act in synergistic action with additional copies of their own SREs, or with the SREs of other steroids, or with the elements of transcription factors. These synergistic combinations act as strong acting arrays called "Steroid Response Units" (SRU). In contrast to the SREs, the SRUs can act in an orientation- and distance-independent manner.[81] It is interesting that two or more SREs for GR have been found in MMTV, lysozyme gene, rat uteroglobin gene, rat tyrosine aminotransferase (TAT) gene, and rat tryptophan oxygenase (TO) gene and for the ER in the xenopus and chicken vitellogenin genes.[82] In many instances, a synergistic action for two of these SREs in a gene is found. Additional SREs (*i.e.*, greater than two) have no further effect on gene transcription.[87,88] Interestingly, two different steroid receptors, GR and ER, have also been shown to play a synergistic role in the regulation of the chicken vitellogenin II gene transcription.[89,90] The synergism between 2 SREs for progesterone and/or glucocorticoid were shown to be partly due to an increase in binding affinity of the SRs to these elements.[88] The binding affinity for purified PR was 100-fold greater for a double GRE/PRE than for a single element as measured by gel shift assays. The binding to the direct repeats or to monomer elements might well involve the interaction of the receptors with other proteins possibly involving heterodimer formation with other factors, as described in the next section. There is evidence for a leucine zipper, a typical motif for DNA binding proteins, in the ER which could be the site of receptor homodimerization or even heterodimerization.[85]

Interestingly, past theoretical studies of the structure of the DNA binding domains[91,92] supported by actual NMR studies [30] strongly suggest that the two zinc finger motifs do not have the typical structures as found in the DNA-binding transcription factors. Instead, the 2 zinc fingers are folded into a single domain whose structure is a helix-turn-helix motif found in many DNA-binding proteins including transcription factors. This structure appears to bind to the large groove of the DNA. Lastly, there have even been reports that the second zinc finger might be involved in receptor–nonreceptor protein interactions.

Role of Transcription Factors and Their DNA-binding Elements in Steroid Action

Recent studies have revealed the presence of DNA regions composed of not only the SREs, but also the elements for binding other transcriptional factors. As mentioned above, these domains which significantly affect steroid-mediated transcription have been termed steroid-response units (SRUs); they can modulate steroid action at great distances from genes. Interestingly, there is evidence that the second zinc finger (closest to the C-terminal end of the receptor) may be involved in the binding to other proteins.[1,76] It should also be noted that zinc finger structures are known to also be involved in protein-protein interactions.[93] Indeed, a role for other nuclear proteins in the nuclear interactions of SR with the DNA and/or the nuclear acceptor sites on the interphase chromatin has long been supported.[1,76,99,108]

Over the past several years there has been an increasing number of reports describing SR interactions with other proteins including transcription factors (TF).[81,94] In one study, the chicken lysozyme gene promoter[95] and the chicken ovalbumin gene promoter[96] were transfected, with reporter genes, into different cell lines containing glucocorticoid and progesterone receptors. Interestingly, these genes responded to steroid in certain cell types but not others, although all cell types contained the receptors.[96] These studies implicate a role for tissue-specific regulatory proteins (transcription factors) in the mediation of steroid action on gene expression. Further, the N-terminal domain (Domain I) of the receptors was found to play a role in this tissue-specific action by interacting with these factors. For example, when transcription was induced with glucocorticoids, the transcription factors were shown to bind within minutes of the steroid treatment as specific sites within the glucocorticoid/progesterone-sensitive promoter of the mouse mammary tumor virus-long terminal repeat (MMTV-LTR).[97] These particular factors are present before hormonal stimulation, but do not bind to the MMTV-LTR DNA until the steroid is added. In the chicken vitellogenin gene, a factor was shown to bind to a 14 base pair element in the third intron and to stimulate transcription of the gene *in vitro.*[98] This intron-binding transcription factor appears to be present in the unstimulated cells, but the addition of estrogen somehow activates the factor to bind to the DNA domain (Jost *et al.*, 1987). The factor is active in E_2-stimulated rooster liver, but not in non-E_2–treated liver.

The cell type specific gene regulation described above has received more attention with additional studies on the interactions between the steroid receptors and transcription factors.[82,99] Some of these studies demonstrated that other sequences besides the SREs are involved in the steroid regulation of gene transcription. Sequences neighboring GREs, *e.g.*, GREs next to the TO gene (a CACCC binding site) or in the MMTV promoter (a NF-1–binding site), are required for steroid regulation and demonstrated the importance of non-DNA–binding sites for steroid induction of gene transcription. A computer search of known transcription factor–binding sites which neighbor known GREs near known glucocorticoid-regulated genes has shown that most genes contain steroid response units (discussed above), *i.e.*, have transcription factor elements within 50 bp of their GREs.[82] These studies have demonstrated that the strength of many SREs is provided not only by the steroid receptor–binding element (SRE) but by non-receptor binding elements which bind other proteins, *i.e.*, transcription factors. These different transcription factor elements and their binding proteins act synergistically with SREs. For instance, studies by Renkawitz *et al.*[100] and Schüle *et al.*[94] demonstrated that the placement of any one of a number of transcription factor binding elements (CACCC, NF-1, CBP, SP-1, OTF) or even another SRE for progesterone (PRs) near a PRE in a CAT reporter gene enhanced the transcription of the CAT gene.[82] Further, the relative orientation and arrangement of the PRE and the CACCC box had no effect on this functional cooperativity.[101] Interestingly, there is evidence for a requirement for a stereo-specific alignment of each of the 2 factors (GRE and CACCC box) since an insertion or deletion in 5 bp increments which displace the factors around one-half turn of the double helix, disrupts their synergism in the transcriptional activation.[94,100,101] These results support a direct receptor-protein-transcription factor interaction.

The spatial distances between two SREs or between an SRE and a transcription-factor element appear to be important. However, such distances are not a factor when considering SREs and the TATA boxes located in the promoter regions of steroid-regulated genes. This is thought to be due to the DNA looping encouraged by protein-protein interactions possibly involving non-DNA–binding proteins.[102] One protein which may represent a "DNA loop-protein" (*i.e.*, "folding-protein or adaptor-protein")

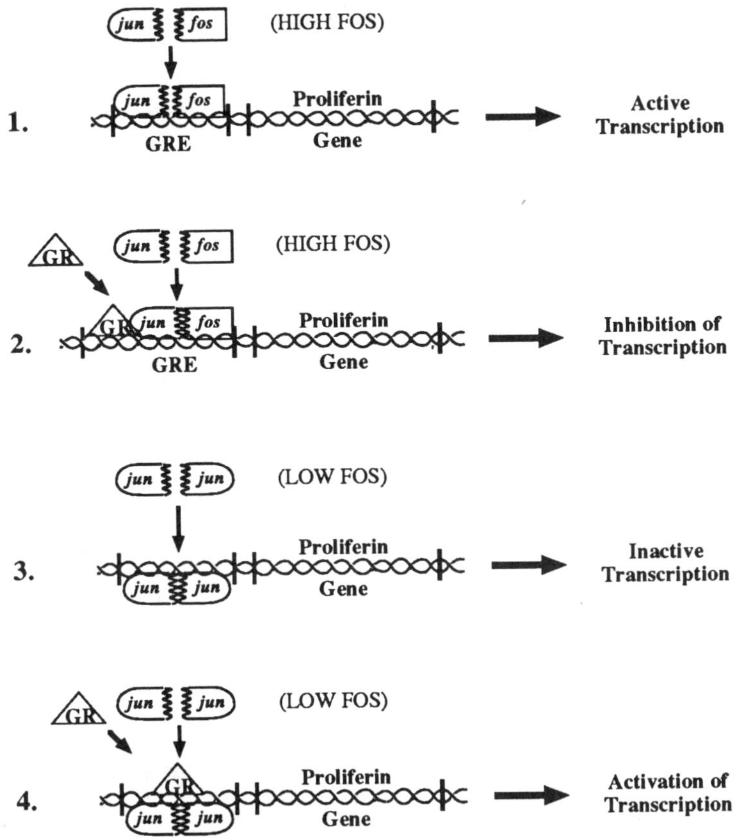

FIGURE 5. Model of the GR interaction with the AP-1 complex to regulate the proliferin gene. Jun and Fos represent oncoproteins making up the AP-1 transcription factor complex. The data upon which this model is based were taken from Diamond *et al.*[106a]

is the S300-II transcription factor in the avian oviduct ovalbumin gene.[103] The S300-II is a non-DNA–binding protein required for transcription of the ovalbumin gene *in vitro.* It stabilizes the binding of COUP-TF (chicken oviduct upstream promoter-transcription factor) to the COUP sequence, and is speculated to bridge a DNA loop binding COUP-TF with the factors bound to the TATA box.

Recently the *jun* and *fos* proteins, bound together as an AP-1 transcription-factor heterodimer, have been shown to play a major role in the steroid receptor interaction with the DNA and in the steroid regulation of gene expression. An example of this is depicted in FIGURE 5. Recent work by Weisz *et al.*,[103b] has shown that estrogen increases the *c-jun* transcription by three- to four-fold in the rat uterus and presented evidence that the transcriptional activation of this proto-oncogene is a primary response to the hormone. Further, four copies of the AP-1 element, cloned in front of the reporter gene, were shown to be sufficient to bring about transcription by estrogen in

MCF-7 cells. These studies demonstrate that SREs are not even required for this estrogen regulation of the *c-jun* and that AP-1 elements can substitute for the SREs in the steroid regulation of gene transcription. The regulation of the human *c-fos* gene expression by steroids may actually involve the estrogen response element located upstream of the promoter. This element has been shown to bind ER as well as the AP-1 transcription factor and has been shown to regulate transcription when placed with a heterologous promoter and examined for estrogen regulation.[104] It is interesting that estrogen response element (ERE) from the ovalbumin gene binds the AP-1 transcription factor complex, *i.e.*, the heterodimer composed of *c-fos* and *c-jun*.[105] Transfection experiments have shown that *c-fos*, *c-jun* and ER (ER) coactivate the ovalbumin promoter through these sequences.[105]

As depicted in FIGURE 5, recent findings have shown that a 25 base pair glucocorticoid response element (GRE) that resides upstream of the mouse proliferin promoter is recognized by both GR and AP-1 factors which are responsible for the positive and negative regulation by glucocorticoids.[106a] A model by Diamond *et al.*[106b] in which the glucocorticoids interact with AP-1 transcription heterodimer (*fos/jun*) or homodimer (*jun/jun*) to either inhibit or activate transcription of the proliferin gene is also outlined in FIGURE 5. The levels of *fos* onco-protein thus determines whether the steroid inhibits or induces the gene. In another system, Jonet *et al.*[106a] and Yang-Yen *et al.*[107] have also demonstrated that glucocorticoids interfere with the AP-1 transcription-factor complex, the essential enhancer factor of the collagenase promoter, to inhibit transcription of the collagenase gene.

The Chromatin Acceptor Proteins/Acceptor Sites

Intact (native) nuclei or chromatin displays highly specific binding sites for a variety of steroid receptors. Using a different approach from the SRE studies described above, we and others (for reviews see refs. 1 and 108) investigated the direct binding of steroid receptors to the native nuclei, the nuclear chromatin, or chromatin fractions, as well as the nuclear matrix. These studies revealed the presence of nuclear "acceptor" sites which display a saturable, high affinity, specific binding of steroid receptors with binding affinities of $K_D \sim 10^{-10}$ to 10^{-8}M. Each species of steroid receptor has its own unique class of nuclear acceptor sites. These nuclear acceptor sites for steroid receptors in chromatin or nuclear matrix have been shown to involve specific nuclear proteins, *i.e.*, acceptor proteins.[69,108–120] An acceptor protein has also been identified for the thyroid receptor.[121]

The chromatin acceptor sites for the avian oviduct PR have been studied extensively. These sites display high affinity binding of steroid receptors *in vivo* and *in vitro* and appear to consist of specific chromatin acceptor proteins bound to DNA, with evidence for specific DNA sequences.[1] Initially the binding of [^{3}H]progesterone *in vivo* in the avian oviduct was characterized and a cell-free binding assay was developed to mimic the former. The cell-free binding of [^{3}H]PR to avian-oviduct chromatin and to a dehistonized chromatin preparation, termed nucleoacidic protein (or NAP), is saturable, with high affinity ($K_D \sim 10^{-9}$ M), and receptor-dependent.[1,122] Besides these *in vivo*-like binding properties, the cell-free binding yields similar numbers of receptor molecules bound per cell as measured *in vivo*.[122] Further, the receptor must be activated and bound with the steroid ligand to display a specific binding to these chromatin acceptor sites *in vitro*. Chuknyiska *et al.*[123] and Spelsberg *et al.*[122] using two separate steroid target tissue systems, were able to show comparable binding *in vivo* to nuclear acceptor sites and *in vitro* in isolated nuclei. Many properties between the sites on chromatin and those on the nuclear matrix appear to be similar.[1,124] Further, the chromatin acceptor sites for PR and the nuclear matrix sites for PR appear to represent one and the same class of acceptor sites.[125] Common properties of these sites are their DNase resistance, their high affinity binding of steroid receptors, and their composition of proteins tightly bound to DNA. Lastly, all the PR binding sites in oviduct chromatin have been localized in the nuclear matrix.[125]

Recently Spelsberg and coworkers[1,108,124] have purified one acceptor protein for the avian oviduct PR. Two, and possibly other, candidate chromatin acceptor proteins for PR, termed receptor binding factors (RBF), have been identified. As these proteins are removed from the chromatin (along with other proteins), a loss of the specific PR binding sites for PR is observed. When bound to avian DNA, both impure and pure fractions of these proteins generate high affinity, saturable, receptor-dependent binding of the PR to DNA. One of these proteins, RBF-1, has been purified over 10^5-fold to apparent homogeneity.[124] It has been partially sequenced and monoclonal antibodies (MAb) prepared against it. RBF-1 is a unique 10 kDa, hydrophobic protein with a pI ~5.5 and is species- and tissue-specific. The RBF-1 and the PR nuclear binding sites were both localized to the oviduct nuclear matrix using MAb in Western blot analyses and cell-free binding assays respectively. Recently studies using Southwestern blot (and DNA gel shift) analyses indicate that these sequences may reside in or near the steroid regulated genes but not the nonregulated genes. The RBF-1 is localized in the oviduct nucleus and specifically to the nuclear matrix where all of the avian oviduct PR nuclear binding sites are localized.[125] FIGURE 6 depicts a nuclear matrix model based on the above data with the RBF-1 protein bound by the avian oviduct PR at specific sequences in the promoter domain of the *c-myc* gene.

The PR binding remaining with the chromatin after the removal of RBF-1, *i.e.*, on the NAP, was classified as RBF-2. Since monoclonal antibodies against RBF-1 do not recognize any proteins in the crude RBF-2 preparations by Western immuno-

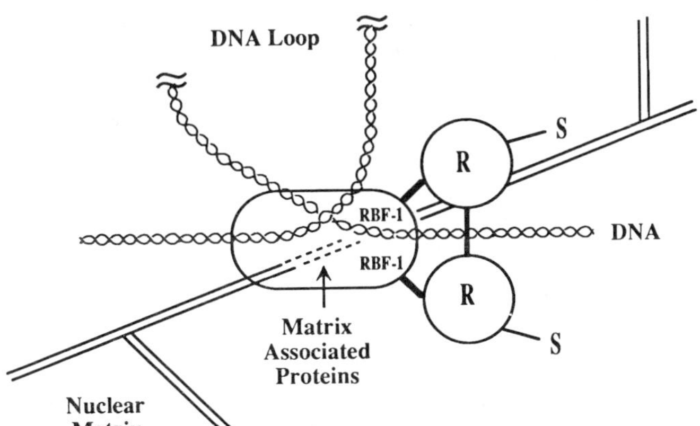

FIGURE 6. Model of the nuclear matrix as the locale for the chromatin acceptor sites for steroid receptors. RBF-1 = Receptor Binding Factor; SR = steroid receptor.

blotting, the PR binding activity remaining with the NAP (4M Gdn-HCl–extracted chromatin) is believed to be structurally distinct. The RBF-2 class of PR-binding activity in the NAP has received significant attention by researchers in our laboratory over the past 6 years.[1,108,122] However, since RBF-1 has been recently purified and found to be associated with the highest affinity PR-binding activity in whole chromatin, this factor and its DNA binding elements are receiving the greatest attention. When RBF-1 and associated proteins are removed from the whole chromatin by 0.2% (v/v) Triton X-100 extraction, the highest affinity class of sites measured in oviduct chromatin is abolished. The binding of [^{3}H]PR to the RBF-1 (chromatin) class of sites can be competed with nonradiolabeled PR but not with nonradiolabeled ER in cell-free and in intact-cell binding assays. These acceptor sites thus display a similar steroid receptor specificity in the cell-free binding assays as is found *in vivo* in the avian oviduct and in other steroid-target tissue systems.[1,108] The exact function for the two classes of PR acceptor sites in avian oviduct chromatin are not known.

It should be noted in concluding this section that small candidate chromatin "acceptor" proteins have been identified which are required for specific ER binding[126–128] or which are bound by androgen receptors *in vivo.*[129] The 12 kDa candidate acceptor protein for ER in rabbit uterine chromatin has very similar properties to the 10 kDA RBF-1 for avian oviduct PR identified by this laboratory. Like RBF-1, this candidate acceptor protein identified by Ruh and coworkers[128] can be recombined with genomic DNAs to regenerate the specific steroid binding to these DNAs. The methods used were similar to those used by this laboratory for the avian oviduct PR. Thus, evidence for the chromatin acceptor sites and acceptor proteins is extensive and their presence is almost universal in the animal kingdom. Their exact role in steroid receptor binding to the chromatin-gene structures is unclear, but it appears that they help guide the receptors to specific acceptor sites.

Role of the Early Genes as Regulatory Genes

Recognition of the distinct early and late transcriptional responses in midge salivary glands following administration of the steroid ecdysone led to the proposal that some of the early genes code for regulatory or transcription factors which are required for transcription of the late genes.[130a,130b] This model has been applied to the steroid-gene regulation systems by the authors[1,68,122] and is described in the following section. The model is appealing since it can explain the variable lag times observed for steroid induction of transcription.

As described above, there are now studies confirming the steroid-induced synthesis of transcription factors, and of steroids regulating the activity of endogenous transcription factors. The *fos/jun* transcription factors are a good example. These factors could be "activated" by enzymatic modifications coded by the regulatory genes or their binding to chromatin might be facilitated by steroid-induced changes in chromatin. A possible example of a "regulatory gene" in steroid regulation of transcription factors comes from recent studies in this laboratory on the effects of progesterone on *c-myc* proto-oncogene expression in the avian oviduct,[131] glucocorticoid action on *c-myc* in the avian oviduct,[132] as well as estrogen regulation of the *c-jun* gene.[133,134] Progesterone and/or glucocorticoids reduce the *c-myc* mRNA levels by 5 minutes in the avian oviduct by a maximum of 70% to 90% within 20 minutes after injection of steroid. The *c-myc* gene codes for a nuclear protein which is now thought to positively regulate the genes involved in the initiation of DNA replication.[135-137] Thus, a possible role of *c-myc* in the steroid regulation of cell proliferation exists. This system also could serve as an example of a steroid-regulated "regulatory" gene with the *c-myc* protein itself acting as a transcription factor, or possibly as an activator of transcription factors which regulate the expression of genes involved in the control of cell division and growth.

Support for this concept comes from other studies showing that *c-myc* is induced by estrogens (inducers of cell proliferation) in human breast cancer cells within 15 minutes after addition to the culture media.[138] Further, the mRNA of *N-myc* (another related proto-oncogene) was found to be induced by estrogens in the rat uterus by 15 minutes post-injection; however, changes in uterine *c-myc* mRNA were not observed until several hours later.[139,140] Similarly, glucocorticoids have been shown to markedly inhibit the *c-myc* gene expression in a lymphosarcoma cell line, in which glucocorticoids repress cell proliferation.[141] These data support the existence of early regulated "regulatory" genes of which the nuclear proto-oncogenes could well be members.

Cascade Model of Steroid Action

Based on the existence of early versus late genes, and the fact that steroids often regulate structural gene expression at post-transcriptional levels, as shown in FIGURE 7, we have formulated a model for ovarian steroid action (shown in FIG. 8). The basic format for this model is similar to that described by Clever and Romball[130a,130b] for the ecdysone-chromosome puff system. Recently, the protein products of the early gene (early puff) responses to the ecdysone steroid were shown to be members of the steroid receptor superfamily. Further, these genes are now identified as nuclear proto-oncogenes coding for transcription factors.[24] This model has been developed to be in accord with the data presented in the preceding section. The model, presented in FIGURE 8, is an extension of a similar model for steroid hormone action

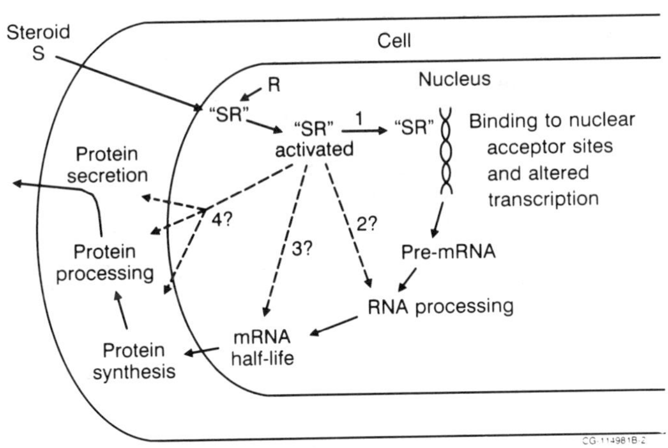

FIGURE 7. Mechanism of steroid action: model for the levels of regulation (*i.e.*, transcriptional and post-transcriptional) of gene expression by steroid hormones. S = steroid; R = receptor. (From Rories & Spelsberg, 1989,[1] used with permission.)

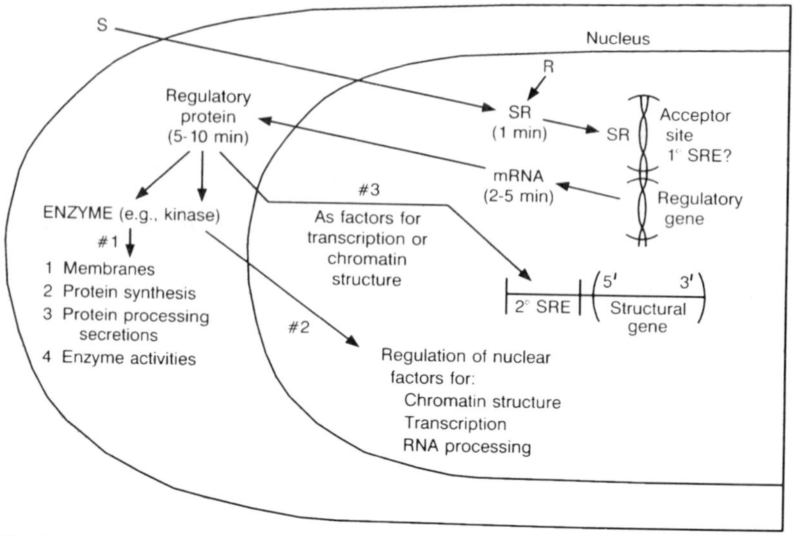

FIGURE 8. Cascade model for steroid action showing the different classes of regulatory genes. The regulatory gene represents an early gene and the structural gene represents a late gene. The times represent estimated time of occurrence after the steroid enters the cell. The 1° SRE represents the primary steroid regulatory element; 2° SRE represents the secondary SRE. (From Rories & Spelsberg, 1989,[1] used with permission.)

presented previously.[68,122] Beginning at the top left side of this figure and following the arrows, steroid hormones enter target cells, bind to their receptors, and the resulting complex binds to the nuclear acceptor sites. These sites are located on a primary (1°) steroid regulatory element, neighboring an early "regulatory" gene (early gene) in the 5′ flanking domain (or even within) the gene. This binding regulates the transcription of the "regulatory" gene within minutes after the steroid enters the target cell. At any given time, within a given target cell, there may be a few dozen of these regulatory genes responding to the steroid.

Each of the regulatory genes codes for a regulatory protein which could alter the expression of a multitude of genes via one of several possible pathways as outlined in FIGURE 8. As shown in Pathway 1, some regulatory proteins could have important cytoplasmic/plasma membrane enzymatic activities (*e.g.*, phosphorylation) which in turn cause changes in membrane transport, protein synthesis, protein processing, or protein secretion. Some of these regulatory proteins could be specific proteases involved with protein processing. An example of the latter comes from the work of Wieben and coworkers[142] who have reported that androgens regulate the production of guinea pig seminal vesicle secretory proteins solely at the level of protein processing. They found that androgens regulate the expression of an elastase-like enzyme that functions in the processing of the secretory proteins. The rapid induction of the elastase gene (regulatory gene) expression results in the equally rapid synthesis of elastase to modulate the secretory protein processing and secretion. Alternatively, as shown in Pathway 2 (FIG. 8), the enzymatic regulatory proteins could modify nuclear factors which in

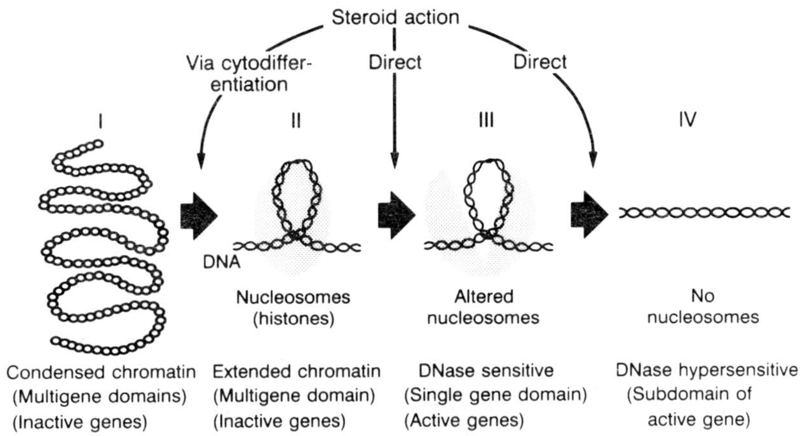

FIGURE 9. Model depicting steroid action on chromatin structure.

turn could regulate chromatin structure, gene transcription (through action as transcription factors), or possibly, RNA processing. Evidence for the existence of steroid-regulated proteins involved in mRNA half-life has been reported.[143-145]

Lastly, as depicted in Pathway 3 of FIGURE 8, the regulatory proteins could, themselves, represent nuclear factors which directly regulate chromatin structure or gene transcription as transcription factors. The steroid regulation of genes coding for transcription factors (*e.g.*, *fos/jun*) has been well documented.[1,131,133,134] The transcription factors would bind to the secondary (2°) steroid regulatory elements residing either in the 5′ flanking domains or within the steroid-regulated structural genes (late genes). Thus, the SREs residing near or within "late" genes would function as secondary SREs which bind transcription factors in addition to or instead of the steroid receptors, as per the previous discussion under transcription factors.[81,82,94-101,105-107] The regulation of structural ("late") gene transcription would occur 2 to 4 hours after steroid entrance into the cell, as opposed to minutes for the early regulatory gene. Lastly, as depicted in FIGURE 9, there are studies supporting the steroid-induced changes in chromatin structure including nucleosome positioning and generation of DNase sensitive domains.[146]

Through these three pathways, each steroid-controlled regulatory gene could regulate the expression of a multitude of genes via transcription and/or post-transcriptional events. This simplified model explains some of the mystery related to steroid regulation of gene expression, including the lengthy lag phase between steroid treatment and nuclear binding of the SR, the changes in structural gene transcription of the early genes versus late genes, and the steroid regulation of post-transcriptional steps.

Model for Direct Steroid Receptor Action on "Early" (Regulatory) Gene Transcription

On the basis of the above cited recent literature, we have attempted to design a model to describe how steroids might directly regulate the early "regulatory" gene

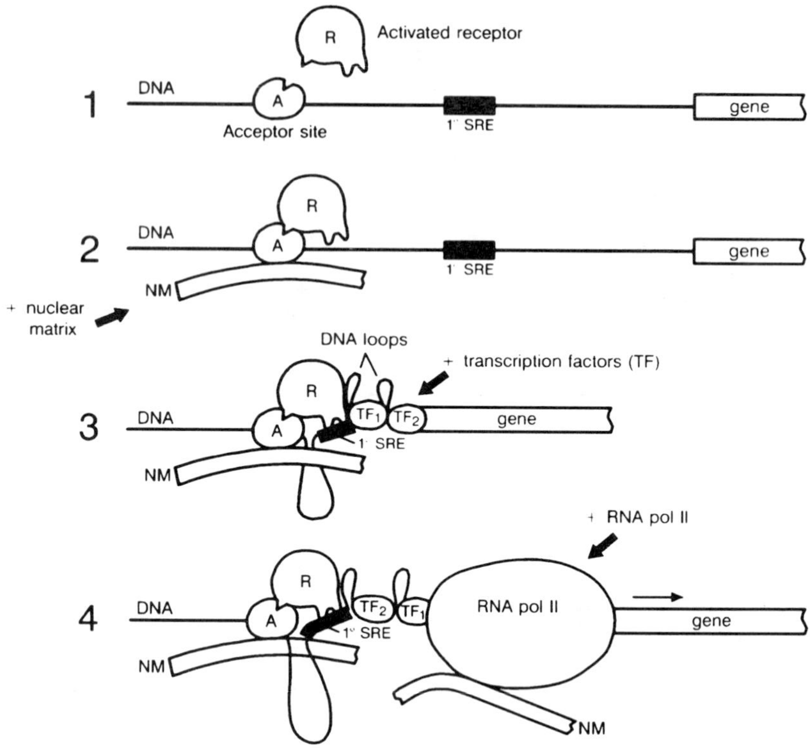

FIGURE 10. Model of SR action to initiate gene transcription. R = receptor; A = acceptor protein; NM = nuclear matrix; TF_1/TF_2 = transcription factors; 1° SRE = primary SRE; RNA pol II = RNA polymerase II. (From Rories & Spelsberg,[1] used with permission.)

transcription. The acceptor site may be located at a site distant to the SRE enhancer sequence, as shown in FIGURE 10, Step 1. The activated steroid receptor complex binds to the acceptor site with high affinity, and the receptor-acceptor complex then becomes associated with the nuclear matrix (FIGURE 10, Step 2). Alternatively, the active receptor may bind to an acceptor site protein that is already attached to the nuclear matrix.[125,147] The DNA binding domain of the matrix-bound receptor could then interact with the SRE, possibly displacing a negative regulatory factor[148] and facilitating the binding of transcription factors to specific sites in the promoter (FIG. 10, Step 3).

Transcription factors which have been shown to interact with steroid receptors and their DNA-binding sites may be tissue-specific and combinations of these may bind DNA in a cooperative fashion. Since some of the regulatory DNA elements which bind these factors are at some distance from the genes, the DNA is probably looping out between the protein-DNA complexes[102,149,150] (see Step 3 and 4 of FIG. 10). The protein-DNA complex formed at the promoter is then recognized by RNA polymerase II (FIG. 10, Step 4), and additional transcription factors bind to give rise to an active "transcription complex," with transcription of the gene ensuing.[151] The nuclear matrix is shown in contact with RNA polymerase (FIG. 10, Step 4) to reflect the evidence that actively transcribed genes are associated with nuclear matrix.[152,153] The active receptor-acceptor complex is shown to be in continuous contact with the SRE (FIG. 10, Steps 3 and 4).

CONCLUSIONS

In the past six years, the area of steroid action on gene expression has been exciting because of many significant advances. The receptors have been purified, genomic clones of their genes have been isolated, and their primary structure determined. The molecular events involved in "receptor activation" and in the regulation of gene expression by the steroid receptor complexes are now being pursued. The role of the steroid regulatory elements (SRE) and transcription factors in the steroid regulation of gene expression are also under investigation and represent potential areas for new breakthroughs. The chemical composition and locale of the nuclear acceptor sites (with respect to steroid-regulated genes) has been controversial and represents another area of investigation. Data in the literature indicate important roles for both the chromatin "acceptor" sites, and the DNA sequences they bind, which function to help guide the steroid receptor complexes to the correct binding sites on the DNA. A model is proposed whereby these acceptor proteins represent chromatin (*i.e.*, nuclear matrix) proteins that are bound to the genomic DNA at specific acceptor site DNA sequences involving SREs which neighbor regulatory genes. These "early" regulatory genes in turn code for regulatory proteins which have several possible functions described in the model. One of these functions is to regulate transcription factor binding to steroid regulatory elements resulting in the regulation of structural (late) gene expression; another regulatory gene might code for a protein which regulates mRNA half-life or protein processing. Candidates for at least one class of the regulatory genes are the nuclear proto-oncogenes *c-jun/c-fos*, and *c-myc.*

ACKNOWLEDGMENTS

Special thanks to Dr. David Toft for his helpful suggestions and to Ms. Jackie House for excellent clerical assistance.

REFERENCES

1. RORIES, C. & T. C. SPELSBERG. 1989. Ovarian steroid action on gene expression: Mechanisms and models. Ann. Rev. Physiol. **51:** 653–681.
2. CARSON-JURICA, M. A., W. T. SCHRADER & B. W. O'MALLEY. 1990. Steroid receptor family: Structure and Functions. Endocrin. Rev. **11:** 201–220.
3. PARKER, M. G., ED. 1991. Nuclear Hormone Receptors. Academic Press. New York.
4. GORSKI, J., D. O. TOFT, G. SHYAMALA, D. SMITH & A. NOTIDES. 1968. Hormone receptors: Studies on the interaction of estrogens with the uterus. Recent Prog. Horm. Res. **24:** 45–80.
5. JENSEN, E. V., T. SUZUKI, T. KAWASHIMA, E. W. STUMPF, P. W. JUNGBLUT & E. R. DESOMBRE. 1968. A two step mechanism for the interaction of estradiol with rat uterus. Proc. Natl. Acad. Sci USA **59:** 632–638.
6. KATZENELLENBOGAN, B. S. 1980. Dynamics of steroid hormone receptor action. Ann. Rev. Physiol. **42:** 17–35.

7. Moudgil, V. K., Ed. 1987. Recent Advances in Steroid Hormone Action. Walter de Gruyter & Co. New York.
8. Carlstedt-Duke, J., P.-E. Stromstedt, O. Wrange, T. Bergman, J. Gustafsson & H. Jornvall. 1987. Domain structure of the glucocorticoid receptor protein. Proc. Natl. Acad. Sci. USA **84:** 4437–4440.
9. Conneely, O. M., W. P. Sullivan, D. O. Toft, M. Birnbaumer, R. Cook, B. Maxwell, T. Zarucki-Schulz, G. Greene, W. Schrader & B. O'Malley. 1986. Molecular cloning of the chicken progesterone receptor. Science **233:** 767–770.
10. Walter, P., S. Green, G. Greene, A. Krust, J.-M. Bornert, J.-M. Jeltsch, A. Staub, E. Jensen, G. Scrace, M. Waterfield & P. Chambon. 1985. Cloning of the human estrogen receptor cDNA. Proc. Natl. Acad. Sci. USA **82:** 7889–7893.
11. Loosfelt, H., M. Atger, M. Misrahi, A. Guiochon-Mantel, C. Meriel, F. Logeat, R. Benarous & E. Milgrom. 1986. Cloning and sequence analysis of rabbit progesterone-receptor cDNA. Proc. Natl. Acad. Sci. USA **83:** 9045–9049.
12. Danielsen, M., J. P. Northrop & G. M. Ringold. 1986. The mouse glucocorticoid receptor: Mapping of functional domains by cloning, sequencing and expression of wild-type and mutant receptor proteins. EMBO J. **5:** 2513–2522.
13. Hollenberg, S. M., C. Weinberger, E. S. Ong, G. Carelli, A. Oro, R. Lebo, E. Thompson & R. M. Evans. 1985. Primary structure and expression of a functional human glucocorticoid receptor. Nature **318:** 635–641.
14. Miesfeld, R., S. Rusconi, P. J. Godowski, B. A. Maler, S. Okret, A.-C. Wikstrom, J.-A. Gustafsson & K. R. Yamamoto. 1986. Genetic complementation of glucocorticoid receptor deficiency by expression of cloned receptor cDNA. Cell **46:** 389–399.
15. Green, S., V. Kumar, A. Krust & P. Chambon. 1987. The oestrogen receptor: Structure and function. *In* Recent Advances in Steroid Hormone Action. V. K. Moudgil, Ed.: 161–183. Walter de Gruyter & Co. Berlin/New York.
16. Krust, A., S. Green, P. Argos, V. Kumar, P. Walter, J.-M. Bornert & P. Chambon. 1986. The chicken oestrogen receptor sequence: Homology with v-erbA and the human oestrogen and glucocorticoid receptors. EMBO J. **5:** 891–897.
17. White, R., J. A. Lees, M. Needham, J. Ham & M. Parker. 1987. Structural organization and expression of the mouse estrogen receptor. Mol. Endocrinol. **1:** 735–744.
18. Weiler, I. J., D. Lew & D. J. Shapiro. 1987. The *Xenopus laevis* estrogen receptor: Sequence homology with human and avian receptors and identification of multiple estrogen receptor messenger ribonucleic acids. Mol. Endocrinol. **1:** 355–362.
19. Pakdel, F., C. Le Guellec, C. Vaillant, M. G. L. Roux & Y. Valotaire. 1989. Identification and estrogen induction of two estrogen receptors (ER) messenger ribonucleic acids in the rainbow trout liver: Sequence homology with other ERs. Mol. Endocrinol. **3:** 44–51.
20. Petkovich, M., N. J. Brand, A. Krust & P. Chambon. 1987. A human retinoic acid receptor which belongs to the family of nuclear receptors. Nature **330:** 444–450.
21. Weinberger, C., C. C. Thompson, E. S. Ong, R. Lebo, D. J. Gruol & R. M. Evans. 1986. The *c-erb-A* gene encodes a thyroid hormone receptor. Nature **324:** 641–646.
22. Wang, L.-H., S. Y. Tsai, I. Sagami, M.-J. Tsai & B. W. O'Malley. 1987. Purification and characterization of chicken ovalbumin upstream promoter transcription factor from HeLa cells. J. Biol. Chem. **262:** 16080–16086.
23. Feigelson, P. & D. T. Kurtz. 1978. Hormonal modulation of α_{2u}globulin mRNA: Sequence measurements using a specific cDNA probe. Cold Spring Harbor Symp. Quant. Biol. **42:** 659–663.
24. Segraves, W. A. & D. S. Hogness. 1990. The E75 ecdysone-inducible gene responsible for the 75B early puff in *Drosophila* encodes two members of the steroid receptor superfamily. Genes Dev. **4:** 204–219.
25. Pignoni, F., R. M. Baldarelli, E. Steingrimsson, R. J. Diaz, A. Patapoutian, J. R. Merriam & J. A. Lengyel. 1990. The Drosophila gene tailless is expressed at the embryonic termini and is a member of the steroid receptor superfamily. Cell **62:** 151–163.
26. Mlodzik, M., Y. Hiromi, U. Weber, C. S. Goodman & G. M. Rubin. 1990. The Drosophila seven-up gene, a member of the steroid receptor gene superfamily, controls photoreceptor cell fates. Cell **60:** 211–224.
27. Evans, R. M. & S. M. Hollenberg. 1988. Zinc fingers: Gilt by association. Cell **52:** 1–3.

28. Berg, J. M. 1990. Zinc fingers and other metal-binding domains. J. Biol. Chem. **265:** 6513–6516.
29. Schwabe, J. W. R., D. Neuhaus & D. Rhodes. 1990. Solution structure of the DNA-binding domain of the oestrogen receptor. Nature **348:** 458–461.
30a. Härd, T., E. Kellenbach, R. Boelens, R. Kaptein, K. Dahlman, J. Carlstedt-Duke, L. P. Freedman, B. A. Maler, E. I. Hyde, J-A. Gustafsson & K. R. Yamamoto. 1990. ^{1}H NMR studies of the glucocorticoid receptor DNA-binding domain: Sequential assignments and identification of secondary structural elements. Biochemistry **29:** 9015–9023.
30b. Green, S. & P. Chambon. 1987. Oestradiol induction of a glucocorticoid-responsive gene by a chimaeric receptor. Nature **325:** 75–78.
31. Hollenberg, S. M., V. Giguere, P. Segui & R. M. Evans. 1987. Colocalization of DNA-binding and transcriptional activation functions in the human glucocorticoid receptor. Cell **49:** 39–46.
32. Adler, S., M. L. Waterman, X. He & M. G. Rosenfeld. 1988. Steroid receptor-mediated inhibition of rat prolactin gene expression does not require the receptor DNA-binding domain. Cell **52:** 685–695.
33. Mader, S., V. Kumar, H. de Verneuil & P. Chambon. 1989. Three amino acids of the oestrogen receptor are essential to its ability to distinguish an oestrogen from a glucocorticoid-responsive element. Nature **338:** 271–274.
34. Rusconi, S. & K. R. Yamamoto. 1987. Functional dissection of the hormone and DNA binding activities of the glucocorticoid receptor. EMBO J. **6:** 1309–1315.
35. Simons, S. S., Jr., F. D. Sistare & P. L. Chrakraborti. 1989. Steroid binding activity is retained in a 16-kDa fragment of the steroid binding domain of rat glucocorticoid receptors. J. Biol. Chem. **264:** 14493–14497.
36. Gronemeyer, H., B. Turcotte, C. Quirin-Stricker, M. T. Bocquel, M. E. Meyer, Z. Krozowski, J. M. Jeltsch, T. Lerouge, J. Garnier & P. Chambon. 1987. The chicken progesterone receptor: Sequence, expression and functional analysis. EMBO J. **6:** 3985–3994.
37. Kumar, V., S. Green, A Staub & P. Chambon. 1986. Localization of the oestradiol-binding and putative DNA-binding domains of the human estrogen receptor. EMBO J. **5:** 2231–2236.
38. Picard, D., S. J. Salser & K. R. Yamamoto. 1988. A movable and regulable inactivation function within the steroid binding domain of the glucocorticoid receptor. Cell **54:** 1073–1080.
39. Webster, N. J. G., S. Green, J. R. Jin & P. Chambon. 1988. The hormone binding domains of the estrogen and glucocorticoid receptors contain an inducible transcription activation function. Cell **54:** 199–207.
40. Tora, L., J. White, C. Brou, D. Tasset, N. Webster, E. Scheer & P. Chambon. 1989. The human estrogen receptor has two independent nonacidic transcriptional activation functions. Cell **59:** 477–487.
41. Willmann, T. & M. Beato. 1986. Steroid-free glucocorticoid receptor binds specifically to mouse mammary tumour virus DNA. Nature **324:** 688–691.
42. Klein-Hitpass, L., S. Y. Tsai, G. Greene, M.-J. Clark & B. W. O'Malley. 1989. Specific binding of estrogen receptor to the estrogen response element. Mol. Cell Biol. **9:** 43–49.
43. Lees, J. A., S. E. Farrell & M. G. Parker. 1989. Identification of two transactivation domains in the mouse oestrogen receptors. Nucl. Acids. Res. **17:** 5477–5488.
44. Murdoch, F. E., D. A. Meier, D. Furlow, D. Grunwald & J. Gorski. 1990. Estrogen receptor binding to a DNA response element *in vitro* is not dependent upon estradiol. Biochemistry **29:** 8377–8385.
45. Brown, M. & P. A. Sharp. 1990. Human estrogen receptor forms multiple protein-DNA complexes. J. Biol. Chem. **65:** 11238–11243.
46. Rodriquez, R., M. A. Carson, N. L. Weigel, B. W. O'Malley & W. T. Schrader. 1989. Hormone-induced changes in the *in vitro* DNA-binding activity of the chicken progesterone receptor. Mol. Endocrinol. **3:** 356–362.
47. Pratt, W. B., D. J. Jolly, D. V. Pratt, S. M. Hollenberg, V. Giguere, F. M. Cadepond, G. Schweizer-Groyer, M.-G. Catelli, R. M. Evans & E.-E. Baulieu. 1988. A region in the steroid binding domain determines formation of the non-DNA binding 9S glucocorticoid receptor complex. J. Biol. Chem. **263:** 267–273.
48. Kost, S. L., D. Smith, W. Sullivan, W. J. Welch & D. O. Toft. 1989. Binding of heat shock proteins to the avian progesterone receptor. Mol. Cell. Biol. **9:** 3829–3838.
49. Bagchi, M. K., S. Y. Tsai, M.-J. Tsai & B. W. O'Malley. 1990. Progesterone-dependent

cell free transcription: Identification of a functional intermediate in receptor activation. Nature **345:** 547–550.
50. SCHAUER, M., G. CHALEPKAIS, T. WILLMANN & M. BEATO. 1989. Binding of hormone accelerates the kinetics of glucocorticoid and progesterone receptor binding to DNA. Proc. Natl. Acad. Sci. USA. **86:** 1123–1127.
51. BEATO, M., D. BARETTINO, U. BRUGGEMEIER, G. CHALEPAKIS, R. J. G. HACHE, M. KALFF, B. PINA, M. SCHAUER, E. P. SLATER & M. TRUSS. 1991. Characterization of DNA receptor interactions. *In* Nuclear Hormone Receptors. M. G. Parker, Ed.: 197–215. Academic Press. New York.
52. BRESNICK, E. H., F. C. DALMAN & W. B. PRATT. 1990. Direct stoichiometric evidence that the untransformed M_r 300,000, 9S, glucocorticoid receptor is a core unit derived from a larger heteromeric complex. Biochemistry **29:** 520–527.
53. PRATT, W. B. 1987. Transformation of glucocorticoid and progesterone receptors to the DNA-binding state. J. Cell. Biochem. **35:** 51–68.
54. BAULIEU, E.-E. 1987. Steroid hormone antagonists at the receptor level: A role for the heat-shock protein MW 90,000 (hsp 90). J. Cell. Biochem. **35:** 161–174.
55. BRESNICK, E. H., F. C. DALMAN, E. R. SANCHEZ & W. B. PRATT. 1989. Evidence that the 90-kDa heat shock protein is necessary for the steroid binding conformation of the L-cell glucocorticoid receptor. J. Biol. Chem. **264:** 4992–4997.
56. GODOWSKI, P. J., S. RUSCONI, R. MIESFELD & K. R. YAMAMOTO. 1987. Glucocorticoid receptor mutants that are constitutive activators of transcriptional enhancement. Nature **325:** 365–368.
57. HOUSELY, P. R., E. R. SANCHEZ, M. DANIELSON, G. M. RINGOLD & W. B. PRATT. 1990. Evidence that the conserved region in the steroid binding domain of the glucocorticoid receptor is required for both optimal binding of hsp90 and protection from proteolytic cleavage. J. Biol. Chem. **265:** 12778–12781.
58. SCHOWALTER, D. B., W. P. SULLIVAN, N. J. MAIHLE, A. DOBSON, O. M. CONNEELY, B. W. O'MALLEY & D. O. TOFT. 1991. Characterization of progesterone receptor binding to the 90 and 70 kDa heat shock proteins. Submitted.
59. CADEPOND, F., G. SCHWEIZER-GROYER, I. MAUREL-SEGARD, N. JIBARD, S. M. HOLLENBERG, V. GIGUERE, R. M. EVANS & E.-E. BAULIEU. 1991. Heat shock protein 90 as a critical factor in maintaining glucocorticosteroid receptor in a nonfunctional state. J. Biol. Chem. **266:** 5834–5841.
60. CHAMBRAUD, B., M. BERRY, G. REDEUILH, P. CHAMBON & E.-E. BAULIEU. 1990. Several regions of human estrogen receptor are involved in the formation of receptor-heat shock protein 90 complexes. J. Biol. Chem. **265:** 20686–20691.
61. ROTHMAN, J. E. 1989. Polypeptide chain binding proteins: Catalysts of protein folding and related processes in cells. Cell **59:** 591–601.
62. ELLIS, J. 1987. Proteins as molecular chaperones. Nature **328:** 378–379.
63. SMITH, D. F., L. E. FABER & D. O. TOFT. 1990. Purification of unactivated progesterone receptor and identification of novel receptor-associated proteins. J. Biol. Chem. **265:** 3996–4003.
64. TAI, P.-K. Y. MAEDA, K. NAKAO, N. WAKIM, J. DUHRING & L. E. FABER. 1986. A 59-kilodalton protein associated with progestin, estrogen, androgen, and glucocorticoid receptors. Biochemistry **25:** 5269–5275.
65. SMITH, D. F., D. B. SCHOWALTER, S. L. KOST & D. O. TOFT. 1990. Reconstitution of progesterone receptor with heat shock proteins. Mol. Endocrinol. **4:** 1704–1711.
66. HORWITZ, K. B. 1987. The structure and function of progesterone receptors in breast cancer. J. Steroid Biochem. **27:** 447–457.
67. SULLIVAN, W. P., D. F. SMITH, T. G. BEITO, C. J. KRCO & D. O. TOFT. 1988. Hormone-dependent processing of the avian progesterone receptor. J. Cell. Biochem. **36:** 103–119.
68. SPELSBERG, T. C., B. A. LITTLEFIELD, R. SEELKE, G. MARTIN-DANI, H. TOYODA, P. BOYD-LEINEN, C. THRALL & O. KON. 1983. Role of specific chromosomal proteins and DNA sequences in the nuclear binding sites for steroid receptors. Recent Prog. Hormone Res. **39:** 463–517.
69. EDWARDS, D. P., B. KUHNEL, P. A. ESTES & S. K. NORDEEN. 1989. Human progesterone receptor binding to mouse mammary tumor virus deoxyribonucleic acid: Dependence on hormone and non-receptor nuclear factors. Mol. Endocrinol. **3:** 381–391.
70. SMITH, A. C., M. S. ELSASSER & J. M. HARMON. 1986. Analysis of glucocorticoid receptor

activation by high resolution two-dimensional electrophoresis of affinity-labeled receptor. J. Biol. Chem. **261:** 13285–13292.

71. Dalman, F. C., E. R. Sanchez, A. L.-Y. Lin, F. Perini & W. B. Pratt. 1988. Localization of phosphorylation sites with respect to the functional domains of the mouse L cell glucocorticoid receptor. J. Biol. Chem. **263:** 12259–12257.

72. Orti, E., D. B. Mendel, L. I. Smith & A. Munck. 1989. Agonist-dependent phosphorylation and nuclear dephosphorylation of glucocorticoid receptors in intact cells. J. Biol. Chem. **264:** 9728–9731.

73. Dingwall, C. & R. A. Laskey. 1986. Protein import into the cell nucleus. Ann. Rev. Cell Biol. **2:** 367–390.

74. Picard, D. & K. R. Yamamoto. 1987. Two signals mediate hormone-dependent nuclear localization of the glucocorticoid receptor. EMBO J. **6:** 3333–3340.

75. Arriza, J. L., C. Weinberger, G. Cerelli, T. M. Glaser, B. L. Handelin, D. E. Housman & R. M. Evans. 1987. Cloning of human mineralocorticoid receptor complementary DNA: Structural and functional kinship with the glucocorticoid receptor. Science **237:** 268–275.

76. Green, S. & P. Chambon. 1991. The oestrogen receptor: From perception to mechanism. *In* Nuclear Hormone Receptors. M. G. Parker, Ed.: 15–38. Academic Press. New York.

77. Trapman, J., P. Klaassen, G. Kuiper, J. van der Korput, P. W. Faber, H. van Rooij, A. Geurts van Kessel, M. Voorhorst, E. Mulder & A. O. Brinkmann. 1988. Cloning, structure and expression of a cDNA encoding the human androgen receptor. Biochem. Biophys. Res. Commun. **153:** 241–248.

78a. Guiochon-Mantel, A., H. Loosfelt, P. Lescop, S. Sar, M. Atger, M. Perrot-Applanat & E. Milgrom. 1989. Mechanisms of nuclear localization of the progesterone receptor: Evidence for interaction between monomers. Cell **57:** 1147–1154.

78b. Danielsen, M., J. P. Northrop, J. Jonklaas & G. M. Ringold. 1987. Domains of the glucocorticoid receptor involved in specific and nonspecific deoxyribonucleic acid binding, hormone activation, and transcriptional enhancement. Mol. Endocrinol. **1:** 816–822.

79. Freedman, L. P., B. F. Luisi, Z. R. Korszun, R. Basavappa, P. B. Sigler & K. R. Yamamoto. 1988. The function and structure of the metal coordination sites within the glucocorticoid receptor DNA binding domain. Nature **334:** 543–546.

80. Urda, L. A., P. M. Yen, S. S. Simons & J. M. Harmon. 1989. Region-specific antiglucocorticoid receptor antibodies selectively recognize the activated form of the ligand-occupied receptor and inhibit the binding of activated complexes to deoxyribonucleic acid. Mol. Endocrinol. **3:** 251–260.

81. Martinez, E. & W. Wahli. 1991. Characterization of hormone response elements. *In* Nuclear Hormone Receptors. M. G. Parker, Ed.: 125–153. Academic Press. New York.

82. Muller, M., C. Baniahmad, C. Kaltschmidt, R. Schule & R. Renkawitz. 1991. Cooperative transactivation of steroid receptors. *In* Nuclear Hormone Receptors. M. G. Parker, Ed.: 155–174. Academic Press. New York.

83. Kumar, V. & P. Chambon. 1988. The estrogen receptor binds tightly to its responsive element as a ligand-induced homodimer. Cell **55:** 145–156.

84. Tsai, S. Y., J. Carlstedt-Duke, N. L. Weigel, K. Dahlman, J.-A. Gustafsson, M.-J. Tsai & B. W. O'Malley. 1988. Molecular interactions of steroid-hormone receptor with its enhancer element: Evidence for receptor dimer formation. Cell **55:** 361–369.

85. Fawell, S. E., J. A. Lees, R. White & M. G. Parker. 1990. Characterization and colocalization of steroid binding and dimerization activities in the mouse estrogen receptor. Cell **60:** 953–962.

86. Forman, B. M. & H. H. Samuels. 1990. Interactions among a subfamily of nuclear hormone receptors: The regulatory zipper model. Mol. Endocrinol. **4:** 1293–1301.

87. Strähle, U., W. Schmid & G. Schütz. 1988. Synergistic action of the glucocorticoid receptor with transcription factors. EMBO J. **7:** 3389–3395.

88. Tsai, S. Y., M.-J. Tsai & B. W. O'Malley. 1989. Cooperative binding of steroid hormone receptors contribute to transcriptional synergism at target enhancer elements. Cell **57:** 443–448.

89. Cato, A. C. C., P. Skroch, J. Weinmann, P. Butkeraitis & H. Ponta. 1988a. DNA sequences outside the receptor-binding sites differentially modulate the responsiveness of the mouse mammary tumour virus promoter to various steroid hormones. EMBO J. **7:** 1403–1410.

90. Ankenbauer, W., U. Strahle & G. Schutz. 1988. Synergistic action of glucocorticoid and

estradiol responsive elements. Proc. Natl. Acad. Sci. USA **85:** 7526–7530.

91. Harris, L. F., M. R. Sullivan & D. F. Hickok. 1990a. Conservation of genetic information between regulatory protein DNA binding alpha-helices and their cognate operator sites—a simple code for site-specific recognition. Computer Math Appl. **20:** 1–23.
92. Harris, L. F., M. R. Sullivan & D. F. Hickok. 1990b. Genetic sequences of hormone response elements share similarity with predicted alpha helices within DNA binding domains of steroid receptor proteins—A basis for site specific recognition. Computer Math Appl. **20:** 25–48.
93. Frankel, A. D. & C. O. Pabo. 1988. Fingering too many proteins. Cell **53:** 675.
94. Schüle, R., M. Muller, C. Kaltschmidt & R. Renkawitz. 1988a. Many transcription factors interact synergistically with steroid receptors. Science **242:** 1418–1420.
95. Renkawitz, R., H. Beug, T. Graf, P. Matthias & M. Grez. 1982. Expression of a chicken lysozyme recombinant gene is regulated by progesterone and dexamethasone after microinjection into oviduct cells. Cell **31:** 167–176.
96. Tora, L., H. Gronemeyer, B. Turcotte, M.-P. Gaub & P. Chambon. 1988. The N-terminal region of the chicken progesterone receptor specifies target gene activation. Nature (London) **333:** 185–188.
97. Cordingley, M. G., H. Richard-Foy, A. Lichter & G. L. Hager. 1987a. The hormone response element of the MMTV LTR: A complex regulatory region. *In* DNA: Protein Interactions and Gene Regulation. E. B. Thompson & J. Papaconstantinou, Eds.: 233–243. University of Texas Press. Austin, TX.
98. Jost, J.-P., H. Saluz, J. Jirleny & B. Moncharmont. 1987. Estradiol-dependent transacting factor binds preferentially to a dyad-symmetry structure within the third intron of the avian vitellogenin gene. J. Cell Biochem. **35:** 69–82.
99. Tsai, S. Y., M.-J. Tsai & B. W. O'Malley. 1991. The steroid receptor superfamily: Transactivators of gene expression. *In* Nuclear Hormone Receptors. M. G. Parker, Ed.: 103–124. Academic Press. New York.
100. Renkawitz, R., R. Schüle, C. Kaltschmidt, A. Baniahmad, J. Altschmied, Ch. Steiner & M. Muller. 1989. Clustered arrangement and interaction of steroid hormone receptors with other transcription factors. *In* Proceedings of the 40th Colloquium Mosbach.: 21–28. Springer-Verlag. Heidelberg.
101. Schüle, R., M. Muller, H. Otsuka-Murakami & R. Renkawitz. 1988. Cooperativity of the glucocorticoid receptor and the CACCC-box binding factor. Nature **332:** 87–90.
102. Ptashne, M. 1988. How eukaryotic transcriptional activators work. Nature **335:** 683–689.
103a. Tsai, S. Y., I. Sagami, H. Wang, M.-J. Tsai & B. W. O'Malley. 1987. Interactions between a DNA-binding transcription factor (COUP) and a non-DNA binding factor (S300-II). Cell **50:** 701–709.
103b. Weisz, A., L. Cicatiello, E. Persico, M. Scalona & F. Bresciani. 1990. Estrogen stimulates transcription of c-jun protooncogene. Mol. Endocrinol. **4:** 1041–1050.
104. Weisz, A. & R. Rosales. 1990. Identification of an estrogen response element upstream of the human c-fos gene that binds the estrogen receptor and the AP-1 transcription factor. Nucl. Acids Res. **18:** 5097–5106.
105. Gaub, M. P., M. Bellard, I. Scheuer, P. Chambon & P. Sassone-Corsi. 1990. Activation of the ovalbumin gene by the estrogen receptor involves the fos-jun complex. Cell **63:** 1267–1276.
106a. Diamond, M. I., J. N. Miner, S. K. Yoshinaga & K. R. Yamamoto. 1990. Transcription factor interactions: Selectors of positive or negative regulation from a single DNA element. Science **249:** 1266–1272.
106b. Jonat, C., H. J. Rahmsdorf, K.-K. Park, A. Cato, S. Gebel, H. Ponta & P. Herrlich. 1990. Antitumor promotion and antiinflammation: Down-modulation of AP-1 (fos/jun) activity by glucocorticoid hormone. Cell **62:** 1189–1204.
107. Yang-Yen, H.-F., J-C. Chambard, Y.-L. Sun, T. Smeal, T. J. Schmidt, J. Drouin & M. Karin. 1990. Transcriptional interference between c-jun and the glucocorticoid receptor. Mutual inhibition of DNA binding due to direct protein-protein interaction. Cell **62:** 1205–1215.
108. Spelsberg, T. C., C. Rories, J. Rejman, A. Goldberger, K. Fink, C. K. Lau, D. Colvard & G. Wiseman. 1989. Steroid action on gene expression: Possible roles of regulatory genes and nuclear acceptor sites. Biol. Reprod. **40:** 54–69.
109. Bagchi, M., J. Elliston, S. Tsai, D. Edwards, T. Tsai & B. W. O'Malley. 1988. Steroid

hormone–dependent interaction of human progesterone receptor with its target enhancer element. Mol. Endocrinol. **2:** 1221–1229.

110. JOST, J.-P., M. SELDRAM & M. GEISER. 1984. Preferential binding of estrogen-receptor complexes to a region containing the estrogen-dependent and hypomethylation site preceding the chicken vitellogenin II gene. Proc. Natl. Acad. Sci. USA **81:** 429–433.

111. OKAMOTO, K., F. ISOHASHI, K. UEDA, I. KOKUFU & Y. SAKAMOTO. 1988. Purification and characterization of an adenosine triphosphate-stimulated factor that enhances the nuclear binding of activated glucocorticoid-receptor complex from rat liver. Endocrinology **123:** 2752–2761.

112. SIMONS, S. S., JR., H. M. MARTINEZ, R. L. GARCEA, J. D. BAXTER & G. M. TOMKINS. 1976. Interactions of glucocorticoid receptor steroid complexes with acceptor sites. J. Biol. Chem. **251:** 334–343.

113. RUH, T. S., P. ROSS, D. M. WOOD & J. L. KEENE. 1981. The binding of [^{3}H]oestradiol receptor complexes to calf uterine chromatin. Biochem. J. **200:** 133–142.

114. RUH, M. F., R. K. SINGH, T. S. RUH & G. SHYAMALA. 1987. Binding of glucocorticoid receptors to mammary chromatin acceptor sites. J. Steroid Biochem. **28:** 581–586.

115. CHUKNYISKA, R. S., M. HAJI, R. H. FOOTE & G. S. ROTH. 1985. Age associated changes in nuclear binding of rat uterine estradiol receptor complexes. Endocrinology **116:** 547–551.

116. CUSHING, C. L., R. A. BAMBARA & R. HILF. 1985. Interactions of estrogen-receptor and antiestrogen receptor complexes with nuclei *in vitro.* Endocrinology **116:** 2419–2429.

117. DEBOER, W., L. SNIPPE, G. AB & M. GRUBER. 1984. Interaction of calf uterine estrogen receptors with chicken target cell nuclei. J. Steroid Biochem. **20:** 387–390.

118. FRANKEL, F. R. & M. B. SENIOR. 1986. The estrogen receptor complex is bound at unusual chromatin regions. J. Steroid Biochem. **24:** 983–988.

119. OGLE, T. F. 1987. Nuclear acceptor sites for progesterone-receptor complexes in rat placenta. Endocrinology **121:** 28–35.

120. PAVLIK, E. J., J. R. VAN NAGELL, K. NELSEN, H. GALLION, E. S. DONALDSON, D. E. KENADY & J. BARANOWSKA-KORTYLEWICZ. 1986. Antagonism to estradiol in the mouse: Reduced entry of receptors complexed with 4-hydroxytamoxifen into a Mg^{2+}-soluble chromatin fraction. Endocrinology **118:** 1924–1934.

121. MURRAY, M. B. & H. C. TOWLE. 1989. Identification of nuclear factors that enhance binding of the thyroid hormone receptor to a thyroid hormone response element. Mol. Endocrinol. **3:** 1434–1442.

122. SPELSBERG, T. C., M. HORTON, K. FINK, A. GOLDBERGER, C. RORIES, B. GOSSE & K. RASMUSSEN. 1987. A new model for steroid regulation of gene transcription using chromatin acceptor sites and regulatory genes and their products. *In* Recent Advances in Steroid Hormone Action. V. K. Moudgil, Ed.: 31–48. Walter de Gruyter, Co. Berlin-New York.

123. CHUKNYISKA, R. S., M. HAJI, R. H. FOOTE & G. S. ROTH. 1984. Effects of *in vivo* estradiol administration of availability of rat uterine nuclear acceptor sites measured *in vitro.* Endocrinology **115:** 836–838.

124. SCHUCHARD, M., J. REJMAN, D. MCCORMICK, B. GOSSE, T. RUESINK & T. C. SPELSBERG. 1991. Characterization of purified chromatin acceptor protein (Receptor Binding Factor-1) for the avian oviduct progesterone receptor. Biochemistry. In press.

125. SCHUCHARD, M., M. SUBRAMANIAM, T. RUESINK & T. C. SPELSBERG. 1991. Nuclear matrix localization and specific matrix DNA binding by Receptor Binding Factor-1 of the avian oviduct progesterone receptor. Submitted.

126. ROSS, P. & T. S. RUH. 1984. Binding of the estradiol-receptor complex to reconstituted nucleoacidic protein from calf uterus. Biochim. Biophys. Acta **782:** 18–25.

127. SINGH, R. K., M. F. RUH, & T. S. RUH. 1984. Binding of [^{3}H]estradiol and [^{3}H]H1285 receptor complexes to rabbit uterine chromatin. Biochim. Biophys. Acta **800:** 33–40.

128. SINGH, R. K., M. F. RUH, W. B. BUTLER & T. S. RUH. 1986. Acceptor sites on chromatin for receptor bound by estrogen versus antiestrogen in antiestrogen-sensitive and -resistant MCF-7 cells. Endocrinology **118:** 1087–1095.

129. RENNIE, P. S., J.-F. BOWDEN, N. BRUNCHOVSKY, P.-S. FRENETTE, J. A. FOEKENS & H. CHEN. 1987. DNA and protein components of nuclear acceptor sites for androgen receptors in the rat prostate. J. Steroid Biochem. **27:** 513–520.

130a. CLEVER, U. 1964. Actinomycin and puromycin: Effects on sequential gene activation by ecdysone. Science **146:** 794–795.

130b. Clever, U. & C. G. Romball. 1966. RNA and protein synthesis in the cellular response to a hormone ecdysone. Proc. Natl. Acad. Sci. USA **56:** 1470.

131. Fink, K. L., E. D. Wieben, G. E. Woloschak & T. C. Spelsberg. 1988. Rapid regulation of c-myc proto-oncogene expression by progesterone in the avian oviduct. Proc. Natl. Acad. Sci USA **85:** 1796–1800.

132. Rories, C., C. K. Lau, K. L. Fink & T. C. Spelsberg. 1989. Rapid inhibition of c-myc gene expression by a glucocorticoid in the avian oviduct. Mol. Endocrinol. **3:** 991–1001.

133. Lau, C. K., M. Subramaniam, K. Rasmussen & T. C. Spelsberg. 1990. Rapid inhibition of the c-jun proto-oncogene expression in avian oviduct by estrogen. Endocrinology. **127:** 2595–2597.

134. Lau, C. K., M. Subramaniam, K. Rasmussen & T. C. Spelsberg. 1991. Rapid induction of the c-jun proto-oncogene in the avian oviduct by the antiestrogen tamoxifen. Proc. Natl. Acad. Sci. USA **88:** 829–833.

135. Gonda, T. J., D. K. Sheiness & J. M. Bishop. 1982. Transcripts from the cellular homologs of retroviral oncogenes: Distribution among chicken tissues. Mol. Cell. Biol. **2:** 617–624.

136. Kelley, K. & U. Siebenlist. 1986. The regulation and expression of c-myc in normal and malignant cells. Ann. Rev. Immunol. **4:** 317–338.

137. Studzinski, G. P., Z. S. Brelvi, S. C. Feldman & R. A. Watt. 1986. Participation of c-myc protein in DNA synthesis of human cells. Science **234:** 467–470.

138. Dubik, D., T. C. Dembinski & R. P. C. Shiu. 1987. Stimulation of c-myc oncogene expression associated with estrogen-induced proliferation of human breast cancer cells. Cancer Res. **47:** 6517–6521.

139. Murphy, L. J., L. C. Murphy & H. G. Friesen. 1987. Estrogen induction of n-myc and c-myc proto-oncogene expression in the rat uterus. Endocrinology **120:** 1882–1888.

140. Travers, M. T. & J. T. Knowler. 1987. Oestrogen-induced expression of oncogenes in the immature rat uterus. FEBS Letters **211:** 27–30.

141. Forsthoefel, A. & E. A. Thompson. 1987. Glucocorticoid regulation of transcription of the c-myc cellular proto-oncogene in P1798 cells. Mol. Endocrinol. **1:** 899–907.

142. Hagstrom, J. E., S. E. Harvey & E. D. Wieben. 1989. Regulation of secretory protein production by androgens in the guinea pig seminal vesicle epithelium. J. Cell Biol. **109**(4) Part 2: 117a (abstract 627).

143. Leibold, E. A., A. Landino & Y. Yu. 1990. Structural requirements of iron-responsive elements for binding of the protein involved in both transferrin receptor and ferritin mRNA post-transcriptional regulation. Nucl. Acids Res. **18:** 1819–1824.

144. Nielsen, D. A. & D. J. Shapiro. 1990. Estradiol and estrogen receptor-dependent stabilization of a mini-vitellogenin mRNA lacking 5,100 nucleotides of coding sequence. Mol. Cell. Biol. **10:** 371–376.

145. Cochran, A. & R. G. Deeley. 1989. Detection and characterization of degradative intermediates of avian apo very low density lipoprotein II mRNA present in estrogen-treated birds and following destabilization by hormone withdrawal. J. Biol. Chem. **264:** 6495–6503.

146. Hager, G. L. & T. K. Archer. 1991. The interaction of steroid receptors with chromatin. *In* Nuclear Hormone Receptors. M. G. Parker, Ed.: 217–234. Academic Press. New York.

147. Barrack, E. R. & D. S. Coffey. 1982. Biological properties of the nuclear matrix: Steroid hormone binding. Recent Prog. Horm. Res. **38:** 133–195.

148. Cordingley, M. G., A. T. Riegel & G.L. Hager. 1987b. Steroid-dependent interaction of transcription factors with the inducible promoter of mouse mammary tumor virus *in vivo.* Cell **48:** 261–270.

149. Ptashne, M. 1986. Gene regulation by proteins acting nearby and at a distance. Nature **322:** 697–701.

150. Schleif, R. 1987. Why should DNA loop? (Commentary) Nature **327:** 369–370.

151. Dynan, W. S. & R. Tjian. 1985. Control of eukaryotic messenger RNA synthesis by sequence-specific DNA-binding proteins. Nature **316:** 774–778.

152. Jackson, D. A. & P. R. Cook. 1985. Transcription occurs at a nucleo-skeleton. EMBO J. **4:** 919–925.

153. Zehnbauer, B. A. & B. Vogelstein. 1985. Supercoiled loops and the organization of replication and transcription in eukaryotes. BioEssays **2:** 52–54.

154. TOFT, D. O., D. SMITH & D. SCHOWALTER. 1990. Heat shock proteins and steroid receptor activity. *In* Contributions to Cellular and Molecular Endocrinology, Nichols Institute Symposium on Cellular and Molecular Endocrinology. Henry, H. L. & A. W. Norman, Eds.: 89–100. University of California, Riverside.
155. JENSEN, E. V. 1991. Overview of the nuclear receptor family. *In* Nuclear Hormone Receptors. M. G. Parker, Ed.: 1–14. Academic Press. New York.
156. SPELSBERG, T. C., C. RORIES, J. J. REJMAN, A. GOLDBERGER, K. FINK, C. K. LAU, D. S. COLVARD & G. WISEMAN. 1989. Steroid action on gene expression: Possible roles of regulatory genes and nuclear acceptor sites. Biol. Reprod. **40:** 54–69.

Molecular Analysis of the Androgen Receptor

ELIZABETH M. WILSON,[a] JORGE A. SIMENTAL, FRANK S. FRENCH, AND MADHABANADA SAR

Departments of Pediatrics, Biochemistry, and Cell Biology and Anatomy
University of North Carolina
Chapel Hill, North Carolina 27599

The androgen receptor (AR) plays a central role in male sexual development. It acts as a ligand-activated transcription factor to induce genes critical in the physiological processes of male development. Cloning of the AR cDNA has provided new approaches with which to address the structure-function relationships of the receptor. This article highlights some recent work on the AR using site directed mutagenesis techniques and transient expression systems. The focus of the studies has been the identification of functional domains in the receptor for phosphorylation, nuclear transport and transcriptional activation.

The full-length AR cDNA cloned in a eukaryotic expression vector, pCMV, allows for the study of receptor properties using the transiently expressed protein. FIGURE 1 is a schematic drawing of an expression vector used in these studies. Indicated in the figure are several unique restriction sites which were useful in creating mutant forms of the receptor. Expression of the AR sequence in this vector is driven by the cytomegalovirus early gene promoter facilitating high level expression. The vector contains the human growth hormone transcription termination and polyadenylation signals and an SV40 origin of replication for high level expression in monkey kidney COS cells, a permanent cell line transformed with SV40.

TRANSCRIPTIONAL ACTIVATION DOMAINS OF THE AR

A series of truncated mutant forms of the AR was created utilizing several unique restriction sites as well as polymerase chain reaction mutagenesis and exonuclease III digestion. A detailed study of AR mutants was recently published.[1] FIGURE 2 shows a series of NH_2-terminal truncated AR mutant constructs which have increasingly larger deletions created by exonuclease III digestion. These mutant DNA vectors were expressed in monkey kidney CV1 cells by cotransfection with a reporter plasmid containing the chloramphenicol acetyltransferase gene linked to an androgen responsive promoter sequence. As evident in FIGURE 2, loss of transcriptional activity occurs with the deletion of 337 amino acids from the NH_2-terminus (AR4). Smaller deletions, including deletion of 72 (AR2) and 140 (AR3) amino acids from the NH_2-

[a] Address correspondence to Elizabeth M. Wilson, Ph.D., CB 7500 MacNider Bldg., University of North Carolina, Chapel Hill, NC 27599; Tel. (919)966-5159; FAX (919)966-2203.

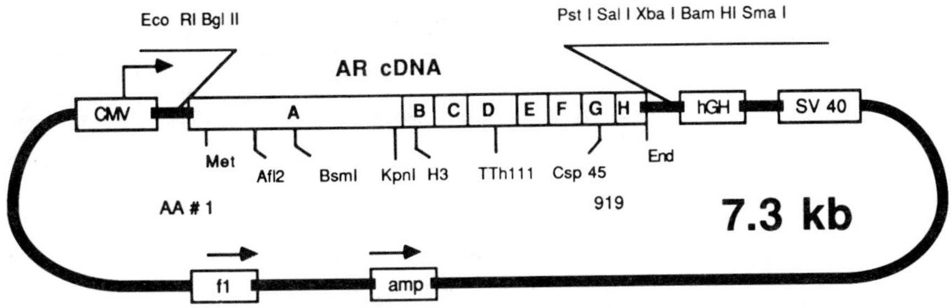

FIGURE 1. Schematic diagram of the full length wild type human AR expression vector. The 3.1 kb coding sequence of the human AR was cloned in the expression vector pCMV5 as previously described.[1] The entire AR expression vector is 7.3 kb in length and restriction sites are indicated that were useful in mutagenesis.

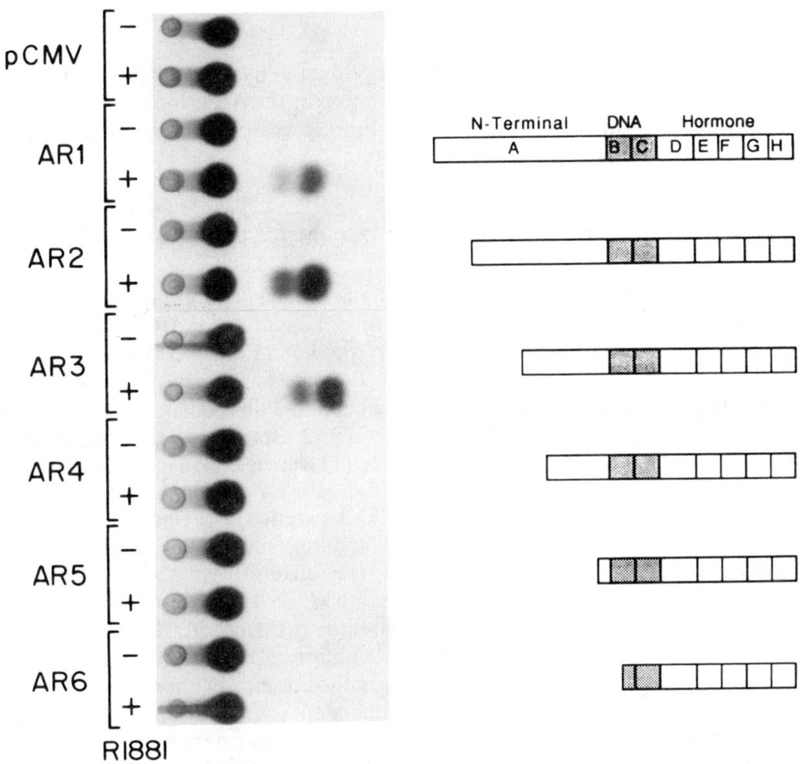

FIGURE 2. Functional analysis of NH_2-terminal deletion mutants of the human androgen receptor. A series of NH_2 terminal deletions was created using unidirectional exonuclease III digestion of wild type human AR. Functional activities were assessed by cotransfection into CV1 cells as previously described.[1] The expression vectors analyzed include the following deletion mutants: pCMV, the parent vector lacking AR sequence; AR1, the full length human AR cDNA; AR2, amino acids 73–919; AR3, amino acids 141 to 919; AR4, amino acids 338–919; AR5, amino acids 507–919; AR6, amino acids 566–919. Shown is the x-ray film autoradiograph of the thin layer chromatogram containing the acetylated forms of ^{14}C-chloramphenicol resulting from the induction of chloramphenicol acetyltransferase gene linked to an androgen responsive promoter.[1]

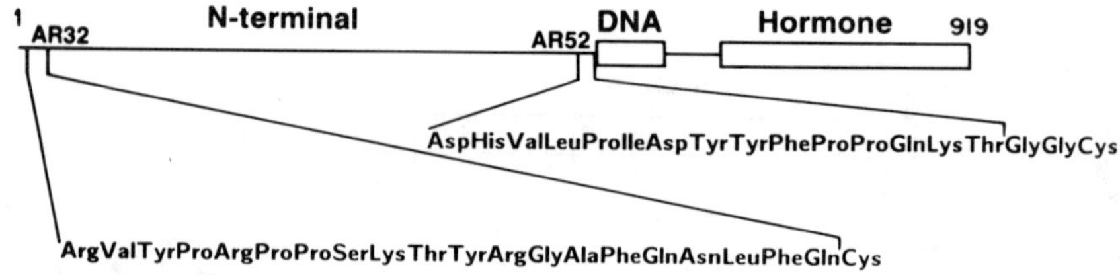

FIGURE 3. Schematic diagram of two synthetic peptide immunogens used in raising antibodies AR32 and AR52. The human AR includes three functional domains, the NH_2-terminal region, and the DNA and steroid binding domains as diagrammed. The peptide used in preparing AR32 begins at amino acid 9 from the NH_2-terminus and contains 20 amino acids derived from human AR. The peptide for AR 52 contains amino acids 544–558 of human AR and amino acids 527–541 of rat AR. The peptides were conjugated to Keyhole limpet hemocyanin and injected into rabbits as previously described.[6]

terminus, did not significantly alter transcriptional activation. These results suggest that a region important in transcriptional activation by the AR is located between amino acids 141 and 338. Studies are ongoing to more precisely identify those sequences required by the receptor for gene activation.

REQUIREMENTS FOR AR NUCLEAR TRANSPORT

High level expression of AR in COS cells facilitates its immunocytochemical detection. Two antipeptide antibodies useful in immunoanalysis of AR were raised against synthetic peptides, the sequences of which are shown in FIGURE 3. The peptide nearest the NH_2-terminus, beginning at amino acid 9, yielded antibody AR32, which reacts with both native and denatured receptor.[2] The peptide with sequence just NH_2-terminal to the DNA binding domain yielded antibody AR52. Both polyclonal antibodies react with endogenous and transiently expressed ARs and were useful in immunocytochemical studies.

Transfection into COS cells of the pCMV5 parent vector lacking AR sequence yielded a low background level of immunostaining, shown in FIGURE 4A, with no influence of androgen addition (FIG. 4B). Expression of full-length AR in the presence of androgen resulted in strong nuclear staining (FIG. 4D) with absence of staining in nucleoli and extranuclear regions. Transient expression of AR in the absence of androgen resulted in a striking punctate distribution in the perinuclear region of the cytoplasm (FIG. 4C). Staining in the nucleus in the absence of androgen was minimal. Thus, in this expression system, androgen-dependent translocation of AR occurs from the perinuclear region to the nucleus. Identical results are obtained when the natural androgens, testosterone and dihydrotestosterone, are used to promote nuclear transport of the AR.

Immunohistochemical staining of endogenous AR in frozen tissue sections was nuclear in the presence of androgen.[4] However, there was loss of receptor staining 48 h after androgen was removed by castration.[4] Interestingly, nuclear staining could be recovered rapidly, within 15 min of androgen treatment. From biochemical studies it is known that AR is present following castration; however, in the absence of androgen the AR apparently cannot be detected immunohistochemically. This lack of AR im-

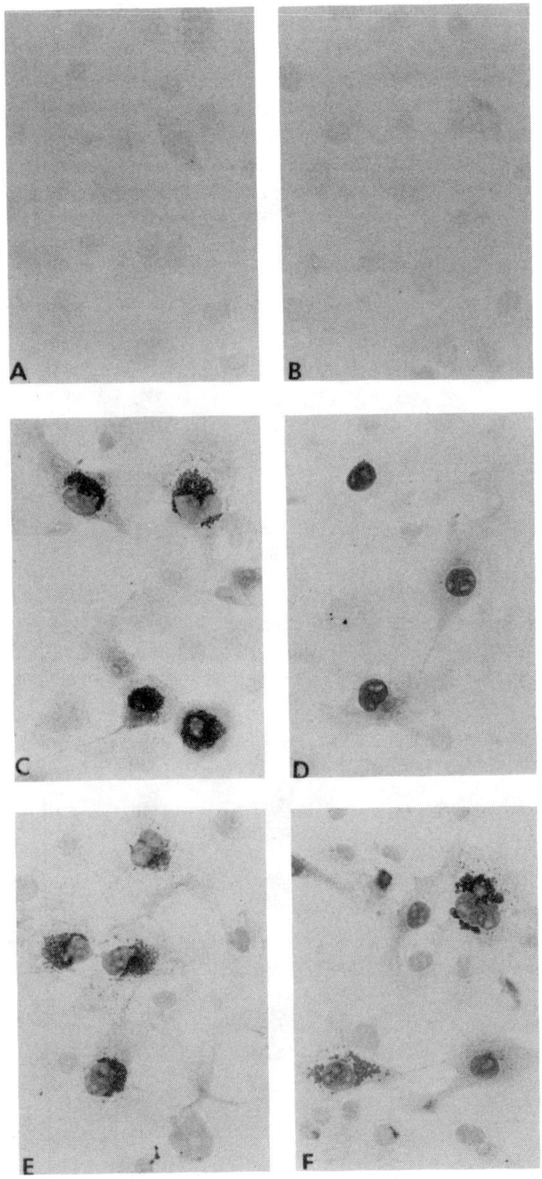

FIGURE 4. Immunocytochemical localization of the human AR in COS cells. COS cells were transfected with the parent pCMV expression vector lacking AR sequence (A & B), the full length AR expression vector (C & D), or a deletion mutant vector lacking a 32 amino acid sequence in the hinge region (E & F). The cells were transfected as previously described[1] and incubated for 48 h in the absence (A,C,E) or presence (B,D,F) of 50 nM of the synthetic androgen, R1881. Cells were fixed and stained using the avidin biotin peroxidase procedure previously described.[1,3,4]

munostaining in tissue sections in the absence of androgen may be attributed to diminished antibody affinity for the unactivated AR as well as to the lower level of endogenous receptor in tissues. In the presence of androgen, nuclear staining of endogenous receptor is intense.[3-5]

When a putative nuclear targeting signal present within a 32 amino acid sequence

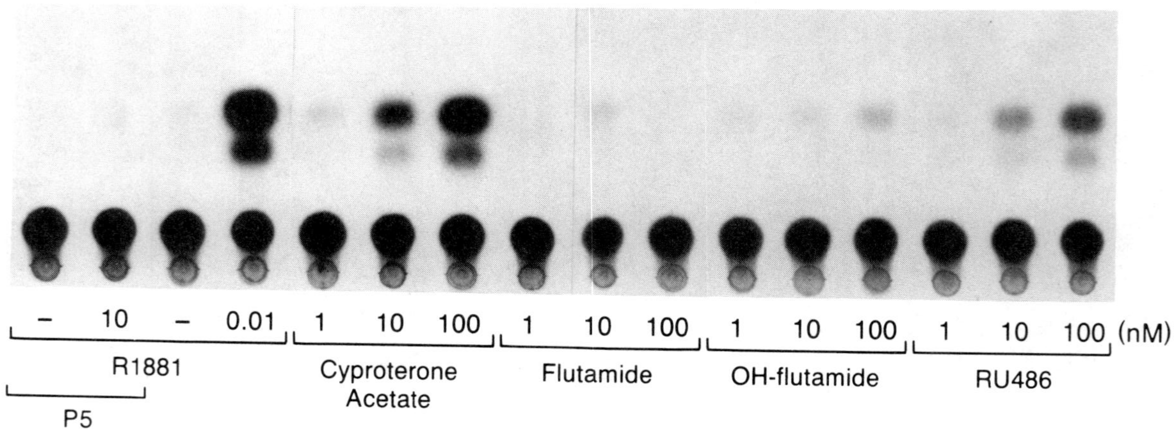

FIGURE 5. Transcriptional CAT activity in the presence of antiandrogens and RU486. Monkey kidney CV1 cells were cotransfected with the full length wild type human AR expression vector and a reporter plasmid containing the chloramphenicol acetyltransferase (CAT) gene linked to an androgen-responsive promoter. CAT activity was determined as previously described[1] in the presence of increasing concentrations of R1881, cyproterone acetate, flutamide, hydroxyflutamide and RU486. The upper spots reflect the presence of acetylated forms of ^{14}C-chloramphenicol and indicates positive transcriptional activity.

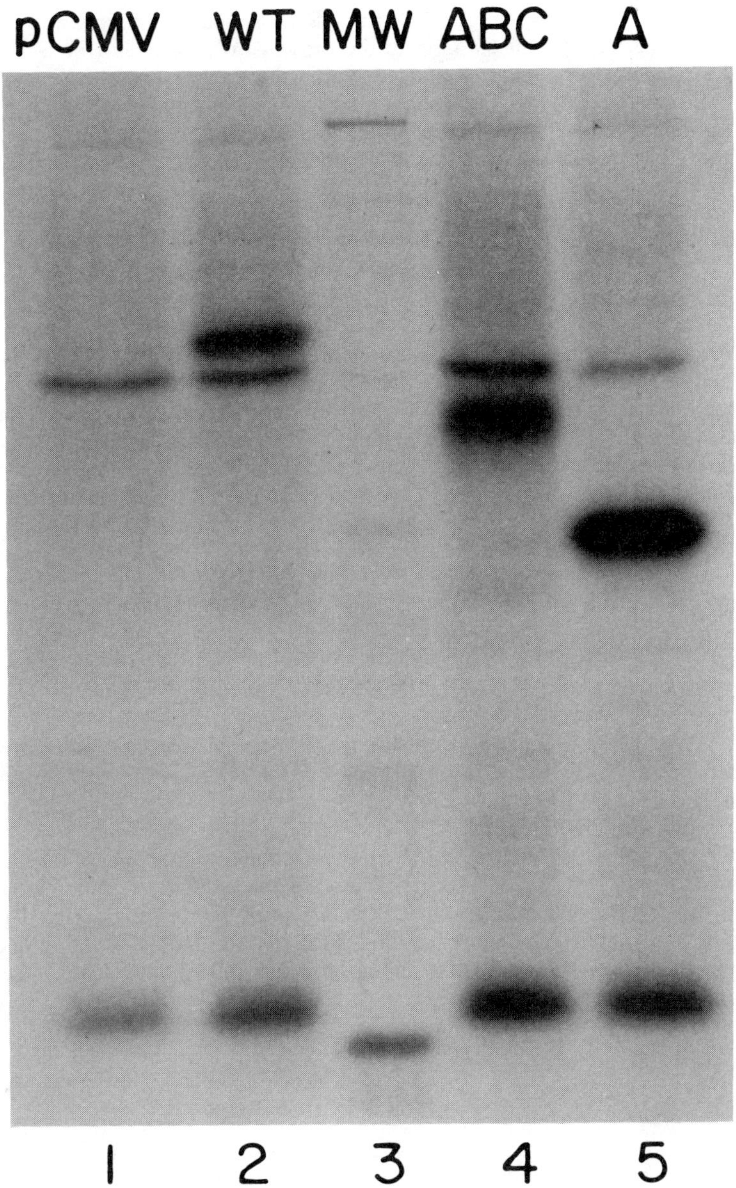

FIGURE 6. Phosphorylation of human AR. COS cells were transfected with the parent pCMV5 expression vector lacking AR sequence (*lane 1*), the full length, wild type AR (*lane 2*), a deletion mutant lacking the steroid binding domain (*lane 4*), and a mutant lacking the DNA and steroid binding domains (*lane 5*). Transfections into COS cells were performed as previously described.[1] Forty-eight h after transfection the cells were placed in phosphate-free media and incubated for 3 h in the presence of 200 μCi of ^{32}P-orthophosphate. The cells were solubilized and incubated with AR32 antipeptide antibody to immunoprecipitate the labeled AR fragments. The extracts were electrophoresed on an 8% SDS polyacrylamide gel, transferred to nitrocellulose paper and exposed to x-ray film.

was deleted from the full-length AR, the AR remained predominantly perinuclear with only minimal nuclear staining in the presence of androgen (FIGS. 4E and F). The nuclear targeting signal is situated within the hinge region between the DNA and steroid binding domains. The decrease in nuclear staining in the presence of androgen of this mutant receptor (FIG. 4F) suggested that a sequence within the 32 amino acid region is important in signaling nuclear transport of AR. Studies on nuclear translocation are ongoing to further evaluate the functional requirements of specific amino acids in this region.

EFFECTS OF ANTIANDROGENS

Cyproterone acetate and hydroxyflutamide were shown previously to inhibit androgen-induced male sexual development and to block the effects of androgen administered to castrated animals.[7,8] It was therefore of interest to examine both agonist and antagonist effects of these antiandrogens in the cotransfection system. Interestingly, cyproterone acetate stimulated an increase in CAT activity at hormone concentrations of 10 and 100 nM (FIG. 5). Similar androgenic activity of other progestins was observed previously *in vivo*.[7] Flutamide and hydroxyflutamide at these concentrations failed to stimulate transcriptional activity by the AR (FIG. 5). A hormone antagonist for the glucocorticoid and progesterone receptors, RU486,[9,10] displayed agonist activity with the AR at concentrations of 10 nM or greater (FIG. 5).

AR PHOSPHORYLATION

The AR is a phosphoprotein which undergoes enhanced phosphorylation in response to androgen treatment. Full-length ^{32}P-labeled AR migrates as 114 kDa molecular weight, shown in FIGURE 6 as wild type receptor (lane 2, WT). When the parent expression vector, pCMV5, which lacks AR sequence, is used in the phosphorylation reaction, no products are observed at this molecular weight (FIG. 6, lane 1). From the data shown in FIG. 6, lanes 4 and 5, there are predominant sites of AR phosphorylation in the NH_2-terminal region of the receptor. The phosphorylated products shown include mutant ARs with deletions of the steroid binding domain (lane 4) and deletions of the steroid plus DNA binding domains (lane 5). Molecular weights of these truncated receptor forms are approximately 87 and 70 kDa, respectively. Phosphorylation was also detected in the hinge region of AR between the steroid and DNA binding domains (not shown). Studies are in progress to identify the sites of phosphorylation in the AR and to determine the functional effects of phosphorylation.

REFERENCES

1. SIMENTAL, J. A., M. SAR, M. V. LANE, F. S. FRENCH & E. M. WILSON. 1991. Transcriptional activation and nuclear targeting signals of the human androgen receptor. J. Biol. Chem. **266:** 510–518.
2. QUARMBY, V. E., J. A. KEMPPAINEN, M. SAR, D. B. LUBAHN, F. S. FRENCH & E. M. WILSON. 1990. Expression of recombinant androgen receptor in cultured mammalian cells. Mol. Endocrinol. **4:** 1399–1407.
3. TAN, J. A., D. R. JOSEPH, V. E. QUARMBY, D. B. LUBAHN, M. SAR, F. S. FRENCH & E. M.

WILSON. 1988. The rat androgen receptor: Primary structure, autoregulation of its messenger RNA and immunocytochemical localization of the receptor protein. Mol. Endocrinol. **2:** 1276–1285.

4. SAR, M., D. B. LUBAHN, F. S. FRENCH & E. M. WILSON. 1990. Immunohistochemical localization of the androgen receptor in rat and human tissues. Endocrinology **127:** 3180–3186.
5. LUBAHN, D. B., D. R. JOSEPH, M. SAR, J. A. TAN, H. N. HIGGS, R. E. LARSON, F. S. FRENCH & E. M. WILSON. 1988. The human androgen receptor: Complementary DNA cloning, sequence analysis and gene expression in prostate. Mol. Endocrinol. **2:** 1265–1275.
6. SMITH, D. F., D. B. LUBAHN, D. J. MCCORMICK, E. M. WILSON & D. O. TOFT. 1988. The production of antibodies against the conserved cysteine region of steroid receptors and their use in characterizing the avian progesterone receptor. Endocrinology **122:** 2816–2825.
7. MOWSZOWICZ, I., D. E. BIEBER, K. W. CHUNG, L. P. BULLOCK & C. W. BARDIN. 1974. Synandrogenic and antiandrogenic effects of progestins: Comparison with nonprogestational antiandrogens. Endocrinology **95:** 1589–1599.
8. NERI, R., E. PEETS & A. WATNICK. 1979. Antiandrogenicity of flutamide and its metabolite Sch 16423. Biochem. Soc. Trans. **7:** 565–569.
9. MEYER, M. E., A. PORNON, J. JI, M. T. BOCQUEL, P. CHAMBON & H. GRONEMEYER. 1990. Agonistic and antagonistic activities of RU486 on the functions of the human progesterone receptor. EMBO J. **9:** 3923–3932.
10. WEBSTER, N. J. G., S. GREEN, J. R. JIN & P. CHAMBON. 1988. The hormone binding domains of the estrogen and glucocorticoid receptors contain an inducible transcription activation function. Cell **54:** 199–207.

Role of Sex Chromosomes in the Control of Male Germ-Cell Differentiation[a]

MARY ANN HANDEL,[b,e] PATRICIA A. HUNT,[c]
MARY C. KOT,[b,d] CYNTHIA PARK,[b] AND
MARK SHANNON[b]

[b] *Department of Zoology and*
Graduate Program in Cellular, Molecular and Developmental Biology
University of Tennessee
Knoxville, Tennessee 37996

[c] *Department of Pathology and Winship Cancer Center*
Emory University
Atlanta, Georgia 30322

INTRODUCTION

Recent cloning of Y-linked genes is providing initial insights into how somatic-cell sex is determined in mammals (R. Lovell-Badge, presented at the XIth North American Testis Workshop). Although we know little about mechanisms of how sex of the mammalian germ line is determined, recognized, and expressed, we are in a position to make some observations about the influence of sex chromosomes on specific aspects of gametogenesis. This review will focus on the role of sex chromosomes in spermatogenesis. We will consider how the male germ cell expresses its genetic sex, which of course is ultimately in the formation of a spermatozoon.

It is useful to keep in mind the sexually dimorphic features of gametogenesis (FIG. 1). The reference point is the laboratory mouse, but the observations are general and can be extended to other species. Germ cells of both sexes reach the fetal gonad at about day 10.5p.c., where they subsequently continue mitotic proliferation. Sex differences are first evident at about day 13.5p.c., when female, but not male, gonadal germ cells enter meiosis. Female cells proceed through meiotic prophase and arrest at the end of prophase, in diplotene. This arrest is lengthy; it is not released until the time of ovulation, sometime after reaching puberty. There is considerable atresia of female germ cells, for reasons not clearly understood. In contrast to the fetal meiosis of female germ cells, male germ cells enter a period of mitotic arrest. This lasts until shortly after birth, when prespermatogonia begin to proliferate mitotically, and stem cells

[a] This work was supported by grants HD-16978 from the National Institutes of Health and DMB-8905117 from the National Science Foundation to MAH, and R29-HD-27393 from the NIH to PAH.

[d] *Present address:* Department of Biology, Kalamazoo College, Kalamazoo, MI 49007.

[e] Address correspondence to Dr. Handel at the Department of Zoology, University of Tennessee, Knoxville, TN 37996-0810; FAX (615)974-0798.

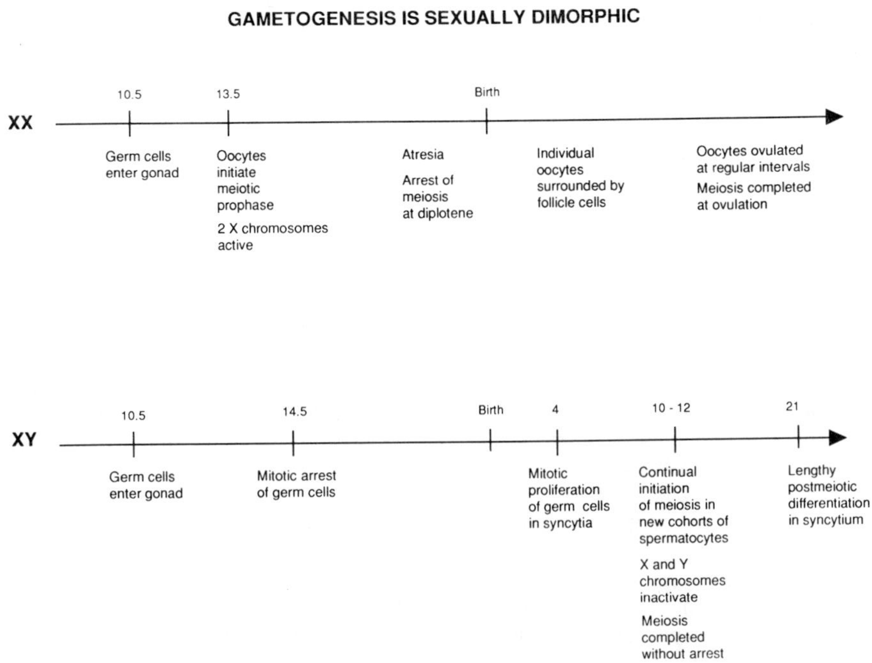

FIGURE 1. Developmental sequence and sexual dimorphism of male and female germ-cell differentiation.

differentiate into spermatogonia, which ultimately give rise, with the onset of puberty, to meiotic spermatocytes. Prophase is long, and there are uniquely spermatogenic aspects of the behavior of sex chromosomes and the response to chromosome anomalies. Meiotic prophase is not characterized by arrest as in female germ cells. Rather, the male germ cells proceed through the two meiotic metaphases immediately upon completion of prophase, and then enter the extended period of post-meiotic, haploid differentiation termed spermiogenesis. Haploid gene expression creates the possibility of genetic differences among gametes, since the postmeiotic gametes can differ in alleles at any genetic locus as well as in their sex-chromosome constitution. This feature of extensive postmeiotic differentiation in a syncytium is a characteristic of male germ cells that is not shared by female germ cells and thus is one more aspect of the sexual dimorphism of gametogenesis.

There are a number of points in this scheme at which behavior and expression of the sex chromosomes differ in male and female gametogenesis, thus characterizing sexually dimorphic differentiative pathways. The first event of sexual differentiation, the fetal decision to undergo meiosis or not, depends on the soma of the testis rather than on the sex chromosome constitution of the gonocytes in the testis. Second, the behavior of sex chromosomes during meiosis is markedly different in male and female germ cells, with X-chromosome inactivation in male meiosis versus X-chromosome activation in female meiosis. The spermatogenic cell has developed mechanisms to cope with the seemingly inconvenient inactivation of its X chromosome. Finally, of considerable interest is the question of the role of the Y chromosome in spermatogenesis.

FETAL MEIOTIC DECISIONS

The first juncture at which the germ-cell sex is evident is at about day 13.5p.c., when XX germ cells in the ovary enter meiotic prophase and XY germ cells in the testis enter a phase of mitotic arrest. It appears that a two-X chromosome constitution is neither necessary nor sufficient to ensure a female meiotic decision, and that while the presence of a Y-chromosome may facilitate embarking on a male path, it is not sufficient. The evidence for these conclusions is as follows.

It has been demonstrated by Zamboni and Upadhyay[1,2] that germ cells in normal individuals of either sex occasionally find themselves in the adrenal cortex instead of their normal destination, the gonad. These misplaced germ cells follow the female path of entering meiosis regardless of their sex. Thus XY germ cells enter meiotic prophase on an appropriate time schedule for female cells; these can even differentiate as oocytes with a zona pellucida! Therefore, an XX chromosome constitution is not necessary for the female developmental path. Additionally, these observations demonstrate that the presence of the Y chromosome does not autonomously ensure a male path and furthermore, that the presence of a Y chromosome does not prevent undertaking a female path. Another inference from these observations is that the female path is the "default" path and the male path of germ-cell differentiation, *i.e.*, fetal mitotic arrest, occurs only in the testis. Thus it must involve communication between the somatic cells (presumably the fetal Sertoli cells) and the germ cells of the testis.

The situation of germ cells in the adrenal gland is admittedly odd. What about germ cells in gonads, and, in particular, in the testis? We have addressed this question by examining the fate of germ cells with two normal X chromosomes and a Y chromosome. These XXY "Klinefelter" mice were produced in a breeding scheme involving an unusual Y chromosome.[3] We were curious to learn if XXY germ cells in a testis follow a female path or a male path. They all appear to follow a male path; they do not enter meiosis (FIG. 2). The morphology of XXY gonocytes is similar to that of XY gonocytes in the testes of control male sibs; there is no evidence of synaptonemal complex, or of the chromatin configuration typical of meiotic prophase nuclei. Thus two X chromosomes are not incompatible with the initiation of a male path of germ-cell development, and the location of the germ cells in testicular seminiferous cords ensures the male decision. However, although two X chromosomes are not incompatible with the initiation of a male germ-cell path of development, they are incompatible with successful progress of male germ-cell differentiation. All germ cells in XXY males fail to proliferate and the gonads are essentially devoid of germ cells within a few days of birth. Why that might be and how it relates to the sexual dimorphism of gametogenesis is not now apparent.

What about XX cells (lacking a Y chromosome) in a testis? This question has been much harder to investigate, as it takes some manipulation to get XX cells into a testis. The condition is met in the case of XX ⟷ XY chimeras, where nearly all germ cells (presumably including XX germ cells) do not initiate meiosis prenatally, and are responding to the sex of the somatic tissue around them. However, it seems that a very few XX cells, in the vicinity of the rete testis, can initiate meiosis.[4,5] The same general observations hold for XX,*Sxr* testes.[6] Although we have sought them,

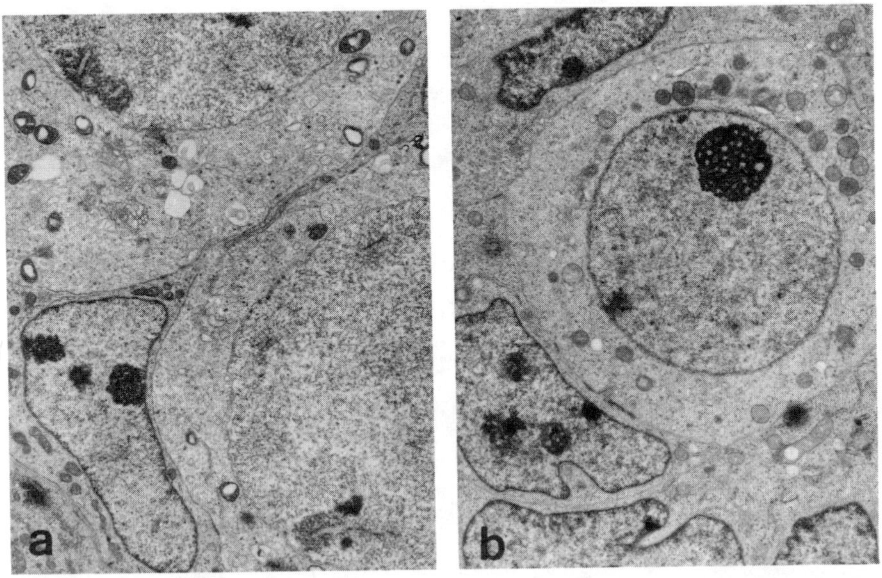

FIGURE 2. a: Two murine oocytes showing profiles of synaptonemal complex. *Magnification:* ×4550. b: Fetal germ cell of XXY testis, showing typical chromatin morphology of an interphase cell, similar to that of XY germ cells of the same developmental age. *Magnification:* ×3900.

we have not found any meiotic XXY germ cells in the testes of our XXY "Klinefelter" mice. It is possible, then, that the presence of the Y chromosome facilitates the male path of differentiation in the XXY germ cells. However, it seems inescapable that the soma of the gonad is critically important in the decision to follow the male path of germ-cell differentiation. The principal role of the Y chromosome at this point might be solely in the somatic cells.

Thus, in this early genetic event of germ-cell differentiation, we find that two X-chromosomes are neither necessary nor sufficient to ensure a female meiotic decision, and the presence of the Y chromosome in the germ cell also is neither necessary nor sufficient to ensure a male path of differentiation. Does germ-cell sex matter at this point? Apparently it does not in the initiation of sexually dimorphic aspects of germ-cell behavior, but in fact, sex chromosome constitution is critically important to male germ-cell survival, since testicular gonocytes that have two X chromosomes begin to die within a few days of this first differentiative event. Although we do not know why they die, it may be related to the sexually dimorphic behavior of sex chromosomes during meiosis, and involve inappropriate activation of the X chromosome.

MALE MEIOSIS–X-CHROMOSOME INACTIVATION

Meiosis is conspicuously dimorphic sexually, and one of the more puzzling aspects of this dimorphism is the behavior of the sex chromosomes during meiotic prophase. As female germ cells enter meiotic prophase, the inactive, heterochromatic X chro-

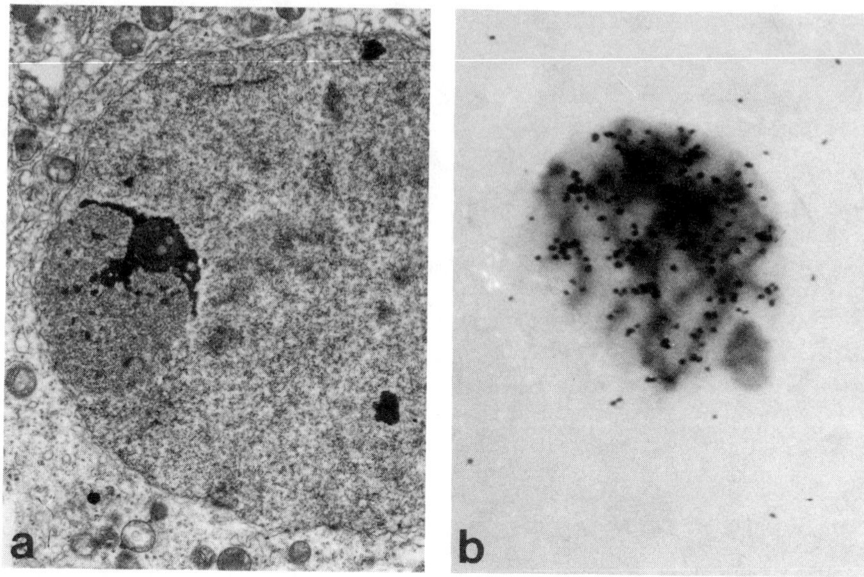

FIGURE 3. **a:** Sex body of a murine pachytene spermatocyte, with closely apposed nucleolus. *Magnification:* ×7110. **b:** Micrograph of murine pachytene spermatocyte with grains revealing incorporation of ^{3}H-uridine, showing incorporation over axes of autosomal chromosomes, but not into the sex body. *Magnification:* ×400.

mosome is reactivated. The evidence for this derives primarily from two kinds of data: the appearance of the heteropolymeric forms of X-encoded isozymes[7] and quantitative differences in amounts of X-encoded proteins in oocytes of XX versus XO individuals.[8]

In striking contrast to this behavior of the X chromosome in female gametocytes, the X chromosome of spermatocytes is inactive at meiotic prophase. Evidence for this derived initially from cytological observations of a heterochromatic sex pair[9,10] and of the sequestration of the X and Y chromosomes to a region of special chromatin structure, the sex body (FIG. 3a), of mammalian pachytene spermatocyte nuclei (originally described by Sachs[11] and Solari[12]). These cytological observations were bolstered by autoradiography (such as that in FIG. 3b) demonstrating no incorporation of ^{3}H-uridine by the meiotic sex chromosomes in insects and mammals (original observations by Henderson,[13] Monesi,[14] and Kierszenbaum and Tres[15]).

We have been interested in the consequences of the inactivation of the single X chromosome in spermatogenic cells, since the X chromosome encodes a number of otherwise ubiquitously expressed housekeeping proteins. How does the germ cell cope with the inconvenient inactivation of its genes for hypoxanthine phosphoribosyl transferase (HPRT), glucose-6-phosphate dehydrogenase (G6PD), and phosphoglycerate kinase (PGK), as well as others? We approached this by studying the developmental pattern of expression of the protein product and the transcript of the *Hprt* gene in mouse spermatogenic cells. We found that HPRT enzyme activity is maintained at constant levels in testes of all developmental stages, with different profiles of germ cells present and, likewise, HPRT activity is at comparable levels in pachytene spermatocytes and round spermatids, but is greatly diminished in mature sperm. Northern-blot analysis revealed that transcripts from the *Hprt* gene are present in testes of all developmental stages; however, the relative abundance is decreased with the appearance in the testis of postmeiotic germ cells. Transcript is present in pachytene spermatocytes and round spermatids, in spite of apparent inactivation of the X chromosome. It has not yet been possible to demonstrate if these transcripts are stable ones synthesized prior to X-chromosome inactivation, or if they are newly transcribed. Consequently, these observations are consistent with either of two hypotheses: the *Hprt* gene may not be inactivated, or transcripts and protein product of the *Hprt* gene may be stable.

Although we cannot exclude the possibility that the *Hprt* gene fails to be inactivated, we find the evidence reviewed above for X-chromosome inactivation to be compelling and we consider it more likely that products of the *Hprt* gene are stabilized. Such stabilization of gene products may well be a strategy that the spermatogenic cell utilizes to cope with the consequences of inactivation of its X chromosome. This is apparently one of at least two strategies that the spermatogenic cell employs. In the case of the *Pgk-1* gene, transcripts and enzyme product of the gene are not as stable. Instead, the spermatocyte and spermatid utilize an alternative gene, *Pgk-2*, on mouse chromosome 17, which is expressed only in meiotic and postmeiotic male germ cells.[16,17] Interestingly, McCarrey and Thomas[18] have found that this gene lacks introns and may have been derived from the X-linked gene by a process of retrotransposition. This is apparently the case also for the gene for the pyruvate dehydrogenase El-α subunit, encoded on the X chromosome, with a testis-specific, postmeiotically expressed form encoded on an autosomal chromosome.[19] Thus there may be at least two strategies by which the male germ cell compensates for the inactivation of its X chromosome: stabilization of gene products, and utilization of an alternative, autosomal, gene. It will be interesting to learn the pattern with respect to the *Gpd* gene.

It should be emphasized that we really know very little about X-chromosome inactivation during spermatogenesis. We don't know why it occurs. It is unlikely that it is a male equivalent to the process of random X-chromosome inactivation that occurs in mammalian female embryos for purposes of dosage compensation. Instead, it is more likely to be related to events of meiosis. It is therefore useful to consider in this context that in oocytes the two homomorphic X chromosomes are in an open chromatin configuration that permits access of enzymes for recombination as well as those for transcription, the two X chromosomes are fully paired along their length, and recombination can occur along the whole chromosome. In contrast, during male meiosis, the heteromorphic sex chromosomes are in a chromatin configuration that seems to prevent access of enzymes for transcription and recombination, the X and Y chromosomes are paired in a very restricted region, and recombination is limited to this region. Pairing and recombination are restricted by lack of homology and, in turn, restricting the opportunity for pairing and recombination, perhaps by chromatin configuration, preserves the differentiation of the X and Y chromosomes. We are likely to reach a more comprehensive understanding of spermatogenic X-chromosome inactivation when we understand sex-specific factors controlling synapsis and recombination between the homomorphic sex chromosome pair in female germ cells and the lack thereof between the heteromorphic sex chromosomes of the male germ cell. Thus we favor the view that transcriptional inactivation of the X chromosome in spermatogenic cells is a consequence of a sex-specific meiotic phenomenon related to chromosome pairing and recombination. However, others[20] consider the possibility that the X chromosome is inactivated because certain X-encoded products are inhibitory to spermatogenesis. Clearly, more research is needed!

Although the Y chromosome appears to be inactivated at the same time as the X chromosome, there has been no definitive documentation of this. We also do not know and have little evidence bearing upon whether the X and Y chromosomes remain inactive throughout postmeiotic spermiogenesis. If, in fact, they do, this would serve to minimize phenotypic differences between the X and Y meiotic segregational products as well as set limits on what we might expect to be the role of the Y chromosome during spermiogenesis. On the other hand, if the X and Y chromosomes are reactivated postmeiotically, this would give rise to the possibility of phenotypic differences between X- and Y-bearing sperm. Andrologists have been attempting for years to separate X-bearing from Y-bearing sperm, and differences in gene expression could facilitate attaining this goal. However, the presence of cytoplasmic bridges joining meiotic segregants might militate against phenotypic differences being expressed by genotypically different spermatids. We have recently demonstrated that transcripts of an autosomal gene can be shared among conjoined spermatids;[21] however, these results do not imply that all gene products are shared. Additionally if the X and Y chromosomes are reactivated postmeiotically, we might then consider a spermiogenic role for the Y chromosome.

ROLE OF THE Y CHROMOSOME IN SPERMATOGENESIS

The Y chromosome might be expected to play a significant role in the sexual dimorphism of gametogenesis. We have already briefly covered the evidence that the Y chromosome of the germ cell plays no role in the early sexual differentiation decisions of the germ cell; germ cells with a Y chromosome can enter fetal meiosis and germ cells without a Y chromosome can at least initiate correct differentiation in the testis.

We were interested in the role of the Y chromosome in later spermatogenic events and used the XO,*Sxr* male mouse as a genetic model to investigate the progress and ultrastructure of spermatogenesis in the absence of a significant portion of the Y chromosome.[22] These mice are progeny of matings between XO females and XY,*Sxr* males. They lack a maternally derived X chromosome and the paternally derived X chromosome is modified by having received a small sex-determining region from the Y*Sxr* chromosome. Thus, XO,*Sxr* mice are phenotypic males; their germ cells survive (since they have only one X chromosome) and differentiate as spermatozoa; however, these males are sterile. Why? We have learned two interesting things about these mice.

First, all sperm-specific structures and modifications, such as acrosome, manchette, condensed nucleus, and the elaborate sperm-tail components, are assembled in a spatially and temporally correct manner.[22] Thus the portion of the Y chromosome missing in these males (which is most of the Y chromosome) cannot encode products specifying or regulating assembly of these structures. This information must be in the small *Sxr* region, or, more likely, encoded on other chromosomes. These observations set limits on the informational content of that portion of the Y chromosome outside the sex-determining region. We must also consider that if the Y chromosome is not reactivated after meiosis, we cannot expect it to function during spermiogenesis (although we cannot exclude the possibility of Y-encoded products synthesized premeiotically and utilized postmeiotically). We have confirmed and extended observations made by others that many spermatozoa from XO,*Sxr* males are morphologically abnormal and the percent of abnormal sperm increases with age.[22] This is consistent with several hypotheses. First, it could be imagined that it is necessary to have a maternally imprinted X chromosome for successful spermatogenesis. However, the finding of normal fertility in male mice who inherit both sex chromosomes from their father[23] argues against this explanation. Second, it is possible that the long arm of the Y chromosome contains a gene or genes that control sperm morphology, already suggested by the data of Krzanowska.[24,25] Third, morphologically abnormal sperm may be a consequence of reduced spermiogenic function. They are found in virtually all conditions where quantitative aspects of spermatogenesis are reduced, as is the case in XO,*Sxr* mice (see below), perhaps because of inadequate germ cell-Sertoli cell signaling. Therefore, the morphological abnormalities of spermatids that we observed may not be an intrinsic property of Y-deficiency, but may be a more general reflection of impaired testicular function due to reduced numbers of differentiating spermatids.

The second interesting feature of spermatogenesis in XO,*Sxr* males is the quantitative reduction of spermatogenesis. Although both Cattanach[26] and Burgoyne[27] had observed reduced spermatogenic output in these mice, it had not previously been analyzed in detail. We have made a careful analysis of quantitative aspects of gametogenesis in XY, XO,*Sxr* and XY,*Sxr* mice.[22] We found that numbers of premeiotic cells normalized to numbers of Sertoli cells in XO,*Sxr* mice were not significantly different from numbers in normal XY mice. Numbers of spermatocytes were somewhat reduced, and there was an 80–90% reduction in the numbers of post-meiotic spermatids. These observations suggest that there is meiotic breakdown in these males. Since the most obvious genetic defect of these males is the lack of an intact Y chromosome, we suggest that meiosis is abnormal and doomed to failure because there is no pairing partner for the X chromosome. There are numerous other examples in the literature that implicate some kind of meiotic quality control mechanism regulating spermatogenic success when pairing failure occurs.[28]

Is the sole spermatogenic role of the Y chromosome that of pairing partner for the X chromosome? Apparently not. Sutcliffe and Burgoyne[29] investigated early features of spermatogenesis in mutant XO,*Sxr*^{b} mice that lack a non-sex-determining portion of the *Sxr* fragment. Here the situation is quite different from XO,*Sxr* in that there is complete failure of spermatogenesis at the early stages of differentiation of Type A and B spermatogonia. These observations implicated a gene, termed *Spy* by Burgoyne, that controls aspects of the onset of spermatogenic function in germ cells. It is not known if this gene acts autonomously in the germ cells or exerts its influence through the testicular soma, in particular, the Sertoli cells.

CONCLUSIONS

Although we have stated at the outset that little is known about how germ-cell sex is determined, recognized and expressed, we can draw some conclusions.

Somatic-cell sex, rather than germ-cell sex, is important in dictating the first evident sexually dimorphic differentiation of gametes. However, soon after the initiation of differentiation, the presence of more than one X chromosome in testicular germ cells acts as a germ-cell-autonomous cell lethal. The X chromosome exhibits sexual dimorphism in its meiotic transcriptive activity in that both X chromosomes are active in XX oocytes, but the X chromosome assumes the form of inactive chromatin in meiotic spermatocytes. This contrast in chromatin configuration may well be an essential feature of homogametic versus heterogametic meiosis and related to chromosome pairing and recombination. Finally, the Y chromosome may not contribute genetic information for sperm-specific structures, but does serve as a pairing partner for the X chromosome as well as to initiate mature spermatogenic function in germ cells.

These observations provide a theoretical and empirical foundation for future investigations. However, it is clear that there are many unanswered and probably unanticipated questions that will keep those fascinated with sex chromosomes and germ cells busy for years!

REFERENCES

1. UPADHYAY, S. & L. ZAMBONI. 1982. Ectopic germ cells: Natural model for the study of germ cell sexual differentiation. Proc. Natl. Acad. Sci. USA **79:** 6584–6588.
2. ZAMBONI, L. & S. UPADHYAY. 1983. Germ cell differentiation in mouse adrenal glands. J. Exp. Zool. **228:** 173–193.
3. HUNT, P. A. & E. M. EICHER. 1991. Fertile male mice with three sex chromosomes: Evidence that infertility in XYY mice is an effect of two Y chromosomes. Chromosoma **100:** 293–299.
4. MYSTKOWSKA, E. T. & A. K. TARKOWSKI. 1970. Behavior of germ cells and sexual differentiation in late embryonic and early postnatal mouse chimaeras. J. Embryol. Exp. Morphol. **23:** 395–405.
5. MCLAREN, A., A. C. CHANDLEY & S. KOFMAN-ALFARO. 1972. A study of meiotic germ cells in the gonads of foetal mouse chimaeras. J. Embryol. Exp. Morphol. **27:** 515–524.
6. MCLAREN, A. 1981. The fate of germ cells in the testis of fetal *Sex-reversed* mice. J. Reprod. Fert. **61:** 461–467.
7. KRATZER, P. G. & V. M. CHAPMAN. 1981. X-chromosome reactivation in oocytes of *Mus caroli*. Proc. Natl. Acad. Sci. USA **78:** 3093–3097.
8. MCLAREN, A. & M. MONK. 1981. X-chromosome activity in the germ cells of *Sex-reversed* mouse embryos. J. Reprod. Fertil. **63:** 533–537.
9. MOHR, O. L. 1916. Studien über die chromatin reifung der mannlichen Geschlechtszellen bei *Locusta viridissima*. Arch. Biol. (Liege) **29:** 579.
10. PAINTER, T. S. 1924. Studies in mammalian spermatogenesis. III. The fate of the chromatin-nucleolus in the opossum. J. Exp. Zool. **39:** 197.
11. SACHS, L. 1954. Sex-linkage and the sex chromosomes in man. Ann. Eugen. **18:** 255–261.
12. SOLARI, A. J. 1974. The behavior of the XY pair in mammals. Int. Rev. Cytol. **38:** 273–317.
13. HENDERSON, S. A. 1964. RNA synthesis during male meiosis and spermiogenesis. Chromosoma (Berl.) **15:** 345–366.
14. MONESI, V. 1965. Differential rate of ribonucleic acid synthesis in the autosomes and sex chromosomes during male meiosis in the mouse. Chromosoma (Berl.) **17:** 11–21.
15. KIERSZENBAUM, A. L. & L. L. TRES. 1974. Transcription sites in spread meiotic prophase chromosomes from mouse spermatocytes. J. Cell Biol. **63:** 923–935.
16. KRAMER, J. M. 1981. Immunofluorescent localization of PGK-1 and PGK-2 isozymes within specific cells of the mouse testis. Dev. Biol. **87:** 30–36.
17. KRAMER, J. M. & R. P. ERICKSON. 1981. Developmental program of PGK-1 and PGK-2 isozymes in spermatogenic cells of the mouse: Specific activities and rates of synthesis. Dev. Biol. **87:** 37–45.
18. MCCARREY, J. R. & K. THOMAS. 1987. Human testis-specific PGK gene lacks introns and possesses characteristic of a processed gene. Nature **326:** 501–505.
19. DAHL, H-H. M., R. M. BROWN, W. M. HUTCHISON, C. MARAGOS & G. K. BROWN. 1990. A testis-specific form of the human pyruvate dehydrogenase E1α subunit is coded for by an intronless gene on chromosome 4. Genomics **8:** 225–232.
20. FOREJT, J. 1982. X-Y involvement in male sterility caused by autosome translocations—a hypothesis. *In* Genetic Control of Gamete Production and Function. P. G. Crosignani & B. L. Rubin, Eds.: 135–151. Academic Press/Grune and Stratton. New York.

21. CALDWELL, K. A. & M. A. HANDEL. 1991. Protamine transcript sharing among post-meiotic spermatids. Proc. Natl. Acad. Sci. USA **88:** 2407–2411.

22. KOT, M. C. & M. A. HANDEL. 1990. Spermatogenesis in XO,*Sxr* mice: Role of the Y chromosome. J. Exp. Zool. **256:** 92–105.

23. HANDEL, M. A. & P. A. HUNT. 1991. Genomic imprinting: Male mice with uniparentally derived sex chromosomes. Mol. Reprod. Devel. **28:** 337–340.

24. KRZANOWSKA, H. 1972. Influence of the Y chromosome on fertility in mice. *In* Proceedings of The International Symposium on Genetics of the Spermatozoon. R. A. Beatty & S. Gluecksohn-Waelsch, Eds.: 370–386. University of Edinburgh, Edinburgh.

25. KRZANOWSKA, H. 1976. Inheritance of sperm head abnormality type in mice—the role of the Y chromosome. Genet. Res. **28:** 189–198.

26. CATTANACH, B. M., G. E. POLLARD & S. G. HAWKES. 1971. Sex-reversed mice: XX and XO males. Cytogenetics **10:** 318–337.

27. LEVY, E. R. & P. S. BURGOYNE. 1986. Diploid spermatids: A manifestation of spermatogenic impairment in XO,*Sxr* and T31H/+ mice. Cytogenet. Cell Genet. **42:** 159–163.

28. HANDEL, M. A. 1988. Genetic control of spermatogenesis in mice. *In* Results and Problems in Cell Differentiation, Spermatogenesis: Genetic Aspects. W. Hennig, Ed. **15:** 1–62. Springer-Verlag, Berlin.

29. SUTCLIFFE, M. J. & P. S. BURGOYNE. 1989. Analysis of the testes of H-Y negative XOSxr^{b} mice suggests that the spermatogenesis gene (*Spy*) acts during the differentiation of the A spermatogonia. Development **107:** 373–380.

Production of Müllerian-inhibiting Substance (MIS) and Sulfated Glycoprotein-2 (SGP-2) Associated with Testicular Differentiation in the XX Mouse Gonadal Graft[a]

TERUKO TAKETO

Urology Research Laboratory and Department of Biology
McGill University
Royal Victoria Hospital
687 Pine Avenue W.
Montréal, Québec, Canada H3A 1A1

SEX REVERSAL OF THE XX GONAD

It has been generally accepted that testicular differentiation is determined by a gene or set of genes on the Y chromosome in mammals (*TDF* in human or *Tdy* in the mouse). A DNA sequence, named SRY (or Sry in the mouse), has been proposed to be a strong candidate for the *TDF* (*Tdy*) gene.[1-3] DNA sequence analysis of SRY has suggested that if SRY proves to be *TDF*, the *TDF* gene product probably functions as a transcription factor which triggers the gene-regulatory cascade participating in testicular differentiation.[3] The mechanism of testis determination down stream of *TDF* remains to be investigated.

In this regard, it would be informative to examine the conditions under which testicular differentiation can be induced in the gonad with the XX chromosomal sex, which normally develops into an ovary. In humans, some XX male patients, who apparently do not carry the SRY or any other Y-encoded sequence, develop testes.[3] In freemartins of cattle, sheep, or goat, the XX fetus is connected to a male twin through the placental anastomosis, and thereby frequently develops testis-like structures in the XX gonad.[4,5] These observations suggest that the XX gonad has the capability to develop testicular components. Müllerian-inhibiting substance (MIS), also known as anti-Müllerian hormone (AMH), has been proposed as the factor responsible for masculinization of the freemartin gonad.[6] Supporting this hypothesis, the same authors have reported that exogenously applied MIS induces development of testis-like cords in the rat XX ovary in culture.[7] Furthermore, chronic expression of MIS in the XX transgenic mouse produces a phenotype similar to the freemartin.[8] On the other hand, it has been reported that the rat ovarian explant develops testis-like cords

[a] This study was partly supported by grants from the National Institutes of Health (USA) (HD-18669) and the Medical Research Council of Canada (MA-9740 and MA-10684).

after long-term culture even without administration of MIS.[9] Therefore, the significance of MIS in inducing testicular differentiation in the XX gonad remains to be verified. Another example of XX sex reversal is the development of testis-like structures in the XX gonad after transplantation into various sites of adult rats[10–15] or mice.[16–18]

Before attempting to interpret these findings with regard to the mechanism of sex determination, the question of whether the reported morphological changes in the XX ovarian primordium reflect true testicular differentiation or not needs to be addressed. It must be pointed out that degeneration of oocytes always precedes development of testis-like structures in the XX gonad. It has been reported that in the XX ovary of W/W^v mutant mice or busulfan-treated rats, in which oogonia are absent or scarce, gonadal epithelial cords become conspicuously like seminiferous tubules under the light microscope, but eventually can be seen to be distinct from true testicular structures under the electron microscope.[19–22] Hence, morphological observations under the light microscope are not sufficient to evaluate testis-specific structures or cellular differentiation in the XX gonad. Although the rat ovarian explant after culture in the presence of MIS has been examined with electron microscopy,[7] the developmental stage was too early to demonstrate characteristics of testicular cell differentiation.

ULTRASTRUCTURAL EVIDENCE FOR TESTICULAR CELL DIFFERENTIATION IN THE XX GONAD

We have previously examined the mouse XX gonadal graft with transmission electron microscopy, and confirmed ultrastructural differentiation of all testicular somatic cell types, *i.e.*, Sertoli, peritubular myoid, and Leydig cells.[17,18] Particularly, the presence of the "intersertoli contact specialization" between epithelial cells inside the seminiferous-like tubules, in contrast to its absence between pregranulosa cells inside the follicles of "transitional" structures, provides strong evidence for Sertoli cell differentiation in the XX gonad. We propose a hypothesis that transformation of pregranulosa cells into Sertoli cells, associated with degeneration of oocytes, plays the key role in formation of testicular structures, and consequently differentiation of other testicular cell types in the XX gonadal graft.

BIOCHEMICAL EVIDENCE FOR TESTICULAR CELL DIFFERENTIATION IN THE XX GONAD

Morphological evidence alone, however, is not sufficient to prove definitively testicular differentiation of the XX gonad. Hence, in the present study, we examined differentiation of Sertoli cells in the mouse XX gonadal graft by immunocytochemical staining for two glycoproteins, MIS and SGP-2, which are uniquely produced by Sertoli cells in fetal and neonatal XY testes. For experiments, fetal ovaries of the NCS (Swiss albino, Rockefeller University) strain at 12 day of gestation (d.g.) were separated from the mesonephros, and transplanted into the subcapsular site of kidney in adult male mice. At 4 to 14 days after transplantation [Day 4–14, equivalent to 16 d.g. to 7 days postpartum (d.pp.)], gonadal grafts were removed from the host kidney, and processed for immunocytochemical staining as described previously.[23] Testes and

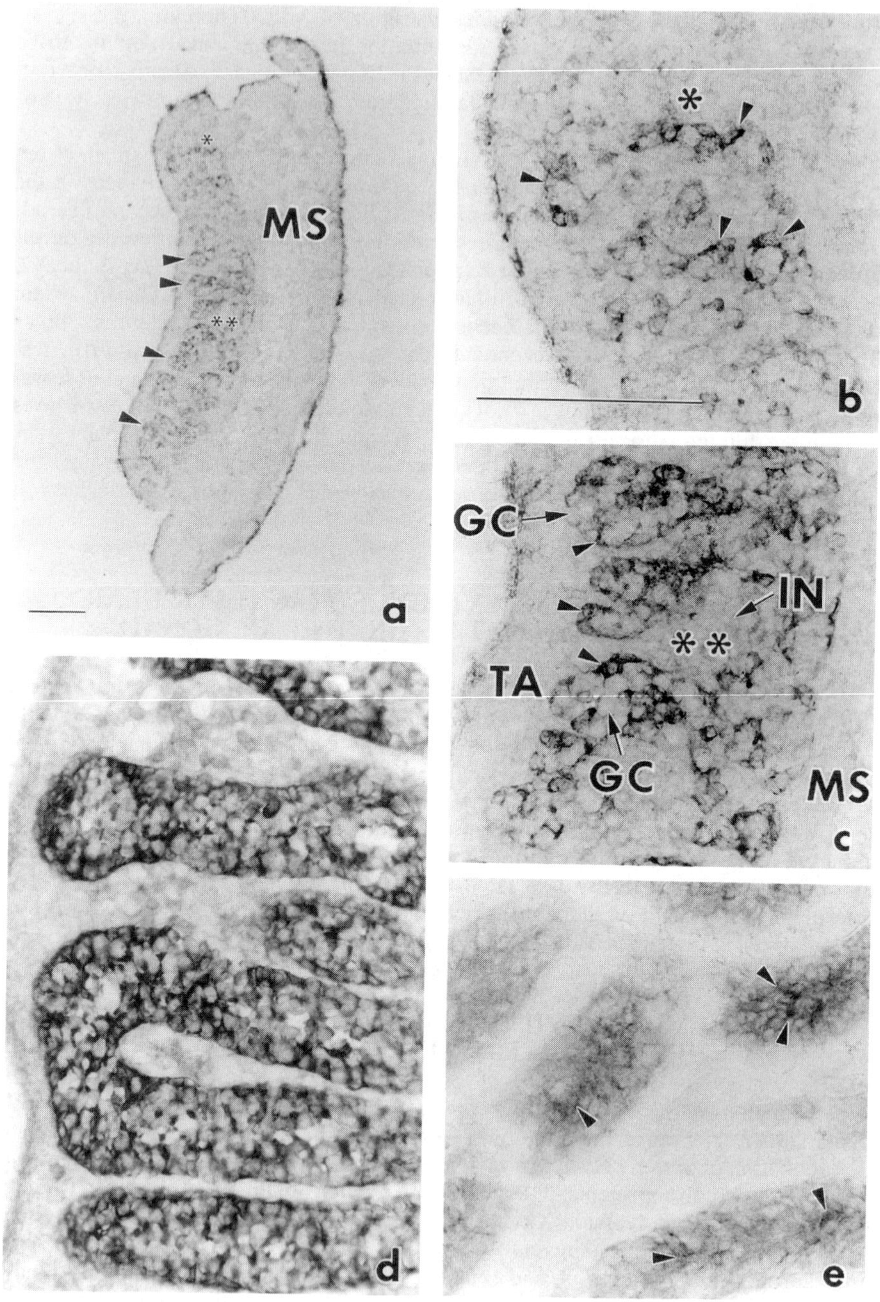

MS
a
b
GC
IN
TA
GC
MS
c
d
e

ovaries were also dissected from fetal and neonatal mice from 11 d.g. to 8 d.pp., and processed for immunocytochemistry to examine the ontogeny of MIS and SGP-2 production during normal gonadal differentiation. The chromosomal sex of fetuses at 11 d.g. and some at later stages after dissection of gonads was determined by dot hybridization with mouse Y chromosome-specific DNA probes as described previously.[24] Otherwise, the chromosomal sex of gonads was judged by the presence or absence of testis cords under a dissecting microscope with transillumination. The results, as outlined below, strongly support the hypothesis that the XX gonadal epithelial cells can develop biochemical characteristics of Sertoli cells.

Müllerian-inhibiting Substance (MIS)

MIS is a glycoprotein, produced by fetal Sertoli cells,[25,26] and causes regression of the Müllerian duct in male fetuses.[27-29] MIS is also produced by granulosa cells of large follicles in postnatal ovaries, but its function is not clarified. Bovine MIS has been purified,[30,31] the human and bovine genes cloned,[32] and the human gene mapped to chromosome 19.[33] We have previously demonstrated that immunocytochemical staining for MIS coincides well with early differentiation of Sertoli cells and testicular organization in the mouse fetal testis.[23] Therefore, MIS is an excellent marker for monitoring the onset of testicular differentiation in the XX gonadal graft.

The present results indicate that the ontogeny of MIS production during normal testicular differentiation in the NCS strain is comparable to that of the C57BL/6J strain reported previously.[23] Briefly, MIS was immunocytochemically detectable in fetal Sertoli cells forming testis cords at 12 d.g., MIS staining remained intense in fetal testes until 19 d.g. (or 1 d.pp.), and then it gradually diminished with progressive testicular development (FIG. 1,a–e). Ovaries were unstained for MIS until 4 d.pp. (data, not shown). At 7 d.pp., granulosa cells of large (probably atretic) follicles in the medullary region were faintly stained for MIS.

In the XX gonadal graft, a few tubular structures composed of MIS-positive cells appeared at Day 7 post-transplantation (FIG. 2a). The ovarian region containing meiotic germ cells was unstained. At Day 9, in addition to a few MIS-positive tubules, small clusters of cells with or without oocytes were stained for MIS with low to intermediate intensities (FIG. 2,b–d). Other oocytes were surrounded by epithelial cells which remained unstained. Both the incidence of XX gonadal grafts containing MIS-positive tubules and the number of MIS-positive tubules per gonadal graft increased

FIGURE 1. Immunocytochemical staining for MIS in the normal testis. **a:** Fetal testis at 12 d.g. Intense staining for MIS is seen inside the testis cords (*arrowheads*), which are well organized in the mid area and less organized at both poles. Ms, mesonephros. The bar indicates 0.1 mm. **b:** The cranial pole of the fetal testis shown in FIGURE 1a (indicated by *). Organization of testis cords is not evident. MIS staining is seen in the cytoplasm of epithelial cells (*arrowheads*), which are connected to each other. The bar indicates 0.1 mm. (Same magnification for FIGURE 1,c–e). **c:** The mid area of the fetal testis shown in FIGURE 1a (indicated by **). Testis cords are well organized near the tunica albuginea (TA), and less so near the mesonephros (MS). Intense staining for MIS is seen in the cytoplasm of fetal Sertoli cells (*arrowheads*) forming testis cords, whereas germ cells (GC) and interstitial tissue (IN) remain at the background level. **d:** Fetal testis at 14 d.g. Intense staining is seen in the cytoplasm of fetal Sertoli cells forming testis cords, which are developed over the entire gonad. **e:** Neonatal testis at 8 d.pp. Intensity of MIS staining is less than at earlier stages, and varies among seminiferous tubules, with the highest activity localized in the center (*arrowheads*).

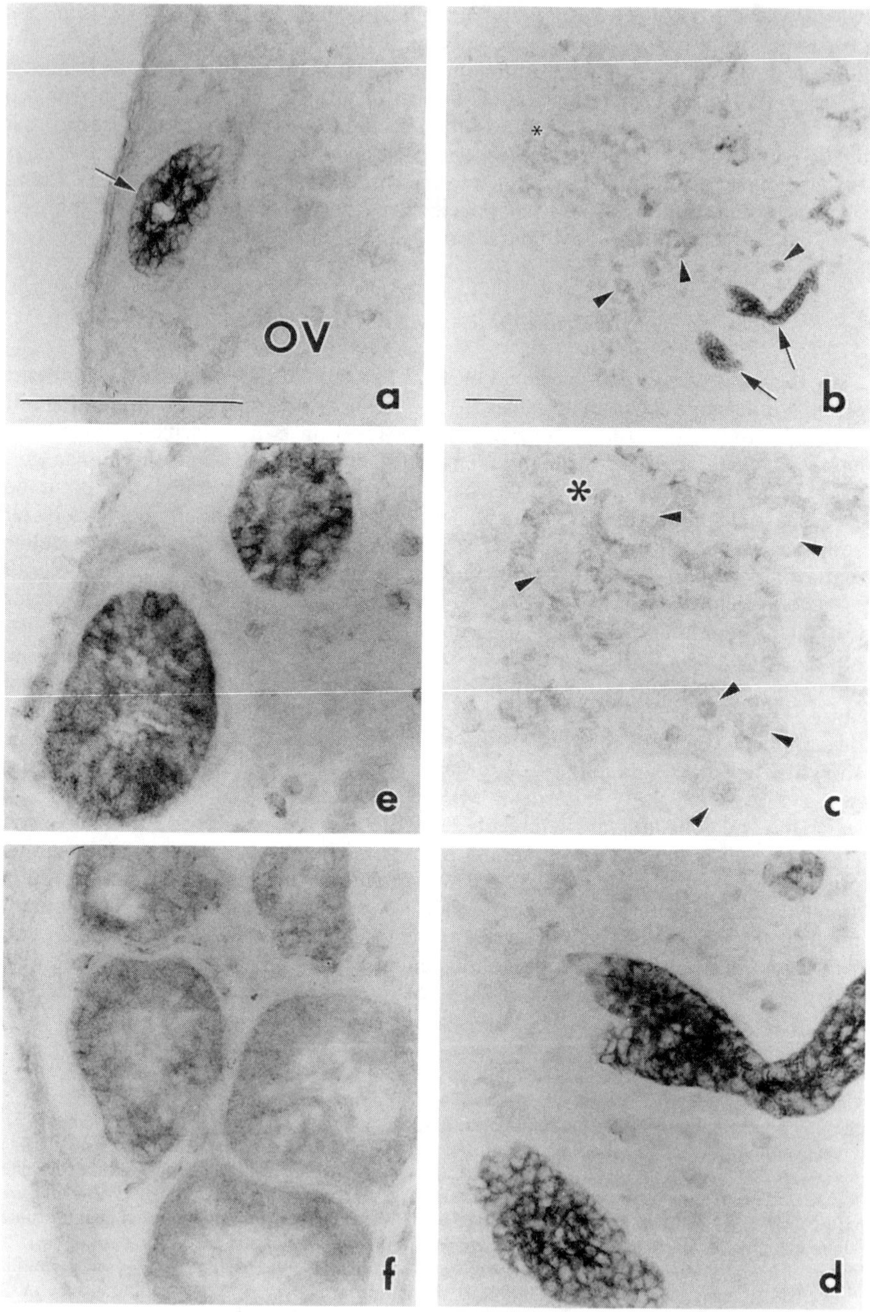
OV
a
b
e
c
f
d

from Day 7 to Day 9, and further to Days 11 and 14 post-transplantation. Therefore, it is conceivable that the small clusters of cells with moderate MIS staining at Days 9 and 11 were undergoing transformation into MIS-positive tubular structures. The MIS-positive tubules at Days 7 and 9 resembled testis cords in the XY fetal testis except for the absence of germ cells. At Day 14, many tubular structures showed characteristics of seminiferous tubules, containing palisade-fashioned arrangement of epithelial cell nuclei along the basement membrane and extension of cytoplasm towards the central area (FIG. 2,e & f). MIS staining in these seminiferous-like tubules was weaker than that of the tubular structures at Day 9 or 11 same as the normal neonatal testis around 7 d.pp. Granulosa cells surrounding oocytes were unstained for MIS at Day 14 (data, not shown). These observations suggest that epithelial cells undergoing ovarian differentiation did not produce MIS in the XX gonadal graft until Day 14, as observed in the cortex region of the normal ovary. Thus, the MIS staining pattern of testicular and ovarian components in the XX gonadal graft was similar to that in the normal XY testis and XX ovary, respectively, although the onset of MIS production varied and was delayed if compared with the XY fetal testis.

Sulfated Glycoprotein-2 (SGP-2)

SGP-2 is a sulfated glycoprotein, originally purified from the spent culture medium of rat prepubertal Sertoli cells.[34] It has been reported that SGP-2 is synthesized in Sertoli cells as a contranslationally glycosylated 64K Da precursor, which is modified to a negatively charged 73K Da form before intracellular cleavage to the mature 47K and 34K Da subunits.[35] Its gene is expressed abundantly in the adult rat epididymis and cultured Sertoli cells, less in the liver, testis, and brain, and minimally in the kidney, spleen, and mammary gland.[36] During testicular development, the level of mRNA is detectable by northern blot analysis at 5 d.pp., steadily increasing until 20 d.pp., and then decreases. Immunocytochemical staining has shown that SGP-2 becomes associated with the acrosome and distal tail portions of spermatozoa after secretion from Sertoli cells in the rat adult testis.[37] It has been claimed that the rat SGP-2 gene is identical to the gene for clusterin,[38] which has been isolated from the ram rete testis fluid, and shown to elicit aggregation of Sertoli cells and erythrocytes *in vitro.*[39,40] The precise ontogeny of SGP-2 (or clusterin) production during normal testicular development has not been determined.

In the present study, immunocytochemical staining for SGP-2 was detectable, concentrated in vesicles, in the cytoplasm of Sertoli cells in the fetal mouse testis at 17 d.g. (FIG. 3a). At 1 d.pp., SGP-2-positive vesicles increased in number, and were

---

FIGURE 2. Immunocytochemical staining for MIS in the XX gonadal graft. **a:** Gonadal graft at Day 7 post-transplantation. MIS staining is seen inside a tubular structure (*arrow*) whereas it is absent in the ovarian region (OV). The bar indicates 0.1 mm. (Same magnification for FIGURE 2,c–f). **b:** Gonadal graft at Day 9 post-transplantation. Intense staining for MIS is seen inside two tubular structures (*arrows*) whereas moderate staining is seen in small clusters of cells (*arrowheads*). The bar indicates 0.1 mm. **c:** The ovarian region shown in FIGURE 2b (indicated by *). Pregranulosa cells around some oocytes (*arrowheads*) are faintly stained for MIS. **d:** The tubular structures shown in FIGURE 2b. Intense staining is seen in the cytoplasm of epithelial cells forming testis-like cords. Germ cells are absent inside these MIS-positive tubules. **e & f:** Gonadal grafts at Day 14 post-transplantation. Seminiferous-like tubules are well organized and stained for MIS with varying intensities.

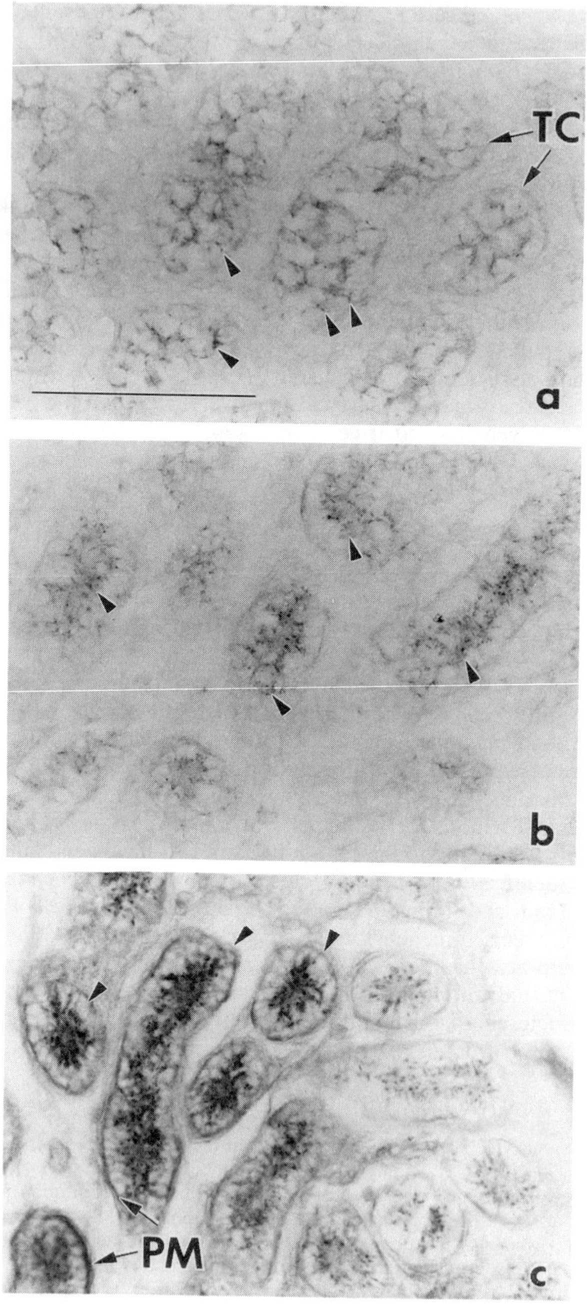
TC
a
b
PM
c

localized on the apical side of Sertoli cell nuclei (FIG. 3b). The distinct staining in vesicular structures may indicate the processing of SGP-2 precursor in the Golgi apparatus, but further examination with electron microscopy is needed for certainty. At 7 d.pp., intensity of SGP-2 staining in the Sertoli cell cytoplasm increased in some, but not all, seminiferous tubules (FIG. 3c). Peritubular myoid cells were also stained considerably. This may reflect active secretion of SGP-2 from Sertoli cells rather than its production in peritubular myoid cells themselves. In contrast, somatic cells in the ovary remained unstained for SGP-2 until 7 d.pp. whereas SGP-2 staining was detectable in the cytoplasm of oocytes at 1 d.pp., and more intense in large oocytes in the medullary region at 7 d.pp. (data, not shown).

In the XX gonadal graft at Day 7, SGP-2 staining was detectable in the cytoplasm, concentrated in vesicles, of epithelial cells forming clusters near the host kidney, but tubular structures were not evident (FIG. 4a). At Day 9, intense staining for SGP-2 was seen in the cytoplasm of epithelial cells forming tubular structures, which resembled fetal testis cords (FIG. 4,b & c), and clusters of cells which were much smaller and thinner in shape than typical testis cords (FIG. 4,b & d). Both structures contained SGP-2-positive vesicles within the cytoplasm (FIG. 4,c & d). Weaker staining was also seen in vesicles inside the cytoplasm of epithelial cells surrounding some oocytes (FIG. 4d). At Day 14, the staining pattern for SGP-2 in some tubular structures strikingly resembled seminiferous tubules in the XY postnatal testis (FIG. 3c), *i.e.*, SGP-2-positive vesicles were localized in the cytoplasm of Sertoli-like cells on the apical side of nuclei (FIG. 4e). No other structures including granulosa cells around oocytes were stained for SGP-2 at Day 14. Thus, the ontogeny and cellular distribution of immunocytochemical staining for SGP-2 in the XX gonadal graft were comparable to those for MIS until Day 11 post-transplantation. Hence, we believe that production of both MIS and SGP-2 represents biochemical differentiation of Sertoli cells in the XX gonadal graft.

Testosterone

Another important testicular product is testosterone, which is produced by Leydig cells in the interstitium and plays essential roles in differentiation of male internal and external genitalia and various testicular functions. We have previously examined the production of testosterone from the XX gonadal graft in culture by radioimmunoassay, and found its positive correlation with the area of testicular structures.[18] This result suggests that steroidogenic cells in the XX gonadal graft function as Leydig cells.

FIGURE 3. Immunocytochemical staining for SGP-2 in the normal testis. **a:** Fetal testis at 17 d.g. SGP-2 staining is detectable in the cytoplasm of fetal Sertoli cells forming testis cords (TC), concentrated in vesicles (*arrowheads*) scattered within the cytoplasm. The bar indicates 0.1 mm. (The same magnification for FIGURE 3,b & c.) **b:** Neonatal testis at 1 d.pp. Many SGP-2-positive vesicles (*arrowheads*) are localized in the cytoplasm of Sertoli cells on the apical side of nuclei. **c:** Postnatal testis at 7 d.pp. Intense staining for SGP-2 is seen in some seminiferous tubules (*arrowheads*) whereas the staining of other tubules is similar to those at 1 d.pp. (FIG. 3b). Peritubular myoid cells (PM) are also stained for SGP-2.

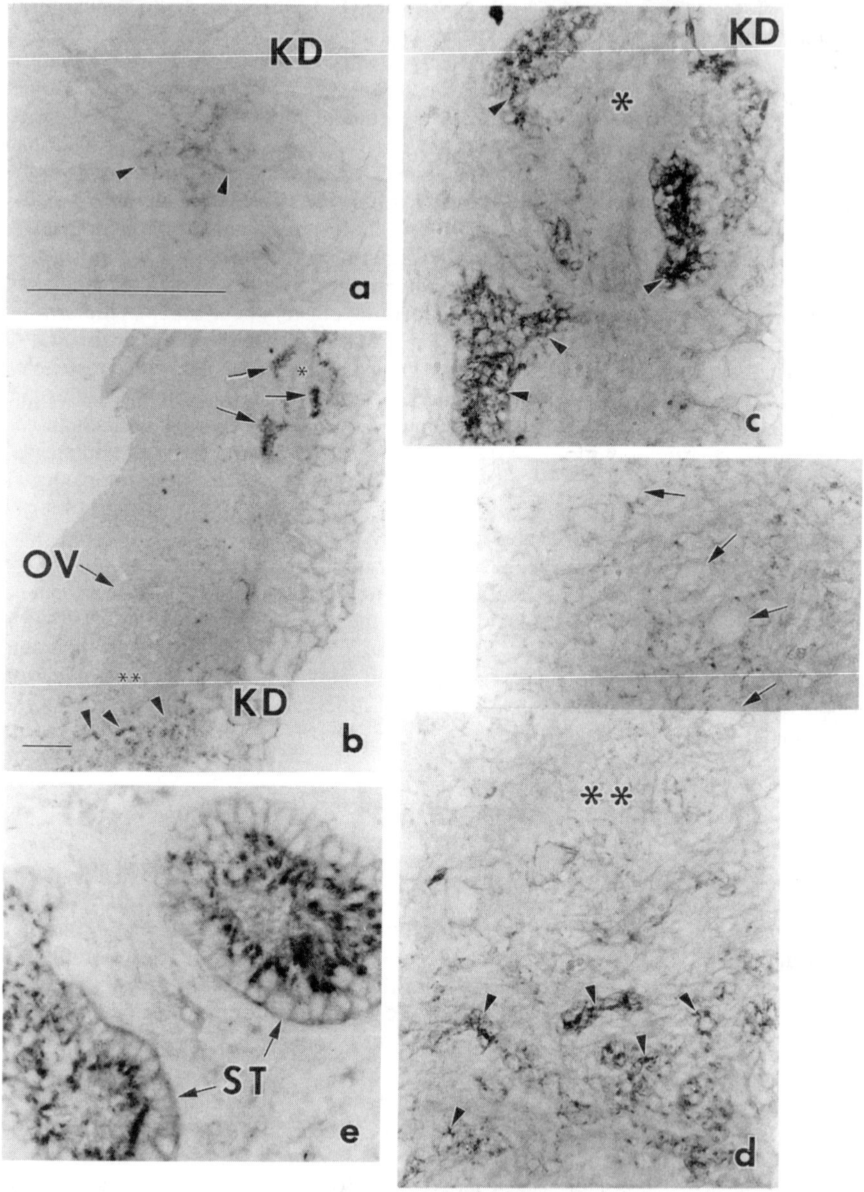

FIGURE 4. Immunocytochemical staining for SGP-2 in the XX gonadal graft. **a:** Gonadal graft at Day 7 post-transplantation. SGP-2 staining is detectable in clusters of cells (*arrowheads*) near the host kidney (KD). More intense staining is localized in vesicles within the cytoplasm. The bar indicates 0.1 mm. (Same magnification for FIGURE 4,c–e). **b:** Gonadal graft at Day 9 post-transplantation. Intense staining for SGP-2 is seen in testis-like cords (*arrows*) and clusters of cells (*arrowheads*) near the host kidney (KD). The ovarian region (OV) is not apparently stained. The bar indicates 0.1 mm. **c:** The upper part of the gonadal graft shown in FIGURE 4b (indicated by *). Intense staining for SGP-2

CONSIDERATION ON THE MECHANISM OF TESTICULAR DIFFERENTIATION IN THE XX GONADAL GRAFT

Thus far, studies in our laboratory using morphological and biochemical markers support the hypothesis that XX gonadal cells can develop characteristics of testicular components. Hence, investigation of the mechanism of testicular differentiation in the XX gonadal graft (termed XX testicular differentiation) should promote our understanding of gonadal sex determination and differentiation. Although great efforts have been made to determine the factors responsible for XX testicular differentiation in the rat, the conclusions were often controversial.[41] Since XX testicular structures have been confirmed under the electron microscope only in the mouse gonadal graft, I will discuss here mainly the conditions required for induction of XX testicular differentiation in the mouse.

Grafting Sites

We have been routinely using the subcapsular site of the kidney for transplantation. According to previous studies in the rat and mouse, testicular components can develop at various grafting sites, although there are quantitative differences in the capacity to induce XX testicular differentiation among different sites.[41] In our laboratory, we have used only the anterior chamber of the eye other than the kidney for successful induction of XX testicular differentiation in the mouse (unpublished observations). However, the frequency of sex reversal at this site was much lower than in the kidney, and therefore, the testicular structures have not been evaluated convincingly.

Mouse Strains

When transplantation was performed within a strain, testicular components developed more frequently in the NCS outbred strain than in the SJL/J (SJL) or C57BL/6J (B6) inbred strain (TABLE 1). Transplantation of the SJL or B6, XX gonadal primordium into the NCS male host produced higher incidence of testicular differentiation than the isogenic grafting. Transplantation of the NCS or SJL, XX gonadal primordium into the B6 male host resulted in gonadal dysgenesis, probably due to the immune response. The NCS, XX gonadal graft was well accepted by the SJL host, and produced high incidence of testicular differentiation. It might be worth noting that both SJL inbred and NCS outbred strains have been developed from a Swiss albino outbred strain. Transplantation of the NCS, XX gonadal primordium into the BALB/c host

---

is seen in the cytoplasm, concentrated in vesicles (*arrowheads*), of epithelial cells forming testis-like cords near the host kidney (KD). **d:** The lower part of the gonadal graft shown in FIGURE 4b (indicated by **). Intense staining for SGP-2 is seen in the cytoplasm, concentrated in vesicles (*arrowheads*), of epithelial cells forming small clusters. Weaker SGP-2 staining is also seen in vesicles within the cytoplasm of epithelial cells surrounding some oocytes (*arrows*). **e:** Gonadal graft at Day 14 post-transplantation. Seminiferous-like tubules (ST) are well developed with palisade-fashioned arrangement of epithelial cell nuclei along the basement membrane and extension of the cytoplasm towards the center. Intense staining for SGP-2 is seen in the cytoplasm of Sertoli-like cells, concentrated in vesicles on the apical side of nuclei.

TABLE 1. Incidence of Testicular Differentiation (%)[a] in the XX Gonad Transplanted into the Adult Male Mouse of Isogenic or Xenogenic Strains

	Graft[b]		
Host	NCS	SJL/J	C57BL/6J
NCS	68 (37)[c]	60 (14)	80 (5)
SJL/J	78 (9)	44 (9)	n.e.[d]
C57BL/6J	0[e] (7)	0[e] (13)	30 (7)
BALB/c	0[e] (8)	n.e.	n.e.
BALB/c, nu/nu	70 (7)	n.e.	n.e.

[a] Examined at Day 14 post-transplantation.
[b] The XX gonadal primordium without mesonephros at 12 d.g. (NCS and C57BL/6J) or 13 d.g. (SJL/J).
[c] Number of grafts examined.
[d] Not examined.
[e] Gonadal dysgenesis in most grafts.

also caused gonadal dysgenesis whereas similar grafts into the thymus-defect nude mouse with BALB/c background produced high incidence of testicular differentiation. These observations suggest that the immune response by the host is not the primary cause for XX testicular differentiation unless the fetal gonad could be recognized as foreign by the adult of the same strain. Furthermore, the genetic background of the host mouse strain does not determine the incidence of XX testicular differentiation. On the other hand, small differences in major histocompatibility appear to facilitate XX testicular differentiation, whereas significant differences probably cause gonadal dysgenesis and therefore prevent both testicular and ovarian differentiation. It is conceivable, if loss of oocytes is indeed responsible for XX testicular differentiation, that oocytes are more vulnerable to minor differences in the histocompatibility than somatic cells, and thereby selective degeneration of oocytes promotes testicular differentiation of somatic cells.

Sex of Hosts/the Adjacent Mesonephros

When the XX gonadal primordium with the adjacent mesonephros is transplanted, the incidence of testicular differentiation is much higher in male hosts than in female hosts.[17,42] In contrast, the XX gonadal primordium separated from the mesonephros develops testicular components more frequently than that with the adjacent mesonephros, and the incidence of testicular differentiation is comparable between male and female hosts.[42] Several other investigators have also reported testicular differentiation in the rat ovarian graft into the female host.[10,11,13] Therefore, the primary host factor responsible for XX testicular differentiation is not necessarily male specific. We have interpreted that the adjacent mesonephros protects the XX gonadal graft from masculinizing stimuli more efficiently in female hosts than male hosts.[42] The male host may have a higher capacity to promote testicular differentiation and, hence, overcome the protecting effect by the mesonephros, or the function of the mesonephros may depend on the female environment. Because the XX gonadal primordium separated from the mesonephros develops only ovarian components in organ culture, the protecting effect by the adjacent mesonephros appears to be important only *in vivo*.[42] At present, we cannot rule out the possibility that the presence of the mesonephros simply prevents invasion of the host tissue or diffusible factor that promotes XX testicular differentiation.

Male Factors Promoting XX Testicular Differentiation

Testosterone in serum appears to be partly responsible for the high incidence of XX testicular differentiation in the male host when the XX gonadal primordium is grafted with the adjacent mesonephros.[43] We have shown that administration of testosterone into the castrated female host produces higher incidence of XX testicular differentiation than in the control female host. However, castration of male hosts does not change the incidence of XX testicular differentiation, suggesting that serum testosterone does not directly influence development of the gonadal graft. It has been generally accepted that steroid hormones do not change the direction of gonadal sex differentiation in mammals.[44,45] Therefore, it is conceivable that serum testosterone modifies host conditions which, in turn, influence the gonadal graft. In any way, it appears that genetic sex of the host plays little role in XX testicular differentiation.

Age of the XX Gonadal Graft

The XX gonadal graft at 11 d.g. (before sexual differentiation occurs) yields the highest incidence of testicular differentiation, and the capacity to form testicular structures diminishes gradually with older gonadal grafts up to 14 d.g.[17,42] Removal of the mesonephros increases the incidence of XX testicular differentiation, most efficiently with gonadal grafts at 12 and 13 d.g., but does not induce testicular differentiation from the fetal ovary grafted at 16 d.g. or later. It should be worth noting that the XX gonadal primordium maintains the bipotentiality for a few days after sexual differentiation is initiated, *i.e.*, testicular organization in the XY gonad at 12 d.g. or differentiation of oocytes in the XX gonad at 13 d.g.

Time Course of XX Testicular Differentiation

The XX gonadal graft at 12 d.g. appears to continue normal ovarian differentiation until, at least, Day 4 post-transplantation.[18] By Day 7, production of MIS and SGP-2 begins in a few tubular structures, but the major part of the graft is still undergoing ovarian differentiation (present results). When these grafts are dissected and cultured *in vitro* for 5 more days, they develop mainly ovarian components.[18] Between Days 7 and 11, the XX gonadal graft loses the majority of oocytes by degeneration. Pregranulosa cells surrounding some oocytes begin to produce both MIS and SGP-2, whereas those around other oocytes remain unstained for either MIS or SGP-2 (present results). Since the number of MIS and SGP-2 positive tubules increases during this period, moderate staining for MIS and SGP-2 in some pregranulosa cells may represent transitional stages of transformation into Sertoli cells. When XX gonadal grafts at Day 11 are excised and cultured *in vitro* for 3–5 more days, they continue to develop both ovarian and testicular components and produce testosterone proportionally to the testicular area.[18] Thus, the critical timing for XX testicular differentiation appears to be between Days 7 and 11 post-transplantation. At Day 14, seminiferous-like tubules are well formed, and production of MIS begins to diminish while that of SGP-2 remains high, comparable to the normal XY testis at 7 d.pp. These observations indicate that although testicular differentiation begins much later in the XX gonadal graft than the normal XY testis and progresses slowly, testicular components in the XX gonadal graft at Day 14 appear to have reached a developmental stage comparable to that of the XY testis. We postulate that ovarian somatic cells, after a certain developmental stage, can transform into testicular cell types without reprogramming the entire differentiation process.

Interaction with the Host Kidney Tissue

To characterize the host factors responsible for XX testicular differentiation, the XX gonadal primordium was microencapsulated in a semipermeable membrane and transplanted into the male host.[46] We found that the gonadal graft that has been completely enclosed in microcapsule membrane, develops only ovarian structures whereas most of the gonadal grafts that have lost microcapsule membranes during or after transplantation develop testicular structures. When the gonadal graft has been partially enclosed in microcapsule membrane, testicular structures develop only in the vicinity of the host kidney. These results suggest that direct interaction between the XX gonadal graft and cells or large macromolecules from the host is essential for XX testicular differentiation. Accordingly, we considered kidney stromal cells, blood vessels, and neurons as probable host factors involved in XX testicular differentiation. We enclosed a piece of adult kidney or fetal metanephros with the XX gonadal primordium inside the microcapsule, but obtained development of only ovarian structures (unpublished data). Hence, we ruled out direct involvement of kidney stromal tissue. We are currently examining the involvement of vascularization and innervation in XX testicular differentiation.

Loss of Oocytes

Whether loss of oocytes secondarily leads to formation of tubular structures in the XX gonad is debatable.[47] We have previously postulated that oocytes are lost in the XX gonadal graft following transformation of adjacent pregranulosa cells into Sertoli cells because we observed occasional healthy-appearing oocytes in contact with Sertoli cells under electron microscopy.[18] However, in the present study, very few germ cells were found in MIS and SGP-2-positive tubules, suggesting that oocytes are lost before biochemical differentiation of Sertoli cells. Since we found faint staining for both glycoproteins in epithelial cells around some oocytes, we cannot rule out the possibility that early phases of Sertoli cell transformation are sufficient to cause degeneration of oocytes. Nevertheless, it is our impression that loss of oocytes is closely associated with biochemical differentiation of Sertoli cells. On the other hand, absence of oocytes alone is not sufficient to induce Sertoli cell differentiation since the oocyte-free ovary of W/W^v mutant mouse develops neither ultrastructural[20-22] nor biochemical characteristics of Sertoli cells (unpublished observations). Therefore, the host environment appears to be required, in addition to the oocyte loss, for induction of Sertoli cell differentiation in the XX gonadal graft.

CLOSING REMARKS

Although we have been accumulating evidence for testicular cell differentiation in the XX gonadal graft, the mechanism of sex reversal still remains to be clarified. From our present and previous studies, we are inclined to hypothesize that degeneration of oocytes plays a crucial role in formation of testicular structures in the XX gonad. However, it seems that loss of oocytes alone is not sufficient to induce ultrastructural and biochemical differentiation of testicular cell types. We postulate that loss of oocytes may provide the precondition for XX testicular differentiation, but the interaction with the host tissue is required for biochemical differentiation of Sertoli cells and organization of seminiferous tubules.

ACKNOWLEDGMENTS

I am grateful to Dr. P. Donahoe for the gift of antibodies against purified human recombinant MIS, to Drs. S. Sylvester and M. D. Griswold for the gift of IgG fractions against SGP-2, to Dr. Y. Nishioka for the mouse Y-specific DNA probes, and to Mrs. E. Sinclair-Thompson and J. Saeed for excellent technical assistance.

REFERENCES

1. GUBBAY, J., J. COLLINGNON, P. KOOPMAN, B. CAPEL, A. ECONOMOU, A. MÜNSTERBERG, N. VIVIAN, P. GOODFELLOW & R. LOVELL-BADGE. 1990. A gene mapping to the sex-determining region of the mouse Y chromosome is a member of a novel family of embryonically expressed genes. Nature **346:** 245–250.
2. KOOPMAN, P., A. MÜNSTERBERG, B. CAPEL, N. VIVIAN & R. LOVELL-BADGE. 1990. Expression of a candidate sex-determining gene during mouse testis differentiation. Nature **348:** 450–452.
3. SINCLAIR, A. H., P. BERTA, M. S. PALMER, J. R. HAWKINS, B. L. GRIFFITHS, M. J. SMITH, J. W. FOSTER, A.-M. FRISCHAU, R. LOVELL-BADGE & P. N. GOODFELLOW. 1990. A gene from the human sex-determining region encodes a protein with homology to a conserved DNA-binding motif. Nature **346:** 240–244.
4. LILLIE, F. R. 1917. The free-martin: A study of the action of sex hormone in the foetal life of cattle. J. Exp. Zool. **23:** 371–452.
5. JOST, A., B. VIGIER & J. PREPIN. 1972. Freemartins in cattle: The first step of sexual organogenesis. J. Reprod. Fertil. **29:** 349–379.
6. VIGIER, B., L. LEGEAI, J. Y. PICARD & N. JOSSO. 1982. A sensitive radioimmunoassay for bovine anti-Müllerian hormone, allowing its detection in male and freemartin fetal serum. Endocrinology **111:** 1409–1411.
7. VIGIER, B., F. WATRIN, S. MAGRE, D. TRAN & N. JOSSO. 1987. Purified bovine AMH induces a characteristic freemartin effect in fetal rat prospective ovaries exposed to it *in vitro.* Development **100:** 43–55.
8. BEHRINGER, R. R., R. L. CATE, G. J. FROELICK, R. D. PALMITER & R. L. BRINSTER. 1990. Abnormal sexual development in transgenic mice chronically expressing Müllerian inhibiting substance. Nature **345:** 167–170.
9. PRÉPIN, J. & N. HIDA. 1989. Influence of age and medium on formation of epithelial cords in the rat fetal ovary in vitro. J. Reprod. Fertil. **87:** 375–382.

10. Buyse, A. 1935. The differentiation of transplanted mammalian gonad primordia. J. Exp. Zool. **70:** 1–41.
11. Moore, C. R. & D. Price. 1942. Differentiation of embryonic reproductive tissues of the rat after transplantation into post-natal hosts. J. Exp. Zool. **90:** 229–265.
12. Holyoke, E. A. 1949. The difference of embryonic gonads transplanted to the adult omentum in the albino rat. Anat. Rec. **103:** 675–699.
13. Torrey, T. W. 1950. Intraocular grafts of embryonic gonads of the rat. J. Exp. Zool. **115:** 37–58.
14. MacIntyre, M. N. 1956. Effect of the testis on ovarian differentiation in heterosexual embryonic rat gonad transplants. Anat. Rec. **124:** 27–41.
15. Mangoushi, M. A. 1975. Scrotal allografts of fetal ovaries. J. Anat. **120:** 595–599.
16. Turner, C. D. & H. Asakawa. 1964. Experimental reversal of germ cells in ovaries of fetal mice. Science **143:** 1344–1345.
17. Taketo, T., H. Merchant-Larios & S. S. Koide. 1984. Induction of testicular differentiation in the fetal mouse ovary by transplantation into adult male mice. Proc. Soc. Exp. Biol. Med. **176:** 148–153.
18. Taketo-Hosotani, T., H. Merchant-Larios, R. B. Thau & S. S. Koide. 1985. Testicular cell differentiation in fetal mouse ovaries following transplantation into adult male mice. J. Exp. Zool. **236:** 229–237.
19. Merchant, H. 1975. Rat gonadal and ovarian organogenesis with and without germ cells. An ultrastructural study. Devel. Biol. **44:** 1–21.
20. Merchant-Larios, H. 1976. The role of germ cells in the morphogenesis and cytodifferentiation of the rat ovary. *In* Progress in Differentiation Research. Muller-Berat, Ed.: 453–462. North Holland Pub. Co. Amsterdam.
21. Merchant-Larios, H. & B. Centeno. 1981. Morphogenesis of the ovary from the sterile W/W^v mouse. *In* Advances in The Morphology of Cells and Tissues. A. Vidrio & C. Galina, Eds.: 383–392. A. R. Liss, Inc. New York.
22. Merchant-Larios, H. & T. Taketo. 1991. Testicular differentiation in mammals under normal and experimental conditions. J. Electr. Micro. Tech. In press.
23. Taketo, T., J. Saeed, Y. Nishioka & P. K. Donahoe. 1991. Delay of testicular differentiation in the B6.Y^{DOM} ovotestis demonstrated by immunocytochemical staining for Müllerian inhibiting substance. Devel. Biol. In press.
24. Taketo-Hosotani, T., Y. Nishioka, C. M. Nagamine, I. Villalpando & H. Merchant-Larios. 1989. Development and fertility in the B6.Y^{DOM} sex-reversed female mouse. Development **107:** 95–105.
25. Tran, D. & N. Josso. 1982. Localization of anti-Müllerian hormone in the rough endoplasmic reticulum of the developing bovine Sertoli cell using immunocytochemistry with a monoclonal antibody. Endocrinology **111:** 1562–1567.
26. Hayashi, H., H. Shima, K. Hayashi, R. L. Trelstadt & P. K. Donahoe. 1984. Immunocytochemical localization of Müllerian inhibiting substance in the rough endoplasmic reticulum and Golgi apparatus in Sertoli cells of the neonatal calf testis using a monoclonal antibody. J. Histochem. Cytochem. **32:** 649–654.
27. Donahoe, P. K., G. P. Budzik, R. Trelstad, M. Mudgett-Hunter, A. Fuller, Jr., J. M. Hutson, H. Ikawa, A. Hayashi & D. MacLaughlin. 1982. Müllerian inhibiting substance: An update. Rec. Prog. Horm. Res. **38:** 279–330.
28. Donahoe, P. K., R. L. Cate, D. T. MacLaughlin, J. Epstein, A. F. Fuller, M. Takahashi, J. P. Coughlin, E. G. Ninfa & L. A. Taylor. 1987. Müllerian inhibiting substance: Gene structure and mechanism of action of a fetal regressor. Rec. Prog. Horm. Res. **43:** 431–462.
29. Josso, N. & J.-Y. Picard. 1986. Anti-Müllerian hormone. Physiol. Rev. **66:** 1083–1090.
30. Budzik, G. P., S. M. Powell, S. Kamagata & P. K. Donahoe. 1983. Müllerian inhibiting substance fractionation by dye affinity chromatography. Cell **34:** 307–314.
31. Picard, J. Y. & N. Josso. 1984. Purification of testicular anti-Müllerian hormone allowing direct visualization of the pure glycoprotein and determination of yield and purification factor. Mol. Cell. Endocrinol. **34:** 23–29.
32. Cate, R. L., R. J. Mattaliano, C. Hession, R. Tizard, N. M. Farber, A. Cheung, E. G. Ninfa, A. Z. Frey, D. J. Gash, E. P Chow., R. A. Fisher, J. M. Bertonis, G. Torres, B. P. Wallner, K. L. Ramachandran, R. C. Ragin, T. F. Manganaro, D. T. MacLaughlin

& P. K. DONAHOE. 1986. Isolation of the bovine and human genes for Müllerian inhibiting substance and expression of the human gene in animal cells. Cell **45:** 685–698.

33. COHEN-HAGUENAUER, O., J. Y. PICARD, M. G. MATTEI, S. SERERO, V. C NGUYEN, M. F. DE TAND, D. GUERRIER, M. C. HORS-CAYLA, N. JOSSO & J. FRÉZAL. 1987. Mapping of the gene for anti-Müllerian hormone to the short arm of human chromosome 19. Cytogenet. Cell. Genet. **44:** 2–6.
34. KISSINGER, C., M. K. SKINNER & M. D. GRISWOLD. 1982. Analysis of Sertoli cell-secreted proteins by two-dimensional gel electrophoresis. Biol. Reprod. **27:** 233–240.
35. COLLARD, M. W. & M. D. GRISWOLD. 1987. Biosynthesis and molecular cloning of sulfated glycoprotein 2 secreted by rat Sertoli cells. Biochemistry **26:** 3297–3303.
36. HUGLY, S., K. ROBERTS & M. D. GRISWOLD. 1988. Transferrin and sulfated glycoprotein-2 messenger ribonucleic acid levels in the testis and isolated Sertoli cells of hypophysectomized rats. Endocrinology **122:** 1390–1396.
37. SYLVESTER, S. R., M. K. SKINNER & M. D. GRISWOLD. 1984. A sulfated glycoprotein synthesized by Sertoli cells and by epididymal cells is a component of the sperm membrane. Biol. Reprod. **31:** 1087–1101.
38. CHENG, C. Y., C.-L. C. CHEN, S.-M. FENG, A. MARSHALL & C. W. BARDIN. 1988. Rat clusterin isolated from primary Sertoli cell-enriched culture medium is sulfated glycoprotein-2 (SGP-2). Biochem. Biophys. Res. Commun. **155:** 398–404.
39. FRITZ, I. B., K. BURDZY, B. SETCHELL & O. BLASCHUK. 1983. Ram rete testis fluid contains a protein (clusterin) which influences cell-cell interactions *in vitro.* Biol. Reprod. **28:** 1173–1188.
40. BLASCHUK, O. W. & I. B. FRITZ. 1984. Isoelectric forms of clusterin isolated from ram rete testis fluid and from secretions of primary cultures of ram and rat Sertoli cell-enriched preparations. Can. J. Biochem. Cell Biol. **62:** 456–461.
41. TAKETO, T. S. S. KOIDE & H. MERCHANT-LARIOS. 1985. Gonadal sex differentiation in mammals. In The Origin and Evolution of Sex. H. O. Halvorson & A. Monroy, Eds.: 271–287. Alan R. Liss, Inc. New York.
42. TAKETO-HOSOTANI, T. & E. SINCLAIR-THOMPSON. 1987. Influence of the mesonephros on the development of fetal mouse ovaries following transplantation into adult male and female mice. Devel. Biol. **124:** 423–430.
43. TAKETO, T. & H. MERCHANT-LARIOS. 1986. Gonadal sex reversal of fetal mouse ovaries following transplantation into adult mice. *In* Progress in Developmental Biology. H. C. Slavkin, Ed. Part A: 171–174. Alan R. Liss, Inc. New York.
44. BURNS, R. K. 1961. Role of hormones in the differentiation of sex. *In* Sex and Internal Secretions. W. C. Young & F. G. W. Corner, Eds. Vol. 1 (edit. 3): 76–158. Williams & Wilkins. Baltimore, MD.
45. SHORT, R. V. 1979. Sex determination and differentiation. Brit. Med. Bull. **35:** 121–127.
46. TAKETO-HOSOTANI, T. 1987. Factors involved in the testicular development from fetal mouse ovaries following transplantation. J. Exp. Zool. **241:** 95–100.
47. BURGOYNE, P. S. 1988. Role of mammalian Y chromosome in sex determination. Phil. Trans. R. Soc. Lond. **B222:** 63–72.

Androgen Regulation of Spermatogenesis in the Rat

KENNETH P. ROBERTS[a] AND BARRY R. ZIRKIN

Division of Reproductive Biology
Department of Population Dynamics
School of Hygiene and Public Health
The Johns Hopkins University
615 N. Wolfe Street
Baltimore, Maryland 21205

INTRODUCTION

The hormonal regulation of spermatogenesis in the rat has been of interest for at least six decades, dating to a report by Smith[1] in which the removal of the rat pituitary gland was shown to result in the suppression of spermatozoa formation. It is now well established that testosterone is produced by Leydig cells in response to luteinizing hormone (LH) and that spermatogenesis is a testosterone-dependent process.[2-5] Indeed, it has become axiomatic that testosterone is required to initiate spermatogenesis at puberty, to maintain spermatogenesis in the adult, and to restore spermatogenesis in the adult after its experimental suppression.

In spite of the impressive accumulation of literature dealing with androgen control of spermatogenesis, there are substantial gaps in our knowledge of the molecular events that are regulated by testosterone, and therefore of the role of testosterone in spermatogenesis.

Our focus in this review will be on what is known of the involvement of testosterone in the maintenance and restoration of spermatogenesis in the adult rat testis, and what is known/believed about the mechanism by which testosterone functions. We will examine the testosterone requirements for the maintenance and restoration of spermatogenesis, and discuss what this tells us about the mechanism by which testosterone may act. We will address the possibility that the modulation of intratesticular steroid concentrations at particular stages of the cycle of the seminiferous epithelium plays a role in the regulatory action of testosterone. We will address whether there are pituitary hormones other than LH, and/or Leydig cell products other than testosterone, that are involved in spermatogenesis, and speculate about how such products might modulate the effects of testosterone. Finally, we will discuss what is known of the testosterone regulation of specific testicular products.

[a] Address correspondence to Dr. Kenneth Roberts at the Department of Population Dynamics.

MAINTENANCE OF ESTABLISHED SPERMATOGENESIS IN THE ADULT RAT TESTIS BY TESTOSTERONE

Over the years, numerous studies have shown that the administration of testosterone to adult rats in which LH is suppressed results in the maintenance of qualitatively normal spermatogenesis (*i.e.*, continued production of all of the cell types that are characteristic of spermatogenesis, though perhaps in diminished numbers compared to controls). Turner *et al.*[6] reported that the average testosterone concentration in rat seminiferous tubule fluid (50 ng/ml) is far higher than that in serum (1–2 ng/ml), and far higher than the concentration required to saturate androgen receptors in the adult rat testis.[7] This suggests that the intratesticular testosterone concentration may be far higher than the concentration that is required to maintain spermatogenesis. Indeed, there is now considerable experimental evidence to suggest that this is so. Cunningham and Huckins[8] first showed that qualitatively complete spermatogenesis can be maintained in rats despite a substantial reduction in intratesticular testosterone concentration from control values. Since that initial publication, a number of workers have reported that qualitatively, and indeed quantitatively, normal spermatogenesis is able to persist despite significant reductions in intratesticular testosterone concentration.[9–11]

To determine the concentration of testosterone required to maintain spermatogenesis, we[11] administered testosterone-containing Silastic implants of 4–40 cm in length to intact, adult rats for 8 weeks. Such treatments resulted in suppression of LH and therefore in inhibition of endogenous testosterone production, but did not affect FSH. We found that advanced spermatid numbers were quantitatively maintained in rats that received implants of sizes that resulted in 20 ng/ml or more testosterone in the seminiferous tubule fluid (FIG. 1); the number of advanced spermatids was reduced as seminiferous tubule fluid testosterone concentration was reduced below this minimally required value of 20 ng/ml. These results demonstrated that despite a reduction

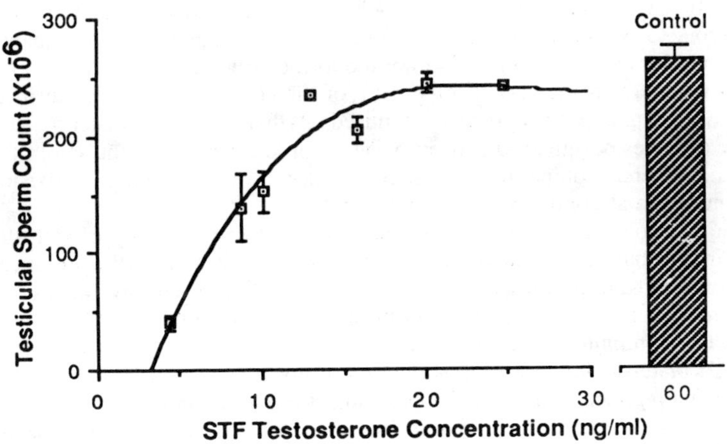

FIGURE 1. Relationship between the mean number of advanced spermatids per testis and the mean testosterone concentration in seminiferous tubule fluid (STF) two months after implantation of testosterone-filled Silastic capsules of increasing sizes into intact adult rats. The bar (right) represents control adult rats. (From Zirkin *et al.*, 1989.[11])

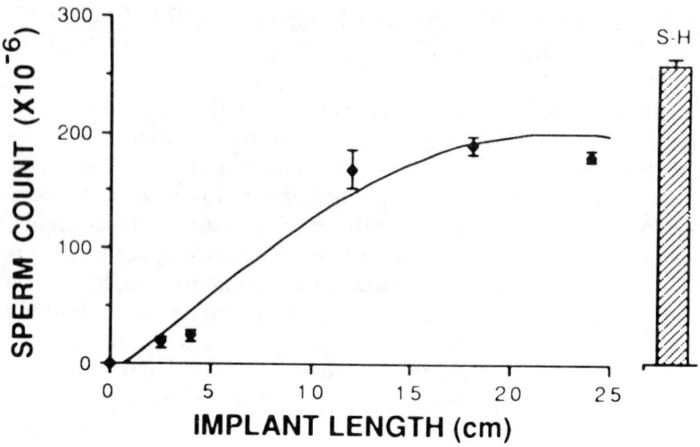

FIGURE 2. Relationship between the length of testosterone-filled Silastic capsules implanted into adult hypophysectomized rats at the time of hypophysectomy and the number of advanced spermatids per testis two months later. The bar (right) represents sham-hypophysectomized control rats. (From Santulli *et al.*, 1990.[14])

of intratesticular testosterone to one-third of the normal concentration, spermatogenesis was quantitatively maintained. However, it should be noted that a testosterone concentration of 20 ng/ml is an order of magnitude greater than that required to saturate testicular androgen receptors.[7] We will return to this important point later in this review.

Numerous studies of hypophysectomized rats have shown that spermatogenesis can be maintained qualitatively if testosterone is administered at the time of hypophysectomy.[2,10,12,13] We[14] demonstrated that although the administration of testosterone via Silastic capsules at the time of hypophysectomy provided as much intratesticular testosterone to hypophysectomized as to intact rats, spermatogenesis was quantitatively maintained in the latter (FIG. 1) but not the former (FIG. 2) rats. Thus, over an eight (or 12) week treatment period, only 60% of the control number of advanced spermatids were maintained in hypophysectomized rats that received testosterone-containing Silastic capsules designed to deliver 20 ng/ml of testosterone to the seminiferous tubule fluid; whereas comparable testosterone concentrations maintained advanced spermatid numbers at control values in intact rats.

The most obvious explanation of the difference in the ability of testosterone to maintain spermatogenesis in intact and hypophysectomized rats is the presence of FSH in the former and its absence in the latter rats. To test this possibility, rats were injected with GnRH conjugated to human serum globulin in Freund's complete adjuvant to induce active immunization against GnRH. Two weeks thereafter, before suppression of GnRH or testicular response, some rats received exogenous testosterone, and all rats began a regimen of biweekly booster injections given in Freund's incomplete adjuvant through week 10. As shown in FIGURE 3, the rats actively immunized against GnRH became azoospermic, whereas spermatogenesis was maintained quantitatively in the immunized rats that received exogenous testosterone. In both groups of rats, serum FSH was undetectable by RIA. These results (Awoniyi and Zirkin, unpublished) provide quantitative data consistent with some previous studies that have concluded

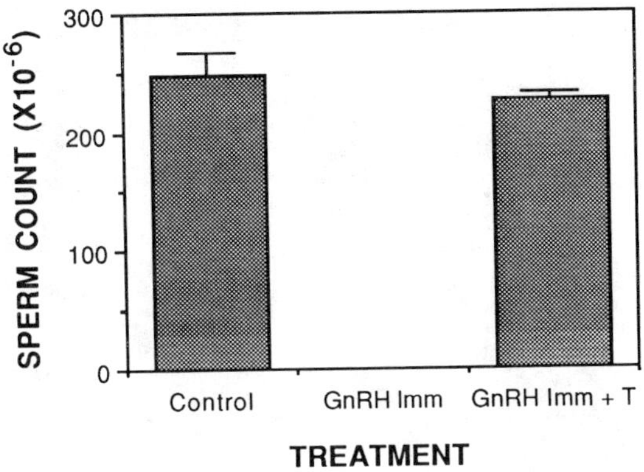

FIGURE 3. Mean number of advanced spermatids per testis in control intact rats, rats actively immunized against GnRH, and rats immunized against GnRH that received testosterone filled Silastic capsules, two months after treatment. (From Awoniyi & Zirkin, unpublished.)

that FSH is not required to maintain spermatogenesis in the adult rat testis.[15] It should be noted, however, that there are reports that testosterone and FSH act synergistically in the adult rat to stimulate germ cell development and/or inhibit germ cell degeneration.[13,16,17] Therefore, at this juncture, the explanation for why testosterone is able to maintain spermatogenesis quantitatively in intact but not in hypophysectomized rats remains elusive.

To this point, the discussion has centered about the involvement of *testosterone* in maintaining spermatogenesis. However, there is good evidence that the administration of steroids other than testosterone to hypophysectomized rats can maintain spermatogenesis qualitatively.[18,19] Can spermatogenesis be maintained quantitatively in the adult rat by androgens other than testosterone? To address this question we administered dihydrotestosterone (DHT) in increasing concentrations to intact rats via Silastic implants of increasing sizes, and then examined advanced spermatid number and intratesticular androgen concentration eight weeks later. FIGURE 4 shows that the larger implants (24–36 cm) maintained spermatogenesis almost quantitatively (Chen

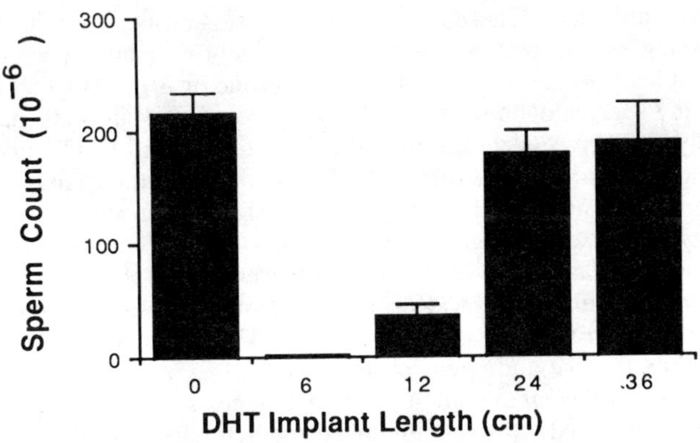

FIGURE 4. Relationship between the mean number of advanced spermatids per testis and the length of DHT-filled Silastic capsules two months after implantation into intact adult rats.

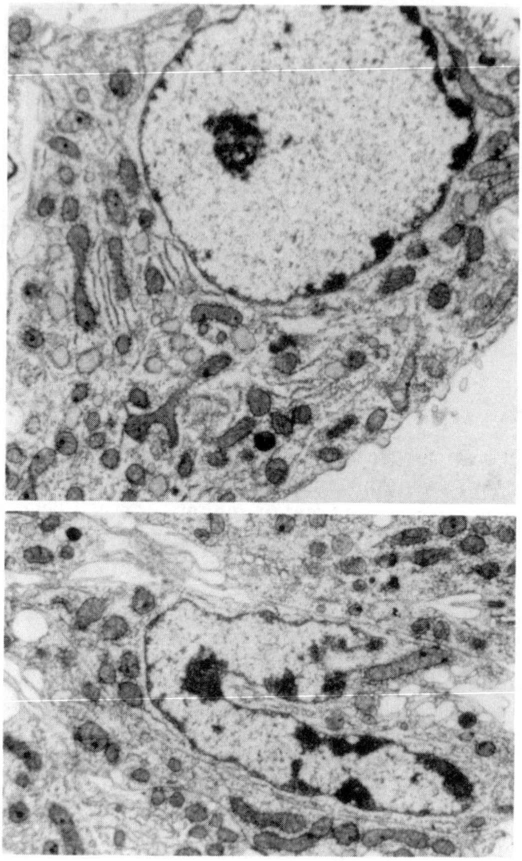

FIGURE 5. Electron micrographs of Leydig cells from a control rat (above) and a rat hypophysectomized for two weeks (below) taken at the same magnification. (From Ewing & Zirkin, 1983.[5])

and Zirkin, unpublished). These results indicate testosterone is not the only androgen receptor-binding steroid that is able to quantitatively maintain spermatogenesis.

This result leads to the question: Is it testosterone or is it DHT that is responsible for maintaining spermatogenesis *in vivo*? Indirect evidence suggests that testosterone is most likely. Turner *et al.*[6] examined the testosterone and DHT concentrations of the interstitial and seminiferous tubule fluids of intact adult rats. Their results indicate that DHT constitutes no more than 5% of the testosterone concentration in either fluid. Testosterone has weaker androgenic potency than DHT as a consequence of its weaker interaction with the androgen receptor.[20] However, when testosterone is present in high concentrations relative to DHT, as is the case in the testis,[6] testosterone displaces DHT at the androgen receptor by mass action.[20] Thus, it seems most likely that testosterone is the effective androgen in the rat testis.

Is testosterone *sufficient* to maintain spermatogenesis in the adult rat testis? In each of testosterone implanted, GnRH-immunized and hypophysectomized rats, LH is suppressed and therefore Leydig cell steroidogenic activity is suppressed; but the Leydig cells, though of considerably smaller volume after LH suppression (FIG. 5), are not

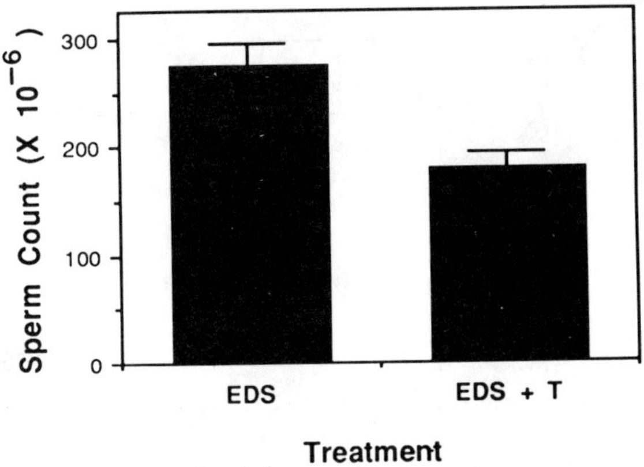

FIGURE 6. Mean number of advanced spermatids per testis two months after a single injection of ethane dimethanesulphonate (EDS) in intact rats or EDS-injected rats implanted with testosterone-filled Silastic capsules at the time of injection (EDS+T). (Drawn from data presented in Sprando *et al.*, 1990.[22])

lost.[21] Examination of the cytoplasm of such cells reveals all of the cytoplasmic organelles of any other cell, including rough endoplasmic reticulum (unpublished). This leads to the question: Are nonandrogenic products from Leydig cells involved in the maintenance of spermatogenesis? We,[22] and others,[23] have addressed this question by treating rats with ethane dimethanesulphonate (EDS), an agent that selectively kills Leydig cells, and simultaneously administering a maintenance dose of testosterone to these rats via testosterone-filled Silastic capsules. The administration of testosterone suppressed LH and thus prevented Leydig cells from repopulating the testis. As shown in FIGURE 6, advanced spermatid number in the EDS injected rats, eight weeks after EDS injection, was the same as the number in vehicle-treated controls. In rats that received EDS plus a high enough dose of testosterone to maintain spermatogenesis in control rats, however, the number of advanced spermatids maintained over the 8-week treatment period was only 60% of, and significantly less than, that in the EDS alone rats. This suggested that Leydig cell products other than testosterone may indeed be required for spermatogenic maintenance. Further examination of this possibility is warranted.

RESTORATION OF SPERMATOGENESIS IN THE ADULT RAT TESTIS BY TESTOSTERONE

Long-term suppression of endogenous LH by any of a number of means will eventually lead to azoospermia. The hormonal requirements for restoring spermatogenesis quantitatively after its experimental suppression will be discussed next.

In adult rats first rendered azoospermic by the implantation of testosterone (T)-containing Silastic implants of 2.5 cm and estradiol (E)-containing implants of 0.1 cm, the administration of additional testosterone via Silastic implants caused restoration of advanced spermatid numbers to control values at an intratesticular testosterone concentration of about 20 ng/ml (FIG. 7) (24). In contrast, in rats rendered azoospermic by hypophysectomy, quantitatively complete spermatogenesis was not achieved by the administration of testosterone (FIG. 7) (24); instead, advanced spermatid numbers plateaued at approximately 20% of the number in the restored testosterone-estradiol rats despite comparable intratesticular testosterone concentrations.

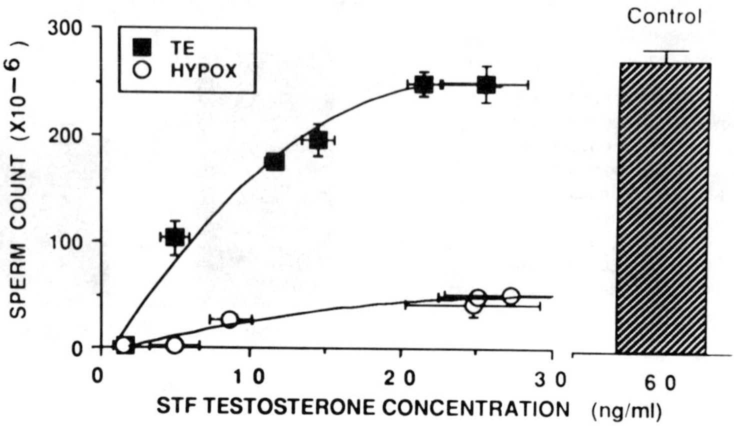

FIGURE 7. Relationship between the mean number of advanced spermatids per testis and the mean seminiferous tubule fluid (STF) testosterone concentration in rats first made azoospermic by implantation with testosterone (T), estradiol (E) Silastic implants (TE), or by hypophysectomy (HYPOX), and subsequently given testosterone-containing Silastic implants of increasing sizes for 8 weeks. (From Awoniyi *et al.*, 1990.[24])

We hypothesized that the difference between the ability of testosterone to restore spermatogenesis in the TE-implanted rats and hypophysectomized azoospermic rats was the presence of FSH in the former and its absence in the latter. To test this, the ability of testosterone to restore spermatogenesis in rats made azoospermic by active immunization either against LH alone or against GnRH was compared.[25] Surprisingly, the administration of testosterone resulted in the complete restoration of spermatogenesis (FIG. 8), despite the fact that FSH was undetectable in the GnRH-immunized

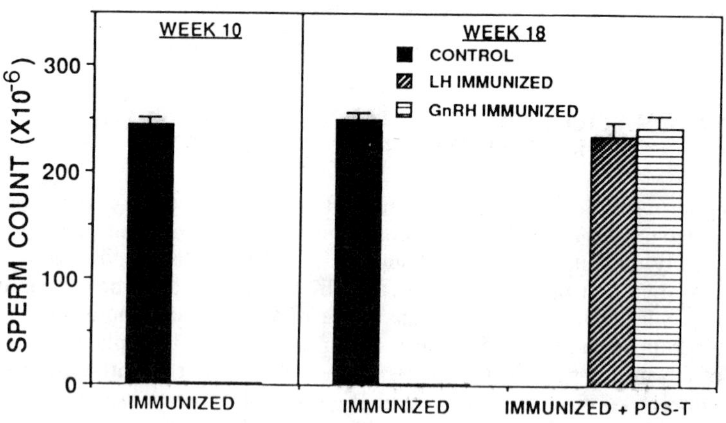

FIGURE 8. Mean number of advanced spermatids per testis in control rats and in LH- and GnRH-immunized rats at weeks 10 and 18 after immunization; and in LH- and GnRH-immunized rats that received testosterone-filled Silastic capsules (PDS-T) from weeks 10–18 post-immunization. (From Awoniyi *et al.*, 1989.[25])

rats. These results suggested that FSH is not required for the restoration of spermatogenesis in either group of immunized rats, and is consistent with the observation that FSH apparently is not required for the maintenance of spermatogenesis. It should be noted that complete restoration of spermatogenesis took place at testosterone concentrations of 20 ng/ml in both the LH- and GnRH-immunized rats.[25]

ANDROGEN ACTION IN THE TESTIS

One important mode by which steroid hormones act on target cells is by regulating the expression of target genes.[26] The basic steps involved are summarized in FIGURE 9. Steroid hormones bind to an intracellular receptor residing within the nucleus (or cytoplasm). The steroid/receptor complex then binds with high affinity to cis acting DNA elements, within or flanking a target gene, where it acts as a transcriptional enhancer. Transcription of the target gene is subsequently enhanced or repressed by steroid/receptor binding, resulting in changes in mRNA synthesis and ultimately protein synthesis.

Although most of the experiments that have given rise to the above model of steroid hormone action were carried out using steroids other than androgens, subsequent work has shown androgens to act according to the same basic model. Recent cloning and sequencing of the androgen receptor cDNA (human and rat) has revealed putative hormone- and DNA-binding domains with significant sequence similarity to other steroid hormone receptors.[27,28] Co-transfection of the androgen receptor cDNA and a reporter gene construct (MMTV-CAT) revealed that the androgen receptor acts as a ligand-activated transcription factor, as do the other characterized steroid receptors.[29]

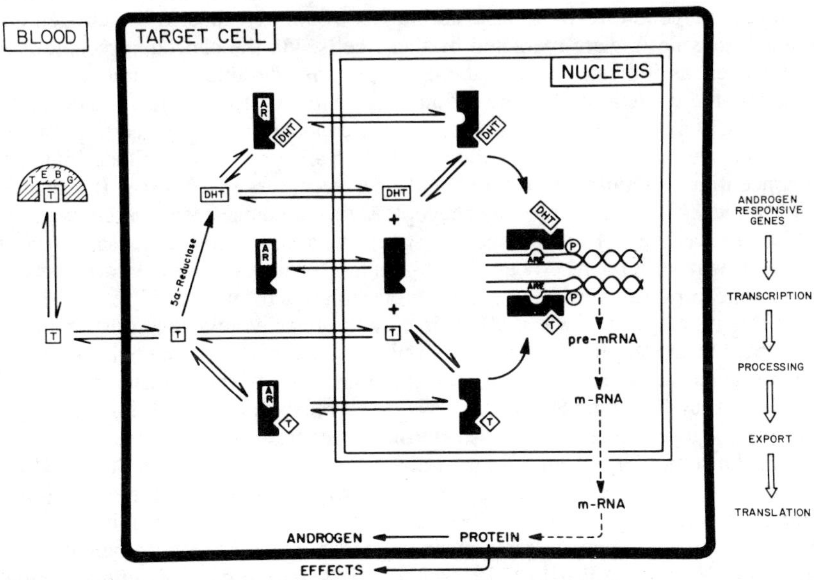

FIGURE 9. Model of transcriptional regulation by androgen in target cells.

Androgens have been shown to regulate the levels of specific mRNAs in many different tissues.[30] Although direct transcriptional regulation has been demonstrated by nuclear run-on experiments for some of these genes,[31,32] mRNA stabilization also contributes to the accumulation of some of these mRNAs and thus may constitute an alternative regulatory mechanism of androgens.[33] In either case, the circulating concentration of androgen required to elicit an effect in organs other than the testis is very low compared to the concentration of testosterone found in the testis.

Several years ago, Lyon *et al.*[34] demonstrated genetically that spermatogenesis took place normally in chimeric mice in which the germ cells could not have contained a functional androgen receptor. This result indicated that direct androgen action on the developing germ cells is not necessary for spermatogenesis, and implicated the somatic cells of the testis as the androgen target cells. This conclusion has been directly confirmed recently by demonstrations that androgen receptor is absent from germ cells;[3] and by localization of the androgen receptor to Sertoli, peritubular myoid and Leydig cells in the prepubertal testis by affinity labeling[35] and in the sexually mature testis by immunohistochemistry.[36] Given the architecture of the seminiferous epithelium,[37] it is most likely that the effects of testosterone on developing germ cells are mediated via the Sertoli cells and/or peritubular myoid cells.

When Sertoli and peritubular myoid cells are exposed to ^{3}H-testosterone in culture, the labeled androgen is accumulated in the nuclei of both cell types.[38] Cultured immature Sertoli cells have been shown to respond to testosterone with an increase in RNA polymerase II activity and increased incorporation of ^{3}H-uridine into RNA.[39,40] Analyses of proteins of testosterone-treated immature Sertoli cells have demonstrated changes in the synthesis of cellular and secreted proteins in response to testosterone.[41,42] Peritubular myoid cells respond to testosterone by secreting P-Mod-S, a protein that stimulates Sertoli cell synthetic activity.[43] These data demonstrate the ability of Sertoli cells and peritubular myoid cells, at least from immature animals, to respond directly to testosterone, as would be expected if androgen effects on spermatogenesis were mediated by these cells, via the androgen receptor.

However, as indicated above, there is now considerable experimental evidence to support the contention that the intratesticular testosterone concentration in intact adult rats (50 ng/ml), and indeed the minimal concentration required to maintain or restore spermatogenesis (20 ng/ml), are at least an order of magnitude higher than the concentration required to saturate androgen receptors in the testis. If testosterone action in the testis is via the androgen receptor, why are the testosterone concentrations required to maintain or restore spermatogenesis so high? How can testosterone regulate androgen-dependent processes in the intact adult testis with an average testosterone concentration within the seminiferous tubules of 50 ng/ml?

At this juncture, it is not at all clear why the testis would require such high testosterone concentrations (20 ng/ml) to maintain or restore spermatogenesis. Several possibilities occur to us. First, it is possible that much of the testosterone within the testis is unavailable to the Sertoli and myoid cell receptors. Second, it is possible that there may be local differences in testosterone concentration at particular stages of the cycle of the seminiferous epithelium. Indeed, there is evidence that Stage VII of the cycle is particularly sensitive to androgen withdrawal.[16] However, there are published reports that such stage-related differences do not occur.[44,45] We examined the possibility of local differences in testosterone concentrations using rats synchronized at Stages VII–VIII and XII–III of the cycle of the seminiferous epithelium[46]; analysis

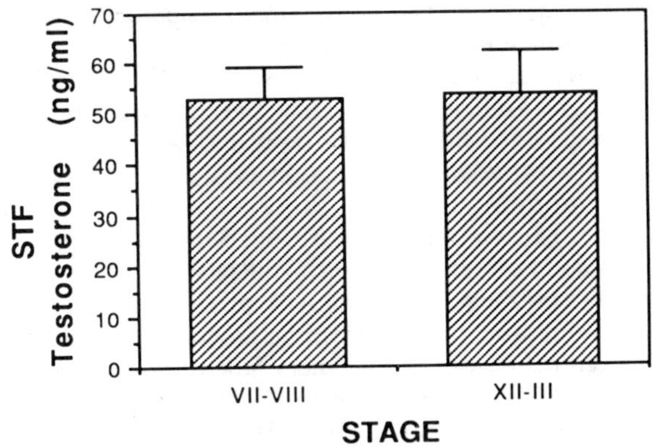

FIGURE 10. Testosterone concentration in seminiferous tubule fluid (STF) of rats synchronized at stages VII–VIII and XII–III of the cycle of the seminiferous epithelium.

of seminiferous tubule fluid isolated from the testes of these rats failed to reveal stage related differences in testosterone concentration (FIG. 10).

A third, possible explanation for high intratesticular testosterone concentrations is that testosterone is acting by an unknown mechanism rather than, or in addition to, its action via the androgen receptor. Fourth, as Yamamoto has suggested,[47] it is possible that genes are regulated by multiple factors that act in concert to give proper regulated expression of the gene. For example, the hormone-bound androgen receptor may be necessary for expression of a target gene in the testis, but other regulatory factors, controlled by other endocrine or paracrine signals, may be required for proper regulated expression. There is physiological evidence for just this type of complex regulation of processes integral to normal, quantitative spermatogenesis. For instance, as indicated above, the administration of high doses of testosterone via Silastic capsules to adult rats at the time of hypophysectomy failed to quantitatively maintain spermatogenesis (FIG. 2), and testosterone alone was insufficient to restore spermatogenesis in hypophysectomy-induced regressed rat testes (FIG. 7). The inability of testosterone to maintain or restore spermatogenesis in hypophysectomized rats is consistent with the inefficient expression of a key gene(s) that requires other regulatory proteins, under the control of other pituitary hormone(s), for optimal expression. It has also been suggested that non-androgenic products from Leydig cells may be involved, along with testosterone, in the maintenance and restoration of spermatogenesis.[22,23]

WHAT DOES TESTOSTERONE REGULATE IN THE TESTIS?

Immature Testis

The effects of testosterone on several of the proteins that are synthesized by Sertoli cells from immature rats has been studied. For example, plasminogen activator and ornithine decarboxylase (ODC) have both been shown to decrease with testosterone treatment of immature Sertoli cells in culture.[48,49] The down regulation of ODC by testosterone occurs at the level of its mRNA, probably as a secondary effect of testosterone since protein synthesis is required.[50] Interestingly, ODC mRNA is increased by testosterone in the mouse kidney, apparently as a result of increased transcription as well as mRNA stabilization.[51]

Three of the most extensively studied Sertoli cell secreted proteins are transferrin, androgen binding protein (ABP) and inhibin. Both transferrin and ABP have been reported to be increased by testosterone *in vivo*, after hypophysectomy of immature rats.[52,53] However, in these studies, the possibility that the responses to testosterone were secondary to changes in germ cell number and type was not considered. Several studies carried out with immature Sertoli cells in culture have failed to demonstrate regulation of transferrin, or its mRNA, by testosterone.[54,55] The results of studies investigating the regulation of ABP production by testosterone in immature Sertoli cells in culture have been conflicting; some studies indicated that ABP synthesis was androgen responsive,[56] but others failed to demonstrate androgen stimulation of ABP production.[55] Similarly, the results of experiments examining the regulation of inhibin secretion by immature Sertoli cells in culture have been conflicting, with some showing a stimulatory effect of testosterone[57] and others not.[58] It is now known that peritubular cells from immature rats, a common contaminant of enriched Sertoli cell cultures, respond to testosterone by secreting P-Mod-S, a factor that stimulates immature Sertoli cells in culture to produce ABP, transferrin and inhibin.[59,60]

Taken together, the above data implicate two possible modes of testosterone action in the seminiferous tubules of the immature rat testis: 1) a direct effect of testosterone on the Sertoli cells, and 2) an indirect effect via the secretion of P-Mod-S by peritubular myoid cells.

Mature Testis

With respect to the adult testis, there is a paucity of information in the literature dealing with the hormonal regulation of Sertoli or myoid cells. For example, to date there have been no published studies dealing with the effect of testosterone alone on adult Sertoli cells in culture. As a result, much of what we know or believe about myoid and Sertoli cell function and their hormonal regulation has been derived from analyses of cells isolated from immature rats. This is unfortunate because, for example, it is becoming clear that Sertoli cell responsiveness to hormones changes with age.[53]

Sertoli cells of adult hypophysectomized rats *in vivo* have been reported to respond to testosterone treatment by a decrease in the synthesis of β-nerve growth factor receptor mRNA.[61] In such *in vivo* studies, however, it is very important to control for the effect of changing germ cell populations that may occur with manipulation of testosterone. For instance, chronic (20-day) testosterone treatment of rats, hypophysectomized during late puberty (40 days), resulted in an increase in transferrin mRNA level.[53] However, the increased level of this mRNA was concomitant with an increase in testicular size and increased numbers of germ cells. Thus the mRNA may have responded to chronic testosterone treatment *or* to increased numbers of germ cells.[55] Indeed, many studies have shown that germ cells influence Sertoli cell function, both in culture and *in vivo*.[62,63] This fact complicates *in vivo* studies of androgen effects because altered populations of germ cells may occur,[11] and must be accounted for.

For example, we have recently investigated the *in vivo* effect of exogenous testosterone administration on the production SGP-2 and transferrin mRNAs by Sertoli cells of hypophysectomized, azoospermic adult rats. Rats that had been hypophysectomized for 4 weeks received testosterone-containing Silastic capsules that rapidly (within 3

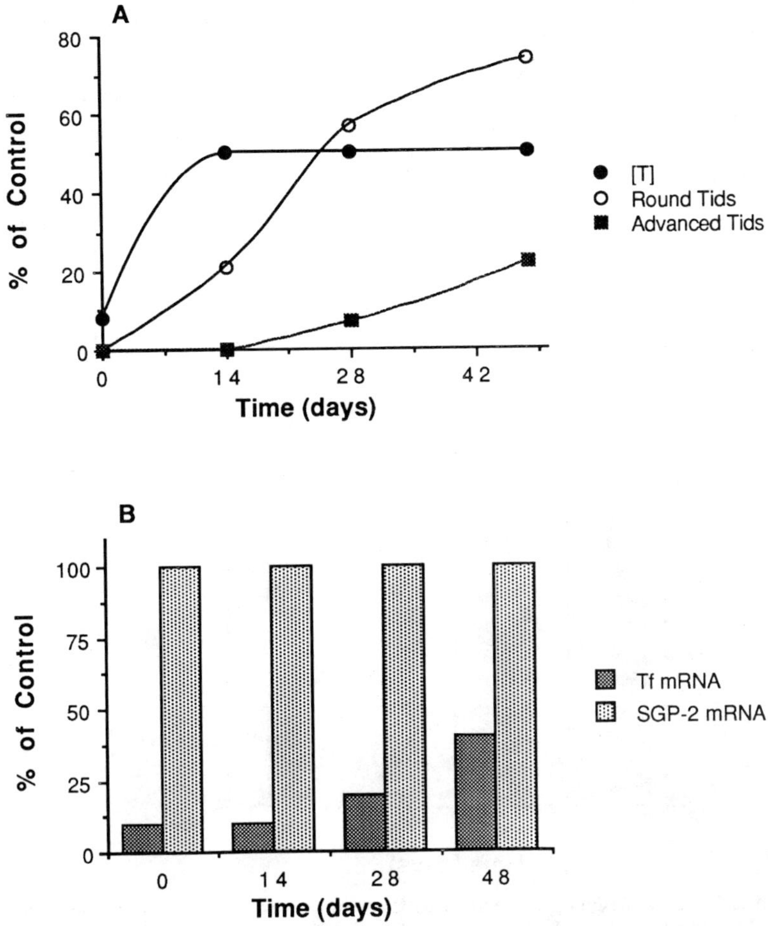

FIGURE 11. Comparison of the increase in testosterone concentration and the restoration of round and advanced spermatids (**A**) to the levels of transferrin (Tf) mRNA and SGP-2 mRNA per testis (**B**) in the testes of rats hypophysectomized for 4 weeks that received exogenous testosterone via Silastic capsules for 0 to 56 days.

days) elevated testosterone in the seminiferous tubule fluid to levels shown previously to restore spermatogenesis quantitatively in intact rats. Through two weeks of testosterone treatment, little change in the germ cell population occurred; but by 4 weeks, large numbers of pachytene spermatocytes and round spermatids, and some elongated spermatids, were restored. As shown in FIGURE 11, transferrin mRNA levels per testis were diminished greatly from control levels by hypophysectomy, and were not elevated above these basal levels until 4 weeks post-testosterone. This result suggested either that chronic testosterone treatment is required for stimulation of transferrin synthesis or, more likely, that germ cells must increase in number before transferrin mRNA

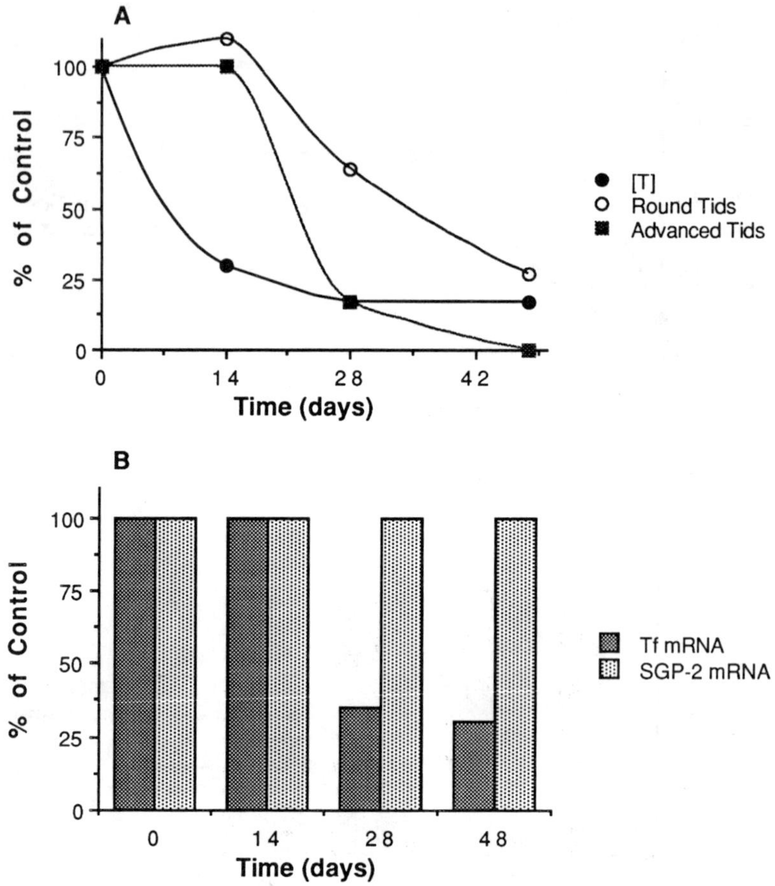

FIGURE 12. Comparison of the decrease in testosterone concentration and the loss of round and advanced spermatids (**A**) to the levels of transferrin (Tf) mRNA and SGP-2 mRNA per testis (**B**) at times (0 to 56 days) after implanting rats with LH-suppressing testosterone and estradiol-filled Silastic capsules.

is increased. In contrast to transferrin mRNA, SGP-2 mRNA levels per testis were unaffected by hypophysectomy or by the reappearance of germ cells that resulted from exogenous testosterone (FIG. 11). This result suggested that SGP-2 is constitutively expressed in adult testes, and is not affected by germ cell number or testosterone levels.

In another study, we examined the effects of diminishing testosterone levels in the adult rat testis on transferrin and SGP-2 mRNA levels per testis. Treatment of rats with LH-suppressing testosterone-estradiol capsules caused testosterone levels to decline from 50 ng/ml to less than 15 ng/ml in two weeks. Germ cells (elongated spermatids, round spermatids and pachytene spermatocytes) began to decline at 4 weeks post-implantation (FIG. 12). Transferrin mRNA levels in these testes declined along the same time course as the germ cell loss, supporting the contention that the levels of this mRNA are sensitive to numbers of germ cells. Again, SGP-2 mRNA levels remained constant throughout the experiment.

Taken together, these two experiments suggest that chronic testosterone treatment affects Sertoli cell transferrin mRNA production indirectly via changes in germ cell numbers, but that SGP-2 mRNA levels are unaffected either by testosterone or germ cell changes. Perhaps more importantly, the experiments indicate that there are *in vivo* models with which the effects or hormonal manipulation can be examined in the absence or presence of a changing germ cell population.

CONCLUSIONS

Spermatogenesis can be quantitatively maintained in intact adult rats at an intratesticular testosterone concentration of 20 ng/ml, one third the physiological concentration but at least an order of magnitude higher than the concentration required to saturate testicular androgen receptors. This high testosterone concentration (20 ng/ml) is also required for maximal maintenance of spermatogenesis in hypophysectomized rats, though spermatogenesis is not maintained quantitatively in these rats. The inability of exogenously administered testosterone to maintain spermatogenesis quantitatively in hypophysectomized rats is not the result of lack of FSH because testosterone will quantitatively maintain spermatogenesis in rats immunized against GnRH. This suggests that other pituitary factors are required. Testosterone administration also failed to maintain spermatogenesis quantitatively in testes in which Leydig cells were eliminated with EDS, suggesting that there may also be non-steroidal Leydig cell products that are required.

Only 20% of advanced spermatid numbers can be restored to regressed testes of hypophysectomized rats by testosterone administration. Lack of FSH is not the reason for the failure to restore spermatogenesis quantitatively because testosterone administration restored spermatogenesis quantitatively in rats immunized against GnRH. Again, intratesticular testosterone concentrations of 20 ng/ml provided the maximal achievable restoration in each of intact, GnRH immunized and hypophysectomized rats.

It is not clear why testosterone concentrations in excess of the concentration of testicular androgen receptors are required for the maintenance and restoration of spermatogenesis. Among the possibilities that occurred to us are: 1) Much of the testosterone within the testis may be unavailable to the androgen receptors of the Sertoli and myoid cells. 2) There may be local differences in testosterone concentration related to different stages of the cycle of the seminiferous epithelium. There is good evidence that argues against this possibility, however. 3) Testosterone may act by an unknown mechanism rather than, or in addition to, its action via the androgen receptor. 4) Genes involved in regulating spermatogenesis may themselves be regulated by multiple regulatory factors that act in concert with androgen receptor. The inability of testosterone to maintain spermatogenesis in hypophysectomized rats and in rats lacking Leydig cells is consistent with this possibility.

REFERENCES

1. SMITH, P. E. 1930. Hypophysectomy and a replacement therapy in the rat. Am. J. Anat. **45:** 205–256.
2. STEINBERGER, E. 1971. Hormonal control of mammalian spermatogenesis. Physiol. Rev. **51:** 1–22.

3. FRITZ, I. B. 1978. Sites of action of androgens and follicle stimulating hormone on cells of the seminiferous tubule. Biochem. Actions Horm. **V:** 249-281.
4. EWING, L. L., J. C. DAVIS & B. R. ZIRKIN. 1980. Regulation of testicular function: A spatial and temporal view. Int. Rev. Physiol. **22:** 41-115.
5. EWING, L. L. & B. R. ZIRKIN. 1983. Leydig cell structure and steroidogenic function. Recent Progr. Horm. Res. **39:** 599-635.
6. TURNER, T. T., C. E. JONES, S. S. HOWARDS, L. L. EWING, B. ZEGEYE, & G. L. GUNSALUS. 1984. On the androgen microenvironment of maturing spermatozoa. Endocrinology **115:** 1925-1932.
7. WRIGHT, W. W., K. CHAN, K. SUNDARAM & C. W. BARDIN. 1982. New observations on androgen action: Androgen receptor stabilization and antisteroid effects of LHRH agonists. *In* Hormones and Cancer. W. W. Leavitt, Ed.: 325-336. Plenum Press. New York.
8. CUNNINGHAM, G. R. & C. HUCKINS. 1979. Persistence of complete spermatogenesis in the presence of low intratesticular concentrations of testosterone. Endocrinology **105:** 177-186.
9. REA, M. A., G. R. MARSHALL, G. F. WEINBAUER & E. NIESCHLAG. 1986. Testosterone maintains pituitary and serum FSH and spermatogenesis in gonadotrophin-releasing hormone antagonist-suppressed rats. J. Endocrinol. **108:** 101-107.
10. SUN, T.-T., D. C. IRBY, D. M. ROBERTSON & D. M. DE KRETSER. 1989. The effects of exogenously administered testosterone on spermatogenesis in intact and hypophysectomized rats. Endocrinology **125:** 1000-1010.
11. ZIRKIN, B. R., R. SANTULLI, C. A. AWONIYI & L. L. EWING. 1989. Maintenance of advanced spermatogenic cells in the adult rat testis: Quantitative relationship to testosterone concentration within the testis. Endocrinology **124:** 3043-3049.
12. CLERMONT, Y. & S. C. HARVEY. 1967. Effects of hormones on spermatogenesis in the rat. Cib Found. Colloq. Endocrinol. **16:** 173-196.
13. BARTLETT, J. M. S., G. F. WEINBAUER & E. NIESCHLALG. 1989. Differential effects of FSH and testosterone on the maintenance of spermatogenesis in the adult hypophysectomized rat. J. Endocrinology **121:** 49-58.
14. SANTULLI, R., R. L. SPRANDO, C. A. AWONIYI, L. L. EWING & B. R. ZIRKIN. 1990. To what extent can spermatogenesis be maintained in the hypophysectomized adult rat testis with exogenously administered testosterone? Endocrinology **126:** 95-101.
15. DYM, M., H. G. M. RAJ, Y. C. LIN, H. E. CHEMES, N. J. KOTITE, S. N. NAYFEH & F. S. FRENCH. 1979. Is FSH required for maintenance of spermatogenesis in adult rats? J. Reprod. Fertil. (Suppl.) **26:** 175-181.
16. RUSSELL, L. D. & Y. CLERMONT. 1977. Degeneration of germ cells in normal, hypophysectomized and hormone treated hypophysectomized rats. Anat. Rec. **187:** 347-355.
17. SHARPE, R. M. 1989. Follicle-stimulating hormone and spermatogenesis in the adult male. J. Endocrinol. **121:** 405-407.
18. AHMAD, N., G. C. HALTMEYER & K. B. EIK-NES. 1973. Maintenance of spermatogenesis in rats with intratesticular implants containing testosterone or dihydrotestosterone (DHT). Biol. Reprod. **8:** 411-419.
19. HARRIS, M. E. & A. BARTKE. 1975. Maintenance of rete testis fluid testosterone and dihydrotestosterone levels by pregnenolone and other C_{21} steroids in hypophysectomized rats. Endocrinology **96:** 1396-1402.
20. GRINO, P. B., J. E. GRIFFIN & J. D. WILSON. 1990. Testosterone at high concentrations interacts with the human androgen receptor similarly to dihydrotestosterone. Endocrinology **126:** 1165-1172.
21. KEENEY, D. S., S. M. L. C. MENDIS-HANDAGAMA, B. R. ZIRKIN & L. L. EWING. 1988. Effect of long-term deprivation of luteinizing hormone on Leydig cell volume, Leydig cell number, and steroidogenic capacity of the rat testis. Endocrinology **123:** 2906-2915.
22. SPRANDO, R. L., R. SANTULLI, C. A. AWONIYI, L. L. EWING & B. R. ZIRKIN. 1990. Does ethane 1,2-dimethanesulphonate (EDS) have a direct cytotoxic effect on the seminiferous epithelium of the rat testis? J. Androl. **11:** 344-352.
23. SHARPE, R. M., S. MADDOCKS & J. B. KERR. 1990. Cell-cell interactions in the control of spermatogenesis as studied using Leydig cell destruction and testosterone replacement. Am. J. Anat. **188:** 3-20.

24. Awoniyi, C. A., R. L. Sprando, R. Santulli, V. Chandrashekar, L. L. Ewing & B. R. Zirkin. 1990. Restoration of spermatogenesis by exogenously administered testosterone in rats made azoospermic by hypophysectomy or withdrawal of luteinizing hormone alone. Endocrinology **127:** 177–184.
25. Awoniyi, C. A., R. Santulli, V. Chandrashekar, B. D. Schanbacher & B. R. Zirkin. 1989. Quantitative restoration of advanced spermatogenic cells in adult male rats made azoospermic by active immunization against luteinizing hormone or gonadotropin-releasing hormone. Endocrinology **125:** 1303–1309.
26. Parker, M. G. 1990. Mechanisms of action of steroid receptors in the regulation of gene transcription. J. Reprod. Fertil. **88:** 717–720.
27. Chang, C., J. Kokontis & S. Liao. 1988. Structural analysis of complimentary DNA and amino acid sequences of human and rat androgen receptors. Proc. Natl. Acad. Sci. USA. **85:** 7211–7215.
28. Lubahn, D. B., D. R. Joseph, M. Sar, J. Tan, H. N. Higgs, R. E. Larson. F. S. French & E. M. Wilson. 1988. The human androgen receptor: complimentary deoxyribonucleic acid cloning, sequence analysis and gene expression in the prostate. Mol. Endocrinol. **2:** 1265–1275.
29. Rundlett, S. E., W.-P. Wu & R. L. Miesfeld. 1990. Functional characterization of the androgen receptor confirm that the molecular basis of androgen action is transcriptional activation. Mol. Endocrinol. **4:** 708–714.
30. Berger, F. G. & G. Watson. 1989. Androgen-regulated gene expression. Ann. Rev. Physiol. **51:** 51–65.
31. Rheaume, C., K. W. Barbour, J. Tseng-Crank & F. G. Berger. 1989. Molecular genetics of androgen-inducible RP2 gene transcription in the mouse kidney. Mol. Cell. Biol. **9:** 477–483.
32. Rheaume, C., C. Schonfeld, C. Porter & F. G. Berger. 1989. Evolution of androgen-regulated ornithine decarboxylase expression in mouse kidney. Mol. Endocrinol. **3:** 1243–1251.
33. Berger, F. G., D. Loose, H. Meisner & G. Watson. 1986. Androgen induction of messenger RNA concentrations in mouse kidney is posttranscriptional. Biochemistry **25:** 1170–1175.
34. Lyon, M. F., P. H. Glenister & M. L. Lamoreux. 1975. Normal spermatozoa from androgen-resistant germ cells of chimeric mice and the role of androgen in spermatogenesis. Nature **258:** 620–622.
35. Anthony, C. T., W. J. Kovacs & M. K. Skinner. 1989. Analysis of the androgen receptor in isolated testicular cell types with a microassay that uses an affinity ligand. Endocrinology **125:** 2628-2635.
36. Sar, M., C. B. Lubahn, F. S. French & E. M. Wilson. 1990. Immunohistochemical localization of the androgen receptor in rat and human tissues. Endocrinology **127:** 3180–3186.
37. de Kretzer, D. M. & J. B. Kerr. 1988. The cytology of the testis. *In* The Physiology of Reproduction. E. Knobil and J. Neill, Eds.: 837–932. Raven Press. New York.
38. Buzek, S. W. & B. M. Sanborn. 1990. Nuclear androgen receptor dynamics in testicular peritubular and Sertoli cells. J. Androl. **11:** 514–520.
39. Lamb, D. J., Y.-H. Tsai, A. Steinberger & B. M. Sanborn. 1981. Sertoli cell nuclear transcriptional activity: Stimulation by follicle-stimulating hormone and testosterone *in vitro*. Endocrinology **108:** 1020–1026.
40. Lamb, D. J., J. R. Wagle, Y.-H. Tsai, L. Lee, A. Steinberger & B. M. Sanborn. 1982. Specificity and nature of the rapid steroid-stimulated increase in Sertoli cell nuclear RNA polymerase activity. J. Steroid Biochem. **16:** 653–659.
41. Roberts, K. & M. D. Griswold. 1989. Testosterone induction of cellular proteins in cultured Sertoli cells from hypophysectomized rats and rats of different ages. Endocrinology **125:** 1174–1179.
42. Cheng, C. Y., J. P. Mather, A. L. Beyer & C. W. Bardin. 1986. Identification of hormonally responsive proteins in primary Sertoli cell culture medium by anion-exchange high performance liquid chromatography. Endocrinology **118:** 480–488.
43. Skinner, M. K. & Z. B. Fritz. 1985. Testicular peritubular cells secrete a protein under androgen control that modulate Sertoli cell functions. Proc. Natl. Acad. Sci. USA **82:** 114–118.
44. Parvinen, M., & I. Huhtaniemi. 1990. Testosterone micromilieu in staged rat seminiferous tubules. J. Steroid Biochem. **36:** 377–381.
45. Bartlett, J. M. S., G. F. Weinbauer & E. Nieschlag. 1990. Stability of spermatogenic syn-

chronization achieved by depletion and restoration of vitamin A. Biol. Reprod. **42:** 603–612.
46. MORALES, C. & M. D. GRISWOLD. 1987. Retinol-induced stage synchronization in seminiferous tubules of the rat. Endocrinology. **121:** 432–434.
47. YAMAMOTO, K. R. 1985. Steroid receptor regulated transcription of specific genes and gene networks. Ann. Rev. Genet. **19:** 209–252.
48. AILENBERG, M., D. MCCABE & I. B. FRITZ. 1990. Androgens inhibit plasminogen activator activity secreted by Sertoli cells in culture in a two-chambered assembly. Endocrinology **126:** 1561–1568.
49. WEINER, K. X. B., B. T. PENTECOST & J. A. DIAS. 1990. Testosterone decreases ornithine decarboxylase messenger RNA levels in primary cultures of rat Sertoli cells. Mol. Endocrinol. **4:** 1249–1256.
50. WEINER, K. X. B., & J. A. DIAS. 1990. Protein synthesis is required for testosterone to decrease ornithine decarboxylase messenger RNA levels in rat Sertoli cells. Mol. Endocrinol. **4:** 1791–1798.
51. WATSON, G. & K. PAIGEN. 1988. mRNA synthesis rates *in vivo* for androgen-inducible sequences in mouse kidney. Mol. Cell. Biol. **8:** 2117–2124.
52. DANZO, B. J., S. N. PAVLOU & H. L. ANTHONY. 1990. Hormonal regulation of androgen-binding protein in the rat. Endocrinology **127:** 2829–2838.
53. HUGLY, S., K. ROBERTS & M. D. GRISWOLD. 1988. Transferrin and sulfated glycoprotein-2 messenger ribonucleic acid levels in the testis and isolated Sertoli cells of hypophysectomized rats. Endocrinology **122:** 1390–1396.
54. HUGGENVIK, J., S. R. SYLVESTER & M. D. GRISWOLD. 1984. Control of transferrin mRNA synthesis in Sertoli cells. Ann. NY Acad. Sci. **438:** 1–7.
55. SKINNER, M. K., S. M. SCHLITZ & C. T. ANTHONY. 1989. Regulation of Sertoli cell differentiated function: Testicular transferrin and androgen-binding protein expression. Endocrinology **124:** 3015–3024.
56. LOUIS, B. G. & I. B. FRITZ. 1979. Follicle-stimulating hormone and testosterone independently increase the production of androgen binding protein by Sertoli cells in culture. Endocrinology **104:** 454–461.
57. VERHOEVEN, G. & P. FRANCHIMONT. 1983. Regulation of inhibin secretion by Sertoli cell-enriched cultures. Acta Endocrinol. **102:** 136–143.
58. MORRIS, P. L., W. W. VALE, S. CAPPEL & C. W. BARDIN. 1988. Inhibin production by primary Sertoli cell-enriched cultures: Regulation by follicle-stimulating hormone, androgens, and epidermal growth factor. Endocrinology **122:** 717–725.
59. NORTON, J. N., & M. K. SKINNER. 1989. Regulation of Sertoli cell function and differentiation through the actions of a testicular paracrine factor P-Mod-S. Endocrinology **124:** 2711–2719.
60. SKINNER, M. K., R. I. MCLACHLAN & W. J. BREMMER. 1989. Stimulation of Sertoli cell inhibin secretion by the testicular paracrine factor PModS. Mol. Cell. Endocrinol. **66:** 239–249.
61. PERSSON, H., C. A. LE LIEVRE, O. SODER, M. J. VILLAR, M. METSIS, L. OLSON, M. RITZEN & T. HOKFELT. 1990. Expression of beta-nerve growth factor receptor mRNA in Sertoli cells downregulated by testosterone. Science **247:** 704–707.
62. STALLARD, B. M. & M. D. GRISWOLD. 1990. Germ cell regulation of Sertoli cell transferrin mRNA levels. Mol. Endocrinol. **4:** 393–401.
63. PINON-LATAILLADE, G., J. F. VELEZ DE LA CALLE, M. C. VIGUIER-MARTINEZ, D. H. GARNIER, R. FOLLIOT, J. MAAS & B. JEGOU. 1988. Influence of germ cells upon Sertoli cells during low-dose rate of gamma-irradiation of adult rats. Mol. Cell. Endocrinol. **58:** 51–63.

Peptide and Steroid Regulation of Spermatogenesis in Primates[a]

GERHARD F. WEINBAUER
AND EBERHARD NIESCHLAG

Institute of Reproductive Medicine of the University and
WHO Collaborating Centre for Research in Human Reproduction
Steinfurter Str. 107
D-4400 Münster, Germany

INTRODUCTION

It is well recognized that mammalian spermatogenesis is dependent on pituitary hormones. A large body of literature provides conclusive evidence that luteinizing hormone (LH) and follicle-stimulating hormone (FSH) are the key regulators of testicular function. Whereas FSH most likely acts directly on the germinal epithelium,[1] LH exerts its stimulatory effects via androgens produced by the Leydig cells.[2]

Rodent studies, however, suggest that factors other than the gonadotropic hormones may be involved in the regulation of male gametogenesis. In the rat model, growth hormone (GH) enhanced the trophic effects of FSH and testosterone on germ cell development.[3,4] Submandibular gland-derived epidermal growth factor has been shown to play an important role in spermatogenesis in mice.[5] To date, however, no evidence has been obtained in primates that extratesticular factors other than LH and FSH are required for normal testis function.

Consequently this chapter will concentrate on the effects of FSH (peptide) and testosterone (steroid) on testicular function in primates. It is generally accepted by now that both hormones must be present to ensure normal testis function. The important question that remains is the relative importance of FSH and testosterone for the spermatogenic process. In other words, do FSH and testosterone have specific spermatogenic targets or do they merely provide a general trophic stimulus leading to germ cell evolution? The relative contributions of FSH and testosterone to testicular function are clinically relevant for the treatment of endocrine infertility and the development of a hormonal male contraceptive. For the latter it is pertinent to know whether FSH must be suppressed entirely and whether the effects of testosterone on spermatogenesis can be separated from its effects on accessory sex organs, reproductive behavior and general metabolic effects on muscle, bone and hematopoiesis.

When dealing with the hormonal regulation of male gametogenesis it is essential to distinguish between initiation, maintenance and reinitiation of the spermatogenic process. *Initiation* refers to the first completion of spermatogenesis, *i.e.*, formation of testicular sperm during puberty. *Maintenance* comprises the requirements of on-

[a] While our earlier work reported here was supported by the Max Planck Society, the current studies are financed by the Deutsche Forschungsgemeinschaft (DFG grant Ni 130/11).

going spermatogenesis in the sexually mature male. *Reinitiation* relates to the restart of gametogenesis once the spermatogenic process has been interrupted. In addition, it is also important to distinguish between qualitatively and quantitatively normal spermatogenesis. *Qualitatively normal* spermatogenesis means that all types of germ cells are present. The term *quantitatively normal* spermatogenesis is used when complete numbers of all germ cell types develop.

For the evaluation of the hormonal dependence of gametogenesis a quantitative analysis of the various germ cells is highly desirable. In men, testicular biopsies, for ethical considerations, cannot be performed without a clinical indication which rarely exists in modern diagnosis. Thus in most instances, studies on the endocrine regulation of spermatogenesis in men must resort to evaluating ejaculated sperm for assessment of the spermatogenic status. In contrast, testicular biopsies can easily be obtained from non-human primates, which are considered appropriate surrogate experimental models[6] for the study of human reproduction. This explains why much of the information relating to peptide and steroid regulation of spermatogenesis in primates derives from non-human primate studies.

INITIATION OF THE SPERMATOGENIC PROCESS

Following the early neonatal rise of gonadotropin and testosterone production the reproductive development of primates is characterized by a period of quiescence of reproductive hormone secretion and arrest of germ cell proliferation lasting over years before the juvenile phase and puberty are reached.[7-10] The relative ability of androgens and FSH to initiate testicular growth and germ cell development during the period of the reproductive hiatus has been the subject of only a few non-human primate studies.

Role of Testosterone

Intratesticular administration of ovine LH caused the appearance of mitotic figures in some germinal cells.[11] Short-term treatment with ovine LH or hCG increased the diameter of seminiferous tubules and testicular weight[12] (TABLE 1). Moreover, spermatocyte-like cells were encountered in the seminiferous tubules. These findings suggest that androgens are involved in initiating the maturation of testicular function.

TABLE 1. Effects of 5-Day (Days 2 to 7) Treatment with Ovine FSH, hCG or PMSG on Seminiferous Tubule Diameter of Immature Monkeys

	Seminiferous Tubule Diameter (μm)	
Treatment	Day 1[a]	Day 7[a]
None	56.9 ± 1.3	59.4 ± 0.9
Ovine FSH (1mg/day)	47.0 ± 1.5	58.3 ± 1.2*
hCG (100 IU/day)	45.2 ± 0.5	52.3 ± 1.1*
PMSG (100 IU/day)	56.8 ± 0.8	65.7 ± 1.0*

[a] Mean values ± SEM of 3–4 animals/group; * $p < 0.01$ *vs.* day 1. (Adapted from Arslan *et al.*, 1981.[12])

However, longer treatment phases are hampered by the formation of antibodies against the foreign peptides.

To assess the role of testosterone alone in the initiation of spermatogenesis in the non-human primate, we treated four immature animals with very high doses of testosterone for a period of one year.[13] Testicular volume increased 5–6-fold (FIG. 1). Germ cell development was markedly stimulated including the appearance of elongated spermatids. The ejaculates of two monkeys contained sperm. The increments of testicular size and germ cell production, however, were far below the range of adult animals. It was concluded that testosterone alone can initiate spermatogenesis in the non-human primate in a qualitative albeit not quantitative manner.

Evidence that testosterone alone may trigger spermatogenic development has also been obtained in the human.[14,15] In boys with a Leydig cell tumor, complete spermatogenesis was found only in the vicinity of the tumorous area, whereas in tumor-free areas spermatogenesis had not been initiated. These observations also support the hypothesis that testosterone can initiate qualitatively normal gametogenesis in primates.

Role of Follicle-stimulating Hormone

Administration of hMG induced some stimulation of spermatogenesis in prepubertal animals but the final interpretation of the results was confounded by the presence of antibodies.[16] Treatment with ovine FSH significantly increased seminiferous tubule diameter (TABLE 1), testicular weight, and the cytoplasm of pre-Sertoli-cells.[12] Pulsatile infusions of synthetic GnRH for a period of twelve weeks induced the formation of (very few) prophase I spermatocytes.[17] The Sertoli cells were large and contained a nucleolus, presumably indicating their maturity.

In a recent investigation we studied the effects of testosterone and/or human FSH on testicular development of juvenile Rhesus monkeys over a period of 12 weeks (Arslan *et al.*, in preparation). Follicle-stimulating hormone alone failed to induce the development of germ cells beyond the spermatogonial stage, whereas combined treatment led to the evolvement of a few primary spermatocytes. Although compelling evidence has been provided for a role of FSH alone in the initiation of the spermatogenic process in non-human primates, further studies are required to ultimately clarify the importance of FSH for the onset of testicular development.

MAINTENANCE OF THE SPERMATOGENIC PROCESS

Role of Testosterone

Immunization against testosterone appears to be an obvious approach to investigate the role of testosterone selectively in the maintenance of spermatogenesis. This strategy, however, did not prove useful since active immunization against testosterone led to increased testosterone production and had no detrimental effects on testicular size.[18]

Therefore, to study the effects of testosterone in the non-human primate model, animals were deprived of endogenous reproductive hormones through hypophysectomy or GnRH antagonist administration followed by testosterone replacement. In earlier studies treatment with hMG or PMSG had only marginal effects on gametogenesis

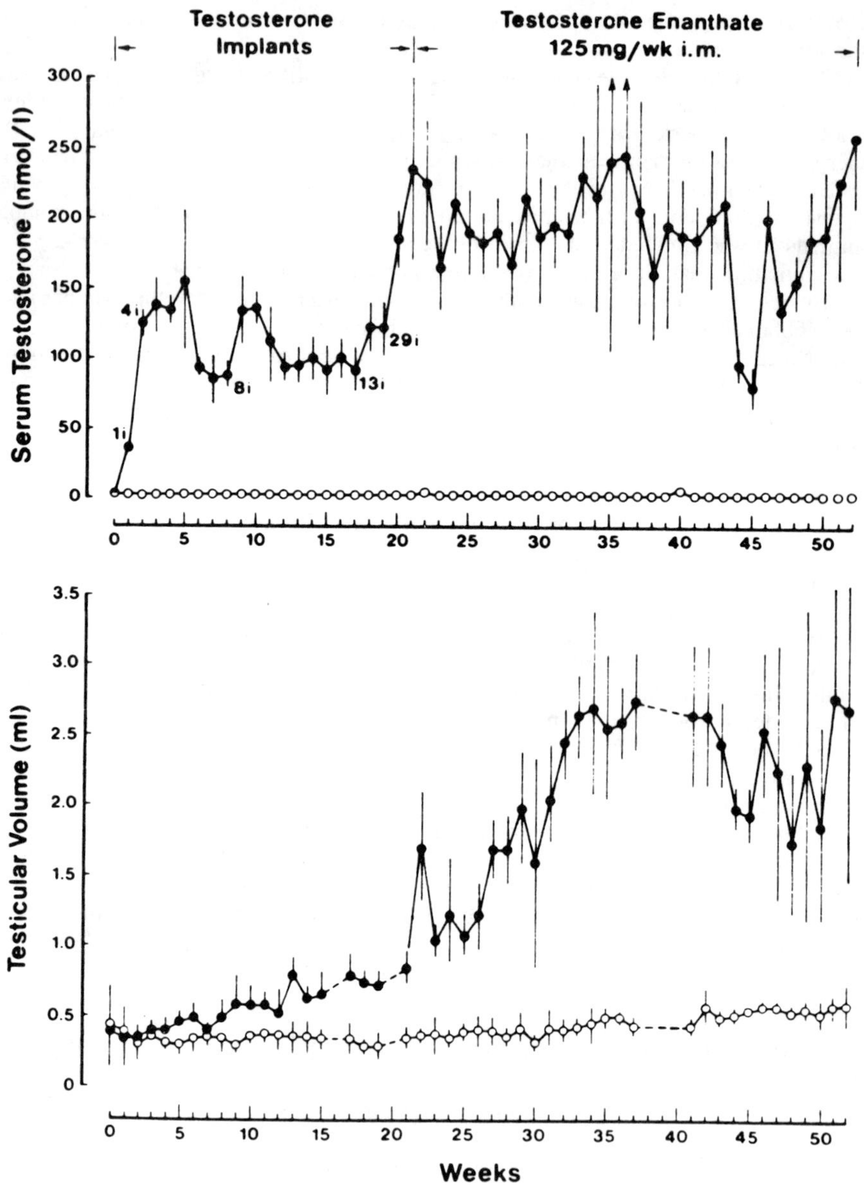

FIGURE 1. Mean (± SD) serum testosterone levels and mean testicular volumes of four untreated (*open symbols*) and testosterone-treated (*solid symbols*) immature monkeys. Numerals followed by letter i indicate additional testosterone-filled capsules. (Reproduced from ref. 13 with permission.)

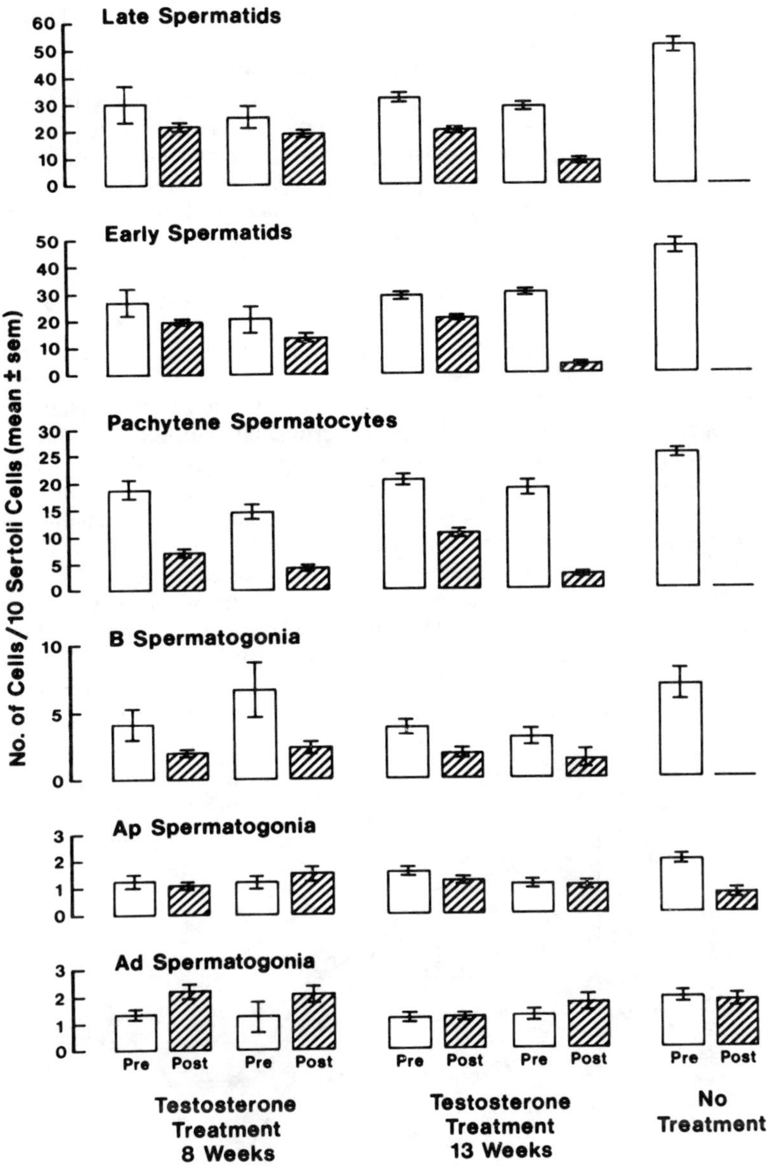

FIGURE 2. Spermatogenic cell types (means ± SD) before (*open bars*) and after (*hatched bars*) hypophysectomy. Two animals each were biopsied after 8 and 13 weeks, respectively, of concurrent high dose testosterone treatment. One monkey received no testosterone treatment. (Reproduced from ref. 20 with permission.)

probably because of formation of antibodies.[16,19] Administration of very high amounts of testosterone via Silastic capsules, which maintained serum testosterone levels 8–10-fold above presurgical levels, maintained spermatogenesis qualitatively for 8 and 13 weeks, respectively.[20] In that study quantitative histological analysis of germ cell numbers was performed prior to and at termination of the study (FIG. 2). In the absence of testosterone supplementation the germinal epithelium, aside from Sertoli cells, contained only Ap- and Ad-spermatogonia. In the presence of testosterone, however, all germ cell types were still found, although the numbers of B-spermatogonia, pachytene spermatocytes, and early and late spermatids were reduced. The numbers of Ad-spermatogonia remained unchanged before and after hypophysectomy. Analysis of spermatogenic efficacy by means of germ cell ratios revealed that spermatogonial transition from type A to type B was impaired while testosterone maintained meiosis and spermiogenesis. From these studies it was concluded that testosterone alone qualitatively maintains spermatogenesis.

Like hypophysectomy,[20,21] administration of a GnRH antagonist completely disrupts spermatogenesis in the primate.[22-24] This experimental approach provides a distinct advantage over hypophysectomy because GnRH antagonists selectively suppress gonadotropin secretion and do not impose the burden and side-effects of brain surgery. In the first experiment GnRH antagonist-treated monkeys were supplemented with testosterone-filled Silastic capsules which maintained serum testosterone concentrations at 50–100% of pretreatment levels.[25] The study lasted for 15 weeks. Under this treatment regimen sperm numbers in the ejaculate were markedly decreased compared to baseline but azoospermia could not be induced, whereas administration of this GnRH antagonist alone induced complete cessation of spermatogenesis within 7–9 weeks.[23]

To evaluate whether these attenuative effects of testosterone on GnRH antagonist-induced inhibition of gametogenesis are dose-dependent, the following experiment

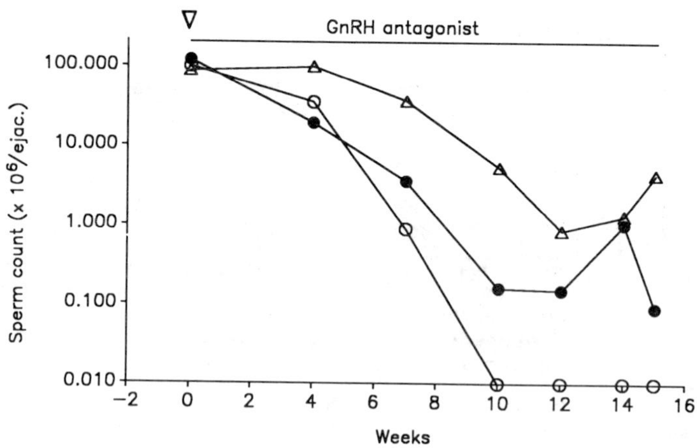

FIGURE 3. Median sperm count of monkeys (n = 5/group) treated for 15 weeks with GnRH antagonist alone (*open symbols*), GnRH antagonist plus 40 mg testosterone ester (*solid symbols*) or GnRH antagonist plus 200 mg testosterone ester (*open triangles*). Sperm numbers in the 200 mg testosterone-treated group are significantly higher compared to the effects of 40 mg testosterone. (Modified from ref. 24.)

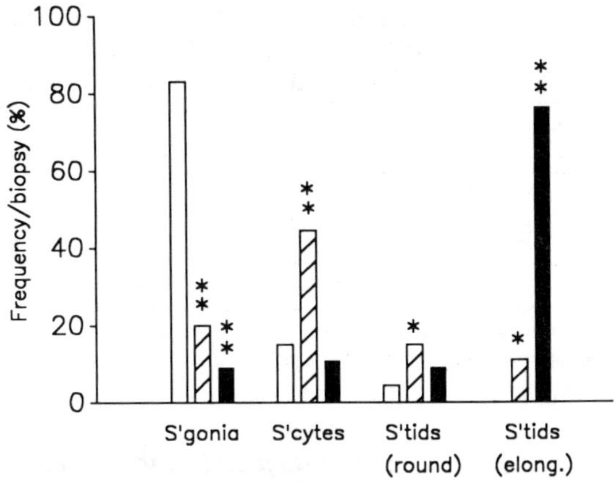

FIGURE 4. Median frequency of seminiferous tubules classified according to the presence of the most advanced germ cell in monkeys (n = 5/group) treated for 15 weeks with GnRH antagonist alone (*open bars*), GnRH antagonist plus 40 mg testosterone ester (*hatched bars*) or GnRH antagonist plus 200 mg testosterone ester (*solid bars*). S'gonia = spermatogonia; S'cytes = spermatocytes; S'tids = spermatids (round or elongated). The asterisk denotes significant differences in relation to GnRH antagonist alone (*open bars*). (Modified from ref. 24.)

was carried out.[24] Animals received treatment with GnRH antagonist alone for 15 weeks or were substituted with testosterone, released from a long-acting testosterone ester,[26] at two doses; the lower dose maintained serum testosterone concentrations within the upper normal range and the higher dose provided serum levels in the supranormal range. Semen samples were collected at regular intervals and a testicular biopsy was obtained before and after 15 weeks of GnRH antagonist treatment.

Within 10–12 weeks of treatment with GnRH antagonist alone all monkeys became azoospermic (FIG. 3). During concomitant administration of testosterone, however, complete suppression of sperm production could not be induced, although sperm numbers were markedly reduced. In addition, the higher dose of testosterone maintained sperm counts at a significantly higher number. This dose-dependent stimulation of germ cell development was also confirmed by quantitative histological analysis (FIG. 4). Following treatment with GnRH antagonist alone spermatogonia were the only germ cell elements left (apart from the Sertoli cells) in about 80% of seminiferous tubules. In contrast, with the lower dose of testosterone approximately 40% of tubules still contained spermatocytes and in 10% of tubules elongated spermatids were present. With the higher dose of testosterone this effect was more pronounced: about 75% of seminiferous tubules contained elongated spermatids. These observations also clearly demonstrate that testosterone alone can qualitatively maintain spermatogenesis in a non-human primate and that these effects of testosterone are dose-dependent.

The main source of information regarding the role of testosterone in the maintenance of human spermatogenesis derives from clinical trials with androgens for male contraception[27–29] and the studies by Matsumoto's group[30] who combined androgens with hCG, LH or FSH to investigate hormonal regulation of spermatogenesis. Administration of androgen alone suppressed gonadotropin secretion but induced azoospermia only in 50–80% of men. Studies involving androgens or hCG administration led to the view that testosterone alone can qualitatively maintain spermatogenesis in the absence of detectable concentrations of immunoreactive FSH.[30] It is also important to note here that in all instances testosterone alone failed to quantitatively maintain the spermatogenic process in primates.

TABLE 2. Correlation between Spermatogenic Status and Testicular Testosterone and Dihydrotestosterone (DHT) Concentrations in GnRH Antagonist-treated and Testosterone-supplemented Monkeys[a]

Testicular Androgen	Spermatogonia	Spermatocytes	Round Spermatids	Elongated Spermatids
Testosterone	−0.09 $p > 0.70$	0.03 $p > 0.90$	−0.04 $p > 0.80$	0.16 $p > 0.50$
DHT	−0.18 $p > 0.50$	0.22 $p > 0.40$	0.25 $p > 0.30$	0.04 $p > 0.80$

[a] Seminiferous tubules were classified according to the presence of the most advanced germ cell type (spermatogonia, spermatocytes, round and elongated spermatids). (Data modified from ref. 24.)

Spermatogenesis and Testicular Testosterone

In two non-human primate studies,[20,24] conducted at our institute, testicular concentrations of androgens were determined in conjunction with evaluation of testicular histology and sperm numbers in the ejaculate. These sets of data enabled us to determine whether a direct relationship exists between intratesticular androgen levels and spermatogenic function in the non-human primate.

Administration of testosterone to hypophysectomized monkeys,[20] as described above, produced a clear-cut stimulatory effect on spermatogenesis which was comparable in all four animals. However, in two monkeys testicular testosterone concentrations were about 50% of baseline, whereas in the remaining two animals testicular testosterone levels were within the baseline range. In GnRH antagonist-treated monkeys[24] testicular testosterone and dihydrotestosterone (DHT) concentrations with and without concomitant testosterone substitution were determined. Within 15 weeks testis

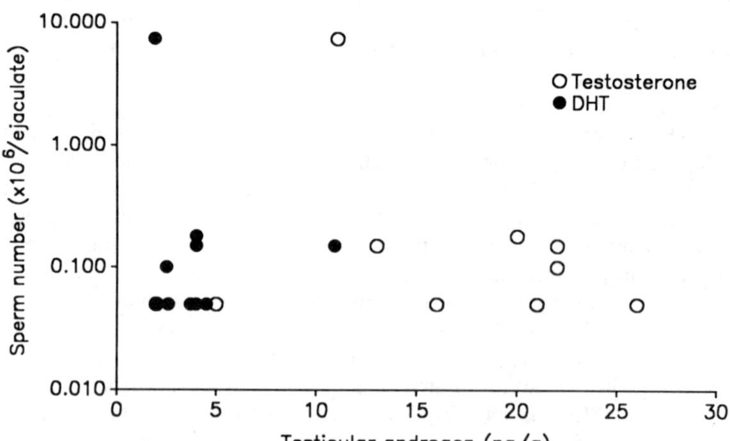

FIGURE 5. Relationship between sperm number in the ejaculate and testicular concentrations of testosterone and dihydrotestosterone (DHT) in monkeys (n = 5/group) treated for 15 weeks with GnRH antagonist or GnRH antagonist plus 40 mg or 200 mg testosterone ester. (Modified from ref. 24.)

levels of testosterone and DHT were reduced to 40–60% and 30–50% of pretreatment irrespective of treatment. Surprisingly, no correlation whatsoever could be found between testicular androgen concentrations and spermatogenic status (TABLE 2) or sperm number in the ejaculate (FIG. 5).

Firstly, these observations demonstrate that qualitative spermatogenesis can occur in the presence of markedly subnormal testicular androgen concentrations in the non-human primate. In this regard the non-human primate is apparently similar to many other non-primate species.[2,31] Secondly, a direct correlation between spermatogenic function and testicular androgen was obviously lacking. This observation is in agreement with findings derived from the rat model which have been reviewed recently.[2] Measurement of testosterone concentrations in testicular interstitial fluid, rete testis fluid, testicular tissue homogenates or seminiferous tubule fluid did not correlate with the degree of spermatogenesis.

Since testosterone is a potent stimulator of the spermatogenic process in many species, a closer relationship between germ cell development and androgens in the testis would be expected. Either our measurements of testicular androgen concentrations are not entirely representative or the trophic effects of exogenously administered testosterone involve additional factors besides androgens.

Role of Follicle-stimulating Hormone

To characterize the relative role of FSH in non-human primate testicular function, monkeys were immunized actively and passively against FSH.[32-35] In terms of endocrine effects it was found that active immunization against FSH specifically neutralized FSH but not LH, and testosterone production overall remained unaltered. Thus, by means of this experimental approach the specific role of FSH in spermatogenesis could be studied. Passive immunization against FSH induced a 50% decrease of testicular size and a pronounced reduction of sperm production within three months[32] (TABLE 3). The diameter of seminiferous tubules was reduced to about 60% of controls. Histological analysis revealed regression of the seminiferous epithelium with spermatogenic arrest in many tubules and some tubules contained only Sertoli cells. Similar effects on testicular parameters were observed following active immunization against FSH.[33,34]

Animals were rendered oligospermic and on several occasions ejaculates were de-

TABLE 3. Effects of Active Immunization with FSH on Testicular Volume and Sperm Number in the Non-human Primate.

Treatment (106 days)	Testicular Size[a] (ml)	Sperm Number[a] (mill./ejaculate)
Control		
pre	26.7 ± 3.3	360 ± 65
after	27.3 ± 5.9	339 ± 54
Immunized		
pre	23.9 ± 3.5	300 ± 23
after	12.2 ± 4.1	31 ± 10

[a] Mean values ± SD of four animals/group. (Modified from ref. 32.)

void of spermatozoa. Moudgal[35] reported that immunization against FSH in the non-human primate induced infertility evidenced by mating tests with females of proven fertility. These findings demonstrate that in the non-human primate FSH plays a pivotal role in the maintenance of the spermatogenic process. It is most important to note that testicular involution of FSH-immunized animals occurred in the presence of normal testosterone concentrations.

To clarify whether FSH is able to maintain testicular function in the absence of testosterone, the GnRH antagonist-treated non-human primate model was used.[36] Monkeys received GnRH antagonist treatment for a period of 16 weeks. During the first 8 weeks a highly purified human FSH preparation devoid of inherent LH bioactivity[37] (Fertinorm, Serono, Freiburg, F.R. Germany) was administered. Follicle-stimulating hormone markedly attenuated the GnRH antagonist-induced decline of testis size and germ cell numbers. Within 8 weeks GnRH antagonist administration alone reduced testis size and numbers of advanced spermatogenic cells to 25 and $<15\%$ of baseline, respectively, whereas in the presence of FSH these parameters were maintained at 60 and 50%, respectively. From these observations it is apparent that FSH alone can qualitatively maintain germ cell development in the non-human primate. The ability of FSH to maintain testicular function in men has not been studied so far.

Concerning the effects of exogenous FSH on non-human primate spermatogenesis it is pertinent to mention that FSH stimulates germ cell numbers even in the intact monkey.[38] Administration of a highly purified human FSH preparation significantly increased the numbers of Ap-spermatogonia, B-spermatogonia, pachytene spermatocytes and round spermatids within 16–28 days of treatment. Thus it would appear that in the intact primate, germ cell production may not be at a maximal level. Assuming that FSH also stimulates gametogenesis in men, therapy with FSH might be beneficial for infertile oligozoospermic patients, although a controlled clinical trial[39] for male infertility with hCG/hMG showed no improvement of seminal parameters. However, the FSH dose used in this trial and commonly used in related studies may not be sufficient to produce sustained circulating bioactive FSH levels since we could demonstrate that following intramuscular injection[40] the half-life in serum of bioactive FSH is much shorter than that of immunoreactive FSH.

REINITIATION OF THE SPERMATOGENIC PROCESS

Role of Testosterone

High doses of testosterone qualitatively restimulated spermatogenesis in the hypophysectomized monkeys as revealed by histological analysis.[41] Similarly, in pituitary stalk-sectioned non-human primates testosterone alone reinitiated testicular growth and the appearance of spermatozoa in the ejaculate.[42] Following a regression period of 10 weeks after transsection of the pituitary stalk, testosterone was administered for a 12-week period. At termination of androgen treatment testicular size was approximately 50% above pretreatment dimensions and the number of sperm/ejaculate increased markedly but did not reach the range of normal intact animals (FIG. 6).

In normal men whose sperm production had been suppressed during treatment with hCG or high doses of testosterone, LH or hCG qualitatively but not quantitatively reinitiated sperm production in the ejaculate.[30] Similarly, in hypogonadotropic patients hCG therapy alone resulted in the appearance of sperm numbers well below the normal

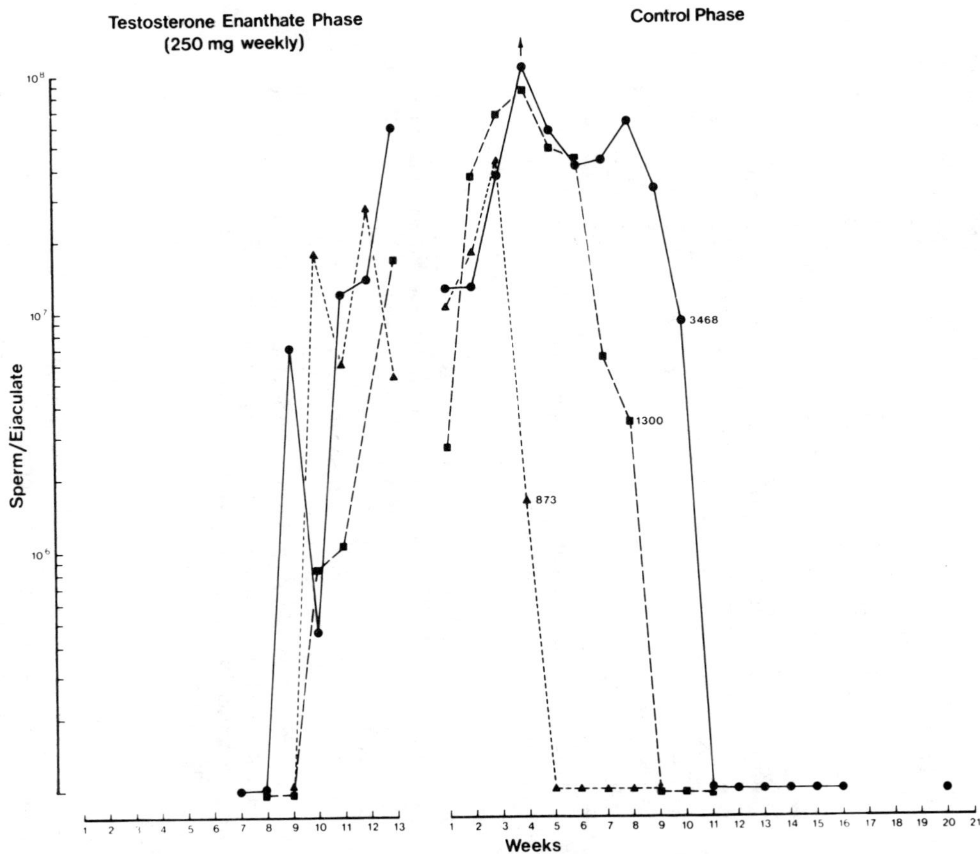

FIGURE 6. Individual sperm counts of pituitary stalk-sectioned monkeys treated with high doses of testosterone after a preceding 10-week period of testicular regression. (Reproduced from ref. 42 with permission.)

range.[43–45] Thus it is evident that testosterone alone can reinitiate spermatogenesis in the primate but not to a normal extent.

Evidence has accumulated indicating that maintenance and reinitiation of non-human primate spermatogenesis have differing androgen requirements. Amounts of testosterone which partially maintained sperm production in GnRH analog-suppressed animals[24,25,46] failed to restimulate the spermatogenic process.[47–49] These findings led us to suggest that a treatment regimen consisting of GnRH antagonist and *delayed* androgen administration might provide a feasible approach towards the development of an endocrine male contraceptive.[49] Two recent clinical male contraceptive trials with GnRH antagonist – based upon this suggestion – reported a high rate of azoospermia achieved with GnRH antagonist and *delayed* substitution of testosterone.[50,51]

Role of Follicle-stimulating Hormone

The ability of FSH alone to restore testicular function in a non-human primate was evaluated in the GnRH antagonist-treated animal model.[36] Human FSH given over a period of eight weeks stimulated germ cell numbers and even induced the formation of a few elongated spermatids. These effects of FSH, however, were much less pronounced when compared to the maintenance of the spermatogenic process.[36] In hCG-suppressed men FSH alone failed to completely reinitiate sperm numbers.[30] Thus it would appear that FSH alone is unable to restimulate primate spermatogenesis to a normal extent. Based on the findings described above that testosterone alone only reinitiates qualitatively normal spermatogenesis it has been inferred that FSH is needed along with androgens to fully normalize the spermatogenic function of the testis.

Several lines of evidence support the validity of this assumption. In out-of-season rhesus monkeys, who are hypogonadotropic and show spermatogenic arrest,[52] pulsatile administration of a GnRH agonist or native GnRH restored testicular function.[53] The beneficial effects of hMG on spermatogenesis were superior to those of LH alone in hypophysectomized patients.[54] That both LH/testosterone and FSH are necessary for reinitiation of complete spermatogenesis in the human is also supported by observations in hypogonadotropic patients subjected to pulsatile GnRH therapy[55] or combined treatment with testosterone/hCG and hMG.[45] It is concluded that in the primate FSH plays an essential role during reinitiation of the spermatogenic process. Consequently, any therapy regimen for hypogonadotropic hypogonadal men should involve both gonadotropic hormones.

CONCLUSIONS

The available information on the hormonal regulation of spermatogenesis in the primate demonstrates that in qualitative terms testosterone alone can initiate, maintain and reinitiate the spermatogenic process. Similarly, FSH alone is also capable of qualitatively maintaining and reinitiating germ cell development. It is likely that FSH alone would initiate complete spermatogenesis; this assumption, however, still awaits proof.

Although based partially on indirect evidence there is considerable support for the view that both androgens and FSH are required for the quantitative aspects of germ cell development. With regard to the effects of testosterone and FSH alone on spermatogenesis, higher doses of either hormone appear necessary for reinitiation as compared to maintenance of testicular function. Finally, the data available so far strongly suggest that the non-human primate is an appropriate surrogate for the study of endocrine regulation of testicular function in the human.

REFERENCES

1. MEANS, A., J. L. FAKUNDING, C. HUCKINS, D. J. TINDALL & R. VITALE. 1976. Follicle stimulating hormone, the Sertoli cell and spermatogenesis. Rec. Prog. Horm. Res. **32:** 477–527.
2. WEINBAUER, G. F. & E. NIESCHLAG. 1990. The role of testosterone in spermatogenesis. *In* Testosterone–Action, Deficiency, Substitution. E. Nieschlag & H. M. Behre, Eds.: 23–50. Springer Verlag. Heidelberg.
3. BOCCABELLA, A. V. 1963. Reinitiation and restoration of spermatogenesis with testosterone propionate and other hormones after long-term post-hypophysectomy regression period. Endocrinology **72:** 787–798.
4. SPITERI-GRECH, J., J. M. S. BARTLETT & E. NIESCHLAG. 1991. Hormonal regulation of epidermal growth factor and insulin-like growth factor-I in adult male hypophysectomized rats treated with ethane dimethane sulphonate. J. Endocrinol. **129:** 109–117.
5. TSUTSUMI, M., H. KURACHI & T. OKA. 1986. Physiological role of epidermal growth factor in male reproductive function. Science **233:** 975–977.
6. NIESCHLAG, E. & E. J. WICKINGS. 1980. Does the rhesus monkey provide a suitable model for human testicular function? *In* Animal Models in Human Reproduction. M. Serio & L. Martini, Eds.: 103–119 Raven Press. New York, NY.
7. ROBINSON, J. A. & W. E. BRIDSON. 1978. Neonatal hormone patterns in the macaque. I. Steroids. Biol. Reprod. **19:** 773–778.
8. STEINER, R. A. & W. J. BREMNER. 1981. Endocrine correlates of testicular development in the male monkey, *Macaca fascicularis*. Endocrinology **109:** 914–919.
9. SWERDLOFF, R. S. & D. HEBER. 1981. Endocrine control of testicular function from birth to puberty. *In* The Testis (Comprehensive Endocrinology). H. Burger & D. M. de Kretser, Eds.: 107–126. Raven Press. New York.
10. BIDLINGMAIER, F., H. G. DÖRR, W. EISENMENGER, U. KUHNLE & D. KNORR. 1983. Testosterone and androstendione concentrations in human testis and epididymis during the first two years of life. J. Clin. Endocrinol. Metab. **57:** 311–315.
11. KAR, A. B., H. CHANDRA & V. P. KAMBOJ. 1966. Effect of non-primate gonadotrophins on the testis of prepuberal rhesus monkeys. Acta Biol. Med. German. **16:** 450–455.
12. ARSLAN, M., P. ZAIDI, F. B. AKHTAR, S. AMIN, T. RANA & M. H. QAZI. 1981. Effects of gonadotrophin treatment *in vivo* on testicular function in immature rhesus monkeys (*Macaca mulatta*). Int. J. Androl. **4:** 462–474.
13. MARSHALL, G. R., E. J. WICKINGS & E. NIESCHLAG. 1984. Testosterone can initiate spermatogenesis in an immature nonhuman primate, *Macaca fascicularis*. Endocrinology **114:** 2228–2233.
14. STEINBERGER, E., A. ROOT, M. FICHER & K. D. SMITH. 1973. The role of androgens in the initiation of spermatogenesis in man. J. Clin. Endocrinol. Metab. **37:** 746–751.
15. CHEMES, H. E., T. PASQUALINI, M. A. RIVAROLA & C. BERGADA. 1982. Is testosterone involved in the initiation of spermatogenesis in humans? A clinicopathological presentation and physiological considerations in four patients with Leydig cell tumors of the testis or secondary Leydig cell hyperplasia. Int. J. Androl. **5:** 299–245.
16. BENNETT, W. I., M. L. DUFAU, K. J. CATT & W. W. TULLNER. 1973. Effect of human menopausal gonadotropin upon spermatogenesis and testosterone production in juvenile rhesus monkeys. Endocrinology **92:** 813–821.
17. ABEYAWARDENE, S. A., W. W. VALE, G. R. MARSHALL & T. M. PLANT. 1989. Circulating inhibin α concentrations in infant, prepubertal, and adult male rhesus monkeys (*Macaca mulatta*) and in juvenile monkeys during premature initiation of puberty with pulsatile gonadotropin-releasing hormone treatment. Endocrinology **125:** 250–256.
18. WICKINGS, E. J. & E. NIESCHLAG. 1978. The effects of active immunization with testosterone on pituitary-gonadal feedback in the male rhesus monkey (*Macaca mulatta*). Biol. Reprod. **18:** 602–607.

19. SMITH, P. E. 1942. Effect of equine gonadotropin on testes of hypophysectomized monkeys. Endocrinology **31:** 1–12.
20. MARSHALL, G. R., F. JOCKENHÖVEL, D. LÜDECKE & E. NIESCHLAG. 1986. Maintenance of complete but quantitatively reduced spermatogenesis in hypophysectomized monkeys by testosterone alone. Acta Endocrinol. **113:** 424–431.
21. SMITH, P. E. 1938. Comparative effects of hypophysectomy and therapy on the testes of monkeys and rats. *In* Les hormones sexuelles. L. Brouha, Ed. Comptes rendues: 601–605. Paris.
22. AKHTAR, F. B., G. F. WEINBAUER & E. NIESCHLAG. 1985. Acute and chronic effects of a gonadotrophin-releasing hormone antagonist on pituitary function in monkeys. J. Endocrinol. **104:** 345–354.
23. WEINBAUER, G. F., F. J. SURMANN, F. B. AKHTAR, G. V. SHAH, B. H. VICKERY & E. NIESCHLAG. 1984. Reversible inhibition of testicular function by a gonadotropin-releasing hormone antagonist in monkeys (*Macaca fascicularis*). Fertil. Steril. **42:** 906–914.
24. WEINBAUER, G. F., E. GÖCKELER & E. NIESCHLAG. 1988. Testosterone prevents complete suppression of spermatogenesis in the gonadotropin-releasing hormone (GnRH) antagonist-treated non-human primate (*Macaca fascicularis*). J. Clin. Endocrinol. Metab. **67:** 284–290.
25. WEINBAUER, G. F., F. J. SURMANN & E. NIESCHLAG. 1987. Suppression of spermatogenesis in a nonhuman primate (*Macaca fascicularis*) by concomitant gonadotropin-releasing hormone antagonist and testosterone treatment. Acta Endocrinol. **114:** 138–146.
26. WEINBAUER, G. F., G. R. MARSHALL & E. NIESCHLAG. 1986. New injectable testosterone ester maintains serum testosterone of castrated monkeys in the normal range for four months. Acta Endocrinol. **113:** 128–132.
27. SWERDLOFF, R. S., A. PALACIOS & R. D. MCCLURE. 1979. Suppression of human spermatogenesis by depot androgen: potential for male contraception. J. Steroid Biochem. **11:** 663–670.
28. NIESCHLAG, E., H. M. BEHRE & G. F. WEINBAUER. 1989. Hormonal methods for the regulation of male fertility. *In* Perspectives in Andrology. M. Serio, Ed: 517–529. Raven Press. New York.
29. BEHRE, H. M., D. NASHAN & E. NIESCHLAG. 1989. GnRH agonists attenuate the 19-nortestosterone-induced suppression of spermatogenesis in a clinical trial for male contraception. 71st Annual Meeting of the Endocrine Society, Seattle, WA. Abstr. 1638.
30. MATSUMOTO, A. M. 1989. Hormonal control of spermatogenesis. *In* The Testis. H. Burger, D. M. de Kretser, Eds. Second Edition: 181–196. Raven Press. New York.
31. CUNNINGHAM, G. R. & C. HUCKINS. 1979. Persistence of complete spermatogenesis in the presence of low intratesticular concentrations of testosterone. Endocrinology **105:** 177–186.
32. WICKINGS, E. J., K. H. USADEL, G. DATHE & E. NIESCHLAG. 1980. The role of follicle stimulating hormone in testicular function of the mature rhesus monkey. Acta Endocrinol. **95:** 117–128.
33. WICKINGS, E. J. & E. NIESCHLAG. 1980. Suppression of spermatogenesis over two years in rhesus monkeys actively immunized with follicle-stimulating hormone Fertil. Steril. **34:** 269–274.
34. SRINATH, B. R., E. J. WICKINGS, C. WITTING & E. NIESCHLAG. 1983. Active immunization with follicle-stimulating hormone for fertility control: a 4.5 year study in male rhesus monkeys. Fertil. Steril. **40:** 110–117.
35. MOUDGAL, N. R. 1981. A need for FSH in maintaining fertility of adult subhuman primates. Arch. Androl. **7:** 117–125.
36. WEINBAUER, G. F., H. M. BEHRE & E. NIESCHLAG. 1991. Effects of human FSH on testicular size and spermatogenesis in the GnRH antagonist-suppressed nonhuman primate. 11th North American Testis Workshop, Abstr. 4.
37. BARTLETT, J. M. S., G. F. WEINBAUER & E. NIESCHLAG. 1989. Differential effects of FSH and testosterone on the maintenance of spermatogenesis in the adult hypophysectomized rat. J. Endocrinol. **121:** 49–58.
38. VAN ALPHEN, M. M. A., H. J. G. VAN DE KANT & D. G. DE ROOIJ. 1988. Follicle-stimulating hormone stimulates spermatogenesis in the adult monkey. Endocrinology **123:** 1449–1455.
39. KNUTH, U. A., W. HÖNIGL, M. BALS-PRATSCH, G. SCHLEICHER & E. NIESCHLAG. 1987. Treatment of severe oligozoospermia with hCG/hMG. A placebo-controlled double-blind trial. J. Clin. Endocrinol. Metab. **65:** 1081–1087.
40. JOCKENHÖVEL, F., U. FINGSCHEIDT, S. A. KHAN, H. M. BEHRE & E. NIESCHLAG. 1990. Bio and immuno-activity of FSH in serum after intramuscular injection on highly purified human FSH in normal men. Clin. Endocrinol. **33:** 573–584.

41. SMITH, P. E. 1944. Maintenance and restoration of spermatogenesis in hypophysectomized rhesus monkeys by androgen administration. Yale J. Biol. Med. **17:** 283–287.

42. MARSHALL, G. R., E. J. WICKINGS & E. NIESCHLAG. 1983. Stimulation of spermatogenesis in stalk-sectioned rhesus monkeys by testosterone alone. J. Clin. Endocrinol. Metab. **57:** 152–159.

43. D'AGATA, R., J. J. HEINDEL, E. VICARI, A. ALIFFI, S. GULIZIA & P. POLOSA. 1984. hCG-Induced maturation of the seminiferous epithelium in hypogonadotropic men. Horm. Res. **19:** 23–32.

44. FINKEL, D. M., J. L. PHILLIPS & P. J. SNYDER. 1985. Stimulation of spermatogenesis by gonadotropins in men with hypogonadotropic hypogonadism. New Engl. J. Med. **313:** 651–655.

45. JOHNSON, S. G. 1978. Maintenance of spermatogenesis induced by hMG treatment by means of continuous hCG treatment in hypogonadotrophic men. Acta Endocrinol. **89:** 763–769.

46. AKHTAR, F. B., G. R. MARSHALL & E. NIESCHLAG. 1983. Testosterone supplementation attenuates the antifertility effects of an LH-RH agonist in male monkeys. Int. J. Androl. **6:** 461–468.

47. AKHTAR, F. B., G. R. MARSHALL, E. J. WICKINGS & E. NIESCHLAG. 1983. Reversible induction of azoospermia in rhesus monkeys by constant infusion of a GnRH agonist using osmotic minipumps. J. Clin. Endocrinol. Metab. **56:** 534–540.

48. WEINBAUER, G. F., M. RESPONDEK, H. THEMANN & E. NIESCHLAG. 1987. Reversibility of long-term effects of GnRH agonist administration on testicular histology and sperm production in the non-human primate. J. Androl. **8:** 319–329.

49. WEINBAUER, G. F., S. KHURSHID, U. FINGSCHEIDT & E. NIESCHLAG. 1989. Sustained inhibition of sperm production and inhibin secretion induced by a gonadotrophin-releasing hormone antagonist and delayed testosterone substitution in non-human primates (*Macaca fascicularis*). J. Endocrinol. **123:** 303–310.

50. SWERDLOFF, R. S., S. BHASIN, W. SALAMEH, L. TOM, M. PETERSON & B. STEINER. 1990. Combined GnRH antagonist and testosterone enanthate for experimental male contraception. Gynecol. Endocrinol. **4:** 28. (Abstract)

51. BASTIAS, M. C., H. KAMIJO & S. N. PAVLOU. 1991. Suppression of spermatogenesis by a GnRH antagonist plus testosterone in normal men does not affect sperm motion parameters (SMP). 16th Annual Meeting American Soc. Androl., Abstr. 39.

52. WICKINGS, E. J. & E. NIESCHLAG. 1980. Seasonality in endocrine and exocrine function of the adult rhesus monkey (*Macaca mulatta*) maintained in a controlled laboratory environment. Int. J. Androl. **3:** 87–104.

53. WICKINGS, E. J., P. ZAIDI, G. BRABANT & E. NIESCHLAG. 1981. Stimulation of pituitary and testicular functions with LH-RH agonist or pulsatile LH-RH treatment in the rhesus monkey during the non-breeding season. J. Reprod. Fertil. **63:** 129–136.

54. MANCINI, R. E. 1969. Effect of different types of gonadotrophins on the induction and restoration of spermatogenesis in the human testis. Acta Eur. Fertil. **1:** 401–429.

55. FINKELSTEIN, J. S., L. S. L. O'DEA, D. I. SPRATT & W. F. CROWLEY, JR. 1987. Pulsatile GnRH therapy in men with idiopathic hypogonadotropic hypogonadism. *In* Highlights on Endocrinology. C. Christiansen & B. J. Riis, Eds.: 333–342. Proceedings of the First European Congress on Endocrinology. Copenhagen.

Thyroid Hormones and Testis Development: A Model System for Increasing Testis Growth and Sperm Production

PAUL S. COOKE[a]

Department of Veterinary Biosciences
University of Illinois, Urbana
2001 S. Lincoln Avenue
Urbana, Illinois 61801

INTRODUCTION

The possible involvement of thyroid hormones in the growth, maturation and function of the testis has been studied extensively, but the precise role of these hormones in the testis remains elusive. In this chapter, we will discuss the previous often conflicting work that attempted to address this problem, and will place special emphasis on recent work which has indicated that thyroid hormones may be important for the early development of the testis. In addition, we will describe a model system we have developed in which pronounced increases in testis size and sperm production in the rat can be obtained by perturbing the thyroid hormone environment during early postnatal life. Our work emphasizes the importance of thyroid hormones for early testicular development, and may be a useful tool to define the precise nature of thyroid hormone-testis interactions. Furthermore, because this experimental system allows unprecedented increases in testicular size and sperm production, it may also be useful for studying the factors which normally control testicular growth and sperm production and may facilitate understanding of how the set-point for these two parameters are normally established.

Thyroid hormones have not been viewed as major factors in the regulation of adult testicular function because of evidence indicating a lack of sensitivity and dependence of this organ on thyroid hormones for normal functioning. For example, early work indicated that thyroxine (T4) did not have a metabolic effect on adult testes,[1] and Oppenheimer *et al.*[2] show that triiodothyronine (T3) receptor concentrations are low in the adult rat. In agreement with these observations are several reports that hypothyroidism in the adult male rat does not affect testicular size or seminiferous tubule morphology,[3,4] but this point is controversial and others[5] have suggested that hypothyroidism in the adult rat causes degenerative changes in seminiferous tubule morphology.

The effects of thyroid hormone deficiency on testicular development in young ani-

[a] Address correspondence to Dr. Paul S. Cooke at the address above; tel. (217) 333–6825.

mals are also controversial. Early work indicated that hypothyroidism in young rats caused only slight decreases in testicular size,[6] while later work[7,8] indicated hypothyroidism during juvenile life severely impairs gametogenesis. However, even assuming that thyroid hormone deficiency does impair testicular growth and spermatogenesis in developing animals, it was not clear from these studies whether thyroid hormones have direct effects on the testis and the process of spermatogenesis or are simply permissive for normal testicular development due to their important role in all aspects of growth, development and metabolism.[9,10]

In contrast to previous reports, recent developments in this field indicate that thyroid hormones may have an important, direct role in early testicular development. This rapidly emerging body of evidence may necessitate a reevaluation of the role of thyroid hormones in testicular development. Jannini *et al.*[11] recently demonstrated that high levels of T3 receptors are present in the developing fetal and neonatal testis, then decline during subsequent development to become virtually absent in the adult. These T3 receptors were present exclusively in the Sertoli cells, the primary regulators of sperm production.[11] Additional evidence supporting a direct role for thyroid hormones in early testicular development comes from the observations that cultured Sertoli cells from young hypothyroid rats produce less insulin-like growth factor I (IGF-I) than do Sertoli cells from euthyroid controls.[12] Furthermore, T3 administration directly stimulated IGF-I production by these cultured Sertoli cells.[12] The involvement of thyroid hormones in the production of IGF-I, which has potent mitogenic and differentiative effects on a variety of cell types, strongly suggests a direct role of these hormones in testicular development and maturation.

We have recently developed a model system which emphasizes the involvement of thyroid hormones in early testicular development,[13,14] and along with the work discussed above may lead to a more complete understanding of the precise role of thyroid hormones in the testis. In this system, transient hypothyroidism during the neonatal period results in increases of 80% and 140% in testis weight and sperm production, respectively, when these animals reach adulthood.[13,14] A brief history of the development of this system will be presented, followed by a discussion of the results obtained to date.

The role of thyroid hormones in the processes of postnatal neuronal maturation and growth are well established. Less studied, however, is the degree to which an animal can recover, both in terms of growth and neuronal maturation, if euthyroidism is reestablished after a period of hypothyroidism early in development. In order to address this question, a model system was developed in which rats were made hypothyroid from birth until day 25 postnatal, then allowed to recover to a euthyroid state.[10,15-17] Their catch-up growth and improved neuronal function during and after the period of recovery to euthyroidism were then documented. While examining growth changes in animals following transient hypothyroidism, Meisami[10] noted that testis size was increased in these rats at 90 days of age.

This unexpected observation that transient hypothyroidism early in development altered testicular size in the adult months later posed many interesting questions. For example, was the increased testicular size due to disease or damage to the testes, or did it represent true growth? Was the increase transitory or permanent, and if it was permanent, what was the ultimate magnitude of the change in testicular size? Was the increase in testicular size also accompanied by changes in functional parameters (*e.g.*, sperm production and testosterone levels)? Finally, the most intriguing question was how could a brief period of neonatal hypothyroidism **increase** testis growth and sperm production? The neonatal period is a time of active testis growth and Sertoli and Leydig cell proliferation,[18-21] but is long before the testicular growth spurt and the onset of spermatogenesis which occurs at puberty. All available literature suggests that hypothyroidism and even hyperthyroidism at all age periods examined had inhibitory effects, if any, on testis growth and function. The observation that transient hypothyroidism increased testis size in the adult was therefore very contraintuitive and no obvious precedent or mechanism for this type of effect presented itself.

In order to fully document and begin to determine the mechanism of this phenomenon, we have examined many aspects of the testicular and endocrine changes which occur in adult animals following transient hypothyroidism early in development. These results are described in detail below.

METHOD FOR INDUCTION OF TESTICULAR ORGANOMEGALY

To induce increased testicular size and sperm production in adult rats, male Sprague-Dawley pups are made hypothyroid from birth to day 25 of life by adding the goitrogen 6-propyl-2-thiouracil (PTU; 0.1%) to the mother's drinking water immediately after birth.[13,14] PTU ingested by the mother is transferred to the pups through the milk, and results in severe hypothyroidism in the pups.[16] PTU is a reversible goitrogen which inhibits iodine uptake and thyroxine synthesis in the thyroid, and also inhibits peripheral deiodination of T4 to T3.[17]

At 25 days of age, the pups are weaned and PTU treatment is discontinued. The pups given PTU, subsequently designated "treated," are then given tap water through the rest of the experiment and allowed to recover to the euthyroid state.

EFFECTS OF PTU TREATMENT ON BODY GROWTH

Growth of treated rats was reduced by approximately 50% during the period of PTU treatment.[10,13] A few days after PTU treatment was stopped, the rats began growing rapidly and their subsequent growth paralleled that of controls (FIG. 1). However, the weight of these animals never equalled that of controls, and remained 15%–25% less at all subsequent ages.[10,13]

TSH, T4 AND T3 LEVELS IN PTU-TREATED AND CONTROL RATS

Administration of PTU to the drinking water of the mother increased blood TSH levels 4- and 10-fold in the mother and pups, respectively, at 25 days of age, while T4 levels in both were completely suppressed.[16] Following the cessation of PTU treatment, TSH levels fell while T4 and T3 levels rose. For example, by 50 days of age, TSH levels in treated rats were not different from controls, T4 levels were slightly reduced (4.24 ± 0.50 μg/100 ml versus 5.67 ± 0.25 μg/100 ml), and T3 levels were normal (86.88 ± 8.85 ng/100 ml in treated vs. 89.32 ± 8.45 ng/ml in controls).[16] By 90 days of age, TSH, T4 and T3 levels were normal in treated rats.[13,16]

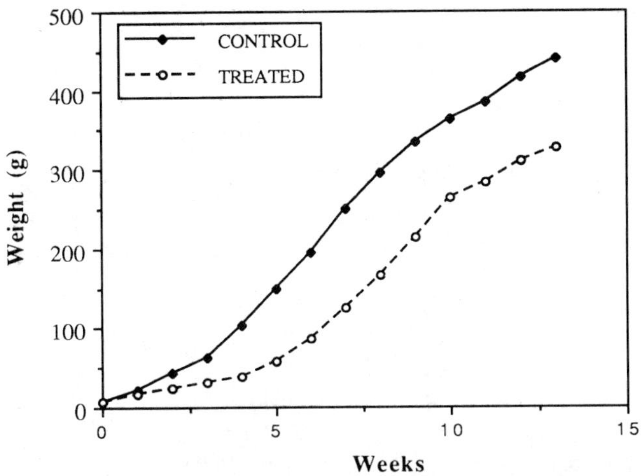

FIGURE 1. Growth of rats that were untreated (control) compared to those given PTU from birth to day 25. Data points are mean values for at least 12 rats in each group. The SEM is not shown but in all cases was less than 6 g. The body weights of treated rats were significantly ($p < 0.05$) lower than controls beginning at one week of age. Body weight decreases in treated animals compared to controls were also seen at 135, 160, and 180 days, and were similar in magnitude to those at 90 days of age.

TESTIS GROWTH IN TREATED RATS

Testis weights of treated rats were 40% greater than control rats at 90 days of age despite a 20% decrease in body weight (FIG. 2).[13] Testicular size normally plateaus in control rats at approximately 90–100 days of age,[13,22] but this was not true for the treated rats. Testis weight in these animals did not plateau until after 135 days in these animals, and by day 160 of age it was over 80% greater than normal[13] (FIG. 2). This increase in testicular weight represented hyperplasia and was accompanied by concomitant increases in testicular DNA content.[13] Non-reproductive organs such as kidney, brain and salivary glands all showed weight decreases similar to that of body weight, and pituitary gland weight was also decreased by about 20%.[13]

MORPHOLOGICAL AND HISTOLOGICAL CHANGES IN THE TREATED TESTES

Testes from treated rats were morphologically normal despite their increased size.[13] Histological examination of the testes from treated rats revealed no overt pathologies, although there were clear histological changes in the treated testes.[23] The overall number of seminiferous tubules per cross section of testis was not increased, but the average diameter of the tubules was increased by approximately 20%.[23] All stages of sperm maturation from spermatogonia to fully formed spermatozoa were present, and preliminary work suggests that the numbers of cells in the different stages of germ cell development per tubule are increased. For example, there was an average of 54%

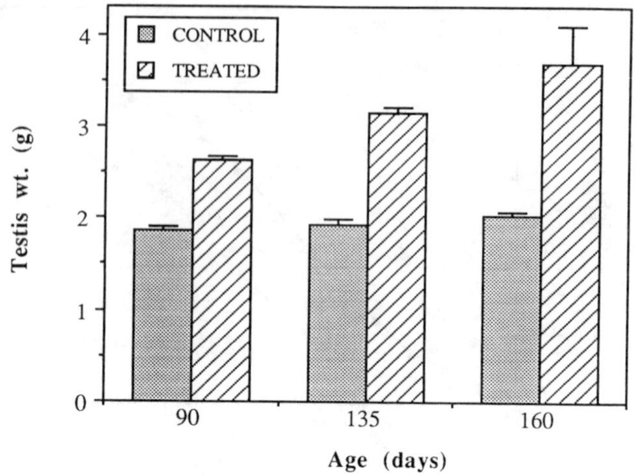

FIGURE 2. Wet weight of testes from control and PTU treated rats at various ages. Bars represent mean ± SEM weights of single testes. The n was ≥24 for all groups. Testis weights were increased 40%, 62%, and 82% at 90, 135, and 160 days, respectively, and were significantly ($p < 0.05$) higher in treated animals at all ages.

more primary spermatocytes per seminiferous tubule cross section in the treated than in the control rats.[23] These findings suggest that the testes of the treated animals are producing sperm, and that the magnitude of that production may be increased compared to controls.

SPERM PRODUCTION IN TREATED ANIMALS

To compare sperm production in treated and control rats, we measured daily sperm production (DSP) and epididymal sperm reserves in both these types of animals using the procedures outlined by Robb *et al.*[22] The increased size of the testes in treated rats is accompanied by increased sperm production.[14] Daily sperm production (DSP) in treated animals increases in concert with the increase in testis size, and peaks at 160 days of age, when DSP is 140% greater than controls (FIG. 3). The greater increase in DSP relative to testes size in the treated animals reflects the fact that the efficiency of sperm production (DSP/g testis) is increased in the treated animals, and the final increase in sperm production therefore represents the multiplicative effect of the increased testicular size and increased efficiency of sperm production.[14]

FERTILITY IN TREATED ANIMALS

The inhibitory effects of hypothyroidism on sperm motility and fertility have been documented in several species.[24] However, it was not known if transient hypothyroidism, in this case before spermatogenesis begins, would have any lasting effects on sperm motility and fertility during adulthood. Our preliminary results indicate that

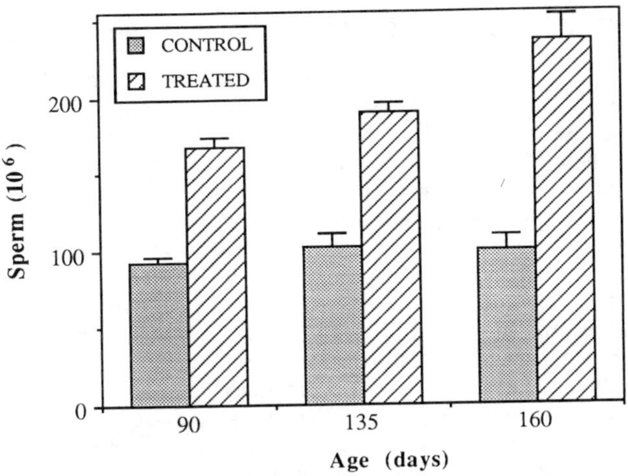

FIGURE 3. Daily sperm production (DSP) in control rats and neonatally hypothyroid rats (treated with PTU from birth to day 25). Data are presented as mean ± SEM. DSP in treated rats was increased 80%, 93%, and 136% compared to controls at 90, 135, and 160 days, respectively. This increase was significant ($p < 0.05$) in the treated compared to the control rats at all ages.

sperm concentration and motility were normal in 90-day treated animals.[13] These treated rats were also fertile, and sired litters of normal size which were without developmental defects.[13] Therefore, transient hypothyroidism in the neonatal period appears to have no deleterious effects on the reproductive ability of these animals when they reach adulthood.

TESTOSTERONE LEVELS IN TREATED ANIMALS

Despite increased testis size and increased sperm production, serum testosterone (T) levels were not increased in the treated animals relative to the controls at any age during adulthood.[13] Therefore, the increased testis growth and function is apparently not dependent on or accompanied by increases in T.

EFFECTS OF DIFFERENT PATTERNS OF PTU EXPOSURE

The PTU treatment protocol used in these studies was originally developed to examine catchup growth and neurological recovery in animals which had been transiently hypothyroid, as described above. The effectiveness of PTU treatments from birth to day 25 raises several additional questions about the possible effects of this drug during other periods of life. For example, is the immediate postnatal period the only time when PTU treatment followed by recovery results in eventual increases in testicular size, or can this phenomenon be obtained by transient PTU treatment at any stage of an animal's life? Is the full 25-day course of PTU treatment necessary to produce this effect, or can shorter treatments produce equal or possibly greater increases in testicular size?

To address these questions, we have recently begun experiments in which rats are treated with PTU for different durations of time starting either at birth or at various postnatal times. Our preliminary results indicate that PTU treatments beginning at birth and continuing for various lengths of time (9, 17 or 25 days) produce gradations of increases in testicular size and sperm production which are proportional to the length of PTU exposure; these gradations are apparent at 90 days of age, but become even more pronounced at 135 days of age. These results suggest that the longer PTU treatment is given during the neonatal period, the greater the adult testis size that is obtained after the animal is allowed to recover to euthyroidism and mature.

When rats are treated with PTU from day 24 to days 32 or 48, no increases in testis size were seen when these animals reached 90 or even 135 days of age, indicating that PTU treatment starting on day 24 postnatal or later appears to be ineffective in increasing adult testicular size. Thus, PTU exposure must occur within the first 25 days of life to be effective in producing eventual increases in testicular size and sperm production. The effects of PTU treatments of various durations and beginning at various ages will be described in detail in a separate paper (Cooke, P. S., J. Porcelli & R. A. Hess. Induction of increased testis growth in the adult rat by transient early hypothyroidism: The critical period. Manuscript submitted to Biol. Reprod.)

ARE THE INCREASES IN TESTIS WEIGHT DUE TO DIRECT PTU EFFECTS?

The drug used to induce hypothyroidism in these studies, PTU, is a potent goitrogen which is somewhat toxic. This raises the possibility that the increased testicular growth seen in the neonatally treated rats might not be a result of hypothyroidism *per se*, but instead could result from direct effects of the PTU on the testis or other structures (*e.g.*, pituitary). To test this possibility, neonatal rats were treated with PTU from birth to day 25 as usual, but were also given T4 and T3 replacement during this period. At 90 days of age, the characteristic increase in testicular growth seen in PTU-treated animals was not observed and testis size was approximately normal.[13] Thus, increases in testicular size caused by neonatal PTU treatment are a result of hypothyroidism rather than a direct effect of the PTU itself.

DISCUSSION

Our results indicate that transient postnatal hypothyroidism dramatically increases testis weight and sperm production in the adult rat.[13,14] The magnitudes of the increases in both these parameters are unique and far greater than can be obtained with other experimental methodologies. The observed increases in testis weight are not accompanied by any pathological changes in the testes, and there are concomitant increases in DNA content which indicate that this weight increase represents true growth.[13] Despite these changes in testicular size and sperm production, sperm motility and concentration in the epididymal fluid were normal, and these males were fertile.[14]

Previous work indicated that early hypothyroidism impaired or did not affect testicular development and spermatogenesis.[6-8] Conversely, our results indicate that **transient** hypothyroidism during the suckling period followed by recovery to the euthyroid state significantly increases testis size and sperm production in the adult. Therefore, it appears that not only can the deleterious effects caused by early hypothyroidism be reversed by allowing the animal to become euthyroid again, but this treatment may actually be stimulatory to testis growth and sperm production in the adult.[13,14]

Extensive progress has been made in the last few decades in establishing the roles that follicle stimulating hormone (FSH), luteinizing hormone (LH), testosterone (T) and other hormones and growth factors play in the processes of testicular growth and spermatogenesis.[20,21] However, many important questions remain. For example, how is adult testis size normally specified and why does the testis stop growing when adult size is reached despite the continued presence of high levels of trophic hormones. Likewise, only fragmentary information exists on the role of thyroid hormones in testicular development and sperm production despite work extending back to the early part of this century indicating they may be involved in testicular development.[6]

If the factors responsible for the increase in testicular growth and sperm production in this system can be determined, they may yield important insights into the normal processes that act during development to specify testis size and levels of sperm production. Similarly, elucidation of the mechanism by which transient hypothyroidism eventually results in marked changes in the testis may be useful for understanding the role of thyroid hormones in normal testicular development and function.

In addition to its possible uses as a model system to study various questions relating to the control of testicular growth and function, this system may also have a more practical application. Owing to the large and unprecedented increases in sperm production which can be produced with this system, it may be useful for increasing reproductive efficiency in economically important animals. In many animals, including the rat, the normal ejaculate contains many times more sperm than are necessary for maximal fertility. Further increases in sperm production in these animals would obviously have no demonstrable benefit for reproduction. However, in animals in which artificial insemination is routinely used, an increase in sperm production of the magnitude seen here may dramatically lower the cost per unit of semen and translate into a significant economic impact. Another advantage of this methodology is that it would allow increased sperm production to be obtained from particularly desirable or valuable males, and here again has the potential for a positive economic impact.

Although the transient hypothyroidism system is the first in which testis size and sperm production can be increased by such a dramatic degree, smaller increases in testicular size and sperm production have been seen with other methodologies. Unilateral castration of rats and a variety of other animals early in postnatal life induces a compensatory hypertrophy in the remaining testicle.[25-27] This system has been used extensively as a model to examine the hormonal and other factors involved in testis growth. Although the magnitude of the increase in the remaining testis following unilateral castration varies with species and the age at which the procedure is performed, the maximal testicular growth increase normally obtained is on the order of about 25%,[25] far less than can be obtained with our system. Likewise, although sperm production in the remaining testicle is slightly increased, overall sperm production is far less than normal, again in contrast to our system in which increases of over 140%

can be obtained. Another complication of the neonatal castration model is that it requires unilateral orchidectomy of neonatal or young animals, a technically demanding operation in laboratory species such as the rat, while our procedure is non-invasive.

Another procedure in which increases in testis growth and sperm production are obtained involves immunizing males against estradiol (E2).[28,29] This system was developed to examine the role of E2 feedback in gonadotropin production and has yielded important information in this area. However, the increases in testis size and sperm production obtained with this methodology are far less than in our system, and the complications of immunizing, assessing titers, giving booster injections, etc. make this methodology more technically difficult than the neonatal hypothyroidism system.

Very little is known about the mechanism by which PTU treatment and the subsequent hypothyroidism early in development results in increased testis growth and sperm production during later life. Our preliminary results in which PTU administration plus thyroid hormone replacement over the first 25 days of life did not result in the increased testis growth when these animals reach adulthood suggests that this effect is caused by hypothyroidism and is not a direct effect of the PTU.[13] The normal T levels in the rats with increased testis size and sperm production also argues that increases in this hormone are not a causative factor in the observed testis changes in these animals.[14]

Despite a lack of any definitive evidence, there are some hormones which are obvious candidates to be involved in some aspect of the testis effect seen in this system. FSH plays important roles in both the perinatal and pubertal development of the testes.[18,20,21] This hormone is also transiently increased in animals following unilateral castration,[25] and is thought to play a role in the compensatory testicular growth which occurs in these animals. Thus, one possible mechanism to explain this effect is that FSH may be increased during the period after hypothyroidism or the responsiveness of target cells to FSH may be increased.

Thyroid hormone receptors are extensively present in the developing testis,[11] and thyroid hormones stimulate IGF-I production in cultured Sertoli cells from young animals,[12] as discussed previously. Although thyroid hormones apparently never exceed normal levels during the period of recovery from hypothyroidism,[13,16] the cells of the testis or other organs may have an increased sensitivity to these hormones as a result of deprivation during the hypothyroidism period, and the resurgence of thyroid hormones in the period after PTU treatment may therefore be responsible for the changes which produce the observed testicular effects. A wide variety of other plausible mechanisms for this effect can also be suggested, and experiments aimed at conclusively determining the mechanism of this effect are presently underway.

SUMMARY

In conclusion, the unique transient hypothyroidism system described here provides a noninvasive means by which testicular size and sperm production can be increased to unprecedented degrees. This system may be useful as a model for understanding the factors which regulate testicular growth and the eventual size that the testes attain, as well as the factors which normally establish and then maintain the amount of sperm produced by an animal.

ACKNOWLEDGMENTS

The author wishes to thank Drs. Essie Meisami and Rex Hess for their collaborative efforts in the studies described here, John Porcelli for his expert technical assistance in all aspects of this work, and Dr. David Bunick for proofreading the manuscript.

REFERENCES

1. BARKER, S. B. & H. W. KLITGAARD. 1952. Metabolism of tissues excised from thyroxine-injected rats. Am. J. Physiol. **170:** 81–86.
2. OPPENHEIMER, J. H., H. L. SCHWARTZ & M. I. SUKS. 1974. Tissue differences in the concentration of triiodothyronine nuclear binding sites in the rat: Liver, kidney, pituitary, heart, brain, spleen and testis. Endocrinology **95:** 897–903.
3. WEISS, S. R. & J. M. BURNS. 1988. The effect of acute treatment with two goitrogens on plasma thyroid hormones, testosterone and testicular morphology in adult male rats. Comp. Biochem. Physiol. **90:** 449–452.
4. VILCHEZ-MARTINEZ, J. A. 1973. Study of the pituitary-testicular axis in hypothyroid adult male rats. J. Reprod. Fertil. **35:** 123–126.
5. AMIN, S. O. & A. S. EL-SHEIKH. 1977. Pituitary-testicular function in hypothyroid male rats. Acta Anat. **98:** 121–129.
6. GOMES, W. R. 1970. Metabolic and regulatory hormones influencing testis function. *In* The Testis. A. D. Johnson, W. R. Gomes & N. L. Vandemark, Eds.: 68–138. Academic Press. New York.
7. CHOWDURY, A. R. & U. ARORA. 1984. Role of thyroid in testicular development of immature rat. Arch. Androl. **12:** 49–51.
8. CHOWDURY, A. R., A. K. GAUTAM & B. B. CHATTERJEE. 1984. Thyroid-testis interrelationship during the development and sexual maturity of the rat. Arch. Androl. **13:** 233–239.
9. COOKE, P. S., C. U. YONEMURA & C. S. NICOLL. 1984. Development of thyroid hormone dependence for growth in the rat: A study involving transplanted fetal, neonatal and juvenile tissues. Endocrinology **115:** 2059–2064.
10. MEISAMI, E. 1984. Complete recovery of growth deficits after reversal of PTU-induced postnatal hypothyroidism in the female rat: A model for catch-up growth. Life Sci. **34:** 1487–1496.
11. JANNINI, E A., M. OLIVIERI, S. FRANCAVILLA, A. GULINO, E. ZIPARO & M. D'ARMIENTO. 1990. Ontogenesis of the nuclear 3,5,3′-triiodothyronine receptor in the rat testis. Endocrinology **126:** 2521–2526.
12. PALMERO, S., M. PRATI, A. BARRECA, F. MINUTO, G. GIORDANO & E. FUGASSA. 1990. Thyroid hormone stimulates the production of insulin-like growth factor I (IGF-I) by immature rat Sertoli cells. Mol. Cell. Endocrinol. **68:** 61–65.
13. COOKE, P. S. & E. MEISAMI, 1991. Early postnatal hypothyroidism causes increases adult size of testis and other reproductive organs but does not increase testosterone levels. Endocrinology **129:** 237–243.
14. COOKE, P. S., R. A. HESS, J. PORCELLI & E. MEISAMI. 1991. Increased sperm production in adult rats following transient neonatal hypothyroidism. Endocrinology **129:** 244–248.
15. TAMASY, V., E. MEISAMI, J.-Z. DU & P. S. TIMIRAS. 1986. Exploratory behavior, learning ability, and thyroid hormonal responses to stress in female rats rehabilitating from postnatal hypothyroidism. Devel. Psychobiol. **19:** 537–553.
16. TAMASY, V., E. MEISAMI, A. VALLERGA & P. S. TIMIRAS. 1986. Rehabilitation from neonatal hypothyroidism: spontaneous motor activity, exploratory behavior, avoidance learning and response of pituitary-thyroid axis to stress in male rats. Psychoneuroendocrinology **11:** 91–103.
17. TAMASY, V., J.-Z. DU, A. VALLERGA, E. MEISAMI & P. S. TIMIRAS. 1984. Suckling ability and maternal prolactin levels in hypothyroid rats. Horm. Behav. **18:** 457–464.
18. ORTH, J. 1984. The role of follicle stimulating hormone in controlling Sertoli cell proliferation in testes of fetal rats. Endocrinology **115:** 1248–1255.
19. HARDY, M. P., B. R. ZIRKIN & L. L. EWING. 1989. Kinetic studies on the development of the adult population of Leydig cells in testes of the pubertal rat. Endocrinology **124:** 762–770.

20. Bellve, A. R. & W. Zheng. 1989. Growth factors as autocrine and paracrine modulators of male gonadal functions. J. Reprod. Fertil. **85:** 771–793.
21. Heindel, J. J. & K. A. Treinen. 1989. Physiology of the male reproductive system: Endocrine, paracrine and autocrine regulation. Toxicol. Pathol. **17:** 411–445.
22. Robb, G. W., R. P. Amann & G. J. Killian. 1978. Daily sperm production and epididymal sperm reserves of pubertal and adult rats. J. Reprod. Fertil. **54:** 103–107.
23. Meisami, E. & P. S. Cooke. 1990. Male reproductive organomegaly in rats recovering from early hypothyroidism. Program of the 72nd Annual Meeting of the Endocrine Society, Atlanta, GA. (Abstract 445).
24. Chandrasekhar, Y., M. K. Holland, M. J. D'Occhio & B. P. Setchell. 1985. Spermatogenesis, seminal characteristics and reproductive hormone levels in mature rams with induced hypothyroidism and hyperthyroidism. J. Endocrinol. **105:** 39–46.
25. Brown, J. L. & P. K. Chakraborty. 1991. Comparison of compensatory pituitary and testicular responses to hemicastration between prepubertal and mature rats. J. Androl. **12:** 119–125.
26. Cunningham, G. R., D. J. Tindall, C. Huckins & A. R. Means. 1978. Mechanisms for the testicular hypertrophy which follows hemicastration. Endocrinology **102:** 16–23.
27. Frankel, A. I. & W. W. Wright. 1982. The hemicastrated rat: definition of a model for the study of the regulation of testicular steroidogenesis. J. Endocrinol. **92:** 225–229.
29. Schanbacher, B. D., J. Pelletier & M. T. Hocherrau-de Reviers. 1987. Follicle stimulating hormone, luteinizing hormone and testicular Leydig cell responses to estradiol immunization in Ile-de-France rams. J. Androl. **8:** 97–102.
29. Monet-Kunz, C., M. T. Hochereau-de Reviers, C. Pisselet, C. Perreau, I. Fontaine & B. D. Schanbacher. 1988. Endocrine parameters, hormone receptors and functions of the testicular interstitium and seminiferous epithelium in estradiol-immunized Ile-de France rams. J. Androl. **9:** 278–283.

The Patterns of LH Secretion in Adult Male Rats Associated with Compensatory Androgen Secretion by the Testis Remaining after Unilateral Orchidectomy

DAVID K. POMERANTZ[a] AND WERNER J. DEBERTIN

Departments of Physiology and Obstetrics & Gynaecology
University of Western Ontario
London, Ontario, Canada, N6A 5C1

BERNARD ROBAIRE

Department of Pharmacology and Therapeutics
Centre for the Study of Reproduction
McGill University
Montréal, Québec, Canada H3G 1Y6

INTRODUCTION

A fundamental concept in regulation of testicular function is the operation of a negative feedback system whereby pituitary gonadotropins stimulate testicular functions, such as secretion of testosterone, which in turn inhibit the secretion of pituitary gonadotropins. The existence of this type of regulation in the hypothalamic/pituitary-testicular axis has been confirmed over the years by ample demonstration of LH stimulation of testosterone secretion and an increase in gonadotropin secretion after orchidectomy. The operation of such a negative feedback system in the regulation of pituitary and gonadal secretions under physiological conditions has been more difficult to demonstrate.

One of the classic methods for investigating the operation of endocrine feedback systems is removal of one member of a pair of endocrine organs and study of the ensuing compensatory responses of the contralateral organ. Such studies have led to descriptions of follicle-stimulating hormone (FSH)-dependent ovarian hypertrophy after unilateral ovariectomy[1,2] and neurally mediated adrenal compensatory hypertrophy after unilateral adrenalectomy.[3] While testicular compensatory hypertrophy does not occur after unilateral orchidectomy of the adult rat, circulating testosterone does return to control levels within 8 h of hemiorchidectomy. This compensatory secretory response is associated with increased concentration of testosterone in the re-

[a] Address correspondence to D. K. Pomerantz, Ph.D. at the Department of Physiology; Tel: (519) 661 3473; FAX: (519) 661 3872.

maining testis as well as an increase in the concentration of testosterone in the testicular venous effluent of the remaining gonad.[4-6] While a negative feedback model for control of androgen secretion would predict a period of relative hypersecretion of LH to elicit the increase in testosterone output by the remaining gonad, this has not been demonstrated in spite of numerous attempts.[7-10] Thus, the mechanism by which the initial increase of testosterone secretion by the surviving gonad is mediated after hemiorchidectomy remains unknown.

As the earlier studies of LH secretion used single blood samples, repeated samples by heart puncture, or repeated samples obtained via indwelling cannulae, but infrequently and in an uncontrolled environment, we felt the data obtained in those studies might not represent the physiological response to unilateral gonadectomy. Therefore, we elected to reinvestigate this issue using the chronically cannulated, freely moving rat in an isolation cage to obtain repeated blood samples during the initial 8 h after unilateral orchidectomy.

MATERIALS AND METHODS

Animals and Housing

Adult male rats (300–325 g, 80 days old) were obtained from Charles River Canada Ltd. (St. Constant, Québec) and were given rat chow and water *ad libitum*. The animals were housed within wire mesh cages suspended within isolation boxes maintained at constant temperature (22°C) and equipped with individual timed fluorescent lights (14 h light: 10 h dark, lights on at 5:00 A.M.).

Catheter Placement

The procedure followed for placing cardiac catheters and keeping them anchored and patent for protracted periods of time has been previously described.[11] Briefly, animals are anesthetized and a Silastic® catheter is inserted into the jugular vein and positioned inside the right atrium. The free end of the catheter is anchored, using dental cement and screws, to the skull of the rat.

Experimental Protocol

Two separate studies were done. In the first experiment, LH secretory patterns were established in three rats which sequentially served as control, sham operated, and hemiorchidectomized individuals. Control animals were sampled for 6 h without any surgical treatment other than catheter emplacement. The sham operation consisted of anesthetizing the animals and doing an abdominal incision and handling of the gonad and replacing it after handling. The sham operations were done five days after the initial sampling at 8:00 A.M. and the animals were sampled for 6 h beginning at 10:00 A.M. Three days later, the animals were hemiorchidectomized at 8:00 A.M. and sampled for at least 6 h beginning at 10:00 A.M. Sham surgery and hemiorchidectomy were done under ether anesthesia; a midline incision was used.

In the second experiment, six control animals were sampled for 7 h beginning at 10:00 A.M. Other than cannulation, these animals had received no other prior treatment. Five days after the initial sampling session, the animals were anesthetized with ether at 8:00 A.M., and the left testicle, epididymis, and fat pad were removed. A second 7-h sampling session was begun 2 h after hemiorchidectomy. As in the control session, the first sample was taken at 10:00 A.M.

Radioimmuno- and Bioassays for LH

Plasma samples were aliquoted into the appropriate amount of assay buffer, frozen at −7°C and shipped on dry ice to London, ON, for both RIA and bioassay. The RIA for LH used a monoclonal antibody (mAb $518B_7$) which was generated against the β-subunit of bovine LH. The validation of this assay system for rat LH was published by the suppliers of the antibody.[12] The reference preparation used was NIH rLH RP-2. The following modifications were used: the antibody was diluted to 2 ng/ml in a solution of 1.5% normal mouse serum and 100 μl was used in each assay tube; the second antibody (goat anti-mouse serum; Antibodies Inc., Davis, California) was diluted 1:300 in 0.05 M sodium phosphate buffer containing polyethylene glycol (7000–9000 MW). The sensitivity and interassay coefficient of variation for the RIAs reported here was 19 pg/tube and 4%, respectively.

The bioactivity of LH in rat plasma was estimated by a mouse interstitial cell assay which was originally described by Ellinwood *et al.*[13] The sensitivity of the assay was increased by the addition of 3-isobutyl-1-methyl-xanthine (0.1 mM) and forskolin (1.5 μM) in the final incubation volume; a preliminary report of these modifications has been presented.[14] This resulted in a sensitivity of 3 pg RP-2 per assay tube. The coefficient of variation for the bioassays reported here was 7.5%. Data were expressed as mean ± SEM.

Data Analysis

A proportion of the samples contained such low amounts of immunoreactive LH that the sensitivity of the RIA was exceeded. No formal analysis of these results was attempted. In some cases the RIA data are plotted for illustrative purposes, and in these cases samples which were below the sensitivity of the assay were arbitrarily assigned a value of 0.4 ng/ml. For all the samples measured in which the RIA result fell in the operating range of the assay, the bioactivity:immunoactivity ratio was calculated; the average was 5.2 ± 0.1. The bioassay data were analyzed for mean concentration, pulse number and pulse amplitude using a modified version of the DC3 iterative, adaptive threshold program described by Clifton *et al.*[15] These computed values were then averaged to discern the performance of similarly treated groups of animals.

RESULTS

Representative patterns of the range of bio- and immunoreactive plasma LH from control, sham-operated, and unilaterally orchidectomized adult male rats are shown for three separate animals in FIGURES 1–3.

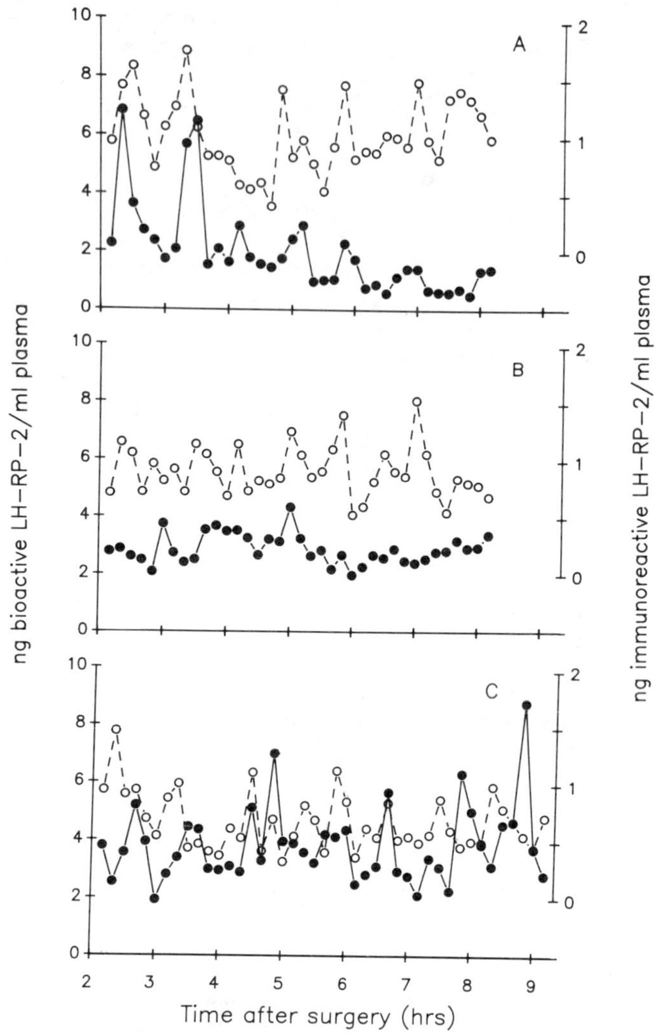

FIGURE 1. Bioactive (*solid circles*) and immunoactive (*open circles*) LH in plasma obtained from a single rat (#2) during successive sampling sessions. The samples were obtained at 10-min intervals. **A** = unoperated control; **B** = sham surgery; **C** = hemiorchidectomy.

Several points can be made by examination of these individual patterns. First, it is clear that the pattern of both bio- and immunoactive LH in these animals is episodic. Second, the ratio of bioassayable:immunoassayable LH is approximately 5.2 under all conditions studied. Third, there appears to be a remarkably good coincidence between the bio- and immunoassayable peaks; however, this coincidence is not perfect in all instances. Fourth, there appears to be no striking effect of sham surgery. Fifth, the effect of unilateral orchidectomy appears to be variable.

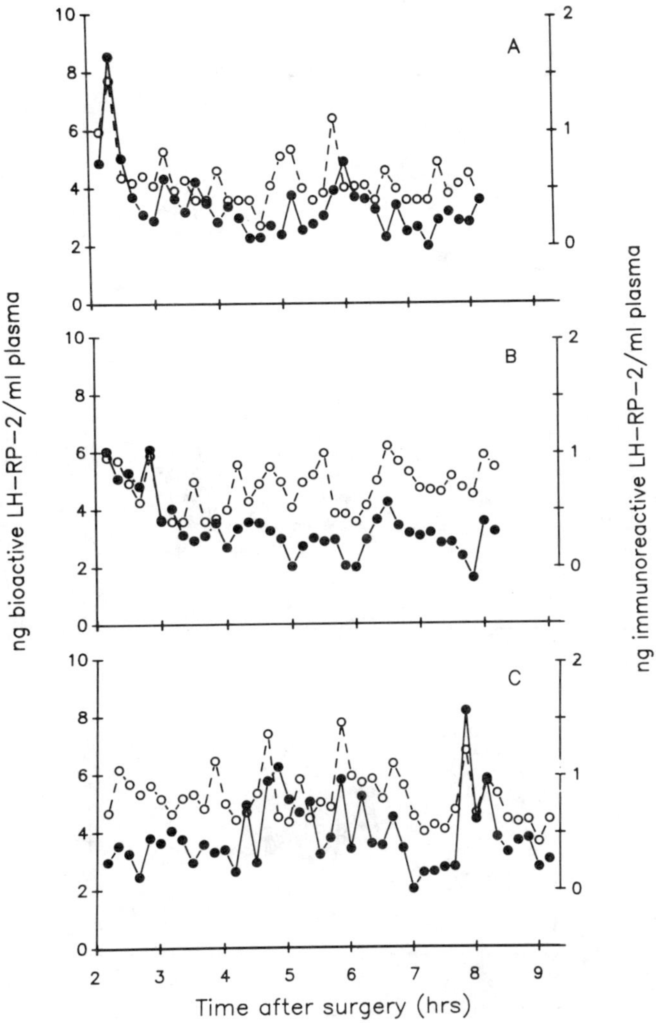

FIGURE 2. Data from an additional rat (#6); see legend for FIGURE 1.

In the animal represented in FIGURE 1, the mean bioactive LH concentration during the sham and hemiorchidectomy sampling periods increased from 2.9 to 3.8 ng/ml, respectively. This increase was achieved by an increase of pulse number from 5 to 9 and mean pulse amplitude from 1.2 to 2.9 ng/ml from the sham to the hemiorchidectomy sessions, respectively. In the animal represented in FIGURE 2 the mean bioactive LH concentration during the sham and hemiorchidectomy sampling periods increased from 3.4 to 4.1 ng/ml, respectively. This increase was achieved without a change in pulse number (n = 5), however the mean pulse amplitude increased from

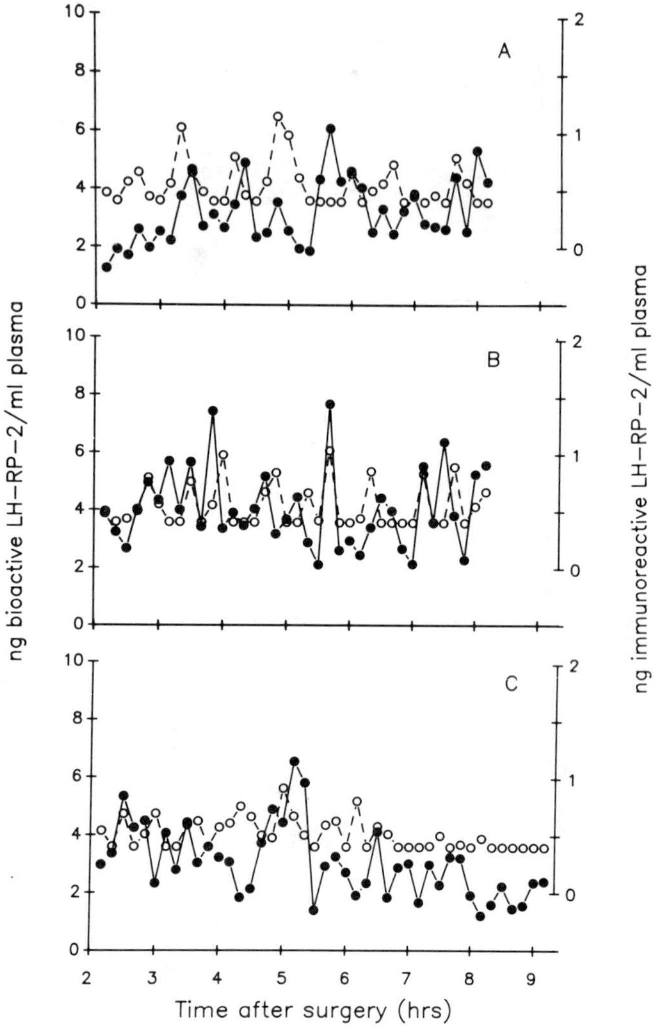

FIGURE 3. Data from an additional rat (#7); see legend for FIGURE 1.

1.5 to 4.5 ng/ml. Quite a different pattern of response was seen in the animal represented in FIGURE 3. In this case hemiorchidectomy resulted in a decrease in mean LH concentration from 4.1 to 3.2 ng/ml. This was achieved by a decrease in mean pulse amplitude from 2.9 to 1.5 ng/ml while pulse number changed little. Thus, in two of the three animals shown here, the average concentration of LH in plasma increased after hemiorchidectomy; this was achieved by increases in pulse amplitude which could or could not be accompanied by an increase in pulse frequency.

The mean and pulse parameter analysis for all the animals used for experiments

TABLE 1. Bioactivity of LH in Six Rats Sampled before and after Hemiorchidectomy[a]

	Mean	Pulse Number	Pulse Amplitude
Before	2.9 ± 0.7	4.0 ± 1.3	2.4 ± 0.7
After	2.9 ± 0.9	4.5 ± 1.3	1.9 ± 0.5

[a] The duration of both sampling periods was 7 hours. The post-hemiorchidectomy sampling period began 2 h after surgery, which was done one week after the presurgical sampling period. Data are mean ± SEM.

TABLE 2. Bioactivity of LH in Three Rats Sampled for 6 h before Surgery, for 6 h after Sham Surgery, and for 7 h after Hemiorchidectomy[a]

	Mean	Pulse	Pulse Amplitude
Control	3.1 ± 0.6	8 ± 1	1.9 ± 0.1
Sham	3.5 ± 0.3	7 ± 2	1.9 ± 0.5
Hemiorchidectomy	3.7 ± 0.3	9 ± 2	3.0 ± 0.9

[a] The post-, sham-, and hemiorchidectomy sampling periods began 2 h after surgery. One week recovery was allowed between each sampling period. Data are mean ± SEM.

1 and 2 are shown in TABLES 1 and 2, respectively. It is apparent that, in the first experiment, the number of pulses, and the amplitude of these LH pulses were not significantly affected, over the sampling period studied, by unilateral hemiorchidectomy. In the second experiment, where each animal served as his own control as well as sham-operated control, neither the mean concentration of serum LH nor the pulse frequency were affected. Mean pulse amplitude was increased by over 50%; however, owing to large inter-animal variation, this increase was not statistically significant (TABLE 2).

Earlier studies[16] had indicated that increased gonadotropin secretion in response to decreased steroid might not be manifested until 6 h after surgery; hence, we analyzed the data in a second way and determined the mean LH concentration in the samples corresponding to 2–4 and 5–7 h after unilateral orchidectomy. Analysis of pulse frequency or amplitude over such short sampling periods would be invalid. There was no discernable effect of hemiorchidectomy on mean LH concentrations at either of the time periods and no difference was detected in the hemiorchidectomized animals between 3 ± 1 and 6 ± 1 h after surgery.

DISCUSSION

The experiments described here are the first to attempt to use the chronically cannulated, freely moving rat to determine the patterns of LH secretion associated with the initial response of the surviving testis after unilateral orchidectomy. The observations were made possible by development of a bioassay for rat LH with sensitivity sufficient to detect circulating LH in plasma from intact rats. The bioactivity:immunoactivity ratio of 5.2 for LH in plasma for intact rats observed in these experiments is consistent with ratios greater than one reported by others.[17] Examination of the secretory patterns of LH illustrated in FIGURES 1–3 are consistent with earlier reports which showed that in intact males LH is released in an intermittent fashion in pigs,[18] monkeys,[19] rams,[20] rabbits,[21] ferrets,[22] mice,[23] and cattle,[24] as well as rats.[25,26]

In the present data there was, generally, good coincidence of peaks of LH bio-and immunoactivity. However, a few striking exceptions were noted (*i.e.*, FIG. 1B at 5 h 50 min and 7 h; FIG. 3A at 5 h 40 min; and FIG. 3C at 4 h 20 min). The bioactive peak could either lead or lag the immunoactive peak, and less commonly one assay detected a peak of activity and the other did not. The cause for such discordance is not apparent, but a potential explanation could be independent release of bio- and immunoreactive LH from the gonadotrophs of the pituitary. Further studies will be required to test such speculation.

A number of investigators have described the endocrine response of the remaining testis after hemiorchidectomy. The circulating concentration of testosterone is normal shortly after hemiorchidectomy; this is thought to be due to increased androgen production by the remaining gonad as reflected in an increase in testosterone concentration in both tissue[4] and testicular venous plasma.[5,6,27] It has, thus far, not been possible to associate the compensatory increase in androgen production with a concomitant increase in LH secretion. Thus, it was believed that the responsiveness of the surviving gonad to existing levels of LH might have increased or that LH-independent mechanisms were involved. Gerendai *et al.*[28] used decapsulated, non-dispersed testicular tissue obtained one week after hemiorchidectomy and found that basal, as well as HCG-stimulated, androgen production was unaltered when compared to bigonadal animals. In a similar study in which observations were made only 24 h after hemiorchidectomy, Frankel and co-workers[29] also found that the loss of one gonad did not affect androgen production, *in vitro*, from the remaining gonad. Testicular responsiveness to LH has not been investigated at intervals less than 24 h after hemiorchidectomy.

Previous investigators have suggested a role for the nervous system in the compensatory responses after unilateral orchidectomy. Studies by Mizunuma *et al.*[9] and Nance and Moger[10] provided evidence for a direct neural involvement in the compensatory increase in FSH secretion occurring 2–3 days after hemiorchidectomy. Neural involvement in the initial increase in testosterone secretion was suggested by Anakwe and Moger[6] who showed that intra-testicular injection of propranolol could interfere with the compensatory increase in androgen secretion.

Although these alternative explanations may account for the compensatory androgen response, the possibility of changes in LH secretion were not thoroughly investigated. In the one earlier study similar to ours,[8] cannulated animals were used to obtain blood samples at 4 h intervals during the first 24 h after unilateral orchidectomy. In that study, no change in LH in hemiorchidectomized rats could be detected. The time interval between samples was too long to be able to ascertain the secretory pattern for LH.

The possibility that frequency or amplitude themselves may not be the only important aspects of LH secretion is suggested by data from Chase and coworkers.[30,31] They have examined the effect of different patterns of LH stimulation *in vivo* on the ability of Leydig cells, isolated from such treated animals, to respond to maximal LH stimuli. Their conclusions, for both sheep and rats, were that exposure to a constant concentration of LH was as effective, in their *in vitro* Leydig cell assessment, as the same amount of LH presented in an intermittent fashion.

The results obtained in the present study suggest a spectrum of responses of LH secretion to unilateral orchidectomy. It appears likely that animals may respond to the removal of one gonad by transiently increasing the mean LH plasma concentration by an increase in pulse amplitude or in both amplitude and frequency. However, it is clear that there is major animal to animal variation, and thus that the nature of the change in pattern and the time "window" during which the gonadotropin pattern may change is not easily predictable.

ACKNOWLEDGMENTS

The authors thank Mr. Vaclav Pitelka and Ms. Judith Pelletier for expert technical assistance. We also wish to acknowledge Dr. A. Parlow and the National Hormone and Pituitary Program for the rat LH used in these studies and Dr. Jan Roser, University of California, Davis and Monoclonal Antibodies, Inc. for the antibody used in the LH RIA. The antibody used in the testosterone assay was supplied by Drs. Armstrong, Seamark, and Ralph, University of Adelaide.

REFERENCES

1. BAST, J. D. & G. S. GREENWALD. 1977. Acute and chronic elevations in serum levels of FSH after unilateral ovariectomy in the cyclic hamster. Endocrinology **100:** 955–966.
2. BUTCHER, R. L. 1977. Changes in gonadotropins and steroids associated with unilateral ovariectomy of the rat. Endocrinology **101:** 830–840.
3. ENGELAND, W. C. & M. F. DALLMAN. 1976. Neural mediation of compensatory adrenal growth. Endocrinology **99:** 1659–1662.
4. LINDGREN, S., J.-E.DAMBER & H. CARSTEN. 1976. Compensatory testosterone secretion in unilaterally orchidectomized rats. Life Sci. **18:** 1203–1206.
5. MOCK, E. J. & A. I. FRANKEL. 1982. Response of testosterone to hemicastration in the testicular vein of the mature rat. J. Endocrinol. **92:** 231–236.
6. MOGER, W. H. & O. O. ANAKWE. 1986. Propranolol inhibits the compensatory increase in androgen secretion after unilateral orchidectomy in rats. J. Reprod. Fertil. **76:** 251–256.
7. ROBAIRE, B. 1979. Effect of unilateral orchidectomy on rat epididymal Δ^4-5α reductase and 3α-hydroxysteroid dehydrogenase. Can. J. Physiol. Pharmacol. **57:** 999–1003.
8. FRANKEL, A. I. & W. W. WRIGHT. 1982. The hemiorchidectomized rat: Definition of a model for the study of the regulation of testicular steroidogenesis. J. Endocrinol. **92:** 213–223.
9. MIZUNUMA, H., L. R. DEPALATIS & S. M. MCCANN. 1983. Effect of unilateral orchidectomy on plasma FSH concentration: Evidence for a direct neural connection between testes and CNS. Neuroendocrinology **37:** 291–296.
10. NANCE, D. M. & W. H. MOGER. 1982. Ipsilateral hypothalamic deafferentation blocks the increase in serum FSH following hemi-castration. Brain. Res. Bull. **8:** 299–302.
11. GROSSER, P. M. & B. ROBAIRE. 1988. Episodic prolactin secretion in the adult male rat is affected by orchidectomy and testosterone replacement. Endocrinology **123:** 2132–2139.
12. MATTERI, R. L., J. F. ROSER, D. M. BALDWIN, V. LIPOVETSKY & H. PAPKOFF. 1987. Characterization of a monoclonal antibody which detects luteinizing hormone from diverse mammalian species. Domest. Anim. Endocrinol. **4:** 157–165.
13. ELLINWOOD, W. E., R. M. BRENNER, D. L. HESS & J. A. RESKO. 1980. Testosterone synthesis in rhesus fetal testes: Comparison between middle and late gestation. Biol. Reprod. **22:** 955–963.
14. DEBERTIN, W J. & D. K. POMERANTZ. 1990. Improved sensitivity of the mouse interstitial cell assay (MICA) for LH and its use in defining the LH response to unilateral orchidectomy (UO) in the adult rat. Biol. Reprod. **42:** 149 (Abstract).
15. CLIFTON, D. K., S. AKSEL, W. J. BREMNER, R. A. STEINER & M. R. SOULES. 1988. Statistical evaluation of coincident prolactin and luteinizing hormone pulses during the normal menstrual cycle. J. Clin. Endocrinol. Metab. **67:** 832–838.
16. DAVIDSON, J. M., D. A. DAMASSA, E. R. SMITH & C. CHEUNG. 1976. Feedback control of gonado-

tropin secretion in the male rat. *In* Regulatory Mechanisms of Male Reproductive Physiology. C. H. Spillman, T. J. Lobl, and K. T. Kirton, Eds.: 151–168. Excerpta Medica. Amsterdam.
17. SOLANO, A. R., M. L. DUFAU & K. J. CATT. 1979. Bioassay and radioimmunoassay of serum luteinizing hormone in the male rat. Endocrinology **105:** 372–381.
18. ELLENDORFF, F., N. PARVIZI, D. K. POMERANTZ, A. HARTJEN, A. KONIG, D. SMIDT & F. ELSAESSER. 1975. Plasma luteinizing hormone and testosterone in the adult male pig: 24 h fluctuation and the effect of copulation. J. Endocrinol. **67:** 403–410.
19. PLANT, T. M. 1981. Time courses of concentrations of circulating gonadotropin, prolactin, testosterone, and cortisol in adult rhesus monkeys (Macaca mulatta) throughout the 24h light-dark cycle. Biol. Reprod. **25:** 244–252.
20. D'OCCHIO, M. J., B. D. SCHANBACHER & J. E. KINDER. 1982. Relationship between serum testosterone concentration and patterns of luteinizing hormone secretion in male sheep. Endocrinology **110:** 1547–1554.
21. ROWE, P. H., C. R. N. HOPKINSON, J. C. SHENTON & T. D. GLOVER. 1975. The secretion of LH and testosterone in the rabbit. Steroids **25:** 313–321.
22. SISK, C. L. & C. DESJARDINS. 1986. Pulsatile release of luteinizing hormone and testosterone in male ferrets. Endocrinology **119:** 1195–1203.
23. COQUELIN, A. & C. DESJARDINS. 1982. Luteinizing hormone and testosterone secretion in young and old mice. Am. J. Physiol. **243:** E257–E263.
24. KATONGOLE, C. B., F. NAFTOLIN & R. V. SHORT. 1971. Relationship between blood levels of luteinizing hormone and testosterone in bulls, and the effects of sexual stimulation. J. Endocrinol. **50:** 457–466.
25. ELLIS, G. B. & C. DESJARDINS. 1982. Male rats secrete luteinizing hormone and testosterone episodically. Endocrinology **110:** 1618–1627.
26. ROBAIRE, B. & S. F. BAYLY. 1989. Testicular signaling: Incoming and outgoing messages. Ann. N. Y. Acad. Sci. **564:** 250–260.
27. FRANKEL, A. I., J. C. CHAPMAN & B. COOK. 1989. Testes are asymmetric in the testicular hemicastration response of the male rat. J. Endocrinol. **122:** 485–488.
28. GERENDAI, I., C. SHAHA, R. THAU & C. W. BARDIN. 1984. Do testicular opiates regulate Leydig cell function? Endocrinology **115:** 1645–1647.
29. FRANKEL, A. I., J. C. CHAPMAN & B. COOK. 1989. The testicular response to hemicastration in the male rat cannot be maintained in vitro. J. Endocrinol. **121:** 43–48.
30. CHASE, D. J., B. D. SCHANBACHER & D. D. LUNSTRA. 1988. Effects of pulsatile and continuous luteinizing hormone (LH) infusions on testosterone responses to LH in rams actively immunized against gonadotropin-releasing hormone. Endocrinology **123:** 816–826.
31. GIBSON-BERRY, K. L. & D. J. CHASE. 1990. Continuous and pulsatile infusions of luteinizing hormone have identical effects on steroidogenic capacity and sensitivity of Leydig cells in rats passively immunized against gonadotropin-releasing hormone. Endocrinology **126:** 3107–3115.

Alterations in the Control and Function of Somatic Cells in the Testis Associated with Suppression of Spermatogenesis in Seasonal Breeders[a]

ANDRZEJ BARTKE,[b] ARTUR MAYERHOFER,[c]
SEAN NEWTON,[d] DORIS MAYERHOFER,[b]
SUBEER MAJUMDAR[e] AND
VARADARAJ CHANDRASHEKAR[b]

[b] *Department of Physiology*
Southern Illinois University
Carbondale, Illinois 62901

[c] *Abteilung Anatomie und Zellbiologie*
Universitaet Ulm
Ulm, Germany

[d] *Department of Anatomy*
University of South Carolina
Columbia, South Carolina 29208

[e] *Department of Physiology*
University of Pittsburgh
Pittsburgh, Pennsylvania 15261

INTRODUCTION

In most animal species, reproductive competence is limited to a rigidly controlled and often quite short annual breeding season. Although timing and duration of the breeding season as well as the amplitude of the circannual rhythm of testicular activity vary widely among species, periods of active spermatogenesis and fertility are generally interspersed with periods of gonadal atrophy and complete suppression of sperm production. Mechanisms responsible for the annual transitions between the states of testicular activity and quiescence attracted considerable attention which focused primarily on the photoperiodic control of gonadal function and on the role of the pineal and its product melatonin in mediating the effects of photoperiod. These studies, including the recent demonstration of specific melatonin receptors in the pars tuberalis, the suprachiasmatic nucleus and other parts of the central nervous system[1,2] are outside the scope of this writing. The general conclusion from these studies appears to

[a] Studies reported in this chapter were supported by NIH through a grant HD20033 and by Deutsche Forschungsgemeinschaft, Ma 1080/1-2, and by the Lalor Foundation.

be that seasonal changes in day length alter the duration and/or timing of the nocturnal rise in melatonin secretion, and that this leads to changes in the function of hypothalamic neurons that control hormone release from the anterior pituitary. Thus changes in testicular function induced by natural or experimentally imposed changes in the photoperiod represent consequences of altered secretion of pituitary gonadotropins. Studies in the Syrian hamster (*Mesocricetus auratus*) Siberian hamster (*Phodopus sungorus*), different breeds of domestic sheep, and many other species provided abundant evidence that seasonal regression of the testis is preceded by suppression of FSH, LH and, in some species, PRL release, while spontaneous or photoperiod-induced recovery of testicular activity is preceded by stimulation of the release of the same hormones[3-7] (reviews in refs. 8–11). Several laboratories addressed the issue of the possible existence of concomitant changes in testicular responsiveness to stimulatory inputs from the pituitary. We have reported that although the atrophic testes of Syrian hamsters exposed to short photoperiod grew rapidly in response to large doses of human chorionic gonadotropin (hCG) and/or pregnant mare serum gonadotropin (PMSG), they appeared unable to respond to once daily injections of moderate doses of LH and/or FSH as assessed by testicular weight, plasma testosterone levels, and number of LH receptors.[12,13] Heindel and his colleagues[14,15] demonstrated that Sertoli cells isolated from gonadally regressed hamsters have increased responsiveness of adenylate cyclase to FSH stimulation. In this chapter we would like to summarize our own studies concerning photoperiod-related changes in the control of Leydig cells, Sertoli cells, and macrophages by pituitary gonadotropins, catecholamines, and other factors, and attempt to relate these changes to seasonal fluctuations in sperm production. For these studies we have used both Syrian and Siberian hamsters. Testicular regression in adult males was induced by transferring the animals from long to short photoperiod (16 h light:8 h darkness versus 6 h light:18 h darkness for 8–12 weeks). Exposure to short photoperiod since birth was used to delay sexual maturation in Siberian hamsters.

LEYDIG CELL FUNCTION

Our early studies resulted in the demonstration that the number of LH and PRL receptors in the regressed testes of short-photoperiod–exposed Syrian hamsters is reduced[12,13,16] and that loss of these receptors is among the earliest changes in testis function after transfer of animals from a long to a short photoperiod.[16,17] Recent morphometric studies allowed us to conclude that a decline in the content of LH receptors in the regressed testes is due primarily to a decrease in the number of LH receptors per Leydig cell.[18] This decrease parallels reduction of Leydig cell surface area with the concentration of receptors per unit of Leydig cell surface remaining unchanged.[18] We have also reported that these changes in testicular LH and PRL binding are due to suppression of pituitary PRL release[12,13,19] and that prolonged treatment with PRL-secreting ectopic pituitary transplants can restore LH binding, plasma testosterone levels, testicular weight, and fertility.[20]

Studies of testicular testosterone secretion *in vitro* in the presence of different doses of hCG provided evidence that Leydig cells of gonadally regressed hamsters continue to respond to gonadotropic stimulation, but have greatly reduced capacity to produce testosterone from endogenous precursors.[21] Subsequently, we have shown that regression of the testes of adult Syrian hamsters exposed to short photoperiods is accompanied by a major decrease in the ratio of testosterone:progesterone released *in vitro* in response to hCG stimulation.[22] Analysis of plasma and testicular levels of progesterone, 17α-hydroxyprogesterone, androstenedione, and testosterone after treatment with different doses of hCG *in vivo* revealed that testicular regression is accompanied by alterations in the ratios of testosterone to its various precursors.[23] Presumably these changes reflect suppression of the activity of 17α-steroid hydroxylase, C_{17-20} steroid lyase and 17β-hydroxysteroid dehydrogenase in the Leydig cells after prolonged exposure to a short photoperiod.[23]

We have also demonstrated that short-photoperiod–induced testicular regression in Syrian hamsters is accompanied by a striking qualitative change in the steroidogenic response to catecholamines *in vitro.*[24] Testicular tissue from gonadally active animals fails to respond to epinephrine, norepinephrine, or a synthetic adrenergic agonist. In contrast, addition of the same compounds to the incubations of testicular parenchyma from gonadally regressed hamsters causes a pronounced and dose-related increase in the accumulation of testosterone in the media.[24] Lack of steroidogenic response to catecholamines in the active testes of long-photoperiod–exposed hamsters resembles previous findings in gonadally active mice and rats.[25,26] Surprisingly, suppression of LH stimulatory input, and testicular LH binding by short photoperiod is accompanied by acquisition of responsiveness to catecholaminergic stimuli. We are not certain whether this unexpected property of regressed testes is due to reduced input from their innervation *in vivo*[24] or to other causes. Regardless of the mechanism(s) involved, we suspect that steroidogenic responsiveness to catecholamines endows the gonadally regressed animals with the ability to respond to stress with a surge of testicular testosterone, in spite of functional suppression of the hypothalamic-pituitary-gonadal axis at this stage of the annual reproductive cycle. The resulting testosterone surges would presumably be transient and thus unlikely to interfere with seasonal suppression of spermatogenesis and fertility. Pharmacological studies *in vitro* revealed that catecholaminergic stimulation of testosterone production by the regressed and active testes (the latter only in the presence of hCG) are mediated via α receptors.[24] This is in contrast to steroidogenic effects in the ovary and the placenta, which are mediated via β receptors[27,28] and to the reported presence of β receptors on rat and mouse Leydig cells.[29] However, in studies of norepinephrine stimulation of cAMP accumulation in the incubations of hamster testes, we found evidence for the presence of functional β receptors in this tissue.[30] Thus, we must conclude that stimulation of adenylate cyclase activity and testosterone production in this system occurs via different mechanisms, and that either hamster Leydig cells possess functional α receptors, or effects of catecholamines on steroidogenesis are due to action on a different cell type, and paracrine influence of this putative target cell on the Leydig cells. We have examined also the effects of short-photoperiod–induced gonadal regression in Syrian hamsters on the ability of their testes to respond to histamine *in vitro.* As was the case with catecholamines, histamine did not affect testosterone accumulation in the incubations of testicular tissue from long-photoperiod–exposed animals, but produced a significant, dose-related increase in testosterone secretion by testicular tissue from short-photoperiod–exposed hamsters.[31] Although the physiological significance of these findings is unclear, they provide another striking example of photoperiod-related seasonal changes in the responsiveness of the testes to regulatory inputs.

Recently, we have obtained preliminary evidence that regressed testes may become responsive to catecholamines and histamine because of the depletion of the germ cells or because of their abdominal position, with seasonal depression of gonadotropin release not being a primary factor. Testicular tissue from adult Syrian hamsters that were maintained in a long (stimulatory) photoperiod but were rendered surgically cryptorchid, responded *in vitro* to both norepinephrine and histamine by increased testosterone output (Bartke, Gow & Mayerhofer, unpublished observations).

The possible significance of photoperiod-related changes in the regulation of Leydig cell function to the seasonal suppression and stimulation of spermatogenesis will be discussed in the concluding section of this chapter.

SERTOLI CELLS

Siberian hamsters born and raised under long photoperiods undergo rapid sexual development and are fertile before attaining the age of 2 months. However, exposure of juvenile males of this species to short photoperiod delays sexual maturation by at least 3 months.[32] In their natural habitat, this response to short photoperiod ensures that animals born late during the breeding season do not reach puberty until the following spring. In order to compare the regulation of Sertoli cell function during "normal" (early) and delayed puberty, we developed a protocol for isolation of Sertoli cells from juvenile Siberian hamsters and for their culture in serum-free media.[33,34] Comparison of Sertoli cells isolated from 12–15, 18–21, 24–27 and 30–33 day-old hamsters born and raised under a long or a short photoperiod allowed us to evaluate the effects of exposure to FSH (and possibly other stimulatory influences) *in vivo* on the ability of the cells to produce lactate and to respond to FSH *in vitro.* Sertoli cell–derived lactate is believed to play a key role in satisfying the energy requirements of dividing and developing germ cells[35] and therefore, we were interested in comparing lactate production by Sertoli cells from animals undergoing early stages of pubertal development (long-day–exposed hamsters) and from animals of the same chronological age in which pubertal development has been postponed (short-day–exposed hamsters). The results revealed that in each of the age groups examined, Sertoli cells from short-photoperiod–exposed hamsters produced more lactate and responded to FSH *in vitro* by a greater increase in lactate production, as compared to Sertoli cells for long-photoperiod–exposed hamsters cultured simultaneously under identical conditions.[34,36] Although this association of increased lactate output with delay of puberty is counter-intuitive, it agrees with previous findings in cultured Sertoli cells from active and regressed testes of adult Syrian hamsters.[14,15] Perhaps enhanced responsiveness to FSH in cultures derived from short-photoperiod–exposed animals represents an increase in the number of FSH receptors or in the responsiveness of post-receptor mechanisms caused by suppression of FSH stimulatory input *in vivo.* It is also possible, that very high levels of plasma FSH in juvenile hamsters exposed to long photoperiods[5,6] can overcome both the low basal lactate production and the modest, although statistically significant decrease in responsiveness to FSH and lead to production of lactate in amounts sufficient to ensure the onset of spermatogenesis. In other words, in contrast to the findings *in vitro*, Sertoli cell lactate production *in vivo* is likely to be greater in long-photoperiod– than in short-photoperiod–exposed juvenile animals owing to differences in plasma FSH levels.

However, we suspect that enhanced responsiveness of Sertoli cells from gonadally quiescent hamsters to FSH may have physiological significance. Presumably it represents maintenance of the ability of the Sertoli cells to respond rapidly to increased requirement of the germ cells for lactate when the annual reproductive rhythm calls for initiation of spermatogenesis. Consistent with this speculation is a remarkably rapid onset of testicular growth in juvenile *Phodopus* upon photostimulation. Transfer of reproductively "delayed" male Siberian hamsters from short to long photoperiods produces rapid stimulation of FSH release with significant increase in testicular weight being detectable as early as seven days after the onset of long photoperiods.[6]

In addition to differences in responsiveness to FSH, Sertoli cells isolated from juvenile *Phodopus* exposed to a long or a short photoperiod differed also in their responses to Vitamin D_3 (Vit D_3). When Sertoli cells were isolated from very young (12–15 day old) hamsters, exposure to Vit D_3 *in vitro* increased lactate secretion into the media only in cultures derived from short-photoperiod–exposed animals.[33] In contrast, in cultures derived from older (18–20 day old) hamsters, Vit D_3 did not affect lactate production by Sertoli cells from short-photoperiod–exposed males, but potentiated the stimulatory effect of FSH on lactate production by cells derived from males exposed to a long photoperiod.[37] These observations require confirmation and extension, but suggest an exciting possibility that Vit D_3 may play a physiological role in the regulation of testicular function and perhaps also in mediating the response of the testes to changes in photoperiod. It has been proposed that the opposing effects of darkness and light on various physiological functions may be mediated by the actions of melatonin and Vit D_3, respectively.[38]

In order to characterize more fully the functional characteristics of the Sertoli cells in relation to seasonal changes in spermatogenesis in Siberian hamsters, we have recently developed a procedure for isolation and culture of Sertoli cells from adult *Phodopus*. A method based on sequential exposure to different concentrations of collagenase at 37°C allows isolation of viable Sertoli cells which are free of Leydig cells and contain less than 1% of peritubular cells.[39] Sertoli cells could be isolated from testes of adult animals with active spermatogenesis with a very good yield and their morphological characteristics *in vitro* were strikingly different from those of Sertoli cells isolated from juvenile animals. Compared to the cells isolated from immature animals, Sertoli cells isolated from adult testes had larger cytoplasmic volume with processes and crypts reminiscent of their structure *in situ*. Preliminary results of electrophoretic analysis of the media from cultured Sertoli cells from juvenile and adult animals suggested that some of the proteins secreted by Sertoli cells from juvenile animals are not produced by Sertoli cells from adult hamsters.[39]

TESTICULAR MACROPHAGES

Recent studies of the interactions between the immune and the endocrine systems provided clear evidence that immune cells can influence the function of the peripheral endocrine organs and neurosecretory neurons, and can themselves produce various hormones and transmitters (reviews in refs. 40 and 41). Specific function of macrophages which are present in testicular interstitium in the control of male gonadal function was suggested by a series of studies by Hutson and his colleagues.[42,43] These investigators provided evidence that rat testicular macrophages bind FSH and respond to FSH *in vitro* by secreting a factor(s) that stimulates steroidogenesis in the Leydig cells.

Seasonal regression of the testes in Syrian hamsters is accompanied by a precipitous decrease in the absolute volume of testicular macrophages.[44] Although the functional significance of seasonal changes in the size and/or number of testicular macrophages is unclear, we were interested in the possibility of concomitant changes in macrophage function or regulation of their activity. The procedure described by Yee and Hutson[42,43] was modified for use in Siberian hamsters and employed for isolation of macrophages from the active and regressed testes of adult animals that, during the preceding 10 weeks, had been exposed to a long or a short photoperiod, respectively. The isolated cells were identified as macrophages by light and electron microscopy, approximately 99% were viable after one day of culture, 85–90% were capable of phagocytosis of polystyrene beads and possessed Fc-receptors. Contamination by Leydig (3β-HSD-positive) cells was less than 3%.[45,46]

Production of lactate, expressed per μg of cell protein, was greater in cultures of macrophages derived from regressed testes than in those derived from active gonads. However, addition of FSH to the cultures stimulated lactate production only by macrophages derived from gonadally active, long-day–exposed males. This effect of FSH was pronounced (greater than twofold) and dose-related in macrophages from active testes and entirely absent in macrophages from regressed testes or in cultures of peritoneal macrophages isolated from the same animals.[45,46] We have also demonstrated that media from cultures of FSH-exposed testicular macrophages were capable of inhibiting testosterone production by testicular tissue from both long- and short-photoperiod–exposed animals. Inhibition of steroidogenesis was not due to the presence of lactate or FSH in the media.[47] The inhibitory effect of macrophage-conditioned media on testicular testosterone production was not expected from previous findings in the rat[42,43] but appeared consistent with the reported ability of products of activated macrophages, including interleukin-1, to inhibit the activity of Leydig cells.[48] However, the latter effects were recently disputed.[49] Regardless of the mechanisms involved, our findings suggest that seasonal transitions between reproductive activity and quiescence in this species are accompanied by alterations in the control of testicular macrophages by FSH, and in their ability to exert paracrine influences on androgen production. Clearly additional studies are required to place these observations in the physiological context and to determine whether testicular macrophages play any part, directly or indirectly, in the control of spermatogenesis by testosterone and FSH.

CONCLUSIONS

In this chapter we have provided a brief review of changes in the function of three types of somatic cells in the testis and in the control of their activity in seasonal breeders. There is little doubt that the seasonal loss and recovery of spermatogenesis and fertility reflect primarily photoperiod-related changes in the release of pituitary gonadotropins. However, it is important to realize that these alterations in FSH, LH and PRL release are associated with changes in the number of testicular FSH, LH and PRL receptors, in the responsiveness of Leydig cells, Sertoli cells and testicular macrophages to gonadotropins and other stimulatory inputs, and in the paracrine influences of different types of somatic cells on each other and on the germ cells. It is interesting that while some of these changes appear to amplify the consequences of suppressed adenohypophyseal activity (*e.g.*, loss of gonadotropin receptors), others may militate against these effects (*e.g.*, increased responsiveness to FSH) or provide novel pathways for stimulation of the testes (*e.g.*, acquisition of responsiveness to catecholamines and histamine). Thus seasonal changes in the milieu of dividing and differentiating germ cells represent net result of very complex alterations in stimulatory inputs received by the testis, in responsiveness of different types of testicular cells to these stimuli, and in the paracrine control mechanisms operating within the testis. We believe that the naturally occurring and fully reversible transitions between the periods of fertility and infertility in seasonal breeders offer a unique opportunity for elucidating the mechanisms that control spermatogenesis in mammals.

ACKNOWLEDGMENT

We thank Mrs. M. Hilt for typing.

REFERENCES

1. Duncan, M. J., J. S. Takahashi & M. L. Dubocovich. 1989. Characteristics and autoradiographic localization of 2-[125I]Iodomelatonin binding sites in Djungarian hamster brain. Endocrinology **125:** 1011–1018.
2. Weaver, D. R., S. A. Rivkees & S. M. Reppert. 1989. Localization and characterization of melatonin receptors in rodent brain by *in vitro* autoradiography. J. Neurosci. **9:** 2581–2590.
3. Turek, F. W., J. A. Elliott, J. D. Alvis & M. Menaker. 1975. Effect of prolonged exposure to nonstimulatory photoperiods on the activity of the neuroendocrine-testicular axis of golden hamsters. Biol. Reprod. **13:** 475–481.
4. Matt, K. S. & M. H. Stetson. 1980. A comparison of serum hormone titers in golden hamsters during testicular growth induced by pinealectomy and photoperiodic stimulation. Biol. Reprod. **23:** 893–898.
5. Yellon, S. M. & B. D. Goldman. 1984. Photoperiodic control of reproductive development in the male Djungarian hamster (*Phodopus sungorus*). Endocrinology **114:** 664–670.
6. Milette, J. J., N. B. Schwartz & F. W. Turek. 1988. The importance of follicle-stimulating hormone in the initiation of testicular growth in photostimulated Djungarian hamsters. Endocrinology **122:** 1060–1066.
7. Lincoln, G. A., M. J. Peet & R. A. Cunningham. 1977. Seasonal and circadian changes in the episodic release of follicle-stimulating hormone, luteinizing hormone and testosterone in rams exposed to artificial photoperiods. J. Endocrinol. **72:** 337–349.
8. Reiter, R. J. 1980. The pineal and its hormones in the control of reproduction in mammals. Endocr. Rev. **1:** 109–131.
9. Lincoln, G. A. & R. V. Short. 1980. Seasonal breeding: Nature's contraceptive. Recent Prog. Horm. Res. **36:** 1–52.
10. Bartke, A. 1985. Male hamster reproductive endocrinology. *In* The Hamster: Reproduction and Behavior. H. I. Siegel, Ed.: 73–98. Plenum Publishing Corp. New York.
11. Steger, R. W. & A. Bartke. 1987. Environmental modulation of neuroendocrine function. *In* Handbook of Endocrinology. G. H. Gass & H. M. Kaplan, Eds. Vol. **II:** 111–141. CRC Press. Boca Raton, FL.
12. Bex, F. J. & A. Bartke. 1977. Testicular LH binding in the hamster: Modification by photoperiod and prolactin. Endocrinology **100:** 1223–1226.
13. Bex, F., A. Bartke, B. D. Goldman & S. Dalterio. 1978. Prolactin, growth hormone, luteinizing hormone receptors, and seasonal changes in testicular activity in the golden hamster. Endocrinology **103:** 2069–2080.
14. Heindel, J. J., A. S. Berkowitz, R. Philo & J. P. Preslock. 1981. FSH stimulation of cAMP accumulation in hamster Sertoli cells: Effect of age and optic enucleation. J. Androl. **2:** 217–221.
15. Heindel, J. J. 1988. Age-related and testicular regression-induced changes in adenosine 3′,5′-monophosphate responses in cultured hamster Sertoli cells. Endocrinology **122:** 475–484.
16. Klemcke, H. G., A. Bartke & K. T. Borer. 1983. Testicular prolactin receptors and serum growth hormone in golden hamsters: Effects of photoperiod and time of day. Biol. Reprod. **29:** 605–614.
17. Bartke, A., B. D. Goldman, H. G. Klemcke, F. J. Bex & A. G. Amador. 1980. Effects of photoperiod on pituitary and testicular function in seasonally breeding species. *In* Functional Correlates of Hormone Receptors in Reproduction. V. B. Mahesh, T. G. Muldoon, B. B. Saxena & W. A. Sadler, Eds.: 171–185. Elsevier, North-Holland. New York.

18. Sinha Hikim, A. P., A. G. Amador, A. Bartke & L. D. Russell. 1989. Structure/function relationships in active and inactive hamster Leydig cells: A correlative morphometric and endocrine study. Endocrinology **125:** 1844–1856.
19. Klemcke, H. G., A. Bartke, K. T. Borer & M. P. Hogan. 1984. Regulation of testicular prolactin and luteinizing hormone receptors in golden hamsters. Endocrinology **114:** 594–603.
20. Bartke, A., M. S. Smith & S. Dalterio. 1979. Reversal of short photoperiod-induced sterility in male hamsters by ectopic pituitary homografts. Int. J. Andrology **2:** 257–262.
21. Bartke, A., K. S. Matt, A. G. Amador, H. G. Klemcke, D. Brown, D. Gonzales & M. P. Hogan. 1985. Effects of inhibitory and stimulatory photoperiods and sexual maturation on the ability of hamster testes to respond to hCG *in vitro*. Int. J. Androl. **8:** 232–242.
22. Bartke, A., V. Chandrashekar & A. G. Amador. 1990. Differential effects of short photoperiod on the release of progesterone and testosterone by hamster testes *in vitro*. J. Biol. Rhythms **5:** 241–246.
23. Chandrashekar, V. & A. Bartke. 1989. The influence of short photoperiod on testicular and circulating levels of testosterone precursors in the adult golden hamster. Biol. Reprod. **40:** 300–306.
24. Mayerhofer, A., A. Bartke & R. W. Steger. 1989. Catecholamine effects on testicular testosterone production in the gonadally active and the gonadally regressed adult golden hamster. Biol. Reprod. **40:** 752–767.
25. Cooke, B. A., M. Golding, C. J. Dix & M. G. Hunter. 1982. Catecholamine stimulation of testosterone production via cyclic AMP in mouse Leydig cells in mono-layer culture. Mol. Cell Endocrinol. **27:** 221–231.
26. Anakwe, O. O. & W. H. Moger. 1986. Catecholamine stimulation of androgen production by rat Leydig cells. Interaction with luteinizing hormone and luteinizing hormone-releasing hormone. Biol. Reprod. **35:** 806–814.
27. Aguado, L. I., S. L. Petrovic & S. R. Ojeda. 1982. Ovarian β-adrenergic receptors during the onset of puberty; Characterization, distribution and coupling to steroidogenic responses. Endocrinology **110:** 1124–1132.
28. Caritis, S. N., R. P. Hirsch & A. J. Zeleznik. 1983. Adrenergic stimulation of placenta progesterone production. J. Clin. Endocrinol. Metab. **56:** 969–972.
29. Anakwe, O. O., P. R. Murphy & W. H. Moger. 1985. Characterization of beta-adrenergic binding sites on rodent Leydig cells. Biol. Reprod. **33:** 815–826.
30. Mayerhofer, A., R. S. Calandra & A. Bartke. 1991. Cyclic adenosine monophosphate (cAMP) does not mediate the stimulatory action of norepinephrine on testosterone production by the testis of the golden hamster. Life Sci. **48:** 1109–1114.
31. Mayerhofer, A., A. Bartke, A. G. Amador & T. Began. 1989. Histamine affects testicular steroid production in the golden hamster. Endocrinology **125:** 2212–2214.
32. Hoffman, K. 1978. Effects of short photoperiods on puberty and moult in the Djungarian hamster (Phodopus sungorus). J. Reprod. Fertil. **54:** 29–35.
33. Newton, S. C., A. Mayerhofer & A. Bartke. 1989. Interaction of photoperiod and vitamin D on FSH-induced lactate secretion in Sertoli cell cultures isolated from Djungarian hamsters (*Phodopus sungorus*). 14th Annual Meeting of ASA (Abstract 96).
34. Newton, S. C. 1989. Lactate production and protein secretion by Sertoli cells isolated from prepubertal Siberian hamsters exposed to long or short photoperiods. Ph.D. dissertation. Southern Illinois University.
35. Mita, M. & P. F. Hall. 1982. Metabolism of round spermatids from rats: Lactate as the preferred substrate. Biol. Reprod. **26:** 445–455.
36. Newton, S. C. 1989. Lactate secretion by Sertoli cells isolated from Djungarian hamsters exposed to different photoperiods. Biol. Reprod. **40**(Suppl.): Abstract 186.
37. Majumdar, S. S., A. Bartke & W. E. Stumpf. 1991. Action of FSH on the Sertoli cells is modulated by vitamin D_3 in immature Siberian hamsters raised in long or short photoperiod. Symposium on the Regulation and Actions of FSH (Molecular mechanisms of FSH action in the testis). Serono Symposia, USA. In press.
38. Stumpf, W. E. & M. E. Denny. 1989. Vitamin D (soltriol), light and reproduction. Am. J. Obst. Gynecol. **161:** 1375–1384.
39. Majumdar, S. S. & F. Brown. 1991. Isolation, culture and characterization of Sertoli cells from

adult testis and a preliminary report on differential secretion of proteins by Sertoli cells from immature and adult Siberian hamsters. Biol. Reprod. **44**(Suppl. 1): 126 (Abstract #296).

40. MARTIN, J. B. 1984. Neuroendocrine regulation of the immune response. *In* Neuroimmunology. P. Behan & F. Spreafico, Eds.: 433–443. Raven Press. New York.
41. KORDON, C. & C. BIHOREAU. 1989. Integrated communication between the nervous, endocrine and immune systems. Horm. Res. **31:** 100–104.
42. YEE, J. B. & J. C. HUTSON. 1983. Testicular macrophages: Isolation, characterization and hormonal responsiveness. Biol. Reprod. **29:** 1319–1329.
43. YEE, J. B. & J. C. HUTSON. 1985. Biochemical consequences of FSH binding to testicular macrophages. Biol. Reprod. **32:** 872–879.
44. SINHA HIKIM, A. P., A. BARTKE & L. R. RUSSELL. 1988. Morphometric studies on hamster testes in gonadally active and inactive states: Light microscope findings. Biol. Reprod. **39:** 1225–1237.
45. MAYERHOFER, D. & A. MAYERHOFER. 1989. Photoperiod-related differences in the function of testicular macrophages of the Siberian hamster, *Phodopus sungorus.* Biol. Reprod. **40**(Suppl. 1): 137. Presented at Society for the Study of Reproduction 22nd Annual Meeting, Columbia, MO, USA.
46. MAYERHOFER, D. E. 1990. Effects of exposure to different photoperiods in vivo on the function of testicular macrophages of the Siberian hamster, *Phodopus sungorus.* M.Sc. Thesis, Southern Illinois University.
47. MAYERHOFER, D., A. MAYERHOFER, A. BARTKE & S. MCGEE. 1990. Inhibition of testicular testosterone production by testicular macrophages conditioned medium in the Siberian hamster, *Phodopus sungorus*. Biol. Reprod. **42**(Suppl. 1): 109. Presented at Society for the Study of Reproduction 23rd Annual Meeting, Knoxville, TN, USA.
48. FAUSER, B. C. J. M., A. B. GALWAY & A. J. W. HSUEH. 1989. Inhibitory actions of interleukin-1β on steroidogenesis in primary cultures of neonatal rat testicular cells. Acta Endocrinol. (Copenhagen) **120:** 401–408.
49. WARREN, D. W., V. PASUPULETI, Y. LU, B. W. PLATTER & R. HORTON. 1990. Tumor necrosis factor and interleukin-1 stimulate testosterone secretion in adult male rat Leydig cells *in vitro.* J. Androl. **11:** 353–360.

Hormonal Control of Leydig Cell Differentiation[a]

MATTHEW P. HARDY,[b,c] SIGRID J. GELBER,[d] ZHIFENG ZHOU,[b] TREVOR M. PENNING,[e] JOSEPH W. RICIGLIANO,[e] VENKATASESHU K. GANJAM,[f] DAN NONNEMAN,[f] AND LARRY L. EWING[b,g]

Departments of [b]Population Dynamics and [d]Pediatrics,
The Johns Hopkins University
Baltimore, Maryland 21205

[e]Department of Pharmacology
University of Pennsylvania School of Medicine
Philadelphia, Pennsylvania 19104

[f]Department of Veterinary Biomedical Sciences
University of Missouri-Columbia
Columbia, Missouri 65211

INTRODUCTION

The development of the Leydig cell has been the subject of extensive review.[1-3] Two major issues remain unresolved: 1) the nature and identity of the progenitors of the adult Leydig cell; and 2) the hormonal stimuli which govern the differentiation of progenitors into Leydig cells. The studies reported herein investigate the endocrine regulation of steroidogenesis in Leydig cell progenitors from 21-day-old rats and immature Leydig cells from 30-day-old rats. For comparison, adult Leydig cells from 90-day-old postpubertal rats will also be examined.

Identity of Leydig Cell Progenitors

Recent studies provide clues regarding the identity of Leydig cell progenitors. In the rat, a small number of Leydig cells (fewer than 200,000 per testis) develop in the fetus and are present at birth.[4,5] These fetal Leydig cells are not progenitors of the adult Leydig cells because they atrophy and do not divide postnatally. Therefore, adult

[a] This work was supported in part by National Institutes of Health grants: R01 HD07204 (L.L.E.); F32 DK08312 (S.J.G.); and R01 GM33464 (T.M.P.).

[c] Address correspondence to M. P. Hardy, The Population Council, 1230 York Ave., New York, NY 10021.

[g] The authors dedicate this paper to the late Dr. Larry L. Ewing, who provided inspirational leadership.

Leydig cells do not arise from pre-existing Leydig cells, but from undifferentiated progenitor cells. A growing body of evidence indicates that interstitial spindle-shaped cells are the undifferentiated progenitors of Leydig cells.[3] These progenitors are referred to as mesenchymal cells because of their morphological similarity to connective tissue cells that originate in the embryonic mesoderm. Adult rat Leydig cells are produced in two phases: 1) between 14 and 28 days postpartum the number of Leydig cells increases from 0.4 to 13.4 million, 10 million of which are derived directly from mesenchymal-like cells; 2) the full population of 25 million Leydig cells per testis is subsequently attained between 28 and 56 days postpartum when the newly derived Leydig cells undergo cell division.[6]

The ultimate origin of the mesenchymal-like progenitor cells has been difficult to define,[2] since they could be derived from peritubular cells,[7,8] mesoephrogenic mesenchyme,[7] neural crest cells,[9] or possibly from a combination of these sources. Two lines of evidence support the hypothesis that Leydig cells are derived from mesenchyme: 1) recent studies (reviewed by Hay[10]) have shown that mesenchymal cells can follow different pathways of differentiation depending on their contact with signaling molecules in the extracellular matrix; 2) Dechelotte *et al.*[11] report that mesenchymal-like cells in the interstitium of the human fetal testis probably comprise a mixed population of progenitor cells for mononuclear phagocytes, peritubular myoid, and Leydig cells.

The identity of progenitor cells can be tested unequivocally only if the cell can be isolated at high purity from the tissue and cultured *in vitro.* If the cell begins without the structural and functional characteristics of the mature Leydig cell type but subsequently acquires these characteristics, then it is a candidate for the progenitor cell. Hardy *et al.*[12] isolated mesenchymal-like cells from the testes of 21-day-old rats, cultured them *in vitro*, and measured a 10-fold increase in testosterone production on day 3 compared to the initial rate.

Immature Leydig Cells

The capacity of Leydig cells to produce testosterone increases gradually between day 14 postpartum, when mesenchymal-like progenitors begin their conversion into Leydig cells, and day 56 postpartum, when puberty is complete. The newly differentiated Leydig cells differ from mature Leydig cells in that they produce predominantly the 5α-reduced androgen, 5α-androstane-3α,17β-diol (3α-DIOL).[13-15] Therefore, prior to day 56 postpartum Leydig cells are considered to be functionally immature.

Hormonal Control of Leydig Cell Differentiation

Studies on Leydig cell differentiation have focused mainly on the roles of pituitary gonadotropins. Hooker[16] proposed that both follicle-stimulating hormone (FSH) and luteinizing hormone (LH) promote Leydig cell differentiation. In Hooker's model, FSH acts to induce differentiation of mesenchymal progenitors into morphologically recognizable Leydig cells, whereupon LH induces the ability of those cells to produce androgen. This model was not tested until recently because most earlier studies used human chorionic gonadotropin (hCG), and did not examine the individual effects of

LH and FSH alone. The effects of these two gonadotropins on Leydig cell differentiation will be reviewed briefly.

Treatment of sexually immature male animals *in vivo* with hCG facilitates differentiation of Leydig cells as evidenced by: increased abundance of Leydig cell smooth endoplasmic reticulum,[17] testosterone production,[18] and increased numbers of Leydig cells relative to other interstitial cells.[19] FSH treatment of immature hypophysectomized rats was found to increase the numbers of steroidogenically active Leydig cells 2.5 times relative to saline-treated controls.[20,21] When a similar study was performed with purified FSH (eliminating LH contamination), FSH caused a twofold increase in Leydig cell numbers that was overshadowed by a larger, 11-fold increase seen with LH.[22] Although neither FSH nor LH increased Leydig cell number to the levels found in intact control rats, both gonadotropins induced Leydig cell–differentiated function as evidenced by control levels of serum testosterone following acute hCG stimulation.

Taken together, these studies indicate that both FSH and LH are important in the control of Leydig cell differentiation. The effects of FSH on Leydig cells are probably exerted indirectly because Sertoli cells are the predominant site of FSH receptors in the testis.[23] To date, three Sertoli cell proteins have been shown to stimulate Leydig cell steroidogenesis: inhibin, transforming growth factor α, and insulin-like growth factor-I (IGF-I).[24] However, because all of these growth factors are also secreted by Leydig cells, it is unclear whether they act in autocrine (Leydig cell-Leydig cell) or paracrine (Sertoli-Leydig cell) fashion. The problem of identifying the regulatory factors that are involved in Leydig cell differentiation again requires the isolation and culture of Leydig cell progenitors *in vitro.* The experiments of Payne and colleagues[25] demonstrating that LH upregulates the expression of cholesterol side-chain cleavage enzyme and 17α-hydroxylase/C17-20 lyase in adult mouse Leydig cells *in vitro* provide a model for such studies.

The present study extends the above findings by addressing the following questions: 1) Do progenitor cells contain androgen receptors?; 2) Does inhibition of dihydrotestosterone (DHT) metabolism to 3α-DIOL increase the DHT-mediated action on progenitor cells?; 3) Does IGF-I promote androgen production by isolated immature Leydig cells?

METHODS

Detailed descriptions of the procedures have been published elsewhere.[12,26] In brief, Leydig cell progenitors and Leydig cells were isolated from the testes of Sprague-Dawley rats by dispersion with collagenase, followed by fractionation using centrifugal elutriation and Percoll density gradient centrifugation. The progenitor cells from 21-day-old testes were collected from the Percoll gradient between densities of 1.064 and 1.070 g/ml. Leydig cells were isolated from the testes of 90-day-old rats and were collected at densities of 1.070 g/ml and greater. Both types of cells were cultured on Cytodex 3 microcarrier beads for three days *in vitro* in the presence of 1 mg/ml bovine lipoprotein and at 5% O_2, 5% CO_2, 34°C. Hormonal treatment was either LH alone, or LH + DHT, for three days. Metabolism of DHT to 3α-DIOL was suppressed in progenitor cells by addition of the suicide substrate of 3α-hydroxysteroid dehydrogenase (3α-HSD), 1-(4′-nitrophenyl)-2-propen-1-ol, to the culture medium at 500 μM. Testosterone, DHT, and 3α-DIOL were measured by radioimmunoassay of HPLC-purified extracts of culture medium.

RESULTS AND DISCUSSION

Androgen Effects on Leydig Cell Differentiation

As androgens inhibit testosterone synthesis in isolated Leydig cells from adult animals,[27-29] the rationale for studying stimulatory effects of androgen on Leydig cell progenitors requires further explanation. Androgen involvement in Leydig cell differentiation was first suggested by Bardin *et al.*[30] in a study of rodents with testicular feminization (tfm), a genetic defect conferring insensitivity to androgen. The testosterone production rate of tfm Leydig cells was approximately 12% of normal, and deficiencies were detected in both the activity of 17β-hydroxysteroid dehydrogenase and the volume of smooth endoplasmic reticulum.

The above observations indicated that androgens are required for Leydig cell maturation. Other evidence of an effect of androgen is found in studies that blocked its action in prepubertal animals either by treatment with ethylene dimethanesulphonate to eliminate Leydig cells and stop androgen production,[31] or with the anti-androgen cyproterone acetate.[32] Either treatment greatly reduced the numbers of Leydig cells that formed during pubertal development.

In an earlier study,[12] Leydig cell progenitors from 21-day-old rats were isolated and cultured *in vitro* for three days in the presence of 0.1 ng/ml ovine LH (LH) and 7.5 μg/ml (26 μM) 5α-dihydrotestosterone (DHT), alone or in combination. A marked increase in differentiated function (*i.e.*, testosterone secretion) occurred when these cells were incubated in LH + DHT. Daily administration of androgen receptor an-

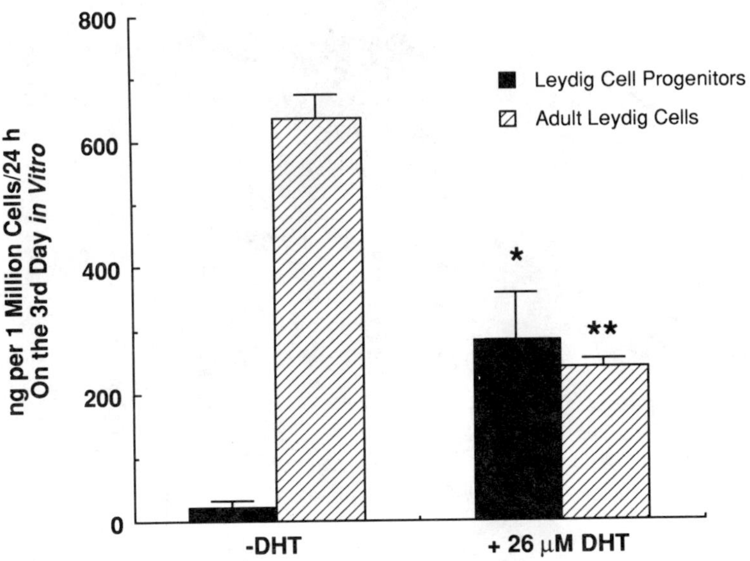

FIGURE 1. Testosterone production in response to exogenous DHT *in vitro*: comparison of Leydig cell progenitors from 21-day-old rats to adult Leydig cells from 90-day-old rats. In the presence of 26 μM DHT, testosterone production by Leydig cell progenitors increased 10-fold, whereas testosterone production by adult Leydig cells decreased by 62%. * = $p < 0.01$; ** = $p < 0.001$.

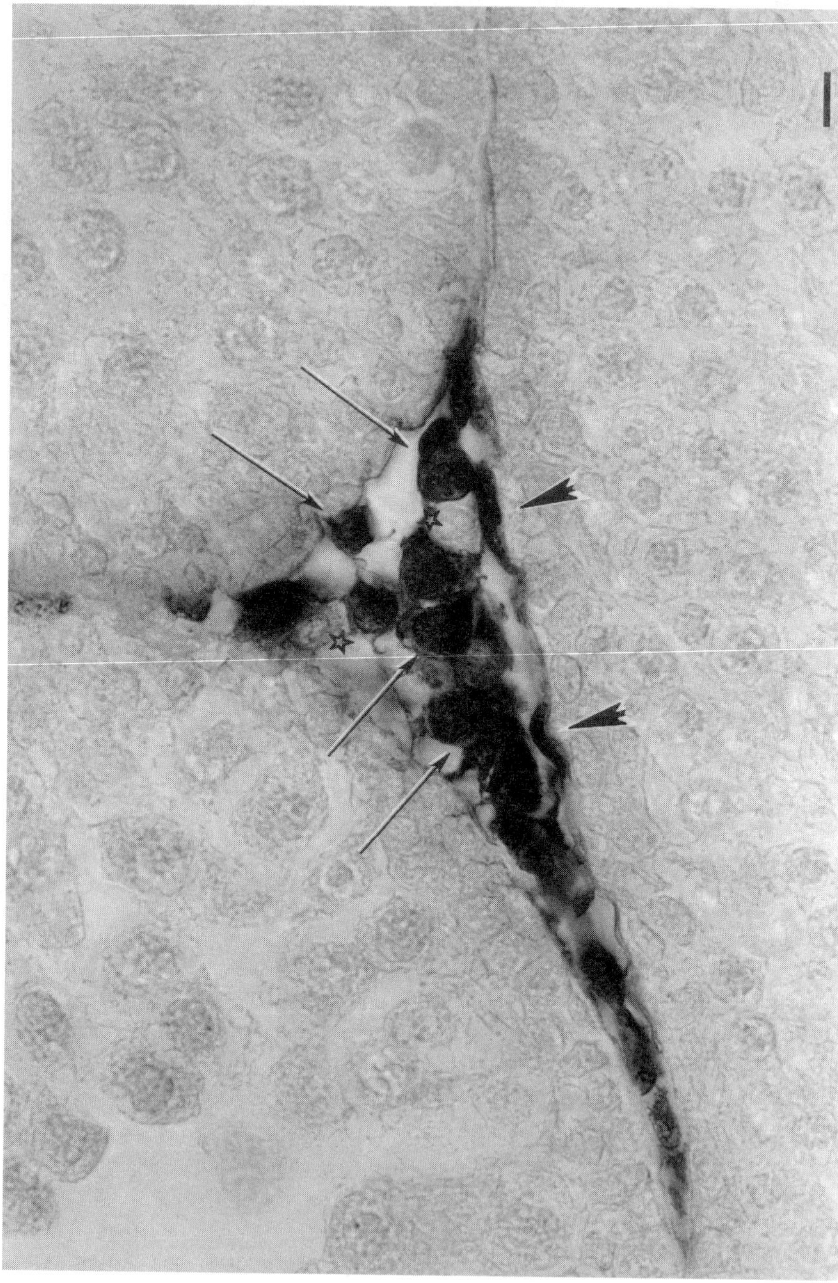

FIGURE 2. Androgen receptors immunocytochemistry. Androgen receptors were localized to interstitial cells in 21-day-old testes (arrowheads = peritubular cells, arrows = putative Leydig cell progenitors, stars = unstained interstitial cells). Scale bar = 10 μm.

tagonists, cyproterone acetate or hydroxyflutamide, inhibited the observed increase in testosterone production by 84% and 67%, respectively. These data indicated that androgen can act in an autocrine fashion on Leydig cell progenitors and, in combination with LH, stimulate their differentiation into Leydig cells. In contrast, when adult Leydig cells from 90-day-old rats were cultured under identical conditions with LH + DHT there was a significant 62% decline in testosterone production compared to cultures that received LH alone (FIG. 1). This indicated that DHT may stimulate conversion of progenitor cells into Leydig cells,[12,33] then inhibit steroidogenesis by fully differentiated, mature Leydig cells as previously reported.[27-29]

Leydig Cell Progenitors Contain Androgen Receptors

Interstitial cells of 21-day-old rat testis were examined for the presence of androgen receptors by immunocytochemistry. The testes were fixed by whole-body vascular perfusion with Bouin's solution. Androgen receptors were identified with a rat monoclonal anti-androgen receptor antibody (clone Anl-15[34]), and were localized to peritubular cells and to interstitial cells that were presumed to be Leydig cell progenitors (FIG. 2). The pattern of androgen receptor localization appeared identical to that seen in the adult testis,[35,36] with the exception that androgen receptors were not detectable in Sertoli cells of the immature testis.

Purified Leydig cell progenitors were analyzed for the presence of androgen receptors by ligand-binding assay. High salt nuclear extracts were prepared from tissue and isolated cells.[37] Specific binding of [^{3}H]-methyltrienolone was determined after separating bound from free ligand by the hydroxylapatite technique.[38] The binding of [^{3}H]-methyltrienolone to testicular androgen receptors from 21-day-old rats was found to be saturable (FIG. 3a). Scatchard analysis of binding data for isolated progenitor cells from 21-day-old rats showed a single class of high-affinity binding sites (FIG. 3b). Similar results were obtained for isolated Leydig cells from 90-day-old rats (FIG. 3c). These results indicate that Leydig cell progenitors contain androgen receptors.

Blocking the Metabolism of DHT Increases the Potency of Its Action on Leydig Cell Progenitors

Despite the presence of high affinity androgen receptors in progenitor cells, >10 μM DHT was required to increase testosterone production *in vitro*. It was hypothesized that the high concentrations of DHT required were attributable to rapid metabolism of DHT by 3α-hydroxysteroid dehydrogenase (3α-HSD) in these cells. That hypothesis was tested by treating Leydig cell progenitors with a nonsteroidal substrate, 1-(4′-nitrophenyl)-2-propen-1-ol ($4NO_2P$, see FIG. 4), which upon oxidation by 3α-HSD irreversibly inactivates the enzyme.[39] The concentrations of DHT and 3α-DIOL in media from cultures of Leydig cell progenitors were measured after 24 h in the presence of 0.1 ng/ml LH and 10 μM DHT ± 500 μM $4NO_2P$. The results indicated that 90% of the added DHT was converted to the weak androgen 3α-DIOL within 24 hours (FIG. 5). An 86% reduction in the activity of 3α-HSD was observed with the addition of $4NO_2P$. Testosterone production increased five-fold in cultures treated with $4NO_2P$ compared to cultures that received LH + DHT alone (FIG. 6). These

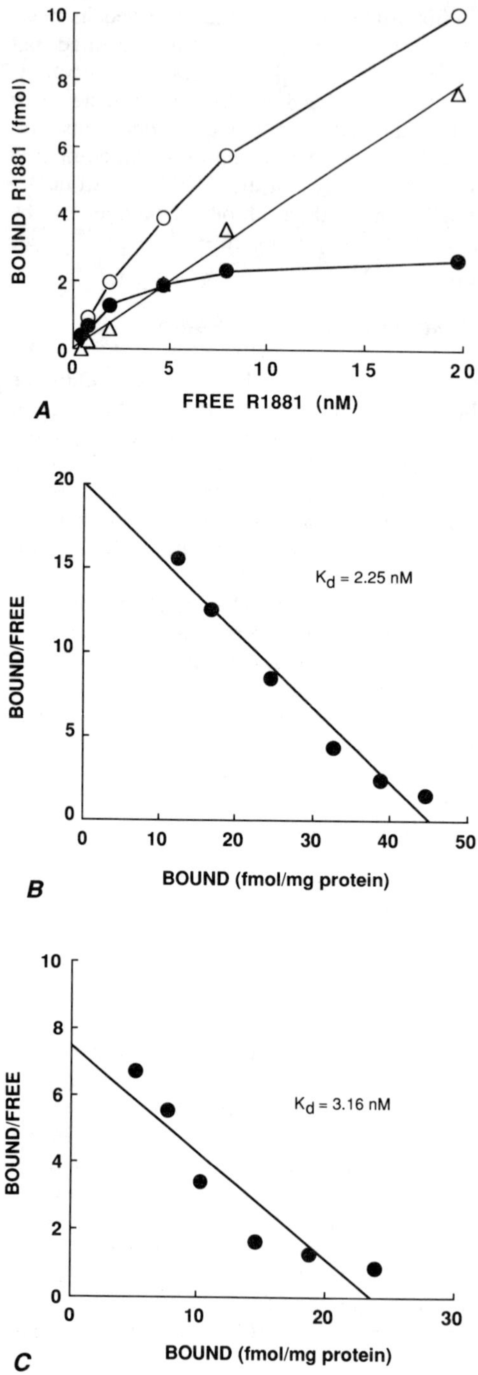

FIGURE 3. Androgen receptor ligand-binding assay. (**A**) Binding of [^{3}H]-methyltrienolone to testicular androgen receptors from 21-day-old rats. Total binding is indicated by the open circles, non-specific binding (200-fold excess unlabeled methyltrienolone) by the open triangles, and specific binding by the filled circles. The binding was saturable. (**B**) Scatchard analysis of binding data for isolated progenitor cells. A single class of high-affinity binding sites was observed. (**C**) Scatchard analysis of binding data for isolated adult Leydig cells. A single class of high-affinity binding sites was observed.

FIGURE 4. Structure of 1-(4′-nitrophenyl)-2-propen-1-ol ($4NO_2P$).

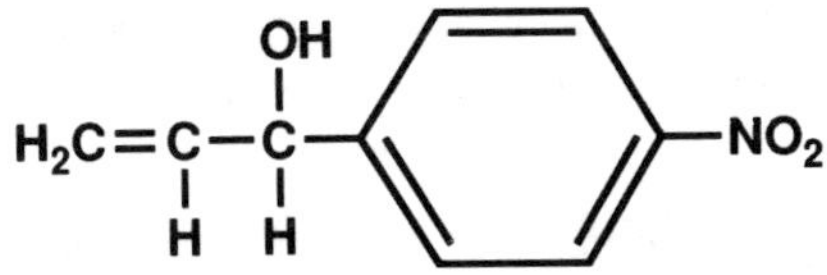

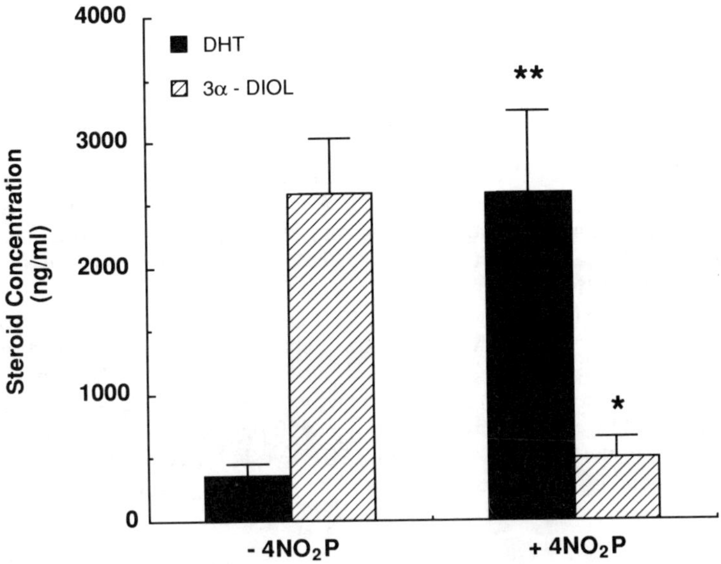

FIGURE 5. Concentrations of DHT and 3α-DIOL in media from cultures of Leydig cell progenitors after 24 h in the presence of 0.1 ng/ml LH and 10 μM DHT ± 500 μM $4NO_2P$, an inactivator of 3α-HSD. The results indicated that 90% of the added DHT was converted to the weak androgen 3α-DIOL within 24 hours. An 86% reduction in the activity of 3α-HSD was observed with the addition of $4NO_2P$. * = $p < 0.01$; ** = $p < 0.001$.

FIGURE 6. Testosterone production by Leydig cell progenitors cultured in the presence of 0.1 ng/ml LH and 10 μM DHT ± 500 μM $4NO_2P$. Testosterone production increased 5-fold in cultures treated with $4NO_2P$ compared to cultures that received LH + DHT alone (101.2 ± 21.5 vs. 19.9 ± 5.3 ng per 10^6 cells/24 hrs. * = $p < 0.01$.

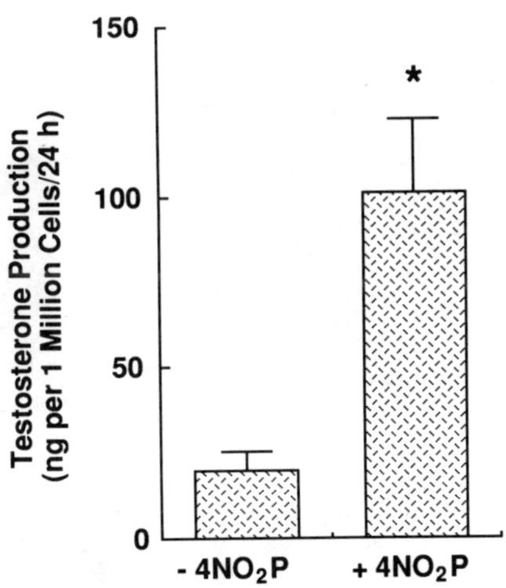

results indicate that the potency of DHT to stimulate increased testosterone production in Leydig cell progenitors increases when its metabolism to 3α-DIOL is blocked.

The Stimulatory Effect of Insulin-like Growth Factor-I on Androgen Production In Vitro *Is Larger for Immature Leydig Cells from Mid-Pubertal Rats than for Adult Leydig Cells*

Insulin-like growth factor-I (also known as somatomedin-C) circulates in the bloodstream, but is also produced locally in many tissues where it acts to promote growth and differentiation. During puberty, serum levels of IGF-I rise concurrently with growth hormone, LH, FSH, and prolactin.[40] Through its binding to specific receptors in target tissues, IGF-I stimulates the uptake of thymidine and amino acids, indicating a role in both proliferation and differentiation.[41] In the testis, IGF-I receptors have been localized to several cell types, including Leydig cells.[42,43] Studies from several laboratories have shown that treatment with IGF-I *in vitro* enhances testosterone production by adult rat Leydig cells.[44,45]

In light of the pubertal rise in serum IGF-I levels, the aim of the present study was to evaluate the stimulatory effect of this peptide on androgen production by immature Leydig cells from 30-day-old, mid-pubertal rats, and to determine whether there is a developmental change in the sensitivity of the Leydig cell to IGF-I stimulation. Purified Leydig cells from both 30- and 90-day-old rats were cultured *in vitro* for three days in the presence of 70 ng/ml IGF-I + low LH (0.1 ng/ml), or low LH alone. At the end of three days the media were changed, and replaced with medium

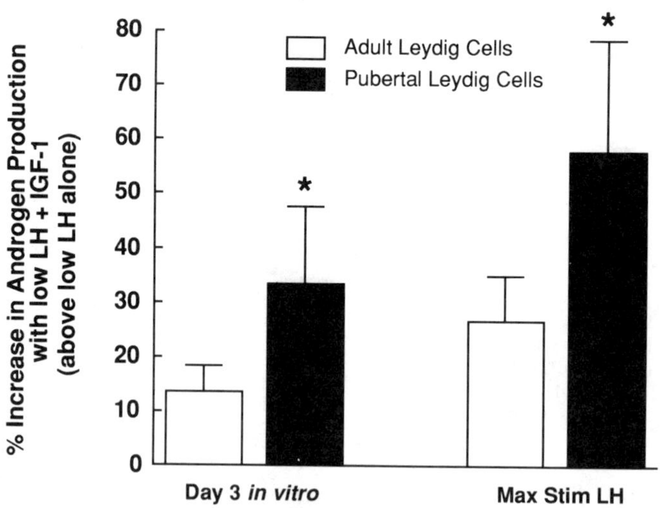

FIGURE 7. IGF-I–induced increase in androgen production: effect of age. Leydig cells from 30-day-old mid-pubertal rats and 90-day-old adult rats were cultured for three days *in vitro*. Androgen concentrations in Leydig cell spent culture media were measured daily and after maximal LH stimulation. IGF-I-mediated androgen production was significantly higher in immature Leydig cells compared to adult Leydig cells ($n = 9$, * = $p < 0.05$).

containing a maximally stimulating dose of 100 ng/ml LH. The results are summarized in FIGURE 7. By day 3 *in vitro*, the increase in androgen production due to IGF-I treatment was 35% (n = 9, $p < 0.05$) for immature Leydig cells (measured as the sum of testosterone + DHT + 3α-DIOL in spent media from IGF-I + low LH cultures compared to low LH alone). In contrast, adult Leydig cells that were treated with IGF-I + low LH produced a lower (though significant) 15% increase in testosterone on day 3 compared to low LH alone (n = 9, $p < 0.05$). Results were similar for cultured Leydig cells that were maximally stimulated with LH at the end of day 3 *in vitro*; IGF-I + low LH treatment again resulted in greater androgen production by immature and adult Leydig cells compared to low LH alone. At 60%, the magnitude of the increase was significantly larger for the immature Leydig cells than for adult Leydig cells, for which the increase was only 25% (n = 9 for 30- vs. 90-day-old, $p < 0.05$). These results demonstrate that IGF-I enhances androgen production by purified immature Leydig cells from mid-pubertal rats. In addition, the results show that immature Leydig cells are more sensitive than adult Leydig cells to IGF-I stimulation.

SUMMARY AND CONCLUSIONS

Leydig cell progenitors contain significant concentrations of androgen receptors. When the metabolism of DHT to 3α-DIOL is blocked, DHT stimulates testosterone production by Leydig cell progenitors, most probably via an androgen receptor dependent mechanism. Rapid metabolism by 3α-HSD may limit the potency of exogenous DHT to stimulate differentiation of Leydig cell progenitors *in vitro.* Insulin-like growth factor-I enhances androgen production by purified immature Leydig cells. The elevated sensitivity of immature Leydig cells versus adult Leydig cells to IGF-I stimulation indicates that this peptide hormone has a role in their differentiation during puberty.

REFERENCES

1. CHRISTENSEN, A. K. 1975. Leydig cells. *In* Handbook of Physiology. R. O. Greep & E. B. Astwood, Eds. **5:** 57–94. American Physiological Society. Washington, DC.
2. BYSKOV, A. G. 1986. Differentiation of mammalian embryonic gonad. Physiol. Rev. **66:** 71–117.
3. DE KRETSER, D. M. & J. B. KERR. 1988. The cytology of the testis. *In* The Physiology of Reproduction. E. Knobil, J. Neill *et al.*, Eds. **1:** 837–932. Raven Press. New York.
4. KERR, J. B. & C. M. KNELL. 1988. The fate of fetal Leydig cells during the development of the fetal and postnatal rat testis. Development **103:** 535–544.
5. KUOPIO, T., J. TAPANAINEN, L. J. PELLINIEMI & I. HUHTANIEMI. 1989. Developmental stages of fetal-type Leydig cells in prepubertal rats. Development **107:** 213–220.
6. HARDY, M. P., B. R. ZIRKIN & L. L. EWING. 1989. Kinetic studies on the development of the adult population of Leydig cells in testes of the pubertal rat. Endocrinology **124:** 762–770.
7. ROSS, M. H. & J. R. LONG. 1966. Contractile cells in human seminiferous tubules. Science **153:** 1271–1273.
8. SCHULZE, C. 1984. Sertoli cells and Leydig cells in man. Adv. Anat. Embryol. Cell Biol. **88:** 1–104.
9. SCHULZE, W., M. S. DAVIDOFF & A.-F. HOLSTEIN. 1987. Are Leydig cells of neural origin? Substance P-like immunoreactivity in human testicular tissue. Acta Endocrinol. (Copenhagen) **115:** 373–377.
10. HAY, E. D. 1989. Extracellular matrix, cell skeletons, and embryonic development. Am. J. Med. Genet. **34:** 14–29.
11. DECHELOTTE, P., J. CHASSAGNE, A. LABBE, M. AFANE, T. SCHEYE, B. DE LAGUILLAUMIE &

D. BOUCHER. 1989. Ultrastructural and immunohistochemical evidence of in situ differentiation of mononuclear phagocyte system cells in the interstitium of the human fetal testis. Early Hum. Dev. **20:** 25–26.
12. HARDY, M. P., W. R. KELCE, G. R. KLINEFELTER & L. L. EWING. 1990. Differentiation of Leydig cell precursors in vitro: A role for androgen. Endrocrinology **127:** 488–490.
13. CHUBB, C. & L. L. EWING. 1981. Steroid secretion by sexually immature rat and rabbit testes perfused *in vitro.* Endocrinology **109:** 199–203.
14. COCHRAN, R. C., A. W. SCHUETZ & L. L. EWING. 1979. Age-related changes in conversion of 5α-androstan-17β-ol-3-one to 5α-androstane-3α,17β-diol and 5α-androstane-3β-17β-diol by rat testicular cells *in vitro.* J. Reprod. Fert. **57:** 143–147.
15. CORPÉCHOT, C., E.-E. BAULIEU & P. ROBEL. 1981. Testosterone, dihydrotestosterone and androstanediols in plasma, testes and prostates of rats during development. Acta Endocrinol. (Copenhagen) **96:** 127–135.
16. HOOKER, C. W. 1948. The biology of the interstitial cells of the testis. Recent Prog. Hor. Res. **3:** 173–195.
17. AOKI, A. 1970. Hormonal control of Leydig cell differentiation. Protoplasma **71:** 209–225.
18. CHEMES, H. E., S. E. GOTTLIEB, T. PASQUALINI, E. DOMENICHINI, M. A. RIVAROLA & C. BERGADA. 1985. Response to acute hCG stimulation and steroidogenic potential of Leydig cell fibroblastic precursors in humans. J. Androl. **6:** 102–112.
19. LEON, M. D., J. C. CALVO, E. H. CHARREAU & H. E. CHEMES. 1990. Developmental changes in testicular interstitial cell populations, LH receptors and in the response to hCG in the rat. Int. J. Androl. **13:** 110–122.
20. KERR, J. B. & R. M. SHARPE. 1985. Follicle-stimulating hormone induction of Leydig cell maturation. Endocrinology **116:** 2592–2604.
21. KERR, J. B. & R. M. SHARPE. 1985. Stimulatory effect of follicle-stimulating hormone on rat Leydig cells. Cell Tiss. Res. **239:** 405–415.
22. TEERDS, K. J., J. CLOSSET, F. F. G. ROMMERTS, D. G. DE ROOIJ, D. M. STOCCO, B. COLENBRANDER, C. J. G. WENSING & G. HENNEN. 1989. Effects of pure FSH and LH preparations on the number and function of Leydig cells in immature hypophysectomized rats. J. Endocrinol. **120:** 97–106.
23. BARDIN, C. W., C. Y. CHENG, N. A. MUSTO & G. L. GUNSALUS. 1988. The Sertoli cell. *In* The Physiology of Reproduction. E. Knobil, J. Neill *et al.*, Eds. **1:** 933–974. Raven Press. New York.
24. SKINNER, M. K. 1991. Cell-cell interactions in the testis. Endocrine Rev. **12:** 45–77.
25. PAYNE, A. H. 1990. Hormonal regulation of cytochrome P450 enzymes, cholesterol side-chain cleavage and 17α-hydroxylase/C_{17-20} lyase in Leydig cells. Biol. Reprod. **42:** 399–404.
26. KLINEFELTER, G. R., P. F. HALL & L. L. EWING. 1987. Effect of luteinizing hormone deprivation in situ on steroidogenesis of rat Leydig cells purified by a multistep procedure. Biol. Reprod. **36:** 769–783.
27. RUIZ DE GALARRETA, C. M., L. F. FANJUL, R. MEIDAN & A. J. W. HSUEH. 1983. Regulation of 3β-hydroxysteroid dehydrogenase activity by human chorionic gonadotropin, androgens, and anti-androgens in cultured testicular cells. J. Biol. Chem. **258:** 10988–10996.
28. HALES, D. B., L. SHA & A. H. PAYNE. 1987. Testosterone inhibits cAMP-induced *de novo* synthesis of Leydig cell cytochrome $P\text{-}450_{17\alpha}$ by an androgen receptor-mediated mechanism. J. Biol. Chem. **262:** 11200–11206.
29. FANJUL, L. F., F. ESTEVEZ, A. DNIZ, I. MARRERO, L. BENITEZ, J. QUITANA, J. GONZALEZ, I. CENTOL & D. M. RUIZ DE GALARRETA. 1989. R1881 regulation of steroidogenesis in cultured testicular cells. Biochem. Inter. **19:** 301–312.
30. BARDIN. C. W., L. P. BULLOCK, R. J. SHERINS, I. MOWSZOWICZ & W. R. BLACKBURN. 1973. Androgen metabolism and mechanism of action in male pseudohermaphroditism: A study of testicular feminization. Recent Prog. Hormone Res. **29:** 65–109.
31. MORRIS, I. D., R. G. LENDON & A. ZAIDI. 1988. Inhibition of testicular and somatic development after treatment of the postnatal rat with the Leydig cell toxic ethylene dimethanesulphonate. J. Endocrinol. **119:** 467–474.
32. HAIDER, S. G., A. URBAN, B. HILSCHER, W. HILSCHER & D. PASSIA. 1983. Cyproterone acetate induced changes in the behaviour of hydroxysteroid dehydrogenases in rat Leydig cells during perinatal development. Andrologia **15:** 498–506.

33. CHEN, Y.-D. I., M. J. SHAW & A. H. PAYNE. 1977. Steroid and FSH action on LH receptors and LH-sensitive testicular responsiveness during sexual maturation of the rat. Mol. Cell. Endocrinol. **8:** 291–299.
34. CHANG, C., C. T. WHELAN, T. C. POPOVICH, J. KOKONTIS & S. LIAO. 1989. Fusion proteins containing androgen receptor sequences and their use in production of poly- and monoclonal anti-androgen receptor antibodies. Endocrinology **125:** 1097–1099.
35. SAR, M., D. B. LUBAHN, F. S. FRENCH & E. M. WILSON. 1990. Immunohistochemical localization of the androgen receptor in rat and human tissues. Endocrinology **127:** 3180–3186.
36. TAKEDA, H., G. CHODAK, S. MUTCHNIK, T. NAKAMOTO & C. CHANG. 1990. Immunohistochemical localization of androgen receptors with mono- and polyclonal antibodies to androgen receptor. J. Endocrinol. **126:** 17–25.
37. TEKPETEY, F. R. & R. P. AMANN. 1988. Regional and seasonal differences in concentrations of androgen and estrogen receptors in ram epididymal tissue. Biol. Reprod. **38:** 1051–1060.
38. WILLIAMS, D. & J. GORSKI. 1974. Equilibrium binding of estradiol by uterine cell suspensions and whole uteri in vitro. Biochemistry **13:** 5537–5542.
39. RICIGLIANO, J. W. & T. M. PENNING. 1989. Synthesis and evaluation of non-steroidal mechanism-based inactivators of 3α-hydroxysteroid dehydrogenase. Biochem. J. **262:** 139–149.
40. DAUGHADAY, W. & P. ROTWEIN. 1989. Insulin-like growth factors I and II. Peptide, messenger ribonucleic acid and gene structure, serum and tissue concentrations. Endocr. Rev. **10:** 68–91.
41. VAN WYK, J. J., S. J. CASELLA, M. HYNES & P. K. LUND. 1988. Indirect actions of growth hormone. *In* Human Growth Hormone, Progress and Challenges. L. E. Underwood, Ed.: 25–55. Marcel Dekker, Inc. New York.
42. HANSSON, H. A., A. NILSSON, J. ISGAARD, H. BILLIG, O. ISAKSSON, A. SKOTTNER, I. K. ANDERSSON & B. ROZELL. 1988. Immunohistochemical localization of IGF-I in the adult rat. Histochemistry **89:** 403–410.
43. PERRARD-SAPORI, M. H., P. G. CHATELAIN, C. JAILLARD & J. M. SAEZ. 1987. Characterization and regulation of SMC/IGF-I receptors on cultured pig Leydig cells. Eur. J. Biochem. **165:** 209–214.
44. LIN, T., J. HASKELL, H. VINSON & J. TERRACIO. 1986. Direct stimulatory effects of IGF-I on Leydig cell steroidogenesis in primary culture. Biochem. Biophys. Res. Commun. **137:** 950–956.
45. MOGER, W. H. & P. R. MURPHY. 1987. Chronic effects of insulin and IGF-I on steroidogenesis by rat Leydig cells. Arch. Exp. Med. Biol. **219:** 591–595.

DNA Attachment to the Hamster Sperm Nuclear Matrix and Nuclear Annulus[a]

JANE E. FARRINGTON

Oncology Center
The Johns Hopkins University
Baltimore, Maryland

RAJESH PATEL AND W. STEVEN WARD[b]

Division of Urology
Robert Wood Johnson Medical School
588 MEB
1 Robert Wood Johnson Place
New Brunswick, New Jersey 08903-0019

INTRODUCTION

The chromatin within the mammalian sperm nucleus is packaged so tightly that conventional thin section electron microscopy reveals only a homogeneous area of very electron dense material throughout the nucleus.[1,2] Given this solid, almost crystalline, highly compacted mass of DNA, it is perhaps surprising to discover that not only is the sperm DNA organized in a very specific manner, but that the sperm nucleus contains a wealth of nuclear structures that mediate the organization.[3]

We examined this organization using hamster sperm nuclei as a model, and our previously reported results are diagrammatically illustrated in FIGURE 1. Hamster sperm DNA is organized into DNA loop domains attached at their bases to the sperm nuclear matrix, at intervals of about 46 Kb (FIG. 1B; ref. 4). This is remarkably reminiscent of the way in which somatic cells are organized in their nuclei,[3,5] and this will be discussed in greater detail in the next section. Sperm DNA packaging differs from somatic cells, however. Pogany *et al.*[6] demonstrated that the mammalian sperm nucleus does not contain enough volume to package its DNA into the nucleosome structures found in somatic cells.[7] Balhorn[8] later proposed a more compact linear, side by side arrangement for the packaging of sperm DNA by protamines (see ref. 3 for a comparison of protamine and nucleosome packaging). In support of this, independent evidence suggests that both in cricket[9,10] and in mammalian[11-12] sperm nuclei, these loop domains are probably arranged in side by side, linear arrays. The fact that the organization into DNA loop domains is preserved during the extreme degree of DNA condensation of spermatogenesis, while the nucleosomal packaging normally

[a] This work was supported in part by National Cancer Institute Grant P30CA06973-27.
[b] Author to whom correspondence should be addressed; tel. (908) 937-7774.

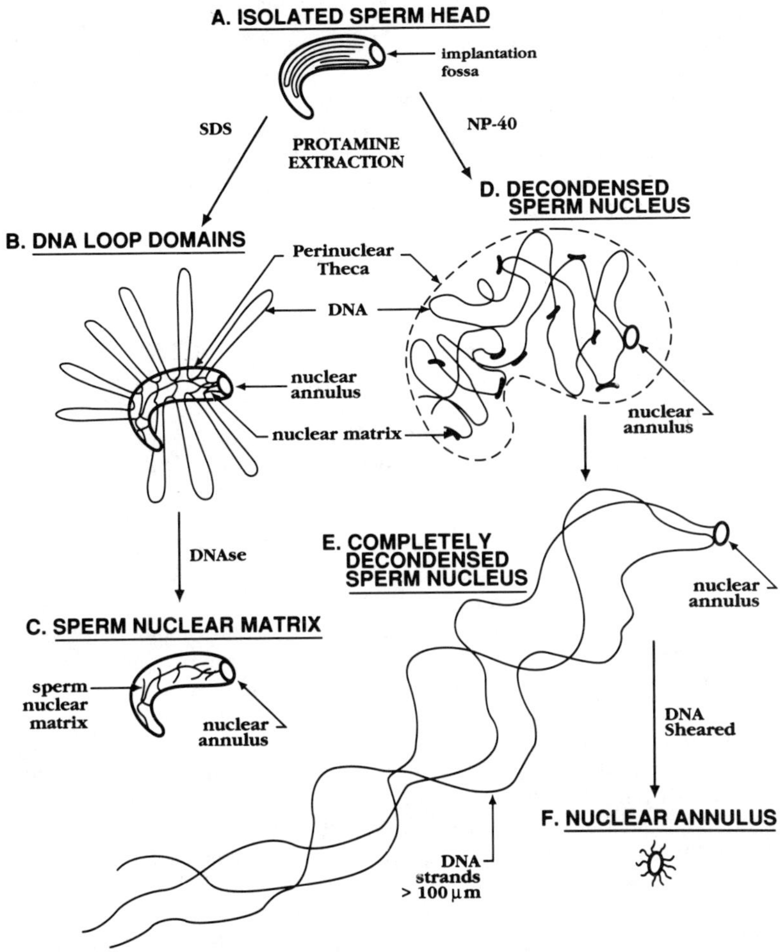

FIGURE 1. Diagrammatic illustration of the DNA organization in the hamster sperm nucleus. The two levels of organization, DNA loop domains (**A–C**, ref. 4) and the anchoring of much larger segments of DNA to the nuclear annulus (**A**, **D–F**, ref. 13), are shown. (Reproduced with permission from *Biology of Reproduction.*[3])

found in somatic cells is sacrificed, suggests that DNA loop domain formation is of fundamental importance in sperm function.

The structural organization of hamster sperm DNA can be further elucidated by allowing the sperm nuclei to decondense, *in vitro* (FIG. 1,D and E; ref. 13). This is done by washing the spermatozoa in the non-ionic detergent NP-40,[13] rather than the ionic detergent SDS.[4] Here, most of the nuclear matrix dissipates, leaving a single structure, the nuclear annulus, intact. The remarkable aspect of the nuclear annulus is that all the sperm DNA appears to remain anchored to the annulus as the rest of the nuclear structure completely dissolves (FIG. 1E), and when the DNA is mechanically sheared to very small pieces, a small amount of DNA remains attached to the annulus (FIG. 1F). This nuclear annulus associated DNA can be visualized with ethidium bromide as a small halo surrounding the annulus.[13] The nuclear annulus is located at the implantation fossa. The function of the annulus is still unknown, but its position and structural association with DNA suggest that it may serve to anchor the paternal genome during the decondensation of the sperm nucleus, and may provide a nucleation site for the formation of the pronucleus during fertilization.

This manuscript focuses on our recent attempts to further understand the specifics of the organization of sperm DNA by the nuclear matrix and the nuclear annulus.

SPERM DNA LOOP DOMAINS ARE ASSOCIATED WITH NUCLEAR MATRIX AT SPECIFIC SITES

DNA in somatic cells has long been known to be organized into loop domains attached at their bases to a structural element termed the nuclear matrix,[3,5,14,15] in a manner similar to that shown for sperm nuclei in FIGURE 1B. In somatic cells the DNA is attached to the matrix at specific sites by specific DNA sequences,[16,17] and these attachment sites are related to function of the DNA; replication origins[18,19] and active genes[16,17] are specifically associated with the nuclear matrix. We therefore examined the specific organization of sperm DNA loop domains for evidence that the sperm nuclear matrix similarly organized DNA in a specific manner. Sperm nuclear matrices with the DNA still attached ("halos," FIG. 1B) were prepared by salt extraction, and treated with restriction endonucleases. The matrix-associated DNA was then isolated from the loop DNA, which was released into the solution, by centrifugation, and the two fractions of DNA were examined by Southern blot hybridization for the presence or absence of specific genes.[20] The results are diagrammatically illustrated in FIGURE 2. All genes tested could be demonstrated to be specifically associated with either the loop fraction or the matrix DNA, suggesting that all sperm nuclei in the sample had the same, specific DNA organization.[20] Kalandadze *et al.*[21] have demonstrated similar results in chicken sperm with one other gene. While these data[20] represent an incomplete mapping of only six genes in the hamster, they suggest that the entire sperm genome is arranged by specific sequences on the sperm nuclear matrix.

THE STRUCTURE AND POSITION OF THE NUCLEAR ANNULUS

Previous work[13] has demonstrated that the nuclear annulus is located at the implantation fossa, inside the nucleus adjacent to the internal nuclear membrane (FIG. 3). It has a distinct morphology, as visualized by scanning electron microscopy,[13] being composed of two rib-like structures joined at their ends to form a bent torus (FIG. 4A). The plate in the center of the torus is thought to be the basal plate, a cytoplasmic structure described by Fawcett,[22] located just outside the nucleus at the implantation fossa. In this image, a few strands of DNA can be visualized (note that the image in FIG. 4A corresponds to the structure drawn in FIG. 1F). FIGURE 4B represents a less commonly obtained image of the nuclear annulus, and may be the nuclear face of the structure. Thin section electron microscopy of one of the ribs of the annulus

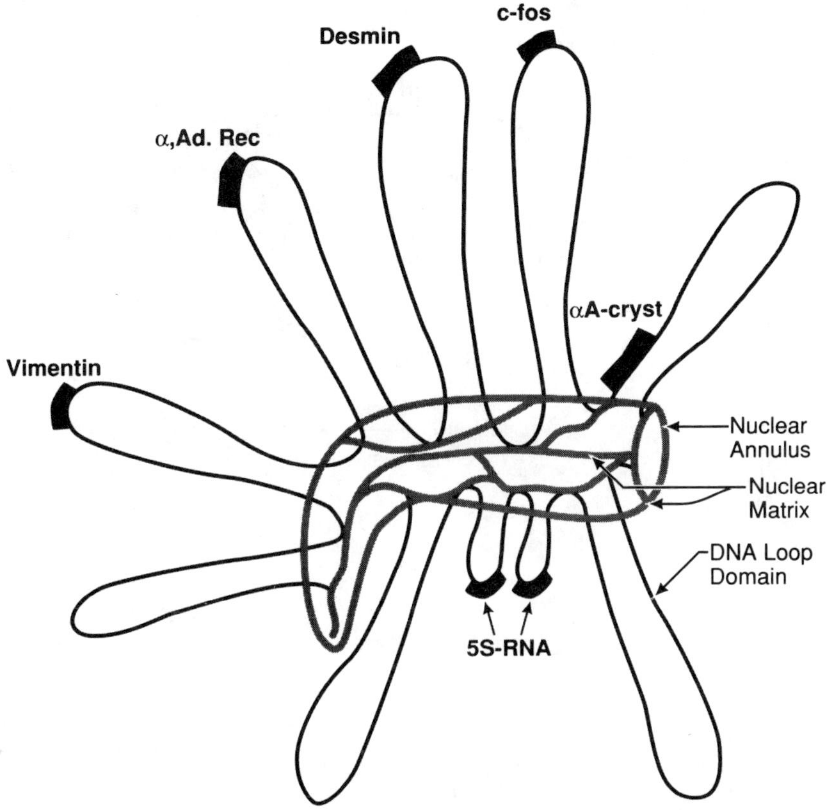

FIGURE 2. Diagrammatic illustration of specific genes' organization in relationship to the sperm nuclear matrix. This diagram is NOT drawn to scale because the exact distances for the genes are not yet known (see ref. 20). What is known is that of the six genes tested, only one, αA-crystallin, was demonstrated to be within 4 Kb of the sperm nuclear matrix. (This diagram is based on the results presented in ref. 20.)

reveals a complex layered structure in the outer edge (FIG. 5). From these studies, it is apparent that the sperm nuclear annulus has a complex, well defined structural composition.

DNA MAY BE ATTACHED TO THE NUCLEAR ANNULUS IN MINI-LOOP DOMAINS

Knowing the structure and the position of the nuclear annulus, we then began to more fully examine the attachment of DNA to the nuclear annulus. Previous (unpublished) work had suggested that the halos of DNA surrounding the isolated nuclear annuli (*i.e.*, FIG. 1F) were actually attached in very small, mini-loop domains. In these

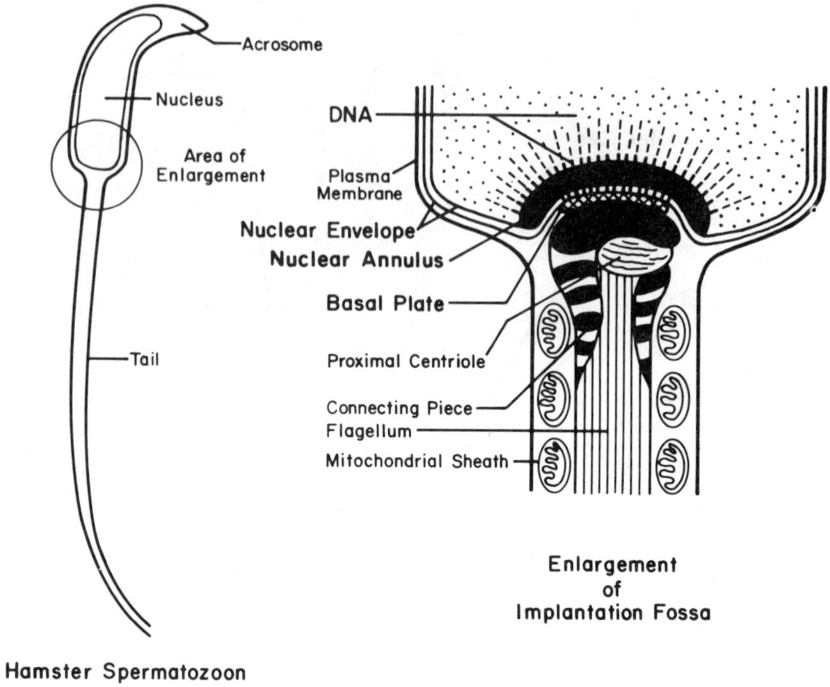

FIGURE 3. Diagram of the position of the nuclear annulus in the hamster sperm nucleus. The nuclear annulus is located just inside the sperm nucleus, adjacent to the inner nuclear membrane. It is probably closely associated with the basal plate, which is juxtaposed to the outer nuclear envelope. (Reproduced with permission from *Biology of Reproduction.*[13])

studies, isolated nuclear annuli were incubated with a high concentration of ethidium bromide and examined by fluorescent microscopy. The halos initially appeared very small, and grew to their full size (about the length of the annulus itself) as they were examined. Since ethidium bromide supercoils DNA when it is topologically constrained,[14,23] this result suggested that they were attached to the nuclear annulus in small, mini-loop domains. The ethidium bromide introduced supercoils into the DNA thereby condensing the loops into tangles, decreasing the size of the halo. As the DNA was visualized with UV light and ethidium bromide, the DNA became nicked, and unwound to its full size.

Because of the minute size of the halos surrounding the nuclear annuli (approximately 2 μm, see ref. 13), this decrease in halo size with ethidium bromide could not be documented with fluorescent microscopy. We have therefore begun rotary shadowing transmission electron microscopy to visualize the DNA emanating from the nuclear annulus. The preliminary results are shown in FIGURE 6. The strands of DNA are barely distinguishable, but it appears that the DNA is associated in loops (arrowheads, FIG. 6,A–C). At higher magnification, it is possible to see a nuclear annulus mini-loop more clearly (FIG. 6,B and C). The technique must be optimized for visual-

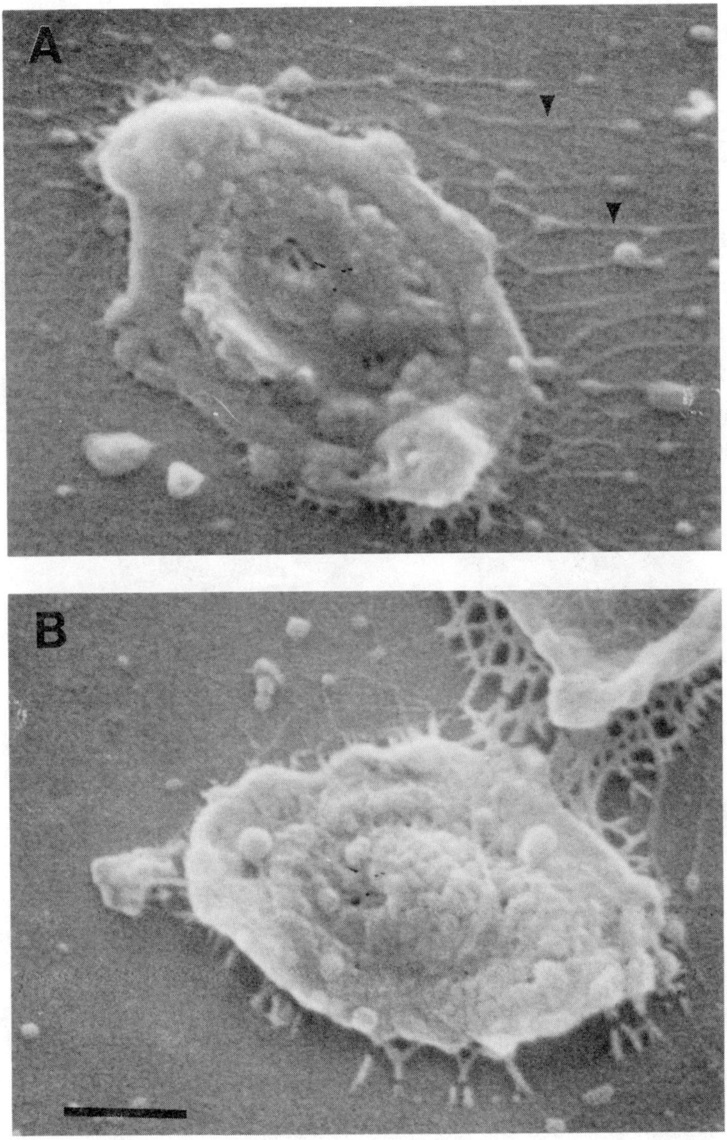

FIGURE 4. Scanning electron microscopy of isolated nuclear annuli. (**A**): One orientation, probably the cytoplasmic face. The center structure is the basal plate. Thin strands of DNA can be seen attached to the annulus (arrowheads). (**B**): A much less frequent orientation of the annulus, probably the nuclear face. Both **A** and **B** were prepared as described.[13] Bar = 0.5 μm.

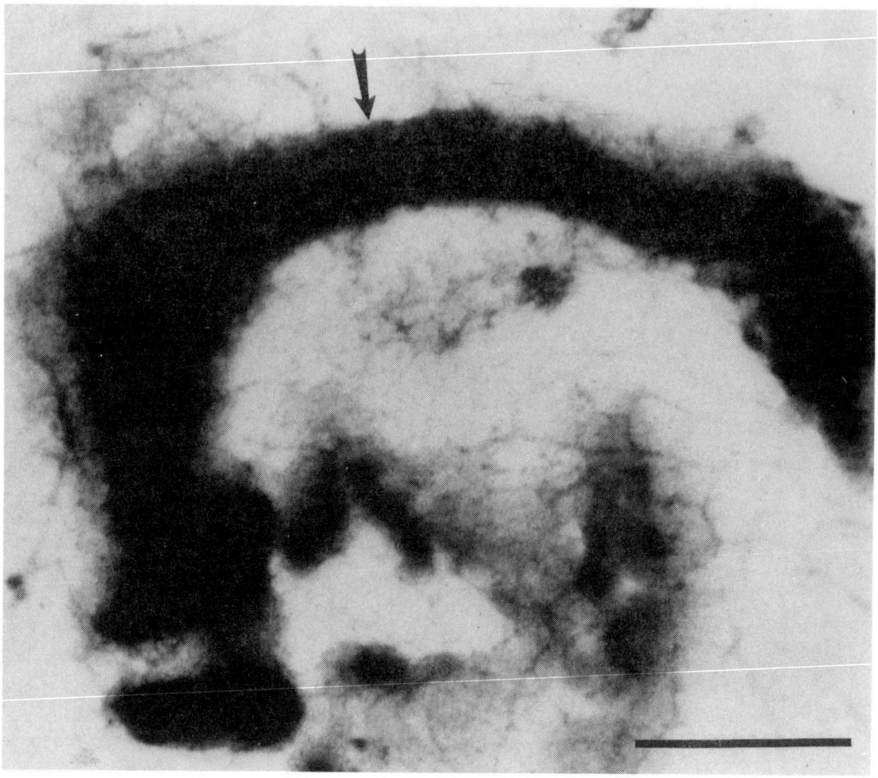

FIGURE 5. Thin section electron micrograph of the nuclear annulus. Nuclear annuli were prepared as described,[13] fixed in 3% glutaraldehyde, and subjected to conventional thin section electron microscopy. The arrow points to a thin ridge seen in all samples. Bar = 0.25 μm.

ization of the DNA before it is possible to say for certain that it is organized into mini-loops, and these experiments are currently underway in our laboratory.

The fact that the DNA may be associated with the nuclear annulus in the form of small loops presents an interesting problem. The original observations[13] demonstrated that the nuclear annulus anchored the entire sperm genome when the nucleus was decondensed. As illustrated in the transmission electron micrograph in FIGURE 6D, the DNA is connected to the annulus in very long strands. But if the DNA on the nuclear annulus is formed into loops, how is it connected with the rest of the DNA?

FIGURE 6. Transmission electron microscopy of the nuclear annulus. Nuclear annuli were prepared as described,[13] incubated for 15 minutes on a grid, and rotary shadowed at 6°. (**A**): Low magnification of the annulus and with its associated DNA. The DNA can barely be seen, and the arrow points to the top of what appears to be a DNA mini-loop. (**B**): Higher magnification of two annuli with emphasis on the DNA attachment. (**C**): Still higher magnification, with emphasis on the sites of attachment of DNA to the annulus. A loop of DNA can be seen in each frame, **A–C** (*arrowheads*). (**D**): A nuclear annulus that was still associated with long strands of DNA (*arrows*). Bar = 200 nm.

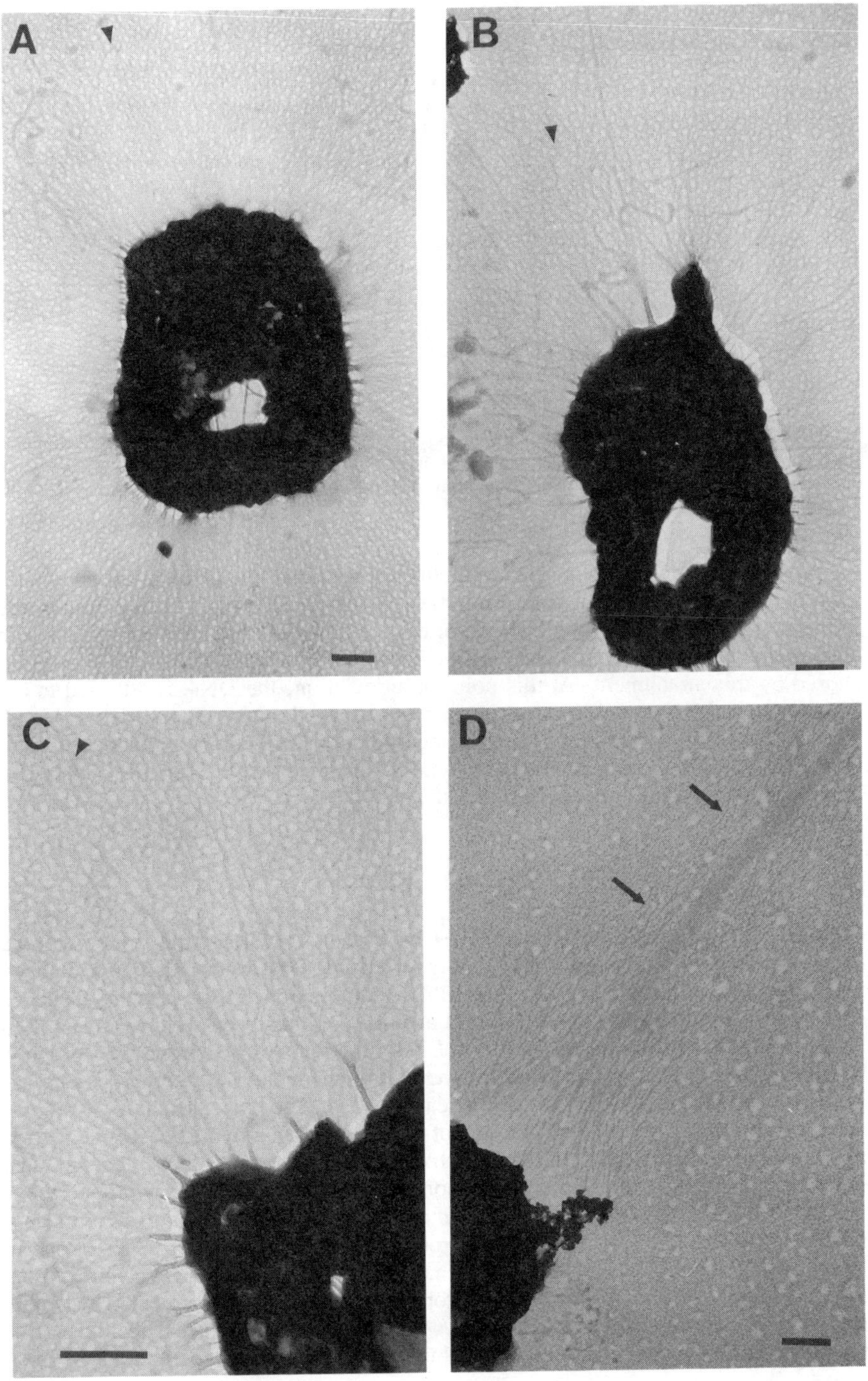
A
B
C
D

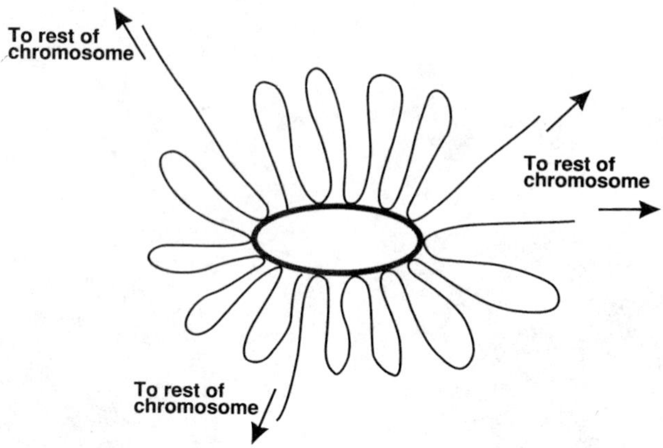

FIGURE 7. Diagrammatic representation of the possible association of DNA with the nuclear annulus. Each chromosome is anchored to the annulus at one or more points along its length. At each point of anchoring, the DNA is attached many times at short (5–10 Kb) intervals, forming mini-loop domains.

We propose a model for the nuclear annulus anchoring all the DNA in the spermatozoon that takes into account both properties, shown in FIGURE 7. Each chromosome in the sperm nucleus is a single strand of double helix DNA, and is associated with the annulus at least at one point along its length with the annulus, thereby being anchored by this attachment. At this point of association, the DNA is attached to the annulus at multiple smaller sites, forming mini-loop domains 5 to 10 Kb in length (FIG. 7). This may serve to render a stronger attachment to the annulus than is necessary for the DNA loop domain attachments of much smaller lengths of DNA to the nuclear matrix (compare FIGS. 2 and 7).

CONCLUSIONS

Mammalian sperm DNA contains at least two orders of complex, very specific organization. In the first level DNA is organized into 46 Kb loop domains attached at their bases to a nuclear matrix (FIG. 1B)[3,4] and these attachment sites are sequence specific.[20,21] This type of DNA structural arrangement has been well documented in somatic cells, and is intimately related to DNA function.[5,16] The second level of DNA organization is unique to spermatozoa, and that is the anchoring of much larger segments of DNA (>10,000 Kb) to the nuclear annulus. The exact structure of this association and its relationship to the rest of the DNA is unknown, but it is suggested by the evidence presented here that the DNA forms mini-loops on the nuclear annulus, indicating a specific, complex organization of DNA at the nuclear annulus.

The specific DNA organization of somatic cell DNA loop domains is intimately related to function,[5,16] and the same is probably true for the higher levels of sperm DNA organization. The function of spermatozoa is to deliver a viable genome to the egg in sufficiently intact form to ensure proper embryologic development. This viable state would include protection from DNA mutation and strand breakage during the transition from the male to the female (thus, the high degree of packaging). But, it may also include the presentation of the paternal genome in the proper tertiary configuration to allow the developing embryo to properly access the genes (thus, the very specific organization). In other words, the paternal part of the "blueprint" for the embryo may not only be the information in the sequence of the DNA, but the information in the organization of loop domains on the nuclear matrix, and the anchoring of the DNA on the nuclear annulus.

Whether or not this is the function of sperm DNA organization, it is clear that mammalian sperm DNA is organized in a very specific fashion. Disruptions in this structure may affect fertility,[24] as well as the first steps in embryonic development.[25] The study of the specific organization of sperm DNA will undoubtedly contribute to the overall understanding of sperm function.

SUMMARY

Hamster sperm DNA is packaged so tightly that it is the most highly condensed eukaryotic DNA known. Nevertheless, the sperm genome is also organized in a very specific fashion by two nuclear structures, the nuclear matrix and the nuclear annulus. The nuclear matrix organizes sperm DNA into loop domains approximately 46 Kb in length by specific attachment sequences. When the sperm nucleus is induced to decondense, the nuclear matrix almost completely dissipates, leaving only the nuclear annulus, a structure located at the implantation fossa within the nucleus. All the DNA remains anchored to the annulus during decondensation. Rotary shadowing transmission electron microscopy of isolated nuclear annuli retaining only a small portion of this anchored DNA suggests that the DNA is anchored to the annulus in a series of mini-loops, 5–10 Kb in length. These data support our previous suggestions that sperm DNA is organized in a very specific manner.

REFERENCES

1. Oko, R. & Y. Clermont. 1988. Isolation, structure and protein composition of the perforatorium of rat spermatozoa. Biol. Reprod. **39:** 673–687.
2. Fawcett, D. W. 1970. A comparative view of sperm ultrastructure. Biol. Reprod. (Suppl)**2:** 90–127.
3. Ward, W. S. & D. S. Coffey. 1991. DNA packaging and organization in mammalian spermatozoa: Comparison with somatic cells (minireview). Biol. Reprod. **44:** 569–574.
4. Ward, W. S., A. W. Partin & D. S. Coffey. 1989. DNA loop domains in mammalian spermatozoa. Chromosoma **98:** 153–159.
5. Getzenberg, R. H., K. J. Pienta, & D. S. Coffey. 1990. The tissue matrix: Cell dynamics and hormone action. Endocr. Rev. **11:** 399–417.
6. Pogany, G. C., M. Corzett, S. Weston & R. Balhorn. 1981. DNA and protein content of mouse sperm: Implication regarding sperm chromatin structure. Exp. Cell Res. **136:** 127–136.
7. McGhee, J. D. & F. Felsenfeld. 1980. Nucleosome structure. Ann. Rev. Biochem. **49:** 1115–1156.
8. Balhorn, R. 1982. A model for the structure of chromatin in mammalian sperm. J. Cell Biol. **93:** 298–305.
9. Suzuki, M. & T. Wakabayashi. 1988. Packaging of DNA in cricket sperm: A compact mode of DNA packaging. J. Mol. Biol. **204:** 653–661.
10. Kierszenbaum, A. L. & L. L. Tres. 1978. The packaging unit: A basic structural feature for the condensation for late cricket spermatid nuclei. J. Cell Sci. **33:** 265–283.
11. Koehler, J. K. 1970. A freeze-etching study of rabbit spermatozoa with particular reference to the head structures. J. Ultrastruct. Res. **33:** 598–614.
12. Livolant, F. 1983. Cholesteric organization of DNA in the stallion sperm head. Tiss. Cell. **16:** 535–555.

13. WARD, W. S. & D. S. COFFEY. 1989. Identification of a sperm nuclear annulus: A sperm DNA anchor. Biol. Reprod. **41:** 361–370.
14. VOGELSTEIN, B., D. M. PARDOLL & D. S. COFFEY. 1980. Supercoiled loops and eucaryotic DNA replication. Cell **22:** 79–85.
15. NELSON, W. G., K. J. PIENTA, E. R. BARRACK & D. S. COFFEY. 1986. The role of the nuclear matrix in the organization and function of DNA. Ann. Rev. Biophys. Chem. **15:** 457–475.
16. MIRKOVITCH, J., S. M. GASSER & U. K. LAEMMLI. 1987. Relation of chromosome structure and gene expression. Philos. Trans. R. Soc. Lond. **317:** 563–574.
17. COCKERILL, P. N. & W. T. GARRARD. 1986. Chromosomal loop anchorage of the kappa immunoglobulin gene occurs next to the enhancer in a region containing topoisomerase II sites. Cell **44:** 273–282.
18. PARDOLL, D. M., B. VOGELSTEIN & D. S. COFFEY. 1980. A fixed site of DNA replication in eucaryotic cells. Cell **19:** 527–536.
19. VAUGHN, J. P., P. A. DIJKWEL, L. H. F. MULLENDER & J. L. HAMLIN. 1990. Replication forks are associated with the nuclear matrix. Nucl. Acids Res. **18:** 1965–1969.
20. WARD, W. S. & D. S. COFFEY. 1990. Specific organization of genes in relation to the sperm nuclear matrix. Biochem. Biophys. Res. Commun. **173:** 20–25.
21. KALANDADZE, A. G., S. A. BUSHARA, Y. S. VASSETZKY, JR. & S. V. RAZIN. 1990. Characterization of DNA pattern in the site of permanent attachment to the nuclear matrix in the vicinity of replication origin. Biochem. Biophys. Res. Commun. **168:** 9–15.
22. FAWCETT, D. W., W. A. ANDERSON & D. M. PHILLIPS. 1971. Morphogenetic factors influencing the shape of the sperm head. Devel. Biol. **26:** 220–251.
23. LIU, L. F. & J. C. WANG. 1975. On the degree of unwinding of the DNA helix by ethidium II. Studies by electron microscopy. Biochim. Biophys. Acta **395:** 405–412.
24. EVANSON, D. 1989. Flow cytometry evaluation of male germ cells. *In* Flow Cytometry: Advanced Research and Clinical Applications. A. Yen, Ed.: 217–246. CRC Press. Boca Raton, FL.
25. BLOW, J. J. & R. A. LASKEY. 1986. Initiation of DNA replication in nuclei and purified DNA by a cell-free extract of Xenopus eggs. Cell **47:** 577–587.

Ectoplasmic ("Junctional") Specializations in Mammalian Sertoli Cells: Influence on Spermatogenic Cells[a]

A. WAYNE VOGL, DAVID C. PFEIFFER, AND
DARLENE M. REDENBACH

Department of Anatomy
Faculty of Medicine
University of British Columbia
Vancouver, British Columbia, Canada V6T 1Z3

INTRODUCTION

Ectoplasmic specializations are unique actin containing structures found in specific regions of intercellular attachment in Sertoli cells. As shown in FIGURE 1, these junction related structures occur in basal regions of Sertoli cells where they lie immediately adjacent to Sertoli-Sertoli junction complexes (sites of the blood-testis barrier), and in more apical regions where they are related to sites of attachment to spermatids. We suspect that the primary function of ectoplasmic specializations is to establish and maintain intercellular adhesion. If this is true, then the controlled disassembly of these structures, and hence of intercellular attachment, would be a requisite for movement of spermatocytes through the basal Sertoli cell junction complexes and for spermiation. In addition to influencing spermatogenic cells directly through a primary role in intercellular adhesion, it is also possible that ectoplasmic specializations may secondarily influence spermatogenic cells through a relationship with cytoskeletal elements positioned deeper in the Sertoli cell cytoplasm.

In this paper, we review the structure of ectoplasmic specializations and discuss evidence supporting the hypothesis that these cytoskeletal complexes are specialized actin associated intercellular adhesion junctions. We also present a model for how ectoplasmic specializations may interact with microtubules and intermediate filaments to translocate and position spermatids in the seminiferous epithelium.

STRUCTURE

Ectoplasmic specializations consist of a layer of actin filament together with regions of the plasma membrane involved with intercellular attachment on one side of

[a] The work reported in this review was supported by grants from the Medical Research Council of Canada (Grant MT-8020) and the British Columbia Health Care Research Foundation (Grants 15(89-2) and 31(88-2)). David Pfeiffer was supported by a predoctoral fellowship from the British Columbia Medical Services Foundation. Darlene Redenbach was supported by an MRC predoctoral scholarship.

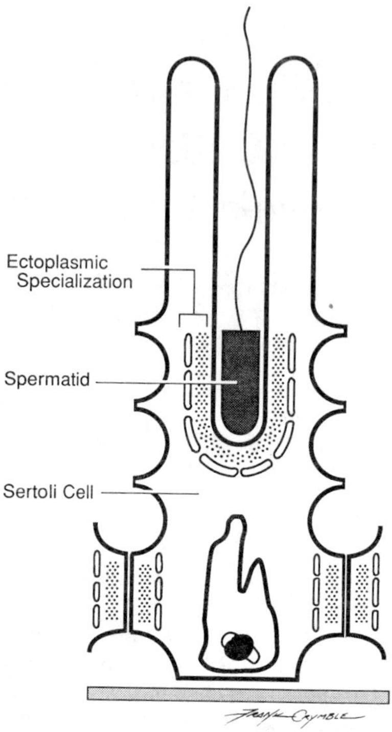

FIGURE 1. A schematic diagram of a Sertoli cell in which the location of ectoplasmic specializations is indicated. Ectoplasmic specializations occur at the base of the cell where they are situated adjacent to Sertoli-Sertoli cell junction complexes and in more apical regions where they occur at sites of attachment to spermatids.

the filament layer and a cistern of endoplasmic reticulum on the other. The ultrastructural appearance of these structures at Sertoli-Sertoli and Sertoli-spermatid contacts is shown in FIGURE 2 parts a and b and c and d, respectively. The morphology of ectoplasmic specializations at these two locations is similar except for the following differences: 1) the cytoplasmic surface of the endoplasmic reticulum in basal locations has ribosomes attached to it whereas that in apical locations generally does not;[8,67]

FIGURE 2. Electron microscopic images of ectoplasmic specializations at basal Sertoli-Sertoli cell junctions (**a & b**) and at apical sites of attachment to spermatids (**c & d**). At each location the structure consists of a layer of hexagonally packed actin filaments sandwiched between the plasma membrane and a cistern of endoplasmic reticulum.

Panel (**a**). A low power micrograph of basal regions of the seminiferous epithelium. Ectoplasmic specializations (*arrowheads*) occur on each side of a basal Sertoli-Sertoli cell junction that is situated apical to a spermatogenic cell in the basal compartment. *Magnification:* ×5800, bar = 1.0 μm.

Panel (**b**). This is a micrograph of a junctional site similar to the one shown in (**a**), but at a higher magnification. Clearly visible are the actin filaments (*arrowheads*) and cisternae of endoplasmic reticulum (asterisks). *Magnification:* ×58,600, bar = 0.25 μm.

Panel (**c**). Shown here is an ectoplasmic specialization associated with the acrosome (*asterisk*) of a spermatid. The hexagonal packing of the actin filaments (*arrowhead*) is evident as are elements of the endoplasmic reticulum (ER). Microtubules (Mt) are also present. *Magnification:* ×140,000, bar = 0.25 μm.

Panel (**d**). This is an image similar to that shown in (**c**), but with the actin filaments shown in longitudinal section. *Magnification:* ×129,000, bar = 0.25 μm.

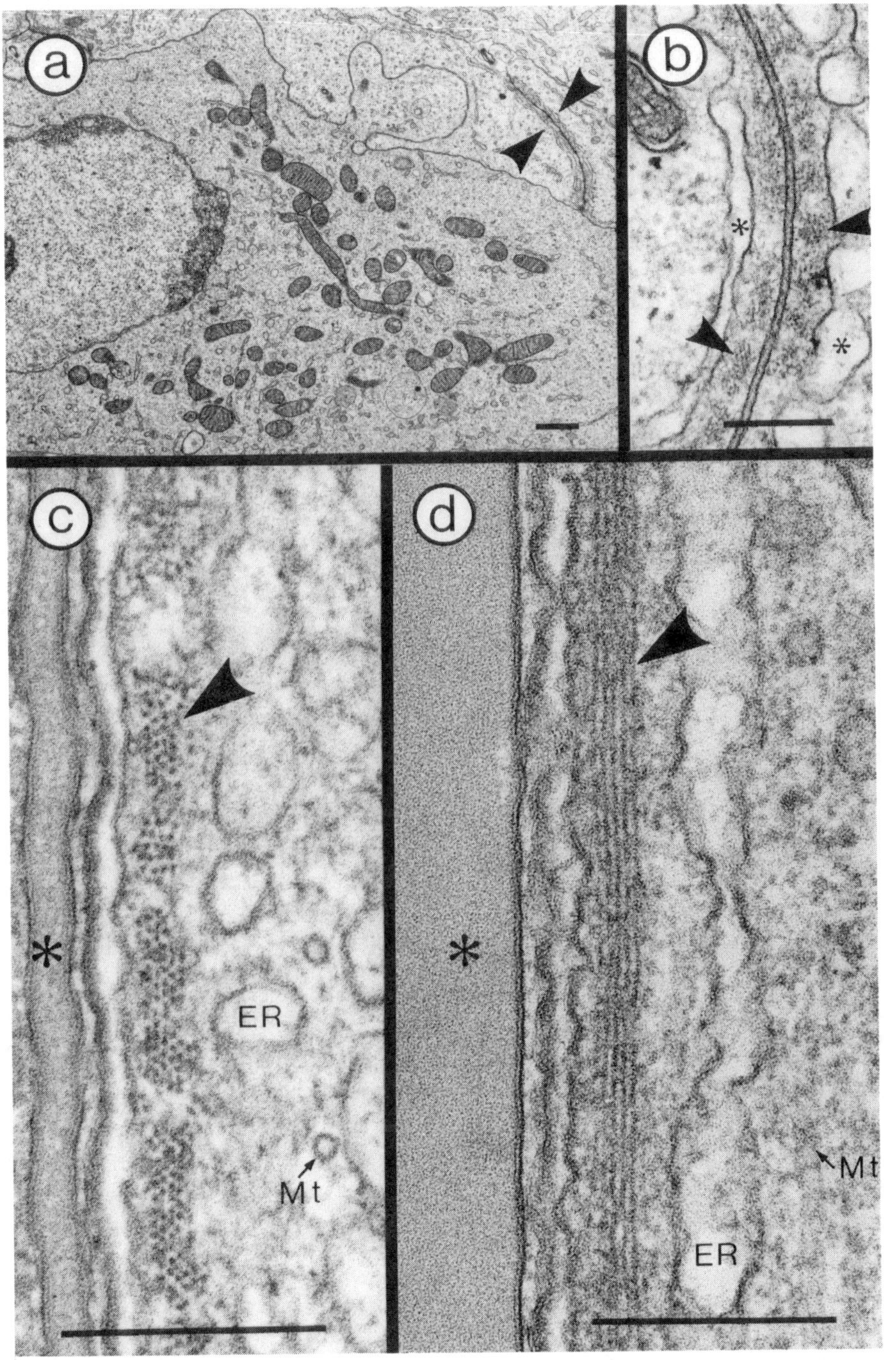
a
b
c
d
ER
Mt
ER
Mt

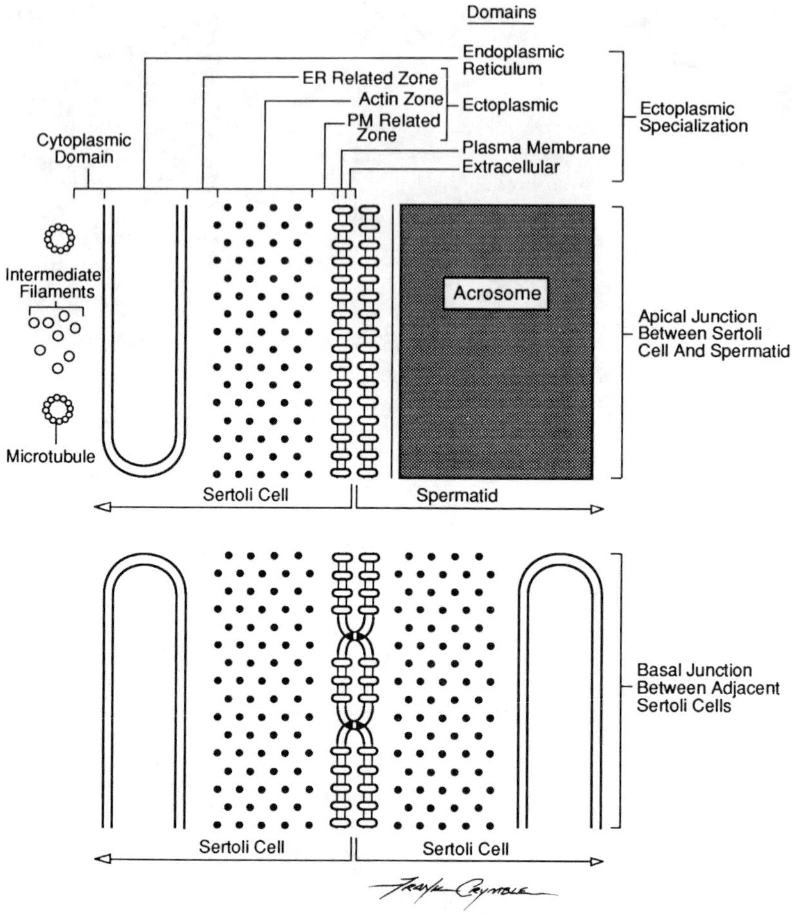

FIGURE 3. Illustrated here is a model of ectoplasmic specialization structure both at basal and at apical locations in the mammalian seminiferous epithelium. Ectoplasmic specializations consist of four major domains. A fifth domain (cytoplasmic) relates the ectoplasmic specialization to other elements, such as microtubules and intermediate filaments, of the Sertoli cell cytoplasm. At basal and apical sites, actin filaments are primarily associated with intercellular adhesion elements (indicated by the ovoid structures) in the plasma membrane. At basal sites they may secondarily be associated with tight junctions (indicated by the two joined black triangles in the area of focal contact between adjacent membranes).

2) the intercellular contact region, characterized by a narrowing of the intercellular space to between 70–100 Å (see refs. 20 and 25), contains prominent gap and tight junctions at basal locations whereas these junctions are not usually observed at apical sites; 3) ectoplasmic specializations in basal locations occur on both sides of the intercellular contact region while those related to spermatids occur only on the Sertoli cell side.

A model of the structure of ectoplasmic specializations is presented in FIGURE 3. Although the model is based on an early model proposed for adhesion junctions in general,[37] the design has been modified to accommodate some of the unique structural features of ectoplasmic specializations. The model consists of four major domains: 1) extracellular; 2) integral membrane (plasma membrane); 3) ectoplasmic; 4) endoplasmic reticulum. Although not defined as part of the structure of ectoplasmic specializations, we have also included a fifth domain (cytoplasmic) in the design because there is some evidence that elements in this region are responsible for relating ectoplasmic specializations, at least in apical locations, to microtubules and intermediate filaments found deeper in the Sertoli cell. Moreover, it may be elements in this region that are responsible for carrying out one of the functions attributed to mammalian ectoplasmic specializations—translocation of spermatids within the seminiferous epithelium.

What is known about each of the domains indicated in FIGURE 3 is summarized in the following sections.

Extracellular Domain

The extracellular domain is situated external to the plasma membrane. Ultrastructurally, fine fibrous linkages have been reported between adjacent plasma membranes in apical locations.[85,87] Although not yet conclusively demonstrated, there are hints in published micrographs that such linkages also may occur at basal sites (see ref. 24, Figs. 67 and 68; ref. 74, Fig. 25; and ref. 116, Fig. 1d).

By analogy with other systems (see ref. 33 for review), this region may contain the extracellular domains of integral membrane components involved with cell-cell attachment. However, at the present time the identity of these components has not been established.

Integral Membrane Domain

As is the case with the extracellular domain, we know very little about the plasma membrane of ectoplasmic specializations. Essential components that we suspect may be present are molecules involved with intercellular adhesion.

At actin-associated intercellular adhesion sites in other systems, actin filaments are thought to be linked to integral membrane elements responsible for intercellular attachment.[33] These elements include members of the cell adhesion molecule (CAM) family.[51] CAM types have been identified as elements of the adhesion domains of a variety of actin-associated adhesion sites including such structurally diverse forms as fascia adherens of cardiac muscle and adherens junctions of the lens.[113-115] The molecules responsible for intercellular attachment at sites of ectoplasmic specializations have not yet been identified.

Ectoplasmic Domain

The ectoplasmic domain is situated between the plasma membrane and the endoplasmic reticulum. More is known about the composition of this region than any other region of ectoplasmic specializations. This region can be subdivided further into three zones: a) plasma membrane–related zone; b) actin zone; c) endoplasmic reticulum–related zone.

Plasma Membrane–related Zone

Among elements present in this zone are molecules involved in linking the actin filaments to the plasma membrane. Morphologically, linkages are present between the actin filaments and the plasma membrane. They appear both as fibrillar strands and as clumps of amorphous material.[29,43,82]

Recent studies, using immunological probes, indicate that one component that is likely present in this region is vinculin. Vinculin is a 130 kD protein that characterizes actin-associated adhesion sites in general and is thought to participate in linking actin filaments to the plasma membrane.[9,11,31,32,34,36–38] Affinity purified antisera to human platelet vinculin reacts with a band of the appropriate molecular weight for vinculin on immunoblots of testicular fractions enriched for ectoplasmic specializations.[43] Moreover, the same probe, when used in conjunction with secondary antibodies conjugated to fluorochromes, labels Sertoli cell regions known to be sites at which ectoplasmic specializations occur in the rat[43,44] and codistributes with actin filament bundles in ectoplasmic specializations of the ground squirrel.[75] Data from similar studies at the ultrastructural level are consistent with the conclusion that vinculin is a component of ectoplasmic specializations.[75]

Immunological probes used at the light level indicate that another element that may be found in this region, at least at basal sites, is ZO-1 (Zonula occludens-1).[12,92] This peripheral membrane protein appears to be specifically associated with tight junctions.[92] Its presence at basal locations in the seminiferous epithelium is not surprising because of the extensive tight junctions found in these regions; however, its relationship to elements of ectoplasmic specializations remains to be established.

Plakoglobin, an 83 kD protein found in the submembrane "plaque" regions of intercellular adhesion junctions both of the actin filament and of the intermediate filament–related types, may be another element present in the plasma membrane–related zone of ectoplasmic specializations.[18] Immunological probes to plakoglobin used at the light microscopic level are reported to label sites corresponding to Sertoli cell junction regions.[18]

Another candidate for inclusion in this region, and/or possibly in the actin region, is the newly described actin-associated adhesion junction–specific peptide, radixin.[100] This 82 kD protein, initially isolated from adhesion junctions of liver cells, apparently has the capacity to bind to the "barbed" end of actin filaments. It is specific to cell/cell actin-associated adhesion junctions and is localized near or in submembrane plaques. Its presence in ectoplasmic specializations has not been determined.

Actin Zone

This region is composed of actin filaments and their associated proteins. The filaments form a layer, approximately four to six filaments deep, situated between the plasma membrane–related zone and endoplasmic reticulum–related zone. Elements in these neighboring zones apparently link the filaments to the adjacent membranes. That the

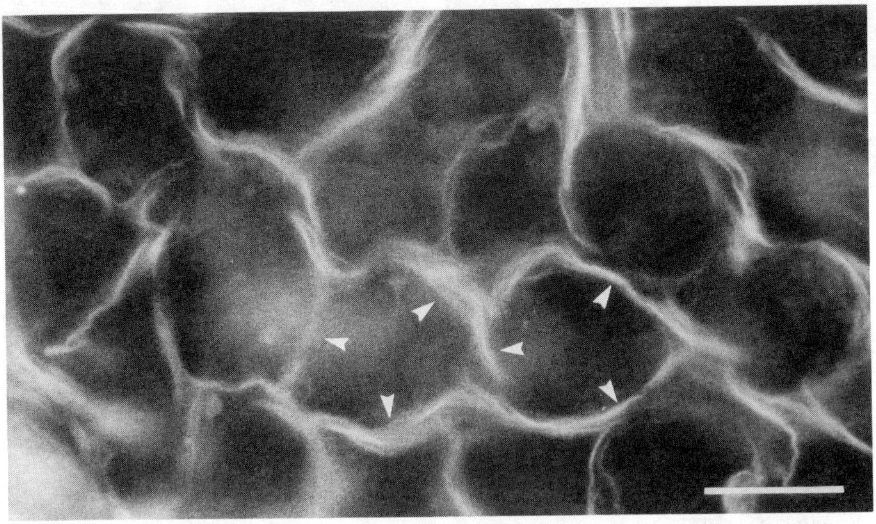

FIGURE 4. Ectoplasmic specializations in basal regions of Sertoli cells. The epithelial fragment shown here was isolated from a seminiferous tubule of the ground squirrel and treated with a fluorescent phallotoxin that labels filamentous actin. The epithelial sheet is viewed *en face*. Actin in ectoplasmic specializations circumscribes the base (*arrowheads*) of each Sertoli cell. *Magnification:* ×800. Bar = 10 μm.

filaments are actin is indicated by their ability to bind fragments of the myosin molecule,[59,99,108,110] anti-actin antibodies,[13,14,26,29] and chemical probes specific for actin (NBD-phallacidin).[94,95,107,109] The filaments are hexagonally packed,[20,29] have a uniform polarity,[99,108,110] and are often arranged in discrete bundles.[29,67,85,107] The interfilament spacing is roughly 10–11 nm and fibrillar linkages are often evident between individual filaments.[43]

At basal locations, the filaments circumscribe Sertoli cells. When isolated sheets of seminiferous epithelium are stained with NBD-phallacidin and are viewed *en face*, a honeycomb pattern is seen[107,109] (FIG. 4). This pattern is characteristic of the staining pattern that results when numerous probes specific for junctions or junction-related elements are used to label epithelia in general.[18,49,53,69,92]

In apical ectoplasmic specializations, the filament bundles form elaborate patterns that change during spermatogenesis.[107,109] These patterns are particularly evident when spermatids together with their attached ectoplasmic specializations are mechanically fragmented from the seminiferous epithelium and stained with fluorescent phallotoxins. Shown in FIGURE 5 is a reasonably complete spermatogenic series of such spermatids that have been isolated from the ground squirrel and labeled for filamentous actin. This series of micrographs nicely confirms that filaments in ectoplasmic specializations occur in bundles, that the filament bundles are organized into elaborate patterns, and that the patterns change during spermatogenesis.

Actin-binding proteins present in this region are just beginning to be identified. One element that is likely to be present is fimbrin or a fimbrin-like protein. Fimbrin is a 68 kD globular protein that cross-links actin filaments into bundles in which all

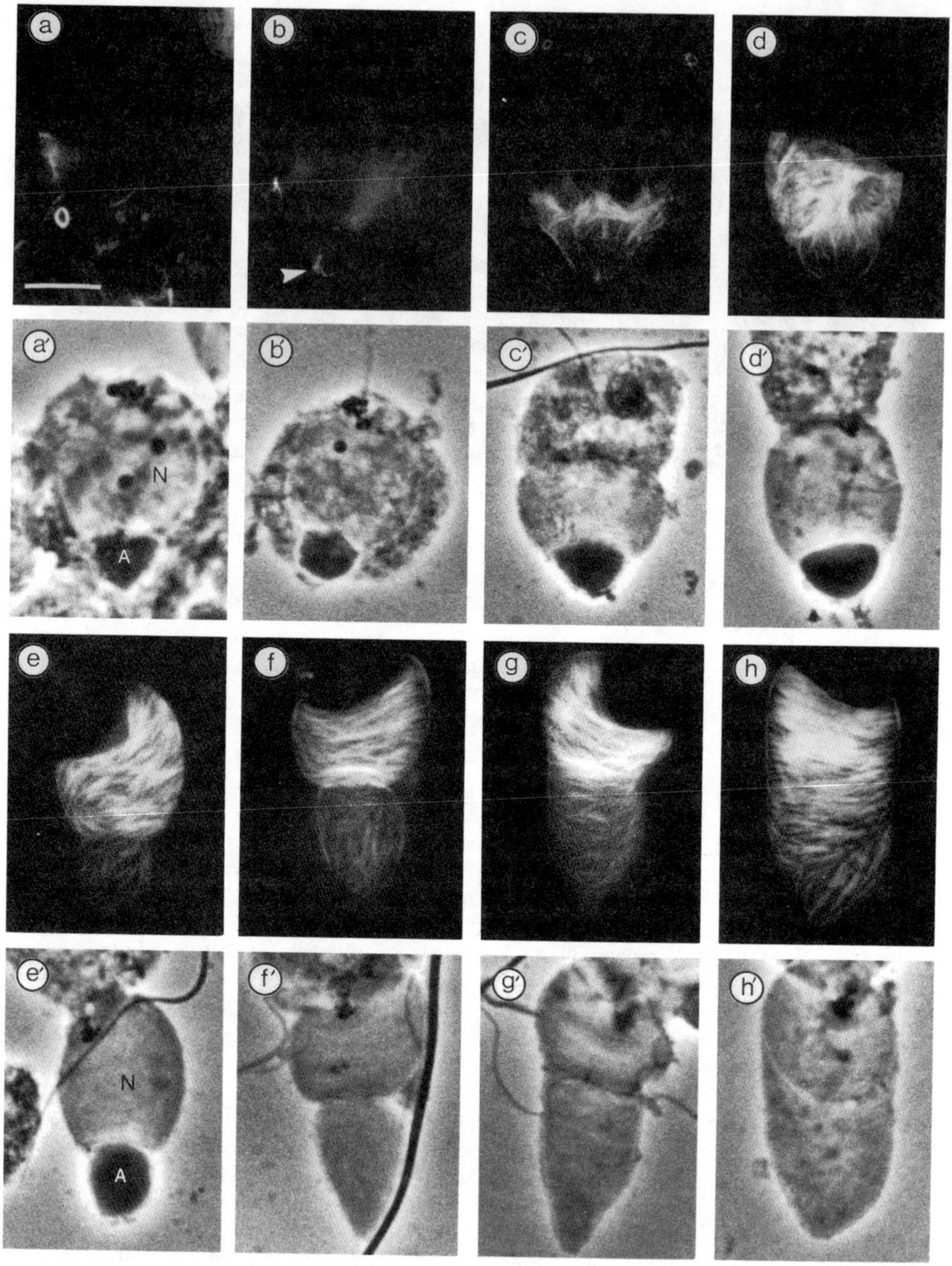

FIGURE 5. Documented in this series of micrographs are changes in filament patterns that occur in apical ectoplasmic specializations of the ground squirrel. The spermatids, with attached ectoplasmic specializations of Sertoli cells, illustrated here have been mechanically fragmented from the seminiferous epithelium and stained with a probe for filamentous actin. The series begins with an unpolarized round spermatid (panel **a**,**a**′) with which an ectoplasmic specialization is not yet detectable. Developing ectoplasmic specializations are first seen in Sertoli cell regions overlying the acrosome as the acrosome moves to the plasma membrane of the spermatid (*arrowhead*, panel **b**,**b**′). From this site, ectoplasmic specializations expand dramatically over regions adjacent to the acrosome and nucleus (panels **c**,**c**′–**h**,**h**′). As spermatid heads flatten, filament bundles on each side of the head course diagonally over the nucleus and acrosome. Seen superimposed, filaments on one side of the head appear oriented perpendicular to those on the other (panel **i**,**i**′). A filament bundle on each side of the spermatid head in panel (**L**,**L**′) is indicated by an arrowhead. As spermiogenesis continues,

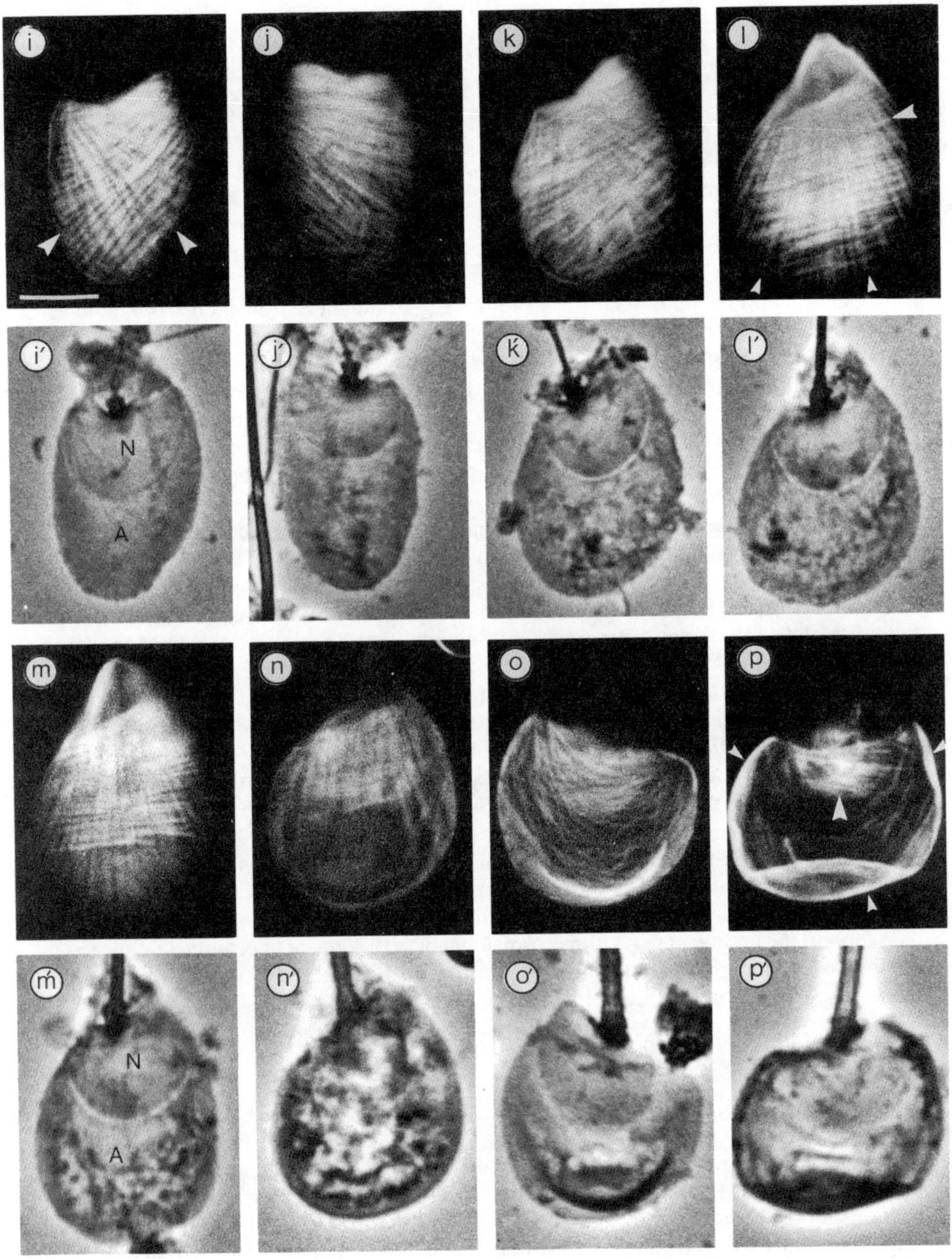

filaments on one side of the head move to a position perpendicular to the axis of the associated spermatid (*large arrowhead* in panel **L**) while those on the other side "fan out" and move to a parallel position (*small arrowheads* in panel **L**). During this period, there appears to be a separation of filament bundles on one side from those on the other. This separation occurs around the perimeter of the head. Following this (panels **m**,**m′**–**p**,**p′**), the perpendicularly oriented filaments are gradually lost in an anterior to posterior direction and remain only in regions over the nucleus (*large arrowhead* in panel **p**). Simultaneously, filaments on the other side of the head assume an arched orientation and are gradually lost in a distal to proximal direction ultimately remaining as a band around the cell margin (*small arrowheads* in panel **p**) in regions overlying a raised fringe of the acrosome. These two filament networks are clearly distinct from one another. N = nucleus. A = acrosome. Bar = 10 μm.

filaments have the same polarity[93] such as in the cores of intestinal microvilli (see ref. 63). Evidence indicating that fimbrin or a fimbrin-like protein may be present in ectoplasmic specializations is indirect. An antibody to fimbrin cross-reacts with a band of similar molecular weight as fimbrin on immunoblots of testicular fractions enriched for ectoplasmic specializations.[43] The presence of fimbrin in these latter structures would be consistent with the observed hexagonal packing and uniform polarity of the constituent actin filaments.

Results of immunofluorescence and preliminary immunoelectron microscopic studies indicate that another actin binding protein that may be present in this zone, and perhaps in neighboring zones, is α-actinin. α-Actinin is a rod-shaped homodimer that links actin filaments into loose bundles.[93] It has also been thought to participate in linking filaments to the plasma membrane (see ref. 6). Franke and coworkers[29] report that antisera raised against α-actinin react at the light level with ectoplasmic specializations. Russell and Goh[86] present some immunofluorescence data consistent with the presence of α-actinin at both apical and basal sites; however, the preliminary ultrastructural data contained in their paper is not sufficient to localize the protein to any particular zone of the ectoplasmic domain.

One actin-binding protein that does not appear to be present in ectoplasmic specializations is myosin II.[94,107] Antisera raised in rabbits against myosin isolated from human platelets does not cross-react with ectoplasmic specializations.[107] Moreover, glycerinated models of ectoplasmic specializations do not contract when exposed to standard contraction buffers.[107] Together these data indicate that, unlike junction-related actin filament networks in other systems,[53,69] filament bundles of mammalian ectoplasmic specializations do not have contractile properties.

Another actin-binding protein that appears absent is villin. In the absence of calcium, villin is an actin-bundling protein. When the concentration of calcium is elevated above micromolar levels, it has actin-severing properties.[93] Villin is localized, together with fimbrin, in intestinal microvilli. Anti-villin antibodies do not cross-react with sections of testis,[79] nor does the appearance of filaments in ectoplasmic specializations change when the isolated structures are exposed to high calcium.[42] These data support the argument that villin is probably not a component of ectoplasmic specializations even though the filament organization in the latter structures is similar in many respects to that in microvilli.

Endoplasmic Reticulum–related Zone

This region lies between the actin filament layer and the associated cistern of endoplasmic reticulum. In electron micrographs of normal or intact tissue, this zone often contains amorphous material that appears to link the filaments to the membrane. In fragmented or extracted material, fibrillar linkages are visible.[29,82] There also is indirect evidence for the presence of firm linkages between the endoplasmic reticulum and the filament layer. In ectoplasmic specializations that have been mechanically separated, together with spermatids, from the seminiferous epithelium, the ectoplasmic membrane of the cistern remains firmly anchored to the filament layer (see ref. 59, Fig. 2a; and ref. 110, Fig. 2c).

Elements in this zone have not been identified.

Endoplasmic Reticulum Domain

This domain consists of the cistern of endoplasmic reticulum that is attached to the ectoplasmic domain. At basal sites, the cytoplasmic membrane has ribosomes on its surface while at apical sites it generally does not, although ribosomes are occasionally reported in the latter location.[29,82,87]

Little is known about this domain; however, some authors have argued that it may serve to control filament-filament and filament-membrane relationships via a pathway that may involve local regulation of calcium levels. Treatment with trifluoroperazine, a calmodulin inhibitor, is reported to disrupt actin networks and junctions in rat testis.[27] Although there have been attempts to localize calcium in the endoplasmic reticulum,[28] the insensitivity of the techniques used has not resulted in convincing data.

Because of a possible role in regulating the function of ectoplasmic specializations, and because the endoplasmic reticulum is anchored to actin filaments on one side and is linked to microtubules on the other, this domain has the potential of being one of the most interesting regions of the entire structure.

Cytoplasmic Domain

This region is not defined as part of the structure of ectoplasmic specializations; nevertheless, it may contribute functional attributes to the system. The cytoplasmic domain lies adjacent to the cytoplasmic membrane of the endoplasmic reticulum and most likely contains elements that relate ectoplasmic specializations to other structures, such as microtubules and intermediate filaments. Shown in FIGURE 6 is a diagrammatic summary of the general arrangement of cytoskeletal elements in Sertoli cell cytoplasm and their relationship to an apical crypt containing an elongate spermatid. The diagram is based on data from the rat system, contained in papers by Vogl, Soucy and Lew,[109] Amlani and Vogl[3] and Vogl,[105] and is modified from a diagram presented elsewhere.[111]

Microtubules are abundant in regions of the Sertoli cell adjacent to apical crypts containing elongate spermatids and are oriented parallel to the long axis of the Sertoli cell.[3,105] These features are dramatically evident in cells that have been immunofluorescently labeled for tubulin (FIG. 7), and are also apparent in electron micrographs of apical regions where the general appearance of cytoplasm has been likened to that of axoplasm.[22] Ultrastructurally, linkages are visible between the microtubules and the endoplasmic reticulum of ectoplasmic specializations lining the apical crypts in which spermatids are embedded.[82] The identity of these linkages is not known; however, they may include mechanoenzymes for microtubule based transport of ectoplasmic specializations.

In addition to being related to microtubules, ectoplasmic specializations also are associated with intermediate filaments[3] (FIG. 8). In the rat, bundles consisting of approximately 8–12 intermediate filaments of the vimentin type extend from perinuclear regions into areas surrounding apical crypts. In these latter regions, the bundles initially lie adjacent to ectoplasmic specializations associated with the dorsal surface of spermatids. As the bundles course further apically, they appear to pass through a defect in the endoplasmic reticulum and through the outer two zones of the ecto-

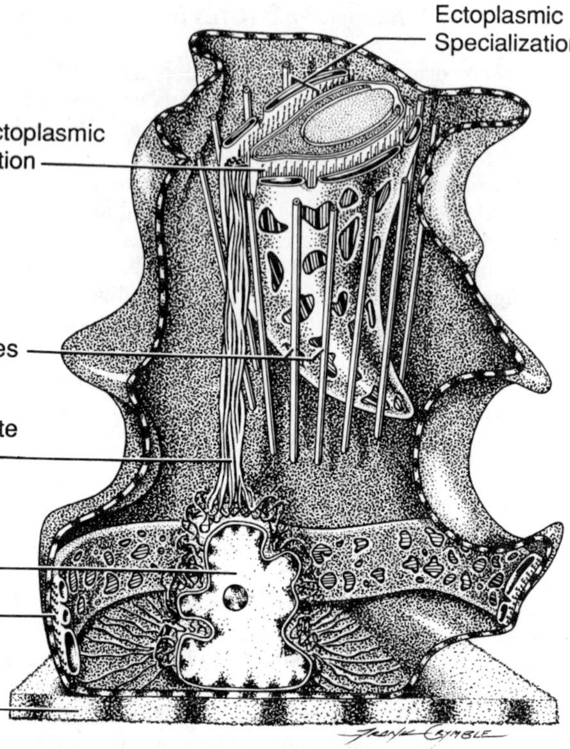

FIGURE 6. Our interpretation of how major concentrations of actin filaments, intermediate filaments and microtubules are arranged in a Sertoli cell of the rat. The diagram is modified after one presented elsewhere[111] and is based on data contained in papers by Vogl *et al.*,[109] Amlani and Vogl,[3] and Vogl.[105] Shown here is the basal half of a Sertoli cell and part of an apical crypt containing an elongate spermatid. Actin filaments are concentrated in ectoplasmic specializations located at basal Sertoli cell junctions and at sites of attachment to spermatids. Intermediate filaments are perinuclear in position. From here, bundles extend to desmosome-like junctions with early spermatogenic cells and to ectoplasmic specializations associated with spermatids. Microtubules are prominent elements of the Sertoli cell cytoskeleton. Most are arranged perpendicular to the long axis of the cell.

plasmic domain to reach the plasma membrane–related zone. None of the components involved in linking the intermediate filaments to various regions of ectoplasmic specializations have been identified.

FUNCTION

Historical Perspective

Many functions have been suggested for ectoplasmic specializations. Of these functions, the most numerous have been those proposing a role in intercellular attachment and the related processes of sperm release and turnover of the blood-testis barrier.

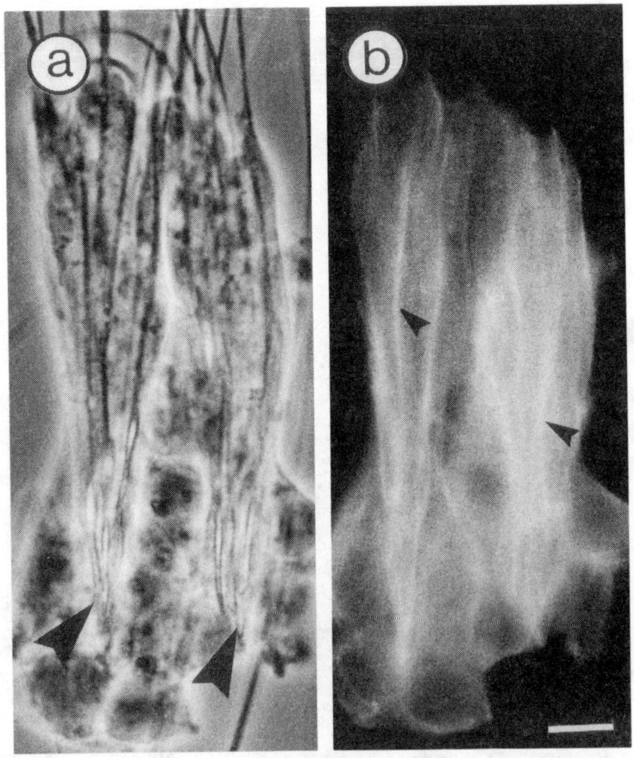

FIGURE 7. These are paired phase (panel **a**) and fluorescence (panel **b**) micrographs of a fragment of rat seminiferous epithelium that has been processed for tubulin immunofluorescence. Linear tracts of fluorescence (*arrowheads* in panel **b**) are oriented parallel to the long axis of the Sertoli cells and surround clusters of spermatids (*arrowheads* in panel **a**). That the staining is mainly in the Sertoli cells and not in the spermatid tails is indicated by the lack of staining in the flagella extending beyond the limits of the epithelium. Controls for specificity are described elsewhere.[105] *Magnification:* ×820, bar = 10 μm.

On the basis of concepts being developed in other systems and on his observations of testicular ultrastructure, Brokelmann[8] suggested two possible functions. First, he suggested the system may facilitate the transfer of "metabolites" between cells. Second, he argued that the structures may be "adhesion plate(s)" that "increase the adhesive forces between the plasma membranes." He observed that the disappearance of ectoplasmic specializations at apical sites was correlated with sperm release.

Like Brokelmann, Nicander[67] argued that the structures are intercellular attachment devices. At basal sites, he observed that the structures appeared reminiscent of the zonula occludens and zonula adherens described in other systems by Farquar and Palade.[21] In fact, he states that "the whole specialized inter-Sertoli junctional complex might represent a modified terminal bar transferred to a deep level of the epithelium." At apical sites, he suggested that the system may have adhesive properties perhaps of a "hemidesmosomal character." He further observed that the loss of ecto-

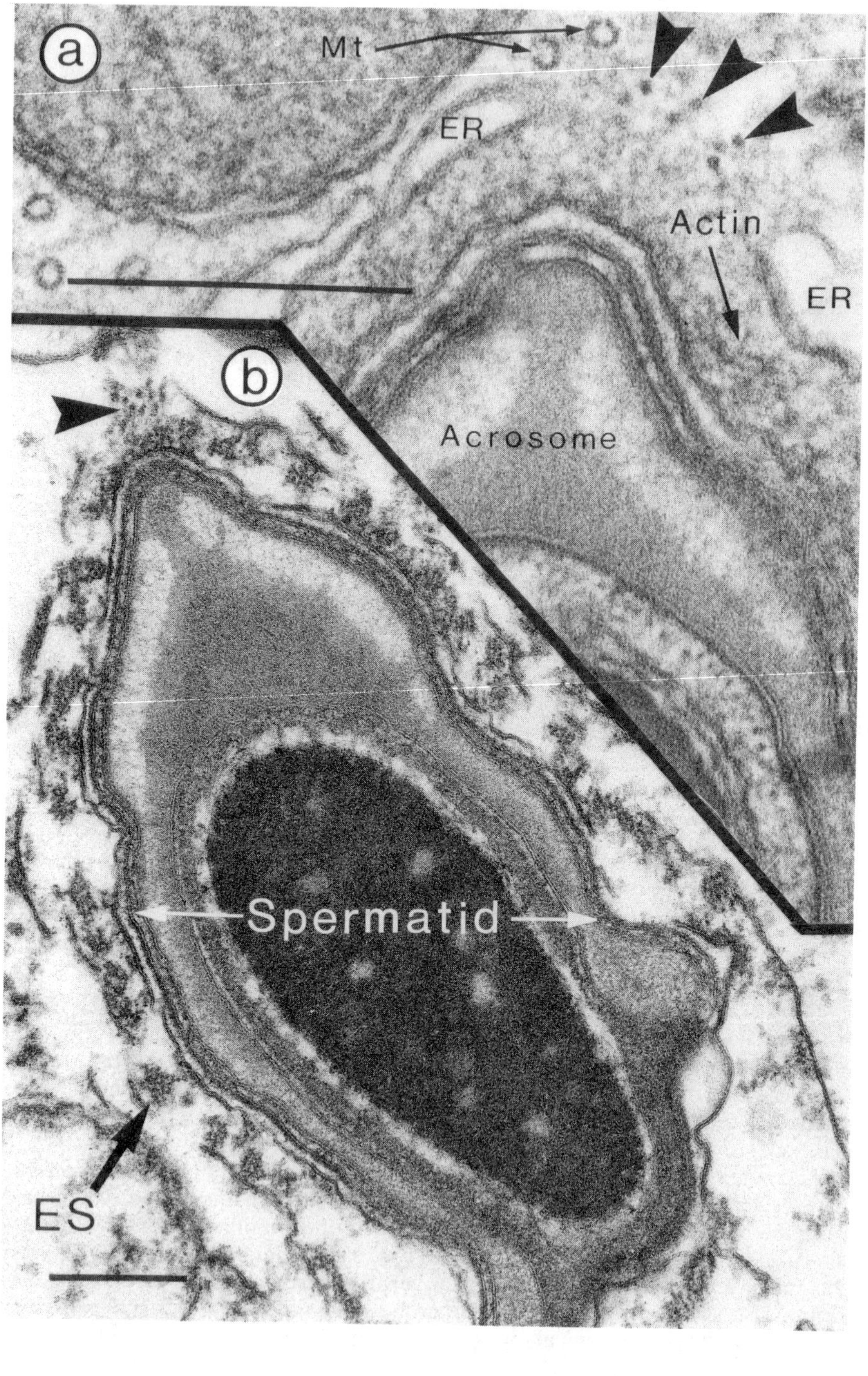
a
Mt
ER
Actin
ER
b
Acrosome
Spermatid
ES

plasmic specializations, at apical sites, was correlated with sperm release and, at basal sites, with movement of spermatocytes through Sertoli-Sertoli junctions.

Flickinger and Fawcett[25] argued against any direct nutritional role for ectoplasmic specializations on grounds that the structures were not found in association with developing spermatogenic cells other than spermatids. They concluded that, although some features of ectoplasmic specializations indicate the system may have some "physiological attributes," their function may not be "fundamentally different from that of desmosomes and zonula adherents" and that, at basal sites, they may be "adaptations to the unusual mechanical problem of maintaining the integrity of the epithelium in the face of constantly changing shape of the sustentacular cells concurrent with the slow escalation of germinal cells."

Another major contribution to the literature on the function of ectoplasmic specializations was published by Ross in 1977.[81] In this study, the author used lanthanum to investigate the permeability of junctional sites both at apical and basal locations. He reported the distance between adjacent plasma membranes at both apical and basal sites to be generally around 90 Å and that permeability junctions were demonstrable only at basal locations. He argued that because ectoplasmic specializations are present and morphologically similar at both apical and basal locations, the structures are most probably related to "maintaining and regulating cell adhesion" and not to establishing permeability junctions.

During the same year, Russell[82] interpreted results of his experiments with hypertonic buffers as providing no convincing evidence for a direct role in cell adhesion. Rather, he suggested that the submembrane filament networks simply "stiffen" the adjacent plasma membrane, thereby forming a reinforcing mantle on which other cytoskeletal elements may act to generate force and movement that, in apical locations, would be responsible for positioning spermatids within the epithelium.

Because the presence of microfilaments was initially viewed as being indicative of contractile activity, ectoplasmic specializations were suggested to carry out their function via some form of contractile mechanism. Dym and Fawcett[20] speculated that contractile force could be part of the mechanism by which ectoplasmic specializations might facilitate the apical movement of spermatogenic cells through Sertoli-Sertoli cell junctions. In apical locations, Toyama[99] suggested that the filament bundles might actually "grip" spermatid heads. The absence of myosin II,[107] the uniform polarity[99,108,110] and hexagonal packing[20] of constituent actin filaments, and the lack of demonstrable contraction by glycerinated models when placed in appropriate buffers[107] argue against a role of contraction in the function of ectoplasmic specializations.

Although other functions, such as influencing the acrosome shape of spermatids,[23] have been suggested for ectoplasmic specializations, it is obvious that the most popular

---

FIGURE 8. Shown here are two electron micrographs in which intermediate filaments are evident in association with ectoplasmic specializations of Sertoli cells. The tissue shown in panel (**a**), was processed using standard techniques for electron microscopy. A group of intermediate filaments (arrowheads) lies in a defect in the endoplasmic reticulum (ER) of the ectoplasmic specialization. Microtubules (Mt), actin, and the acrosome of a spermatid are also indicated. The tissue shown in panel (**b**) was detergent extracted prior to fixation. The position of the intermediate filaments (arrowhead) relative to the spermatid head and surrounding ectoplasmic specialization (ES) is indicated by the large arrowhead. Details of how this material was obtained and evidence that the filaments are of the intermediate type are contained in the paper by Amlani and Vogl.[3] *Magnification:* ×168,000, bar = 0.25 μm.

functions have been those in which the structures are proposed to facilitate intercellular attachment and to assist in positioning spermatogenic cells within the epithelium. In the following sections we present working hypotheses in both of these areas and present the evidence on which each hypothesis is based.

Adhesion Hypothesis

Based on discussions presented in the literature, on what is currently known about the structure of ectoplasmic specializations, and on what is known about junction-related actin complexes in other systems, it is possible to generate the following working hypothesis: *Ectoplasmic specializations are a form of actin-associated intercellular adhesion junction in which the actin filaments function to establish and/or reinforce membrane domains involved with intercellular attachment. Inherent to this concept is some form of linkage between the actin filaments and elements in the membrane responsible for intercellular adhesion. At basal sites, the system secondarily interacts with components of other junction types (tight and perhaps gap) to facilitate establishment of basal junctional complexes. Loss of ectoplasmic specializations, through disassembly and/or internalization, results in a loss of intercellular adhesion. This loss is part of the process by which spermatogenic cells move through the "blood-testis barrier" and the mechanism of sperm release.*

Evidence by Analogy with Other Systems

Filament related adhesion junctions in general can be divided into two general classes: those that, on their cytoplasmic faces, are related to intermediate filaments, and those that are related to filamentous actin. Each of these classes is composed of a spectrum of molecular components that is characteristic of that class.[33,88] Actin-associated adhesion junctions, which are the junctions that concern us in this review, are characterized mainly by the presence of vinculin and, of course, filamentous actin.

Actin associated adhesion junctions are subdivided further into two categories: cell/cell and cell/substratum junctions.[33] In addition to containing the elements that characterize actin associated adhesion junctions in general, each of these subtypes appears to possess its own set of unique components. For example, intercellular adhesion junctions contain radixin,[100] while those present between cells and their substratum contain talin.[10] Both at cell/cell and cell/substratum adhesion sites, actin filaments are thought to be linked to elements in the membrane responsible for adhesion.[11,33,36–38,96] At intercellular sites these elements include the CAMs (cell adhesion molecules). At cell/substratum locations, they include cell/matrix receptors such as the integrins.

Actin-associated adhesion junctions are reasonably widespread in vertebrate cells. Examples of the cell/cell type of junction include the zonula adherens of epithelia[34,35] and the fascia adherens of cardiac muscle.[34,98] Examples of the cell/substratum type include focal contacts of cultured cells,[9,30] dense plaques of smooth muscle,[34,35,112] myotendon junctions of skeletal muscle,[89] and costameres of skeletal muscle and cardiac muscle.[70,71]

If ectoplasmic specializations are a form of actin associated adhesion junction, they should possess both the morphological features and the molecular elements that characterize actin associated junctions in general. The fact that ectoplasmic specializations occur mainly at sites of intercellular attachment is accepted. Moreover, it is firmly established that the filament type present in these structures is actin. Most importantly, recent evidence indicates that vinculin, a molecule characteristically present at actin-associated adhesion sites and not present at tight junctions and desmosomes, is likely present in ectoplasmic specializations.[43,75]

It is perhaps pertinent at this stage in our discussion to point out that there are two major differences between ectoplasmic specializations and the zonula adherens in other epithelia. First, and as mentioned previously, the actin filament bundles do not have contractile properties. Second, the intercellular space is approximately half that reported for typical zonula adherens (see ref. 21). This latter observation may indicate that the types of attachment molecules present in ectoplasmic specializations are different from those at other adhesion junctions or that the extracellular domains of the molecules are different.

In most epithelia, tight and adhesion junctions occur in close proximity to each other as part of the apical junctional complex. There is currently much interest in how the presence of one junction type may influence the formation and placement of the other. Recent data tend to indicate that there is a developmental relationship between the junctions,[47] and at least one model of this relationship indicates that the presence of adhesion junctions may secondarily influence the development and location of tight junctions.[45,46] This latter model fits nicely with what is observed for ectoplasmic specializations of Sertoli cells. Ectoplasmic specializations have similar morphology at both apical and basal sites. The junction type common to both appears to be of the adhesion type. At basal sites, tight junctions are found within, but are not restricted to, ectoplasmic specializations.[20]

Evidence from Morphology

A number of morphological observations indicate that the submembrane filaments and attached cistern of endoplasmic reticulum of ectoplasmic specializations are associated with junctions and that the junction type is of the adhesion variety. First, the complex occurs adjacent to areas where the intercellular space narrows to 70–100 Å.[20,67] Second, fibrous linkages, reminiscent of those demonstrated between adjacent plasma membranes of the zonula adherens in intestinal epithelium,[52] occur in the intercellular space at ectoplasmic specializations.[85,87] Third, ectoplasmic specializations remain firmly attached to spermatids that are mechanically dissociated from the seminiferous epithelium.[29,59,80,82,107,109,110] In fact, treatment with trypsin[80] or exposure to rigorous mechanical force[43] is necessary to separate the two structures in preparations such as these. Because gap and tight junctions do not characteristically occur at apical sites, these two junction types can be eliminated as being responsible for the observed intercellular attachment. Fourth, the normal "disappearance" of ectoplasmic specializations during spermatogenesis is generally correlated with two major events that involve a loss of intercellular attachment—sperm release and movement of spermatocytes through the blood-testis barrier.[83,84]

Evidence from Perturbation Experiments

If actin filaments within ectoplasmic specializations are associated with reinforcing membrane domains involved with intercellular adhesion, then removal of the filaments should result in a weakening or loss of intercellular adhesion. Experiments attempting to verify this prediction are difficult to perform most likely because the heavily cross-linked actin bundles of ectoplasmic specializations, *in vitro*, appear insensitive to cytochalasin.[29] Experiments in which cytochalasin is injected intratesticularly are somewhat more successful, perhaps because the drug interferes with the formation and/or turnover of the structures. In these experiments, disruption of ectoplasmic specializations associated with early elongating spermatids occurs and is correlated with a loss of intercellular adhesion.[87] At basal locations, regional disruption of ectoplasmic specializations also occurs; however, loss of adhesion is difficult to assess at this site because of the presence of other junction types in the same location. What is observed is a change in the morphology (freeze fracture) and permeability of tight junctions.[116] Changes in permeability and morphology of tight junctions have been correlated with submembrane disruption of actin filaments in several epithelia.[15,19,58,61,62] One of a number of possible interpretations of this result in the seminiferous epithelium is that disruption of adhesion elements, which are primarily associated with the actin filaments, secondarily results in a disruption of the associated tight junctions. Alternatively, the observed effects on tight junctions may result from disruption of actin filaments that are directly associated with tight junction elements. Madara[57] has provided compelling evidence that actin filaments, in fact, are associated directly with tight junctions in intestinal epithelial cells.

Results of the few perturbation experiments that have been done are inconclusive, but are consistent with the hypothesis that the filaments are in some way involved with intercellular adhesion.

Involvement of Ectoplasmic Specializations in Positioning Spermatogenic Cells in the Seminiferous Epithelium: Relationship to Microtubules and Intermediate Filaments

In addition to a primary role in intercellular adhesion, there is growing evidence that ectoplasmic specializations found at apical sites interact with microtubules and intermediate filaments to orient, anchor, and translocate spermatids within the seminiferous epithelium.[3,91,105,106]

During spermatogenesis, early elongate spermatids become situated in apical invaginations (crypts) of the Sertoli cell. At the same time, they become oriented with their developing long axis perpendicular to the tubular wall. As spermatogenesis proceeds, the crypts deepen and the attached spermatids appear to "descend" toward the basally situated Sertoli cell nucleus. Some authors have termed this process entrenchment.[82,91] Still later in spermatogenesis, the crypts become shallower and the spermatids assume progressively more apical positions until the cells are finally released from the epithelium during spermiation. Throughout this process of first basal and then apical translocation, regions of the crypts that occur adjacent to the acrosome of the attached spermatids are lined by ectoplasmic specializations.

Microtubule Hypothesis

It is possible that ectoplasmic specializations, together with their attached spermatids, move as units along adjacent microtubule tracts and that the mechanism in-

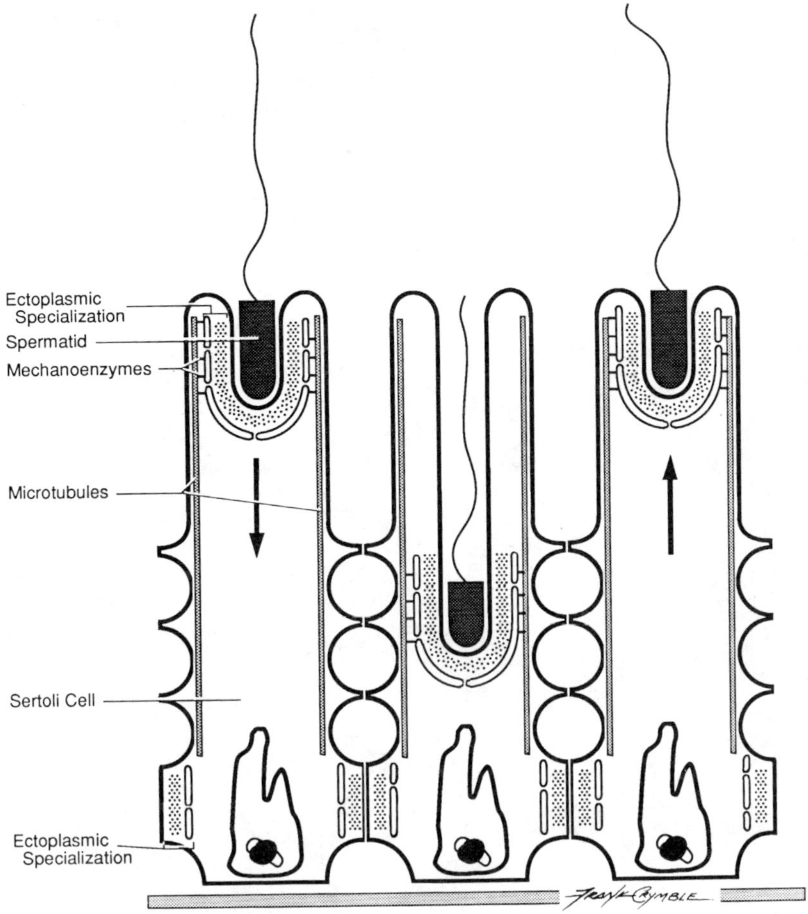

FIGURE 9. Model of microtubule based translocation of spermatids in the mammalian seminiferous epithelium. In this model, it is assumed that ectoplasmic specializations are structural mantles attached to and surrounding the spermatid heads. The ectoplasmic specializations, and hence the attached spermatids, are transported in basal and apical directions along adjacent microtubules by mechanoenzymes similar to those described in other systems.

volved is similar to that proposed for microtubule based vesicular transport in general.[78,82,105,106] This hypothesis, illustrated in pictorial form in FIGURE 9, is consistent with the known morphology of the system, with available information about molecular motors present in Sertoli cells, and with current models of microtubular based intracellular transport in other cell systems. Fundamental to this hypothesis is the prediction that the endoplasmic reticulum of ectoplasmic specializations is moved along microtubule tracts in the Sertoli cell cytoplasm. Because the endoplasmic reticulum is coupled via the layer of actin filaments to the plasma membrane and ultimately to the adjacent spermatid, when the endoplasmic reticulum moves it carries with it

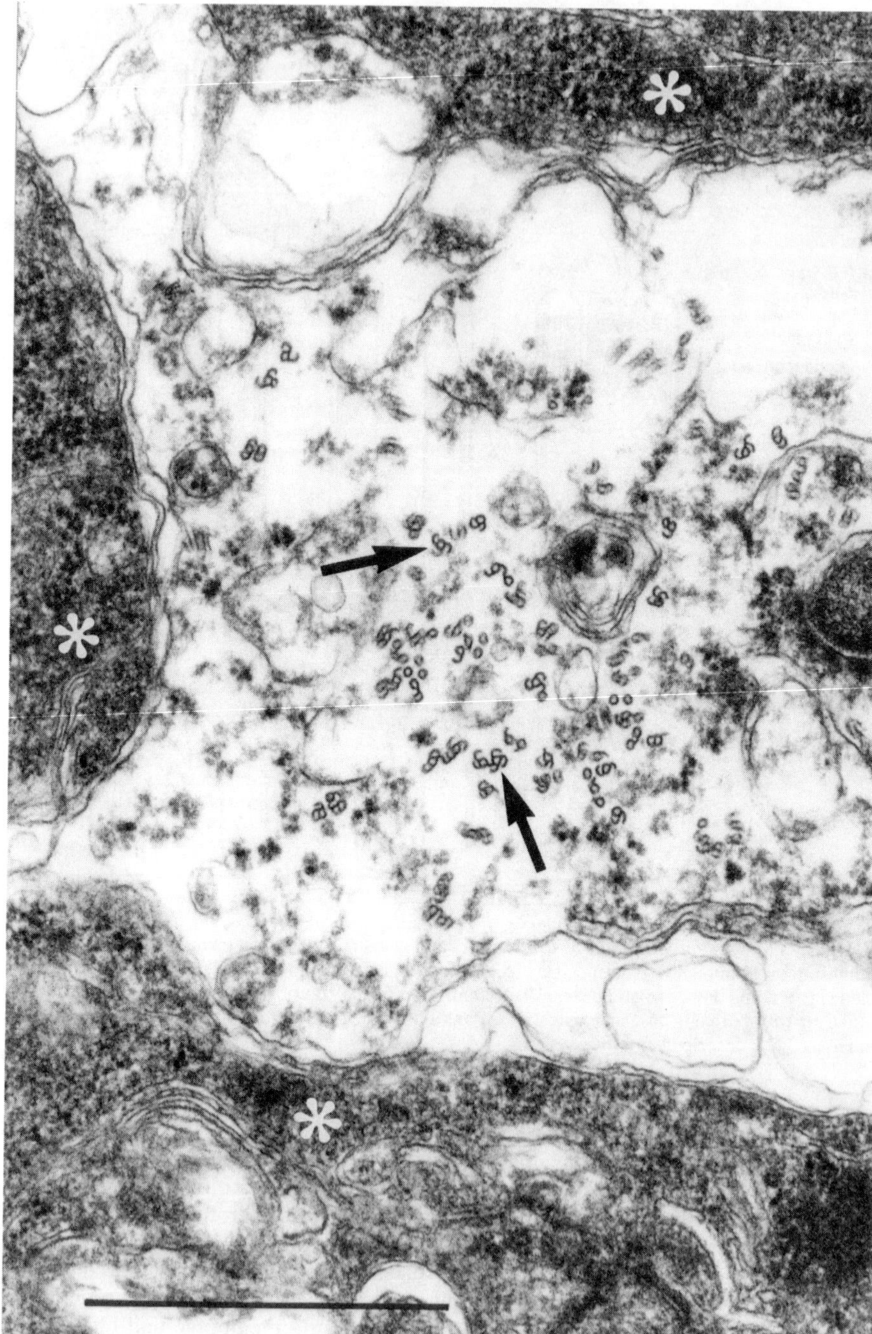

the attached spermatid. Moreover, the occurrence of translocation both in a basal and an apical direction indicates that there may be at least two motors involved in generating the movement.

Evidence by Analogy with Other Systems

In other cell systems, membranous organelles are thought to be moved and/or positioned along microtubule tracts by mechanoenzymes of the dynein and kinesin families.[2,4,7,40,41,50,55,56,60,68,72,73,76,77,97,101–104]

The kinesins are microtubule-activated ATPases that have the capacity to move vesicles along microtubules in an anterograde direction (toward the plus end).[101] The molecules are rod-shaped with two globular domains at one end and a fan-shaped domain at the other.[54] The native proteins are a complex of two heavy and two light chains. Although initially isolated from axoplasm, the proteins have more recently been detected in numerous cell types.[39,66]

Cytoplasmic dyneins, like kinesins, are microtubule-activated ATPases; however, unlike kinesins, they move vesicles along microtubules in a retrograde direction (toward the minus end).[72]

Although the presence of a kinesin in Sertoli cells has not been confirmed, there is evidence that a cytoplasmic dynein (MAPIC) occurs in these cells. The concentration of this motor is high in testis homogenates.[17] Furthermore, cell enrichment studies indicate that it is most probably localized in Sertoli cells.[65]

Recent evidence indicates that microtubules in Sertoli cells are organized with their negative ends positioned apically[78] (FIG. 10). This orientation is consistent with that observed in some other polarized epithelial cells[1,5,64] and with the possibility that cytoplasmic dynein may be the motor responsible for the apical movement of maturing spermatids in the seminiferous epithelium.

Evidence from Morphology

As described in an earlier section, microtubules are abundant in Sertoli cells and the arrangement of these cytoskeletal elements is consistent with the direction of spermatid translocation.[3,105]

Sertoli cell microtubules are concentrated in regions apical to the nucleus and are

---

FIGURE 10. Electron micrograph of a section through the supranuclear cytoplasm of a Sertoli cell and adjacent spermatogenic cells. The spermatogenic cells are less extracted than the Sertoli cell and are indicated by the asterisks. The section was cut perpendicular to the base of the tubule wall and the reader is viewing the section as if standing beneath the section and looking toward the tubule lumen. The material has been processed using a technique, introduced by Heidemann and McIntosh,[48] for determining microtubule polarity. The technique involves decorating microtubules with tubulin. The tubulin polymerizes onto microtubules in the form of curved sheets. In cross section, the curvature of the sheets, visualized as hooks extending off of the microtubules, indicates the polarity of the microtubules. In the field shown here, most of the microtubules are decorated with hooks that curve in a clockwise direction (*arrows*) indicating that the majority of microtubules are oriented with their minus-ends positioned at the apex of the cell (see Redenbach and Vogl[78] for details). *Magnification:* ×48,424, bar = 1.0 μm.

generally oriented parallel to the long axis of the cell.[16] Linkages, similar to those observed between membranous organelles and microtubules in other systems in which microtubule based motility appears to occur,[90] are present between microtubules and the endoplasmic reticulum component of ectoplasmic specializations. These linkages are most evident when tissue is treated with hypertonic solutions which tend to damage (rip open) the cells and "clear" (extract) the cytoplasm.[82] The nature of these linkages is not known; however, their detection formed the basis for the initial suggestion that microtubules may be involved with the movement of ectoplasmic specializations and attached spermatids within the epithelium.[82]

The present evidence for microtubule-based translocation of spermatids in the seminiferous epithelium is scant and indirect. Nevertheless, the evidence that we do have is consistent with the hypothesis.

Intermediate Filament Hypothesis

Intermediate filaments, through a transient association with ectoplasmic specializations, may facilitate anchoring apical crypts in a basal position during stages of spermatogenesis when spermatids are deeply entrenched within Sertoli cells.[3,106]

Evidence from Morphology

Intermediate filaments of the vimentin type are abundant in Sertoli cells. From perinuclear regions, filaments extend over the base of the cell and into more apical regions where they associate with desmosome-like junctions with early spermatogenic cells and with apical crypts containing elongate spermatids.[3] In the latter location they become intimately associated with ectoplasmic specializations and are most obvious when spermatids are at their deepest position within the epithelium. It is tempting to speculate that transient intermediate filament-associated adhesion junctions may form within each apically situated ectoplasmic specialization during these stages of spermatogenesis and that these focal junctions facilitate anchoring the crypts in a basal position. This hypothesis remains to be verified.

CONCLUDING REMARKS

The positions of ectoplasmic specializations and related cytoskeletal elements in Sertoli cells are shown in FIGURE 11. Also shown in this diagram is a summary of how we think that ectoplasmic specializations may participate in some of the fundamental events involving spermatogenic cells that occur in the mammalian seminiferous epithelium during spermatogenesis.

In this paper we have argued that ectoplasmic specializations are primarily a form of intercellular adhesion junction. The presence of actin together with vinculin at these sites is consistent with this hypothesis. Extensive cross-linking and hexagonal packing of the actin filaments may contribute to the reinforcement of membrane adhesion domains. The presence of adhesion elements at basal sites of contact between Sertoli cells may secondarily influence the position of tight junctions at the same locations.

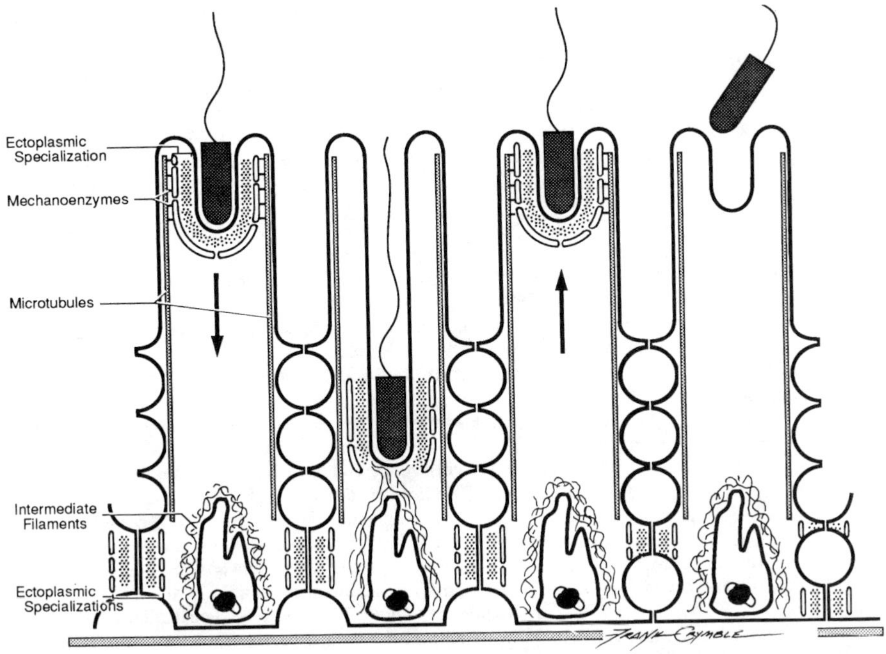

FIGURE 11. Diagram illustrating the possible involvement of ectoplasmic specializations and related intermediate filaments and microtubules to some of the major events involving spermatogenic cells that occur during spermatogenesis in the mammalian seminiferous epithelium. We propose that ectoplasmic specializations are primarily a form of intercellular adhesion junction. The disassembly of these junctions would be a requisite for turnover of the basal junction complex to allow entry of spermatocytes into the adluminal compartment of the epithelium and for the release of spermatozoa from the apices of Sertoli cells. Translocation of spermatids in the epithelium may occur via a microtubule based vesicular transport system in which apical ectoplasmic specializations and attached spermatids are moved as units along microtubule tracts in the Sertoli cell. Bundles of intermediate filaments may facilitate anchoring apical crypts in a perinuclear position at stages of spermatogenesis when spermatids are at their deepest position in the epithelium. Disassembly of these focal attachments would occur prior to the proposed microtubule based translocation of spermatids to an apical position in preparation for spermiation.

Consistent with this possibility is the observation that morphologically similar structures occur both at sites of attachment to spermatids, where tight junctions do not generally occur, and in association with Sertoli-Sertoli contacts, where tight junctions are extensive. In apical locations, ectoplasmic specializations may interact with microtubules and intermediate filaments to position spermatids in the seminiferous epithelium.

ACKNOWLEDGMENT

Frank Grymble provided the excellent artwork.

REFERENCES

1. Achler, C., D. Filmer, C. Merte & D. Drenckhahn. 1989. Role of microtubules in polarized delivery of apical membrane proteins to the brush border of the intestinal epithelium. J. Cell Biol. **109:** 179–189.
2. Allen, R. D., D. G. Weiss, J. H. Hayden, D. T. Brown, H. Fujiwake & M. Simpson. 1985. Gliding movement of and bidirectional transport along single native microtubules from squid axoplasm: Evidence for an active role of microtubules in cytoplasmic transport. J. Cell Biol. **100:** 1736–1752.
3. Amlani, S. & A. W. Vogl. 1988. Changes in the distribution of microtubules and intermediate filaments in mammalian Sertoli cells during spermatogenesis. Anat. Rec. **220:** 143–160.
4. Amos, L. A. & W. B. Amos. 1987. Cytoplasmic transport in axons. J. Cell Sci. **87:** 1–2.
5. Bacallao, R., C. Antomy, C. Dotti, E. Karsenti, E. H. Stelzer & K. Simons. 1989. The subcellular organization of Madin-Darby canine kidney cells during the formation of a polarized epithelium. J. Cell Biol. **109:** 2817–2832.
6. Blanchard, A., V. Ohanian & D. Critchley. 1989. The structure and function of alpha-actinin. J. Muscle Res. Cell Motil. **10:** 280–289.
7. Brady, S. T. 1985. A novel brain ATPase with properties expected for the fast axonal transport motor. Nature (Lond.) **317:** 73–75.
8. Brokelmann, J. 1963. Fine structure of germ cells and Sertoli cells during the cycle of the seminiferous epithelium in the rat. Z. Zellforsch. **59:** 820–850.
9. Burridge, K. & J. R. Feramisco. 1980. Microinjection and localization of a 130K protein in living fibroblasts: A relationship to actin and fibronectin. Cell **19:** 587–595.
10. Burridge, K. & L. Connell. 1983. Talin: A cytoskeletal component concentrated in adhesion plaques and other sites of actin membrane interaction. Cell Motil. **3:** 405–417.
11. Burridge, K., K. Fath, T. Kelly, G. Nuckolls & C. Turner. 1988. Focal adhesions: Transmembrane junctions between the extracellular matrix and the cytoskeleton. Ann. Rev. Cell Biol. **4:** 487–525.
12. Byers, S. W., R. Graham & B. Stevenson. 1988. Distribution of ZO.1 in the mouse testis. Development of the Sertoli cell tight junction. J. Cell Biol. **107:** 170a.
13. Camatini, M., G. Anelli & A. Casale. 1986. Identification of actin in boar spermatids and spermatozoa by immunoelectron microscopy. Eur. J. Cell Biol. **42:** 311–318.
14. Camatini, M., A. Casale & M. Cifarelli. 1987. Immunocytochemical identification of actin in rabbit spermiogenesis and spermatozoa. Eur. J. Cell Biol. **45:** 274–281.
15. Cereijido, M., I. Meza & A. Martinez-Palomo. 1981. Occluding junctions in cultured epithelial monolayers. Am. J. Physiol. **240:** C96-C102.
16. Christensen, A. K. 1965. Microtubules in Sertoli cells of the guinea pig testis. Anat. Rec. **151:** 335a.
17. Collins, C. A. & R. B. Vallee. 1988. MAP 1C (dynein) is a major component of microtubules from rat liver and testis. Int. Congr. Cell Biol. 4th, P2.9.2.
18. Cowin, P., H-P. Kapprell, W. W. Franke, J. Tamkun & R. O. Hynes. 1986. Plakoglobin: A protein common to different kinds of intercellular adhering junctions. Cell **46:** 1063–1073.
19. Duffey, M. E., B. Hainau, S. Ho & C. J. Bentzel. 1981. Regulation of epithelial tight junction permeability by cyclic AMP. Nature (Lond.). **294:** 451–453.
20. Dym, M. & D. W. Fawcett. 1970. The blood-testis barrier in the rat and the physiological compartmentation of the seminiferous epithelium. Biol. Reprod. **3:** 308–326.
21. Farquhar, M. G. & G. E. Palade. 1963. Junctional complexes in various epithelia. J. Cell Biol. **17:** 375–412.
22. Fawcett, D. W. 1975. Ultrastructure and function of the Sertoli cell. *In* Handbook of Physiology. R. O. Greep, Ed. Sect. 7, Vol. 5: 21–55. Williams & Wilkins. Baltimore, MD.
23. Fawcett, D. W. 1979. Comparative aspects of the organization of the testis and spermatogenesis. *In* Animal Models for Research on Contraception and Fertility. N. J. Alexander, Ed.: 84–104. Harper & Row. New York.
24. Fawcett, D. W. 1981. The Cell. W. B. Saunders. Philadelphia, London, Toronto.
25. Flickinger, C. & D. W. Fawcett. 1967. The junctional specializations of Sertoli cells in the seminiferous epithelium. Anat. Rec. **158:** 207–222.

26. FOUQUET, J-P., M-L. KANN & J. P. DADOUNE. 1989. Immunogold distribution of actin during spermiogenesis in the rat, hamster, monkey, and human. Anat. Rec. **223:** 35–42.
27. FRANCHI, E. & M. CAMATINI. 1985. Evidence that a Ca^{2+} chelator and a calmodulin blocker interfere with the structure of the inter-Sertoli junctions. Tissue & Cell **17:** 13–25.
28. FRANCHI, E. & M. CAMATINI. 1985. Morphological evidence for calcium stores at Sertoli-Sertoli and Sertoli-spermatid interrelations. Cell Biol. Int. Rep. **9:** 441–446.
29. FRANKE, W. W., C. GRUND, A. FINK, K. WEBER, B. M. JOCKUSCH, H. ZENTGRAF & M. OSBORN. 1978. Location of actin in the microfilament bundles associated with the junctional specialisations between Sertoli cells and spermatids. Biol. Cell **31:** 7–14.
30. GEIGER, B. 1979. A 130K protein from chicken gizzard: Its localization at the termini of microfilament bundles in cultured chicken cells. Cell **18:** 193–205.
31. GEIGER, B. 1982. Involvement of vinculin in contact-induced cytoskeletal interactions. Cold Spring Harbor Symp. Quant. Biol. **46:** 671–682.
32. GEIGER, B. 1983. Membrane-cytoskeleton interaction. Biochim. Biophys. Acta **737:** 305–341.
33. GEIGER, B. 1989. Cytoskeleton-associated cell contacts. Curr. Opinion Cell Biol. **1:** 103–109.
34. GEIGER, B., K. T. TOKUYASU, A. H. DUTTON & S. J. SINGER. 1980. Vinculin, an intracellular protein localized at specialized sites where microfilament bundles terminate at cell membranes. Proc. Natl. Acad. Sci. USA **77:** 4127–4131.
35. GEIGER, B., A. H. DUTTON, K. T. TOKUYASU & S. J. SINGER. 1981. Immunoelectron microscope studies of membrane-microfilament interactions: Distributions of alpha-actinin, tropomyosin, and vinculin in intestinal epithelial brush border and chicken gizzard smooth muscle cells. J. Cell Biol. **91:** 614–628.
36. GEIGER, B., Z. AVNUR, T. E. KREIS & J. SCHLESSINGER. 1984. The dynamics of cytoskeletal organization in areas of cell contact. *In* Cell and Muscle Motility, Vol. 5, The Cytoskeleton: 195–234. J. W. Shay, Ed. Plenum Press. New York.
37. GEIGER, B., Z. AVNUR, T. VOLBERG & T. VOLK. 1985. Molecular domains of adherens junctions. *In* The Cell in Contact. G. M. Edelman and J. P. Thiery, Eds.: 461–489. Neurosciences Institute Publication, John Wiley and Sons. New York.
38. GEIGER, B., T. VOLK & T. VOLBERG. 1985. Molecular heterogeneity of adherens junctions. J. Cell Biol. **101:** 1523–1531.
39. GELFAND, V. I. 1989. Cytoplasmic microtubular motors. Curr. Opinion Cell Biol. **1:** 63–66.
40. GIBBONS, I. R. 1988. Dynein ATPases as microtubule motors. J. Biol. Chem. **263:** 15837–15840.
41. GILBERT, S. P. & R. D. SLOBODA. 1986. Identification of a MAP2-like ATP-binding protein associated with axoplasmic vesicles that translocate on isolated microtubules. J. Cell Biol. **103:** 947–956.
42. GROVE, B. D. & A. W. VOGL. 1986. The effect of calcium on actin bundles in ectoplasmic specializations of rat Sertoli cells. Anat. Rec. **214:** 45A.
43. GROVE, B. D. & A. W. VOGL. 1989. Sertoli cell ectoplasmic specializations: A type of actin-associated adhesion junction? J. Cell Sci. **93:** 309–323.
44. GROVE, B. D., D. C. PFEIFFER, S. ALLEN & A. W. VOGL. 1990. Immunofluorescence localization of vinculin in ectoplasmic ("junctional") specializations of rat Sertoli cells. Am. J. Anat. **188:** 44–56.
45. GUMBINER, B. 1987. Structure, biochemistry, and assembly of epithelial tight junctions. Am. J. Phys. **253:** C749–C758.
46. GUMBINER, BC& K. SIMONS. 1987. The role of uvomorulin in the formation of epithelial occluding junctions. *In* Junctional Complexes of Epithelial Cells. G. Bock and S. Clark, Eds.: 168–186. John Wiley and Sons. Chichester, UK.
47. GUMBINER, B., B. STEVENSON & A. GRIMALDI. 1988. The role of the cell adhesion molecule uvomorulin in the formation and maintenance of the epithelial junctional complex. J. Cell Biol. **107:** 1575–1587.
48. HEIDEMANN, S. R. & J. R. MCINTOSH. 1980. Visualization of the structural polarity of microtubules. Nature **286:** 517–519.
49. HERGOTT, G. J., M. SANDIG & V. I. KALNINS. 1989. Cytoskeletal organization of migrating retinal pigment epithelial cells during wound healing in organ culture. Cell Motil. Cytoskeleton **13:** 83–93.
50. HEUSER, J. E. 1989. Mechanisms behind the organization of membranous organelles in cells.

Curr. Opinion Cell Biol. **1:** 98–102.

51. Hirano, S., A. Nose, K. Hatta, A. Kawakami & M. Takeichi. 1987. Calcium-dependent cell-cell adhesion molecules (cadherins): Subclass specificities and possible involvement of actin bundles. J. Cell Biol. **105:** 2501–2510.
52. Hirokawa, N. & J. Heuser. 1981. Quick-freeze, deep-etch visualization of the cytoskeleton beneath surface differentiations of intestinal epithelial cells. J. Cell Biol. **91:** 399–409.
53. Hirokawa, N., T. C. S. Keller III, R. Chasan & M. S. Mooseker. 1983. Mechanism of brush border contractility studied by quick-freeze, deep-etch method. J. Cell Biol. **96:** 1325–1336.
54. Hirokawa, N., K. K. Pfister, H. Yorifuji, M. C. Wagner, S. T. Brady & G. S. Bloom. 1989. Submolecular domains of bovine brain kinesin identified by electron microscopy and monoclonal antibody decoration. Cell **56:** 867–878.
55. Kelly, R. B. 1990. Associations between microtubules and intracellular organelles. Curr. Opinion Cell Biol. **2:** 105–108.
56. Kreis, T. E. 1990. Role of microtubules in the organization of the Golgi apparatus. Cell Motil. Cytoskeleton **15:** 67–70.
57. Madara, J. L. 1987. Intestinal absorptive cell tight junctions are linked to the cytoskeleton. Am. J. Physiol. **253:** C171–C175.
58. Madara, J. L., D. Barenberg & S. Carlson. 1986. Effects of cytochalasin D on occluding junctions of intestinal absorptive cells: Further evidence that the cytoskeleton may influence paracellular permeability and junctional charge selectivity. J. Cell Biol. **102:** 2125–2136.
59. Masri, B. A., L. D. Russell & A. W. Vogl. 1987. Distribution of actin in spermatids and adjacent Sertoli cell regions of the rat. Anat. Rec. **218:** 20–26.
60. McIntosh, J. R. & M. E. Porter. 1989. Enzymes for microtubule-dependent motility. J. Biol. Chem. **264:** 6001–6004.
61. Meza, I., G. Ibarra, M. Sabanero, A. Martinez-Palomo & M. Cereijido. 1980. Occluding junctions and cytoskeletal components in a cultured transporting epithelium. J. Cell Biol. **87:** 746–754.
62. Meza, I., M. Sabanero, E. Stefani & M. Cereijido. 1982. Occluding junctions in MDCK cells: Modulations of transepithelial permeability by the cytoskeleton. J. Cell Biochem. **18:** 407–421.
63. Mooseker, M. S. 1985. Organization, chemistry, and assembly of the cytoskeletal apparatus of the intestinal brush border. Ann. Rev. Cell Biol. **1:** 209–241.
64. Morgensen, M. M., J. B. Tucker & H. Stebbings. 1989. Microtubule polarities indicate that nucleation and capture of microtubules occurs at cell surfaces in *Drosophila.* J. Cell Biol. **108:** 1445–1452.
65. Neely, N. D. & K. Boekelheide. 1988. Sertoli cell processes have axoplasmic features: An ordered microtubule distribution and an abundant high molecular weight microtubule-associated protein (cytoplasmic dynein). J. Cell Biol. **107:** 1767–1776.
66. Neighbors, B. W., R. C. Williams, Jr. & J. R. McIntosh. 1988. Localization of kinesin in cultured cells. J. Cell Biol. **106:** 1193–1204.
67. Nicander, L. 1967. An electron microscopical study of cell contacts in the seminiferous tubules of some mammals. Z. Zellforsch. **83:** 375–397.
68. Ogawa, K., H. Hosoya, E. Yokota, T. Kobayashi, Y. Wakamatsu, K. Ozato, S. Negishi & M. Obika. 1987. Melanoma dynein: Evidence that dynein is a general "motor" for microtubule-associated cell motilities. Eur. J. Cell Biol. **43:** 3–9.
69. Owaribe, K., R. Kodama & G. Eguchi. 1981. Demonstration of contractility of circumferential actin bundles and its morphogenetic significance in pigmented epithelium *in vitro* and *in vivo.* J. Cell Biol. **90:** 507–514.
70. Pardo, J., J. D'A. Siliciano & S. W. Craig. 1983. A vinculin-containing cortical lattice in skeletal muscle: Transverse lattice elements ("costameres") mark sites of attachment between myofibrils and sarcolemma. Proc. Natl. Acad. Sci. USA **80:** 1008–1012.
71. Pardo, J., J. D'A. Siliciano & S. W. Craig. 1983. Vinculin is a component of an extensive network of myofibril-sarcolemma attachment regions in cardiac muscle fibers. J. Cell Biol. **97:** 1081–1088.
72. Paschal, B. M. & R. B. Vallee. 1987. Retrograde transport by the microtubule-associated protein MAP 1C. Nature (Lond.) **330:** 181–183.

73. PASCHAL, B. M., H. S. SHPETNER & R. B. VALLEE. 1987. MAPIC is a microtubule-activated ATPase which translocates microtubules *in vitro* and has dynein-like properties. J. Cell Biol. **105:** 1273–1282.
74. PELLETIER, R.-M. 1988. Cyclic modulation of Sertoli cell junctional complexes in a seasonal breeder. The mink (*Mustela vison*). Am. J. Anat. **183:** 68–102.
75. PFEIFFER, D. C. & A. W. VOGL. 1991. Evidence that vinculin is co-distributed with actin bundles in ectoplasmic ("junctional") specializations of mammalian Sertoli cells. Anat. Rec. In press.
76. PRATT, M. M. 1980. The identification of a dynein ATPase in unfertilized sea urchin eggs. Dev. Biol. **74:** 364–378.
77. PRATT, M. M. 1986. Stable complexes of axoplasmic vesicles and microtubules: Protein composition and ATPase activity. J. Cell Biol. **103:** 957–968.
78. REDENBACH, D. M. & A. W. VOGL. 1991. Microtubule polarity in Sertoli cells: A model for microtubule-based spermatid transport. Eur. J. Cell Biol. **54**(2): 277–290.
79. ROBINE, S., C. HUET, R. MOLL, C. SAHUQUILLO-MERINO, E. COUDRIER, A. ZWEIBAUM & D. LOUVARD. 1985. Can villin be used to identify malignant and undifferentiated normal digestive epithelial cells? Proc. Natl. Acad. Sci. USA **82:** 8488–8492.
80. ROMRELL, L. J. & M. H. ROSS. 1979. Characterization of Sertoli cell-germ cell junctional specializations in dissociated testicular cells. Anat. Rec. **193:** 23–42.
81. ROSS, M. H. 1977. Sertoli-Sertoli junctions and Sertoli-spermatid junctions after efferent ductule ligation and lanthanum treatment. Am. J. Anat. **148:** 49–56.
82. RUSSELL, L. D. 1977. Observations on rat Sertoli ectoplasmic ("junctional") specializations in their association with germ cells of the rat testis. Tissue & Cell **9:** 475–498.
83. RUSSELL, L. D. 1977. Movement of spermatocytes from the basal to the adluminal compartment of the rat testis. Am. J. Anat. **148:** 313–328.
84. RUSSELL, L. D. 1984. Spermiation—the sperm release process: Ultrastructural observations and unresolved problems. *In* Ultrastructure of Reproduction. J. Van Blerkom and P. M. Motta, Eds.: 46–66. Martinus Nijhoff Publishers, Boston.
85. RUSSELL, L. D. & R. N. PETERSON. 1985. Sertoli cell junctions: Morphological and functional correlates. Int. J. Cyt. **94:** 177–211.
86. RUSSELL, L. D. & J. C. GOH. 1988. Localization of alpha-actinin in the rat testis: Preliminary observations. *In* Development and Function of the Reproductive Organs. M. Parvinen, I. Huhtaniemi, and L. J. Pelliniemi, Eds.: 237–344. Serono Symp. Rev., Vol. 2. Ares-Serono Symp. Via Ravenna, 8-Rome.
87. RUSSELL, L. D., J. C. GOH, R. M. A. RASHED & A. W. VOGL. 1988. The consequences of actin disruption at Sertoli ectoplasmic specialization sites facing spermatids after *in vivo* exposure of rat testis to cytochalasin D. Biol. Reprod. **39:** 105–118.
88. SCHWARZ, M. A., K. OWARIBE, J. KARTENBECK & W. W. FRANKE. 1990. Desmosomes and Hemidesmosomes: Constitutive molecular components. Annu. Rev. Cell Biol. **6:** 461–491.
89. SHEAR, C. R. & R. BLOCH. 1985. Vinculin in subsarcolemmal densities in chicken skeletal muscle: Localization and relationship to intracellular and extracellular structures. J. Cell Biol. **101:** 240–256.
90. SMITH, D. S. 1971. On the significance of cross-bridges between microtubules and synaptic vesicles. Phil. Trans. Roy. Soc. Lond. B. **261:** 395–405.
91. SPRANDO, R. L. & L. D. RUSSELL. 1987. A comparative study of Sertoli cell ectoplasmic specializations in selected non-mammalian vertebrates. Tissue & Cell **19:** 479–493.
92. STEVENSON, B. R., J. D. SILICIANO, M. S. MOOSEKER & D. A. GOODENOUGH. 1986. Identification of ZO-1: A high molecular weight polypeptide associated with the tight junction (zonula occludens) in a variety of epithelia. J. Cell Biol. **103:** 755–766.
93. STOSSEL, T. P., C. CHAPONNIER, R. M. EZZELL, J. H. HARTWIG, P. A. JANMEY, D. J. KWIATKOWSKI, S. E. LIND, D. B. SMITH, F. S. SOUTHWICK, H. L. YIN & K. S. ZANER. 1985. Nonmuscle Actin-Binding Proteins. Annu. Rev. Cell Biol. **1:** 353–402.
94. SUAREZ-QUIAN, C. A. & M. DYM. 1984. Further observations on the microfilament bundles of Sertoli cell junctional complexes. Ann. N. Y. Acad. Sci. **438:** 476–480.
95. SUAREZ-QUIAN, C. A. & M. DYM. 1988. Detection of microfilaments in rat Sertoli cell ectoplasmic specializations with NBD-phallicidin. Int. J. Androl. **11:** 301–312.
96. TAKEICHI, M. 1988. The cadherins: Cell-cell adhesion molecules controlling animal morphogenesis. Development **102:** 639–655.

97. TERASAKI, M. 1990. Recent progress on structural interactions of the endoplasmic reticulum. Cell Motil. Cytoskeleton **15:** 71–75.
98. TOKUYASU, K. T., A. H. DUTTON, B. GEIGER & S. J. SINGER. 1981. Ultrastructure of chicken cardiac muscle as studied by double immunolabeling in electron microscopy. Proc. Natl. Acad. Sci. USA **78:** 7619–7623.
99. TOYAMA, Y. 1976. Actin-like filaments in the Sertoli cell junctional specializations in the swine and mouse testis. Anat. Rec. **186:** 477–492.
100. TSUKITA, S., Y. HIEDA & S. TSUKITA. 1989. A new 82-kD barbed end-capping protein (Radixin) localized in the cell-to-cell adherens junction: Purification and characterization. J. Cell Biol. **108:** 2369–2382.
101. VALE, R. D. 1987. Intracellular transport using microtubule-based motors. Annu. Rev. Cell Biol. **3:** 347–378.
102. VALE, R. D. & L. S. B. GOLDSTEIN. 1990. One motor, many tails: An expanding repertoire of force-generating enzymes. Cell **60:** 883–885.
103. VALE, R. D., B. J. SCHNAPP, T. S. REESE & M. P. SHEETZ. 1985. Organelle, bead, and microtubule translocations promoted by soluble factors from the squid giant axon. Cell **40:** 559–569.
104. VALE, R. D., T. S. REESE & M. P. SHEETZ. 1985. Identification of a novel force-generating protein, kinesin, involved in microtubule-based motility. Cell **42:** 39–50.
105. VOGL, A. W. 1988. Changes in the distribution of microtubules in rat Sertoli cells during spermatogenesis. Anat. Rec. **222:** 34–41.
106. VOGL, A. W. 1989. Distribution and function of organized concentrations of actin filaments in mammalian spermatogenic cells and Sertoli cells. Int. Rev. Cytol. **119:** 1–56.
107. VOGL, A. W. & L. J. SOUCY. 1985. Arrangement and possible function of actin filament bundles in ectoplasmic specializations of ground squirrel Sertoli cells. J. Cell Biol. **100:** 814–825.
108. VOGL, A. W., Y. C. LIN, M. DYM & D. W. FAWCETT. 1983. Sertoli cells of the golden-mantled ground squirrel (*Spermophilus lateralis*): A model system for the study of shape change. Am. J. Anat. **168:** 83–98.
109. VOGL, A. W., L. J. SOUCY & G. L. LEW. 1985. Distribution of actin in isolated seminiferous epithelia and denuded tubule walls of the rat. Anat. Rec. **213:** 63–71.
110. VOGL, A. W., B. D. GROVE & G. J. LEW. 1986. Distribution of actin in Sertoli cell ectoplasmic specializations and associated spermatids in the ground squirrel testis. Anat. Rec. **215:** 331–341.
111. VOGL, A. W., D. C. PFEIFFER & D. M. REDENBACH. 1991. Sertoli cell cytoskeleton: influence on spermatogenic cells. *In* Proceedings of the VI International Congress on Spermatology. Comparative Spermatology 20 Years After. Serono Symposia. In press.
112. VOLBERG, T., H. SABANAY & B. GEIGER. 1986. Spatial and temporal relationships between vinculin and talin in the developing chicken gizzard smooth muscle. Differentiation **32:** 34–43.
113. VOLK, T. & B. GEIGER. 1984. A 135-kD membrane protein of intercellular adherens junctions. EMBO J. **3:** 2249–2260.
114. VOLK, T. & B. GEIGER. 1986. A-CAM: A 135 kD receptor of intercellular adherens junctions. I. Immunoelectron microscopic localization and biochemical studies. J. Cell Biol. **103:** 1441–1450.
115. VOLK, T. & B. GEIGER. 1986. A-CAM: A 135 kD receptor of intercellular adherens junctions. II. Antibody-mediated modulation of junction formation. J. Cell Biol. **103:** 1451–1464.
116. WEBER, J. E., T. T. TURNER, K. S. K. TUNG & L. D. RUSSELL. 1988. Effects of cytochalasin D on the integrity of the Sertoli cell (blood-testis) barrier. Am. J. Anat. **182:** 130–147.

Biogenesis of Specialized Cytoskeletal Elements of Rat Spermatozoa[a]

RICHARD J. OKO AND YVES CLERMONT

Department of Anatomy
McGill University
3640 University
Montréal, Québec, Canada H3A 2B2

INTRODUCTION

The mammalian spermatozoon is the end product of an extraordinarily intricate process of cell differentiation termed spermiogenesis. Its highly specialized cytoskeletal structure reflects a complex process of structural and biochemical transformation.

During the past few years our laboratory has studied the biogenesis of several structural proteins making up the major cytoskeletal elements of the mammalian spermatozoon, namely the outer dense fibers (ODF), the fibrous sheath (FS), and the perinuclear theca (PT). The proteins composing these elements have the common property of being resistant to solubilization in ionic detergents (*e.g.*, SDS) because of their high content of cystine.[1-5] Many of these proteins are highly phosphorylated, reflecting their high content of serine.[6-8] Recent findings also indicate that some of the major polypeptides of these cytoskeletal elements share similar molecular weights and antigenic determinants.[9,10] Immunocomparative studies show little resemblance between intermediate filaments of somatic cells and the cytoskeletal elements of spermatogenic cells,[11-15] suggesting that the proteins making up the ODF, FS, and PT may be derived from a set of genes which is uniquely expressed during spermatogenesis.

Based on quantification of testicularly incorporated isotopic amino acids, analyzed in epididymal spermatozoa, O'Brien and Bellvé[16] found that the majority of SDS-insoluble proteins, constituting the cytoskeletal elements of the head and tail of spermatozoa are synthesized during spermiogenesis. Our objective has been to define the identity, temporal expression and intracellular distribution of some of these developmentally regulated SDS-insoluble proteins, focusing our attention on the proteins constituting the ODF, FS, and PT.[9,10,17-20] Our approach has been to follow the developmental expression of these proteins in the rat seminiferous epithelium by means of immunoperoxidase and immunogold labeling at the light and electron microscope level. The prerequisite to this approach is to isolate the cytoskeletal element of interest from spermatozoa, determine its protein composition and raise antibodies that are specific against either the whole cytoskeletal element or some of its major proteins. In order to emphasize the variability and complexity that exists in the production and develop-

[a] This work was supported from grants of the WHO Special Program of Research in Human Reproduction, Project 90041 (R.J.O.), Natural Sciences and Engineering Research Council of Canada (R.J.O.), and the Medical Research Council of Canada (Y.C.).

mental regulation of cytoskeletal proteins during spermiogenesis this study will compare the results collected on two cytoskeletal elements of spermatozoa, *i.e.*, the perforatorium of the head and outer dense fibers of the tail.

STRUCTURE OF THE OUTER DENSE FIBERS AND THE PERFORATORIUM

Central to the sperm tail is the axoneme made up of 9 peripheral microtubular doublets surrounding a pair of microtubular singlets. Along the axoneme in the middle piece of the tail, which is characterized by the presence of the mitochondrial sheath, are nine coarse cytoskeletal fibers termed outer dense fibers (ODF) each one being associated to one microtubular doublet (FIG. 8b). In the principal piece of the tail, which is characterized by the presence of the fibrous sheath, the ODF are reduced to seven, ODF 3 and 8 being replaced in their association with the corresponding microtubular doublets by the longitudinal columns of the fibrous sheath. The ODF progressively reduce in diameter distally, disappearing completely in the end piece of the tail. Ultrastructurally each one of the ODF has a characteristic size and shape and is composed of a central medulla and a thin cortex.[5,21]

The perforatorium is part of a rigid capsule, termed the perinuclear theca (PT), that covers the entire nucleus of mammalian spermatozoa, except over the perifossal zone (FIG. 1).[10,19,22,23] The perforatorium has been defined operationally as the region of the PT that underlies the acrosomic system,[19] whereas the postacrosomal sheath, making up the distal part of the PT, begins where the acrosomic system ends and directly underlies the plasmalemma.[21] At the apex of the falciform sperm head, the perforatorium is in the shape of a curved triangular rod and as it passes over the apex of the nucleus it splits into three interconnected prongs – one dorsal and two ventral – that taper off caudally and form the thinner perforatorial layer underlying the acrosomic head cap (FIG. 1). This thinner layer is continuous with the postacrosomal sheath.

ISOLATION OF THE OUTER DENSE FIBERS AND PERFORATORIUM

The isolation of the ODF and perforatorium is based on their differential resistance to commonly used protein solubilizing agents.[3,-5,7,9,10,24] FIGURE 2 presents the respective isolation schemes employed. The first step in the isolation protocol is to separate rat sperm heads and tails by sonication and to subfractionate them on a discontinuous sucrose gradient.[2]

To obtain a pure ODF fraction, the tails are extracted for an hour or more in a buffer containing 1% sodium dodecyl sulfate (SDS) and 2 mM dithiothreitol (DTT). With the exception of the ODF all other tail proteins are solubilized during this time. The resulting suspension is then fractionated on a discontinuous sucrose gradient and the pure ODF fraction collected at the 35–75% sucrose interface (FIGS. 3 and 4).[9]

To obtain a pure perforatorial fraction, the heads are extracted for 30 min in 1N NaOH. This alkaline treatment has the combined effect of keeping the nucleus condensed, solubilizing all the acrosomal and membrane proteins, and partially detaching the intact perforatorium from the nucleus. To assure complete detachment of the perforatorium from the nucleus the suspension is subjected to shear forces by passing

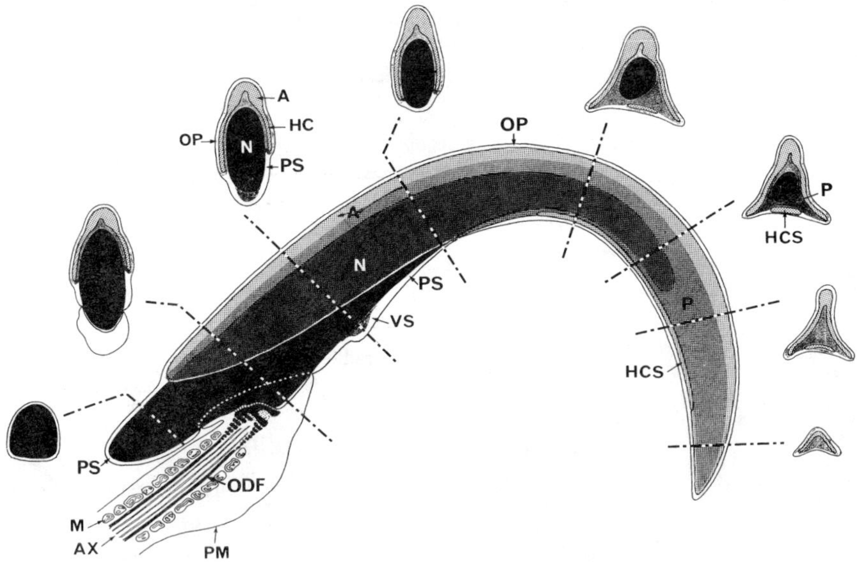

FIGURE 1. Drawing of the head of a rat spermatozoa as seen from the side and accompanied by representative cross-sectional views (modified from Lalli and Clermont, 1981). The region of the perinuclear theca delineated in smooth gray and lying between the acrosomic system (A: stippled in light gray) and the nucleus (N: dark black) represents the perforatorium (P). The region of the perinuclear theca beginning where the acrosomic system ends and lying between the nucleus and the plasmalemma is the postacrosomal sheath (PS). The ventral spur (VS) refers to the ventral prominence of the sperm head, which is due to the ventral thickening of the postacrosomal sheath. The inner part of the ventral spur is colored in smooth gray to convey that this part of the ventral spur is similar in composition to the perforatorium.[10,19] The acrosomic system is composed of the acrosome (A), head cap (HC) and separated head cap segment (HCS). The outer periacrosomic layer (OP), lying between the plasmalemma and the acrosomic system, is continuous structurally with the perforatorium and acrosomal sheath.[10,19] The region of the outer periacrosomal layer adjacent to the acrosomic head cap is denoted in smooth gray to convey that this part of outer periacrosomal layer is similar in composition to the perforatorium. The dashed white line at the base of the nucleus indicates the borderline of the perifossal zone. Labels: PM, plasma membrane; A, axoneme; M, mitochondria; ODF, outer dense fibers.

it through a 22 gauge needle. Perforatoria are then separated from the nuclei on a discontinuous gradient and the pure P fraction collected at the 10–70% sucrose interface (Figs. 5 and 6).[10]

POLYPEPTIDE COMPOSITION OF THE PERFORATORIUM AND OUTER DENSE FIBERS

Polyacrylamide SDS gels of isolated rat perforatorial fractions revealed several polypeptide bands of which the 16, 34 and 43 kDa bands are most prominent (Fig. 7).[10] Previously only the 16 kDa polypeptide was attributed to the perforatorium.[3] Particularly striking is that this polypeptide is rich in cysteine, proline, glutamic acid and serine.[3]

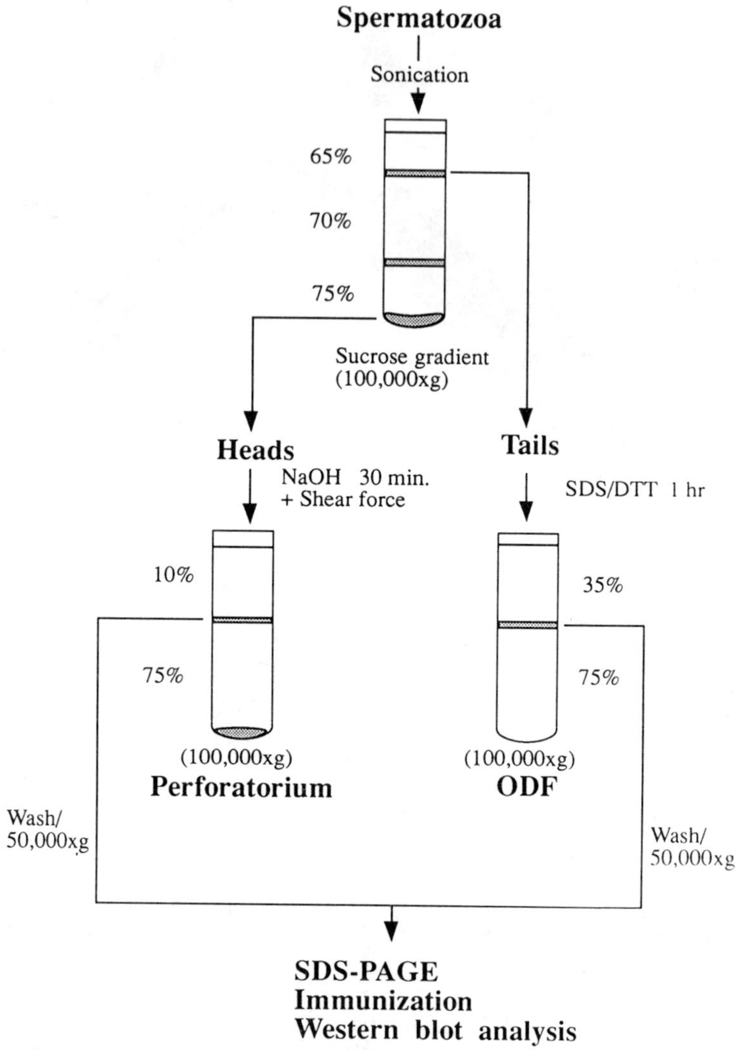

FIGURE 2. Diagrammatic representation of isolation protocol used to obtain perforatoria and outer dense fibers (ODF). For details of isolation protocol refer to text.

Polyacrylamide SDS gels of isolated rat ODF fractions revealed numerous polypeptide bands of which the 14, 20, 27, 80, and 84 kDa bands are major (FIG. 7).[9] This polypeptide pattern is in general agreement with previous studies.[7,24] The 27 kDa polypeptide complex accounts for about 50% of the total protein of the rat ODF and has been shown by amino acid analysis to be composed of two almost identical polypeptides which share histidine at the NH_2-terminal.[7] These two polypeptides are highly enriched in cysteine, proline, aspartic acid, serine, and leucine and are similar but not identical in composition to the 20 and 14 kDa ODF polypeptides.[7]

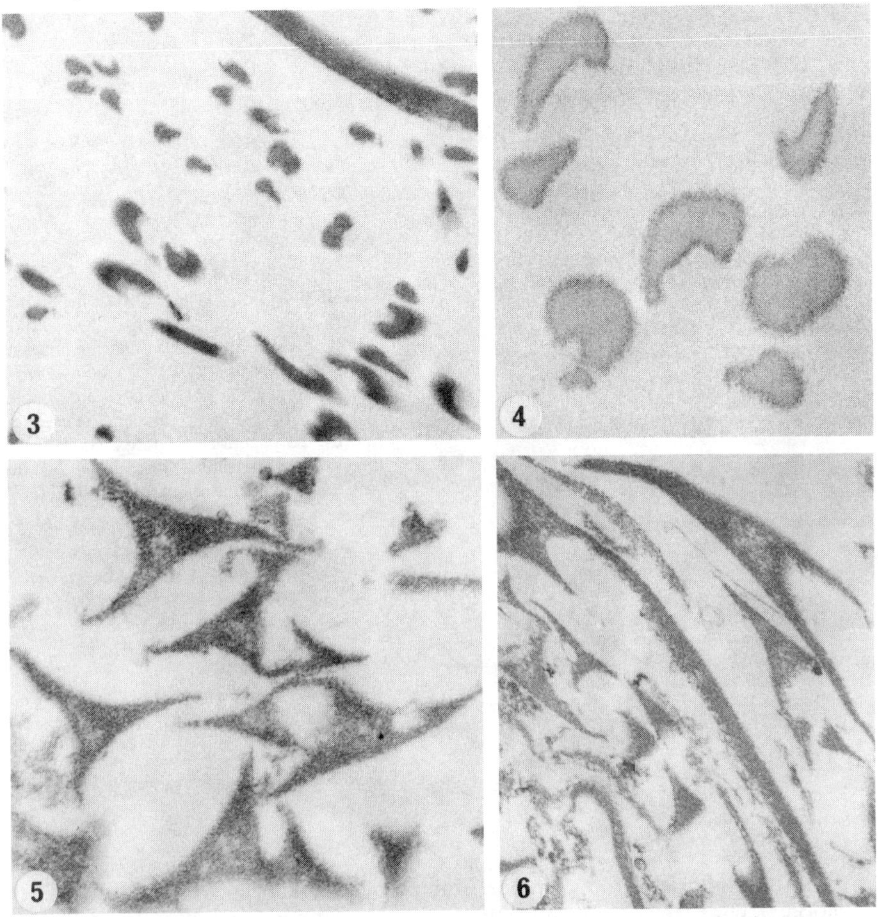

FIGURES 3–6. Electron micrographs of isolated outer dense fibers (FIGS. 3 and 4) and of isolated perforatoria (FIGS. 5 and 6).

SPECIFICITY OF ODF AND PERFORATORIAL ANTIBODIES ON WESTERN BLOTS AND SPERMATOZOA

Anti-ODF serum obtained from rabbits immunized with the isolated ODF fraction reacted strongly with all the major ODF polypeptides on Western blots and specifically immunogold labeled the ODF of rat spermatozoa prepared for electron microscopy (FIG. 8).[9] Using the anti-ODF serum, antibodies were affinity purified from the 27 and 14 kDa ODF polypeptide by the method of Talian *et al.*[25] Both affinity-purified antibodies reacted strongly with their respective polypeptides on Western blots but also cross-reacted with all the major ODF polypeptides. This suggests that the ODF polypeptides are either derived from an individual gene product that has been proteolytically cleaved or that they are derived from a group of genes which are closely related or a combination of these two possibilities.

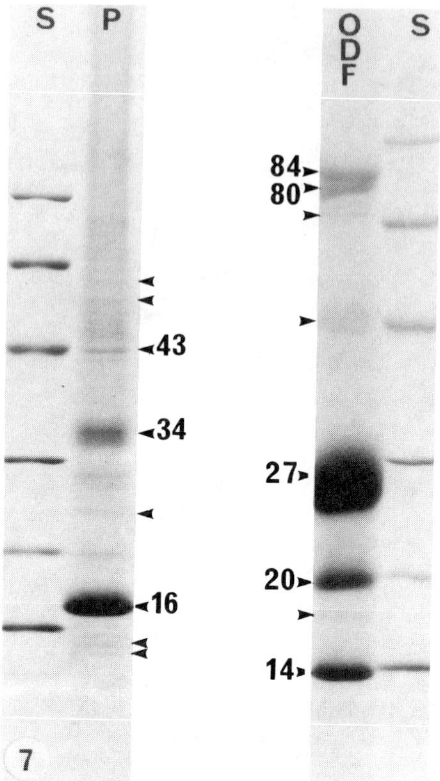

FIGURE 7. Coomassie brilliant blue-stained 8–18% linear gradient sodium dodecyl sulfate (SDS) polyacrylamide gels of perforatorial (P) and outer dense fiber (ODF) fractions. Molecular masses of the polypeptides are denoted by numbers $\times 10^3$ in this and subsequent figures. Polypeptide standards (S) were obtained from Pharmacia (Piscataway, NJ) and have molecular masses of 94, 67, 43, 30, 20, and 14 kDa.

Anti-perforatorial serum obtained from rabbits immunized with the isolated perforatorial fraction reacted strongly with the major perforatorial polypeptides on Western blots and immunogold labeled the perforatorium, inner zone of the ventral spur and the part of the outer periacrosomal layer adjacent to the acrosomal collar (FIG. 9).[10,19] Antibodies affinity purified from the major perforatorial polypeptides reacted strongly with their respective polypeptides on Western blots but also cross-reacted with all the other major polypeptides.[19] This cross-reactivity, reminiscent of the results obtained with the ODF polypeptides, also suggests that the perforatorial polypeptides are either derived from a larger protein that has been proteolytically processed or from a closely related group of proteins. The latter possibility is partly favored because immunogold labeling of spermatozoa with antibodies, affinity purified from the major polypeptides, showed a difference in distribution for the lower (13, 13.4, 16 kDa) and higher (34, 43, 57, 63 kDa) polypeptides.[19] The high molecular weight polypeptides were distributed throughout the perforatorium, within the inner zone of the ventral spur, and along the portion of the outer periacrosomal layer adjacent to the acrosomal collar.[19] The low molecular weight polypeptides were restricted in their distribution to the thicker apical part of the perforatorium, *i.e.*, the apical triangular rod and dorsal and ventral prongs.

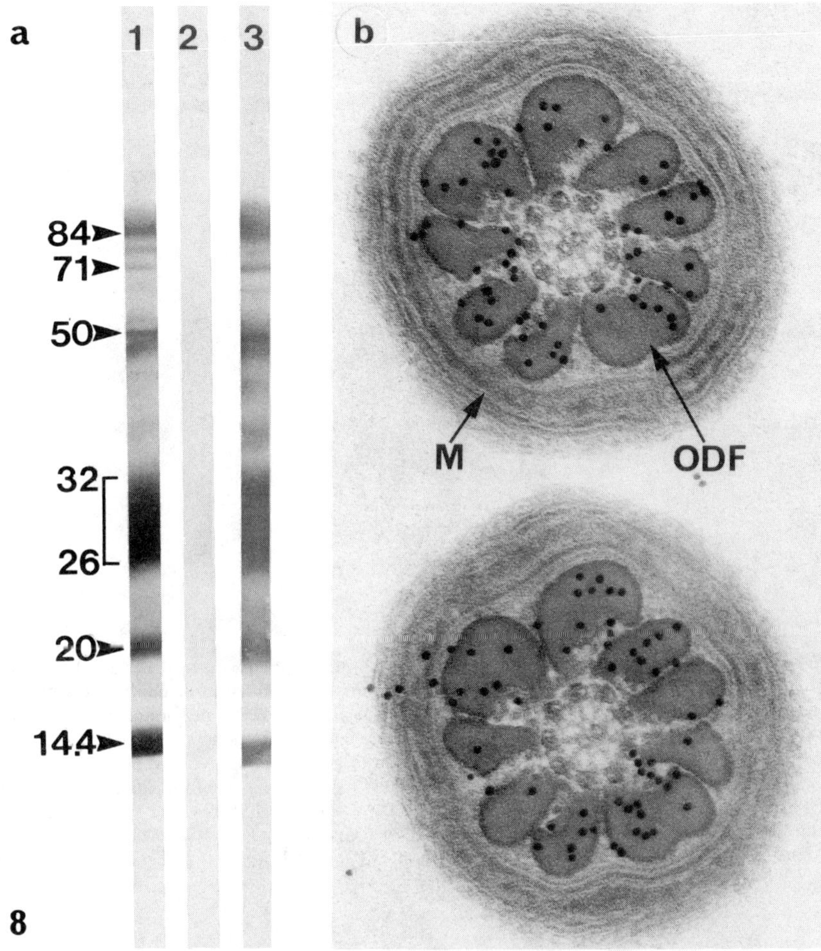

FIGURE 8. **a**: Preparative Western blot of ODF polypeptides. *Lane 1*, colloidal gold stain of transferred ODF polypeptides. *Lane 2*, preimmune serum control. *Lane 3*, ODF polypeptides immunostained with immune serum raised against the whole ODF fraction. **b**: Cross sections through the middle piece of the rat sperm tail immunogold labeled with immune serum against the ODF fraction. Note that the labeling is limited to the ODF. *Magnification:* ×100,000.

DEVELOPMENTAL EXPRESSION OF ODF AND PERFORATORIAL PROTEINS

General Pattern of ODF Protein Distribution in the Seminiferous Epithelium

Immunoperoxidase staining of paraffin embedded testicular tissue, which was reacted with the anti-ODF serum and the anti-14 kDa and anti-27 kDa ODF antibodies (the reaction elicited was identical with these three antibodies), revealed a step-specific

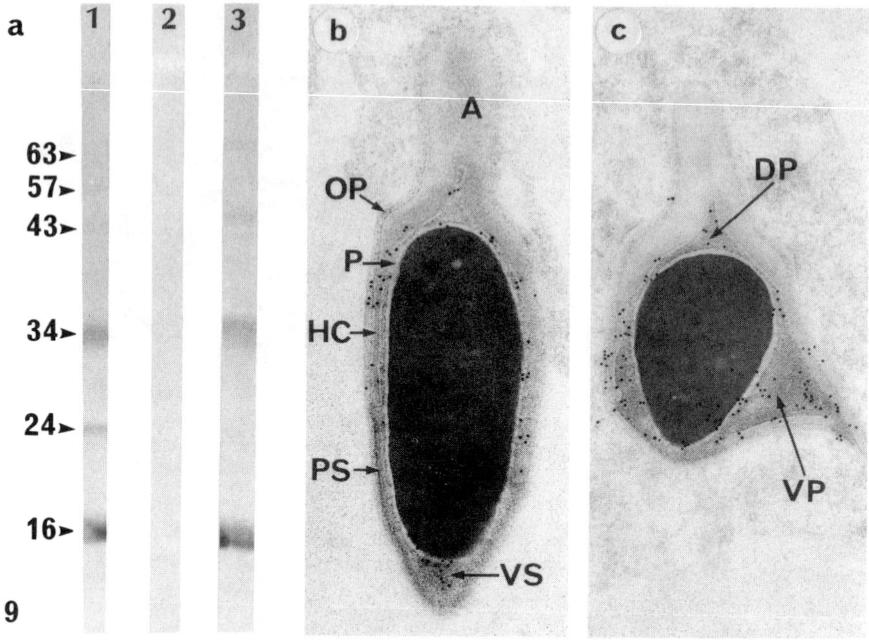

9

FIGURE 9. a: Preparative Western blot of perforatorial polypeptides. *Lane 1*, colloidal gold stain of transferred perforatorial polypeptides. *Lane 2*, preimmune serum control. *Lane 3*, Perforatorial polypeptides immunostained with immune serum raised against the whole perforatorial fraction. **b,c**: Cross sections through the head of step 19 spermatids showing the immunogold labeling distribution obtained with anti-perforatorial antibodies. In addition to gold labeling over the perforatorium, labeling is found over the inner aspect of the ventral spur (VS) and the part of the outer periacrosomal layer (OP) adjacent to the acrosomic head cap (HC).[10,19] **Labels**: A, acrosomic system; OP, outer periacrosomal layer; P, perforatorium; HC, head cap of acrosomic system; PS, postacrosomal sheath; VS, ventral spur; DP, dorsal prong of perforatorium; VP, ventral prong of perforatorium. *Magnification:* ×60,000.

reaction which was restricted to the elongated spermatid population (FIG. 10).[17] Interpretation of the immunoperoxidase results suggest that the ODF proteins are synthesized and assembled in the cytoplasm of step 9–19 spermatids, a period lasting approximately 12 days.[17] The cytoplasmic reactivity to ODF proteins is relatively weak in steps 9–13 spermatids (FIG. 12), moderately increases in steps 14–15 (FIG. 13), reaches a peak in step 16 (FIG. 14) and diminishes in step 19 (FIG. 15). Although the immunoperoxidase reaction is distributed throughout the spermatid's cytoplasm it becomes increasingly granular so that by step 16 (peak activity) large immunoreactive clumps are seen scattered throughout the cytoplasmic lobule (FIG. 14). At this time the immunostaining of the flagellum becomes intense indicating that the assembly of ODF proteins along the axoneme is coordinated with its synthesis (FIG. 14). In step 19, or at the time of spermiation residual ODF cytoplasmic reactivity is eliminated via the residual bodies of the Sertoli cell (FIG. 15). The temporal expression of the ODF proteins during spermiogenesis is diagrammatically summarized in FIGURE 30.

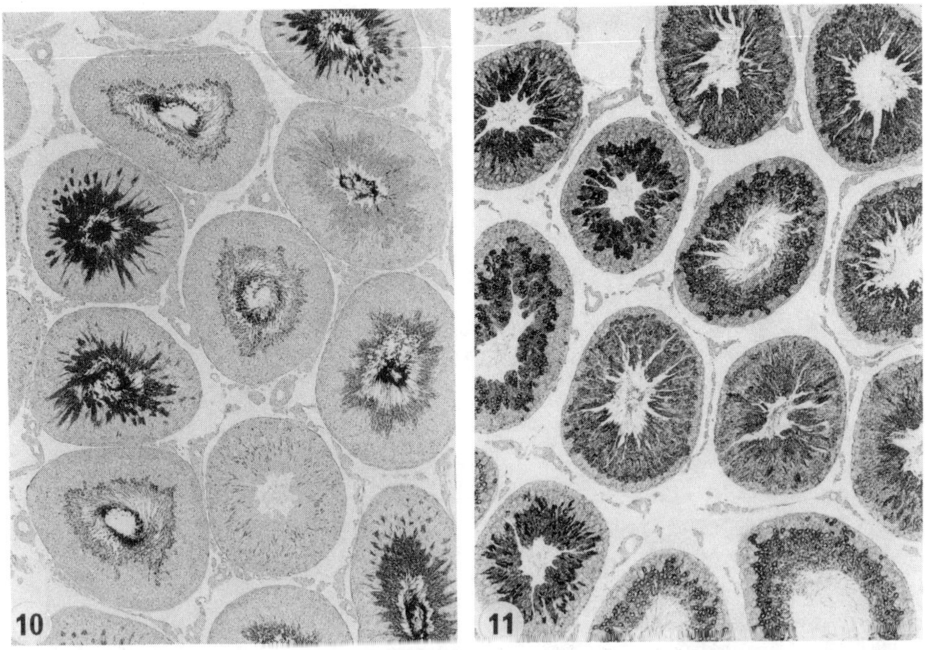

FIGURE 10. Survey section through seminiferous tubules showing the extent and pattern of immunoperoxidase staining obtained with immune serum prepared against the whole ODF fraction. Note that the reaction is restricted to the elongated spermatids. *Magnification:* ×200.

FIGURE 11. Survey section through seminiferous tubules showing the extent and pattern of immunoperoxidase staining obtained with immune serum prepared against the whole perforatorial fraction. Note that the reaction is particularly intense over the spermatids. *Magnification:* ×200.

Intracellular Localization of ODF Proteins

Immunogold labeling at the ultrastructural level revealed that the granular nature of the immunoperoxidase reaction at the light microscope level is attributed to a characteristic type of cytoplasmic granular body (Figs. 16 and 18).[18] These granular bodies are massive, have a coarse granulated texture, are irregular in shape and are numerous. They originate in association with cisternae of endoplasmic reticulum, vesicles containing an electron dense material and fine filamentous spheroidal bodies or "satellites," these three structures are unreactive to the ODF antibodies (Figs. 16 and 17).

The similar immunogold labeling of the ODF and granular bodies, the relatively light labeling in the cytoplasmic matrix of the spermatid and the fact that maximum number and size of the granular bodies is reached at the time of maximal growth in diameter of the ODF (step 16) suggest that the granular bodies are the source of precursor proteins for the assembly of the ODF.[18] Such a transitory storage role has more credence if one considers that by the end of spermiogenesis (step 19) the number and size of these granular bodies is markedly reduced. The length and size of these ODF makes these cytoskeletal structures by far the most massive component of the sper-

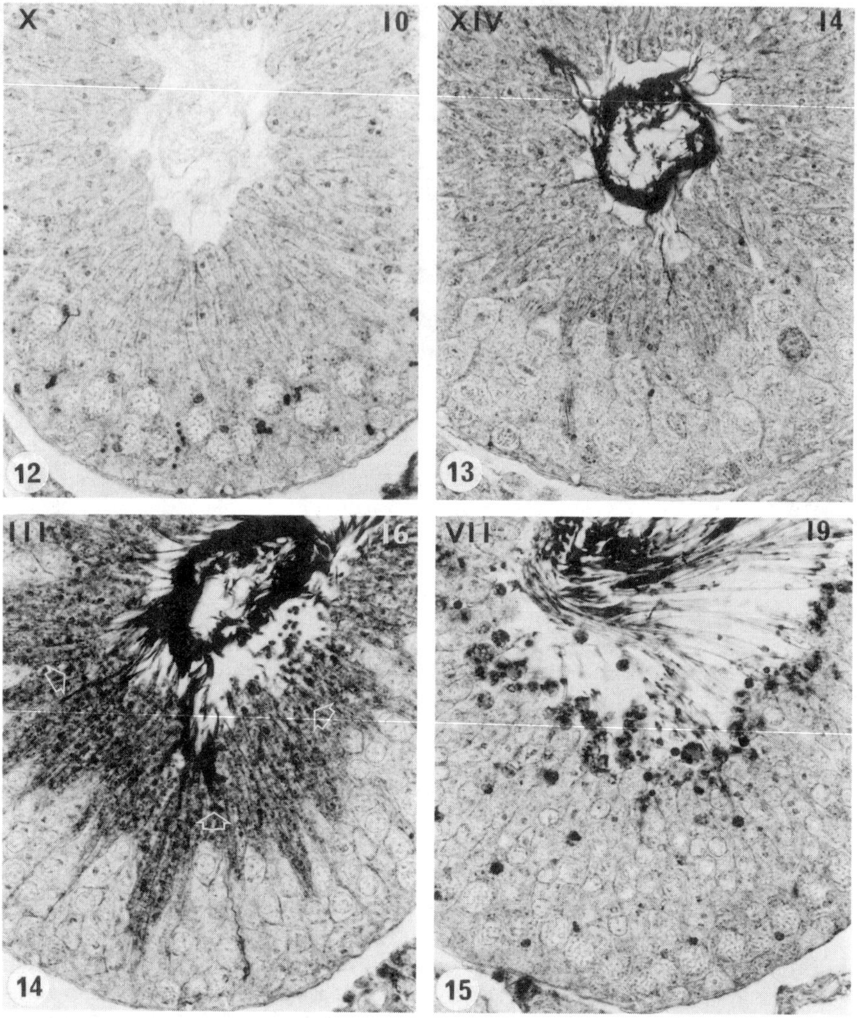

FIGURES 12–15. Immunoperoxidase staining in sections of the seminiferous tubules representing various stages (X, XIV, III, VII) of the cycle of the seminiferous epithelium, as indicated on the top left corner of each photograph, and respective steps (10, 14, 16, 19) of spermiogenesis, as indicated on the top right corner. The sections were reacted with immune serum raised against the whole ODF fraction. The white arrows in FIGURE 14 point to immunoreactive clumps scattered throughout the elongated spermatid cytoplasm. Note the intense immunoreactivity of the tails of the spermatids in the tubular lumina from step 14 of spermiogenesis onward. *Magnification:* ×600.

matozoa and therefore the amount of proteins required for their formation must be correspondingly large. The voluminous amount of protein required for the assembly of the ODF and the lengthy period of time needed for the assembly of ODF proteins along the axoneme (~12 days) may explain the reason for requiring a storage compartment in which synthesized proteins are initially deposited only to be retrieved

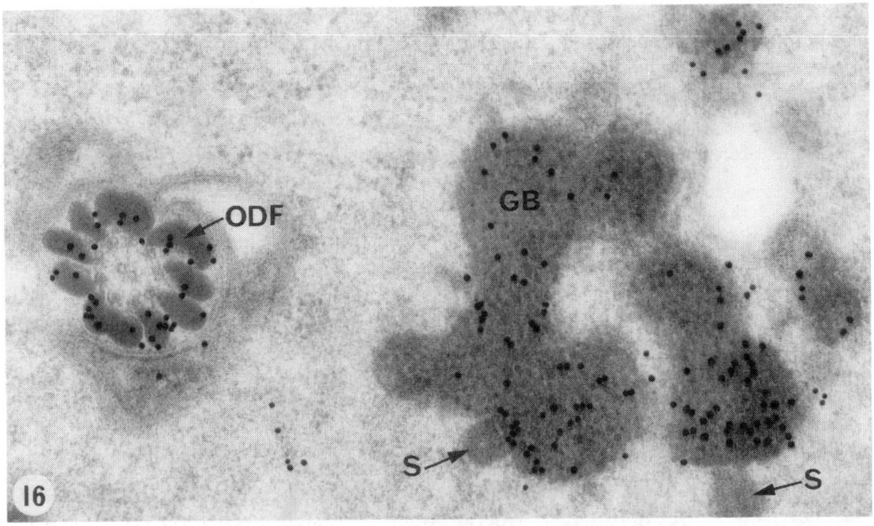

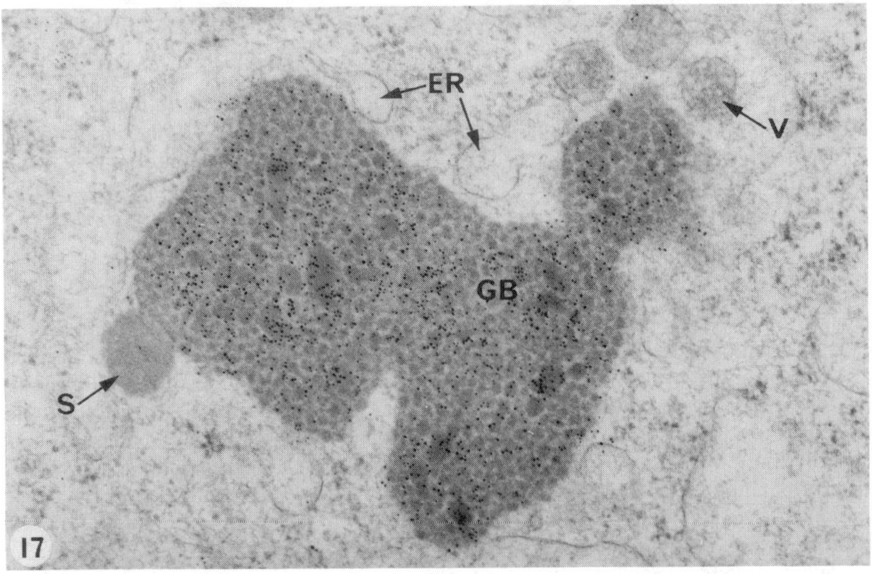

FIGURE 16. Lowicryl embedded section through the cytoplasm of step 16 spermatid immunogold labeled with anti-ODF antibodies. The forming outer dense fibers (ODF) and the granular bodies (GB) are clearly immunoreactive, whereas the satellite bodies (S) and the surrounding cytoplasm appear to be unreactive. *Magnification:* ×70,000.

FIGURE 17. Epon-embedded section through the cytoplasm of a step 16 spermatid showing a granular body immunogold labeled with anti-ODF antibodies. The cisternae of endoplasmic reticulum (ER), the vesicles with a dense content (V), and the fine filamentous satellite bodies (S) are all unreactive to the ODF antibodies whereas the granular body (GB) is well and selectively labeled with the antibody. *Magnification:* ×100,000.

later for their assembly. If granulated bodies indeed serve as transitory storage stations for ODF proteins then mechanisms must exist for protein binding and release from this structure.

General Pattern of Perforatorial Protein Distribution in the Seminiferous Epithelium

Immunoperoxidase staining with anti-perforatorial antibodies (*i.e.*, anti-perforatorial serum, anti-16 and 34 kDa antibodies) elicited an intense reaction in the spermatid population of the seminiferous epithelium regardless of the steps of spermiogenesis (FIG. 11).[20] It is estimated that the perforatorial proteins are present in the seminiferous epithelium for a period of more than 20 days. Based on interpretation of our immunoperoxidase results, regardless of the perforatorial antibodies used, the perforatorial proteins first appear in mid-pachytene spermatocytes (FIG. 20), progressively increase in concentration in late pachytene spermatocytes (FIG. 21) and early spermatids (FIGS. 18 and 19) and reach a peak in concentration in steps 8–9 spermatids (FIG. 20).[20] It is apparent that the perforatorial proteins are present both in the cytoplasm and nuclei of the round spermatid population (steps 1–9; FIGS. 18–20). However after the beginning of spermatid nuclear condensation and elongation in step 9 (FIG. 20) the perforatorial protein concentration in the nuclei rapidly diminishes so that by step 12 most of the protein resides in the spermatid cytoplasm (FIG. 21). Thereafter, in the elongated spermatid population (steps 12–19) the perforatorial protein distribution appears to be entirely cytoplasmic (FIGS. 18 and 19). The temporal expression of the perforatorial proteins during spermatogenesis is diagrammatically summarized in FIGURE 31.

Intracellular Localization of Perforatorial Proteins

Immunogold labeling with the perforatorial antibodies was not observed in Sertoli cells, spermatogonia, and early primary spermatocytes.[20] The gold labeling confirmed the nuclear and cytoplasmic immunoperoxidase localization of perforatorial proteins in late primary spermatocytes (FIG. 22) and round spermatids (FIG. 23).[20] It should be emphasized that this stage-specific nuclear and cytoplasmic immunoreactivity was not only found with the anti-perforatorial serum but was also found with the antibodies affinity purified from the 16 and 34 kDa perforatorial polypeptides.

During nuclear condensation in steps 9–12 spermatids, the immunolabeling distribution indicated that there is a progressive loss of perforatorial proteins in the nuclei and a corresponding increase in the cytoplasm (FIG. 24). The disappearance of these proteins from the nuclei occurs in an apical to caudal direction along the nuclei, in parallel with the direction of chromatin condensation (FIG. 24).[20] Once the chromatin has fully condensed (by step 13) the perforatorial proteins are no longer immunodetected in the spermatid nuclei. The possibility that the antigenic determinants of these proteins are masked after nuclear condensation can be excluded because it has been shown by immunoblot analysis that the isolated nuclei of spermatozoa are devoid of perforatorial proteins.[10] The other two possibilities are that the perforatorial proteins are either degraded in the spermatid nuclei or displaced from the nucleus to the cytoplasm. The latter possibility is favored because the loss of perforatorial proteins from

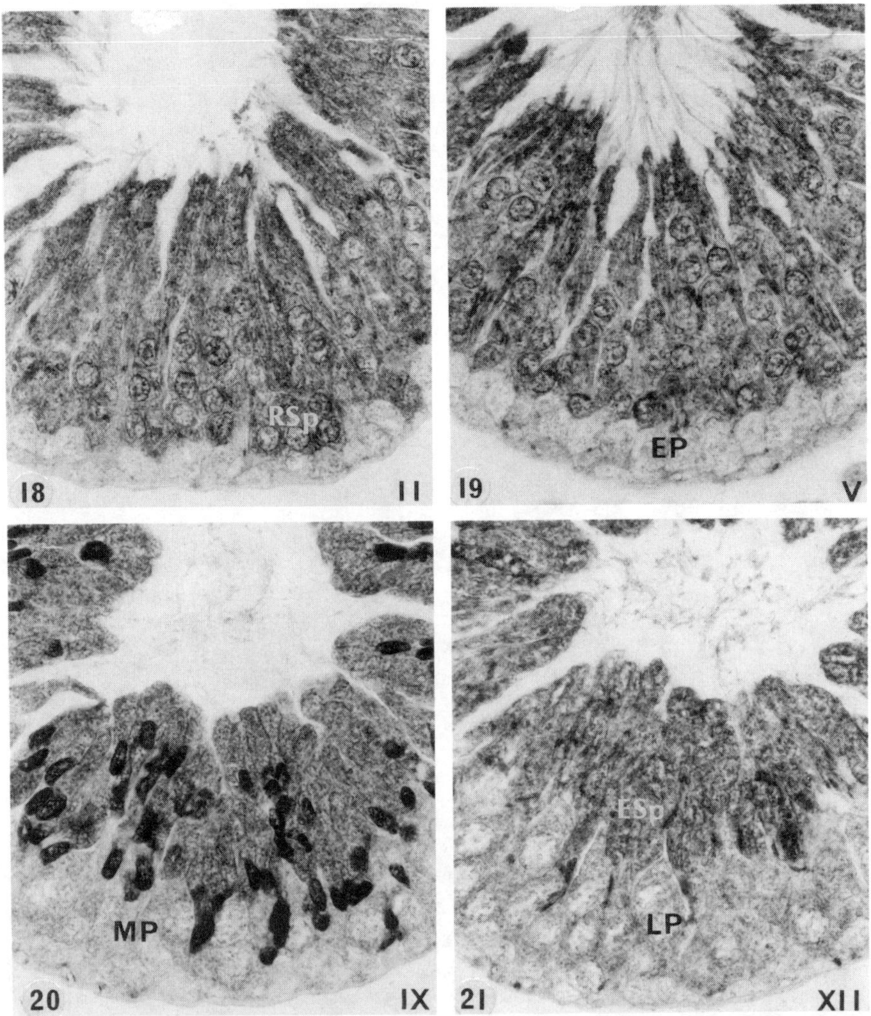

FIGURES 18–21. Immunoperoxidase staining in sections of the seminiferous tubules representing various stages (II, V, IX, XII) of the cycle of the seminiferous epithelium, as indicated on the bottom right corner of each photograph. The sections were reacted with anti-perforatorial antibodies. The mid-pachytene spermatocytes (MP) and the late pachytene spermatocytes (LP) show some immunoreactivity in both the nucleus and cytoplasm. The round spermatids (RSp) and elongated spermatids (ESp) are also immunostained (see detailed description in the text). *Magnification:* ×600.

the spermatid nuclei during condensation of the chromatin in steps 9–12 appears proportional to their increase in the spermatid cytoplasm (FIGS. 24 and 29). The translocation of proteins from the nucleus to the cytoplasm in steps 9–12 spermatids is possible through the numerous pores found in the nuclear envelope at the level of the perifossal zone in the basal compartment of the nucleus.[22,26]

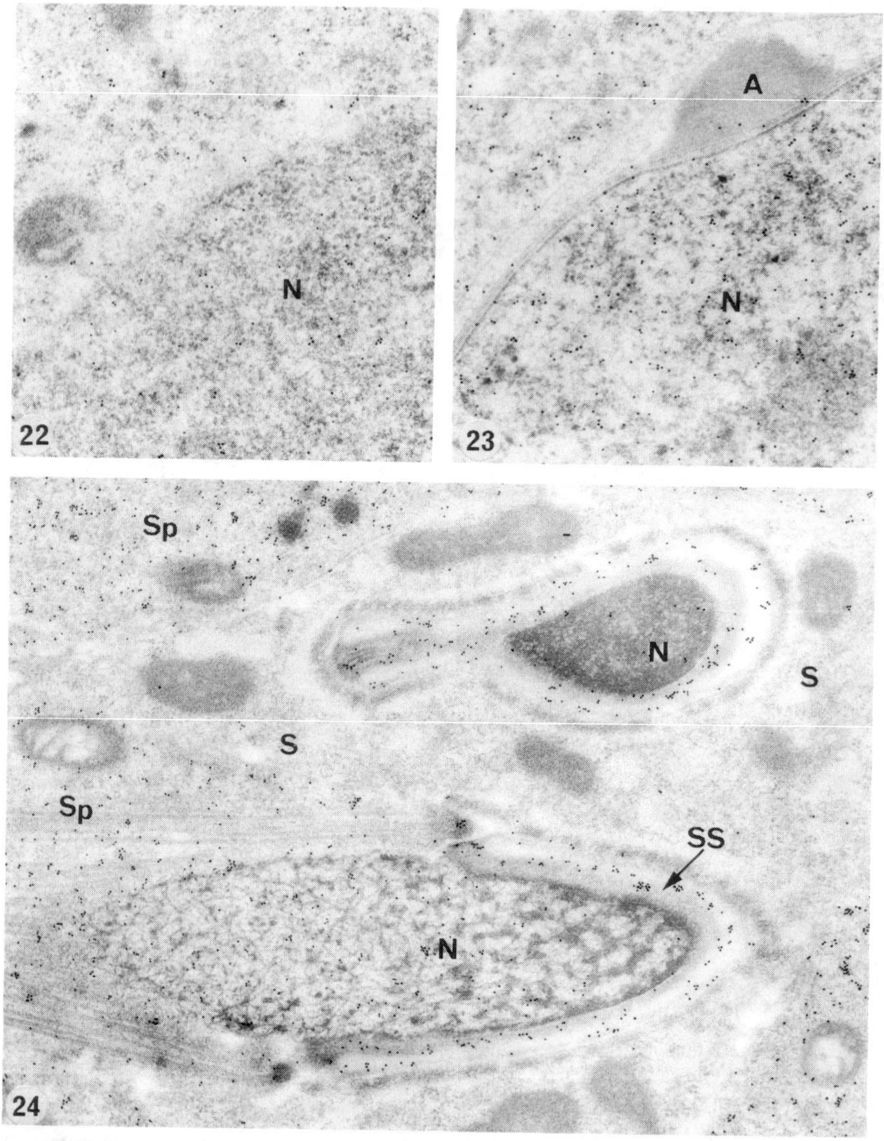

FIGURES 22–24. Immunogold labeling with anti-perforatorial antibodies of sections representing mid-pachytene spermatocytes (FIG. 22) and spermatids in step 6 (FIG. 23) and step 10 (FIG. 24). In pachytene spermatocytes and round spermatids the immunogold labeling is found in both the nucleus (N) and cytoplasm. As the chromatin condenses from the apical to caudal end of the nucleus (N) there is a progressive loss of immunogold labeling in the nucleus of step 10 spermatids. Compare the condensed areas to the relatively uncondensed areas of the nucleus for gold label. The label appears to be restricted to the subacrosomal space (SS) and distal cytoplasm (SP). The spermatid cytoplasm (Sp) in step 10 spermatids is intensely labeled, whereas the Sertoli cytoplasm (S) is free of labeling. **Labels**: A, acrosomic system. *Magnification:* ×35,000.

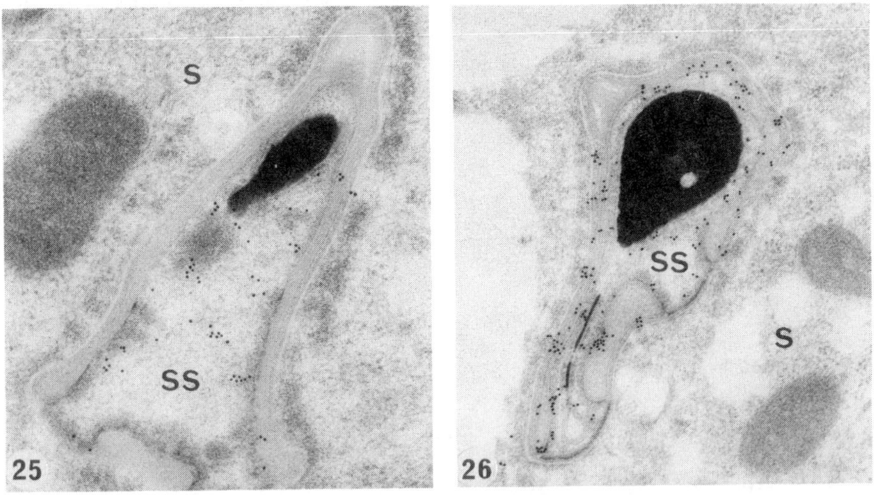

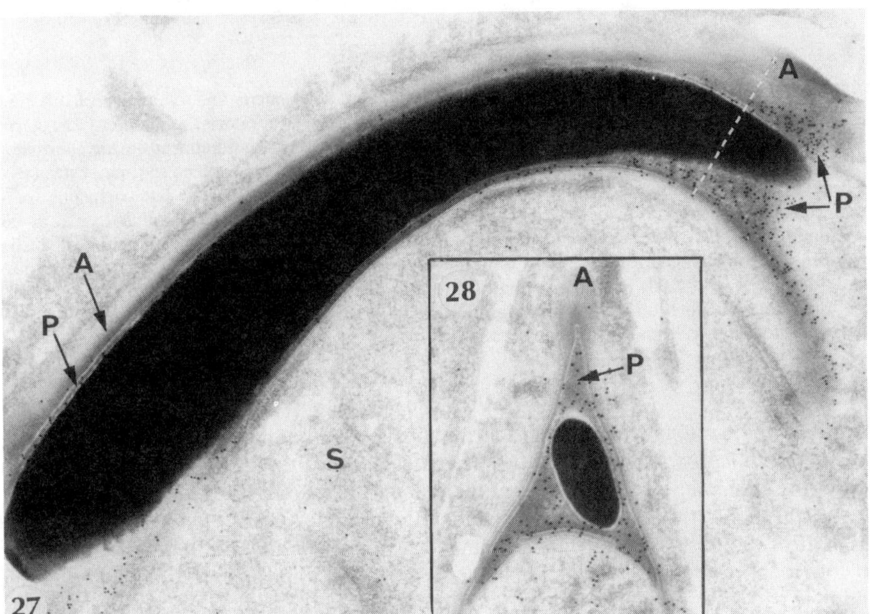

FIGURES 25 and 26. Sections through the apical part of the spermatid head in step 16 of spermiogenesis that were immunogold labeled with anti-perforatorial antibodies. The immunogold label appears in the subacrosomal space (SS) of the yet uncondensed cytoplasmic matrix. There is a tendency for the gold label to accumulate along the inner edge of the acrosomic system (FIG. 26). No labeling is found in the Sertoli cytoplasm (S). *Magnification:* ×35,000.

FIGURES 27 and 28. Longitudinal and cross sections through the spermatid head in step 19 of spermiogenesis that were labeled with anti-perforatorial antibody. The white dashed line in FIGURE 27 indicates the level of the spermatid head at which the cross-section in FIGURE 28 was taken. The perforatorium (P) which condenses at this step of spermiogenesis is intensely reactive with the gold labeled antibody. **Labels**: A, acrosomic system; S, Sertoli cytoplasm. *Magnification:* ×35,000.

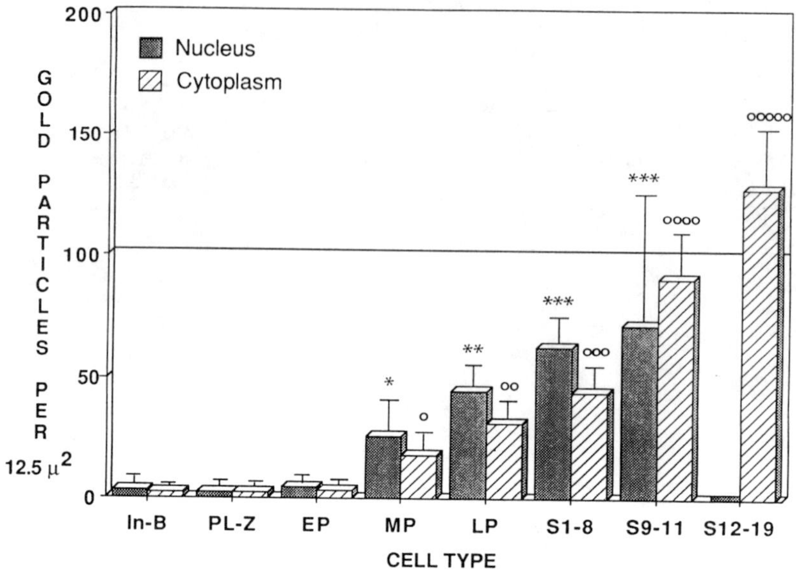

FIGURE 29. Mean concentration (+SD) of gold labeling in the nuclei and cytoplasm of different categories of spermatogenic cells reacted with the anti-34 kDa perforatorial antibodies. The germ cell categories are arranged in the chronological order in which they would appear during spermatogenesis, *i.e.*, intermediate and B spermatogonia (In-B), preleptotene to zygotene spermatocytes (PL-Z), early pachytene spermatocytes (EP), middle pachytene spermatocytes (MP), late pachytene spermatocytes (LP), steps 1 to 8 spermatids (S1–8), steps 9 to 11 spermatids (S9–11) and steps 12 to 19 spermatids (S12–19). Asterisks denote significant differences ($p \leq 0.05$) in gold labeling of nuclei between different cell categories (*e.g.* ** is significantly different from * *etc.*). Circles denote significant differences ($p \leq 0.05$) in gold labeling of cytoplasm between different cell categories. Cell categories without a denotation did not vary significantly in mean gold concentration from control values that were determined with preimmune serum.

After the condensation of the spermatid nuclei a gradual transformation occurs within the subacrosomal space of the spermatid's head (FIGS. 25–28) concomitant with structural and shape changes in the nucleus and acrosomic system.[20,22] By step 16, the apical half of the subacrosomal space, the region destined to form the thicker apical half of the perforatorium, has expanded triangularly and is filled with a material of low electron density except for some denser flocculent material deposited along the inner acrosomal membrane (FIGS. 25 and 26). In the last step of spermiogenesis (step 19) this electron lucent material in the subacrosomal space condenses to form the definitive perforatorium (FIGS. 27 and 28). As would be expected the immunoreactivity to the perforatorial antibodies is much more intense over the condensed perforatorium in step 19 (FIGS. 27 and 28) than over the electron pale subacrosomal matrix of step 16–18 spermatids (FIGS. 25 and 26). During steps 16–18, however, the buildup of immunogold label over the denser cytoplasmic material located on the inner edge of the acrosomic system suggests that the inner acrosomal membrane, rather than the nuclear membrane, may serve as the nucleation site for the deposition and condensation of perforatorial proteins.

Immunogold Quantitation of Perforatorial Protein Distribution

The mean concentration of gold labeling found in the nuclei and cytoplasm of different categories of spermatogenic cells that were reacted with the anti-34 kDa perforatorial antibody is presented in FIGURE 29. A similar statistical trend was found with the anti-perforatorial serum and with the anti-16 kDa perforatorial antibody.[20]

Statistical evaluation shows that the first significant rise ($p \leqslant 0.5$) in the concentration of gold label, from control values, in both the nuclei and cytoplasm is in the mid-pachytene spermatocytes. Beginning with early pachytene spermatocytes there is a significant upward trend in the concentration of gold labeling, such that there are successive increments in gold concentration ($\leqslant 0.5$) in both the nuclei and cytoplasm of mid-pachytene spermatocytes, late pachytene spermatocytes and steps 1–8 spermatids. In these germ cells the gold particle concentration is significantly higher ($p \leqslant 0.001$) in the nuclei than in the cytoplasm and reaches a peak in the nuclei of steps 1–8 spermatids (FIG. 29). During nuclear condensation and elongation in steps 9–11 spermatids a transition in gold labeling concentration occurs so that by step 12 spermatids the gold labeling becomes entirely cytoplasmic. The amount of gold labeling lost in the nuclei during this transition period appears to correspond to the amount of cytoplasmic labeling gained, suggesting that perforatorial proteins are displaced from the nucleus to the cytoplasm during spermatid nuclear condensation. On the premise that there is truly a displacement of perforatorial proteins from the nucleus to the cytoplasm a nuclear storage role for these proteins can be proposed in pachytene spermatocytes and early spermatids. It may be speculated that the efflux of perforatorial proteins from the nucleus is necessary to assure that the concentration of these proteins in the subacrosomal cytoplasm is sufficiently dense.

SUMMARY AND CONCLUSION

Our results on the formation of the ODF and perforatorium are diagrammatically summarized in FIGURES 30 and 31. The developmental expression of proteins making up these two cytoskeletal elements differs in timing, duration and intracellular localization. The ODF proteins are synthesized exclusively during the latter part of spermiogenesis, well after transcriptional activity in the haploid germ cell nucleus has ended.[27-29] This implies that these major integral proteins of the tail are translationally regulated and that mechanisms must exist for the storage and eventual release of the mRNAs encoding these proteins. The perforatorial proteins, on the other hand, begin to be synthesized during the meiotic prophase reaching a peak of production in early spermiogenesis just before the initiation of the condensation of the spermatid's nucleus, at which time RNA synthesis stops.[27-30]

Another major difference between ODF and perforatorial protein production is that there seems to be a coordinated activity between the synthesis and the assembly of the ODF proteins, whereas there appears to be an almost 25 day delay between the initial meiotic synthesis and final condensation of perforatorial proteins in the subacrosomal space at the end of spermiogenesis.

As for the intracellular localization of ODF and perforatorial proteins both have unprecedented distributions. The ODF proteins appear to be concentrated in a particular type of granular body which is especially abundant in the elongated spermatid at the time of peak ODF assembly. The perforatorial proteins, on the other hand,

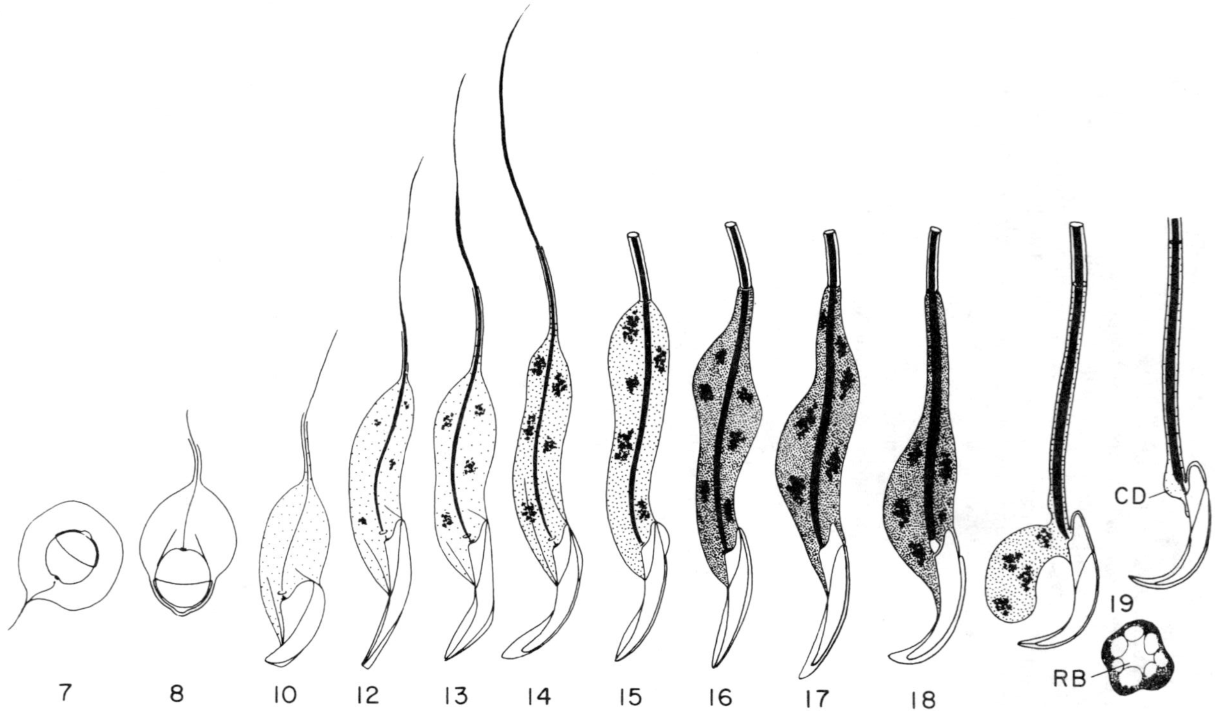

FIGURE 30. Diagrammatical summary of the reactivity of rat spermatids to immune serum raised against the whole ODF fraction (taken from the authors' previous publication[17]). The cytoplasmic reactivity to the immune serum is relatively weak in steps 9–13 spermatids and moderate in steps 14 and 15. The immunoreactivity reaches a peak in step 16, remains elevated in step 17 and 18, and diminishes in step 19. Although the reactivity is distributed throughout the cytoplasm of elongated spermatids, as indicated by the stippling, it becomes increasingly concentrated over numerous cytoplasmic granular bodies (GB) in steps 12–16. Flagellar reactivity to ODF antiserum begins in the proximal part of the axoneme in step 12, covers the entire axoneme by step 14, and markedly increases in intensity in steps 15 and 16. The elimination of the residual ODF reactive material is through the residual bodies (RB).

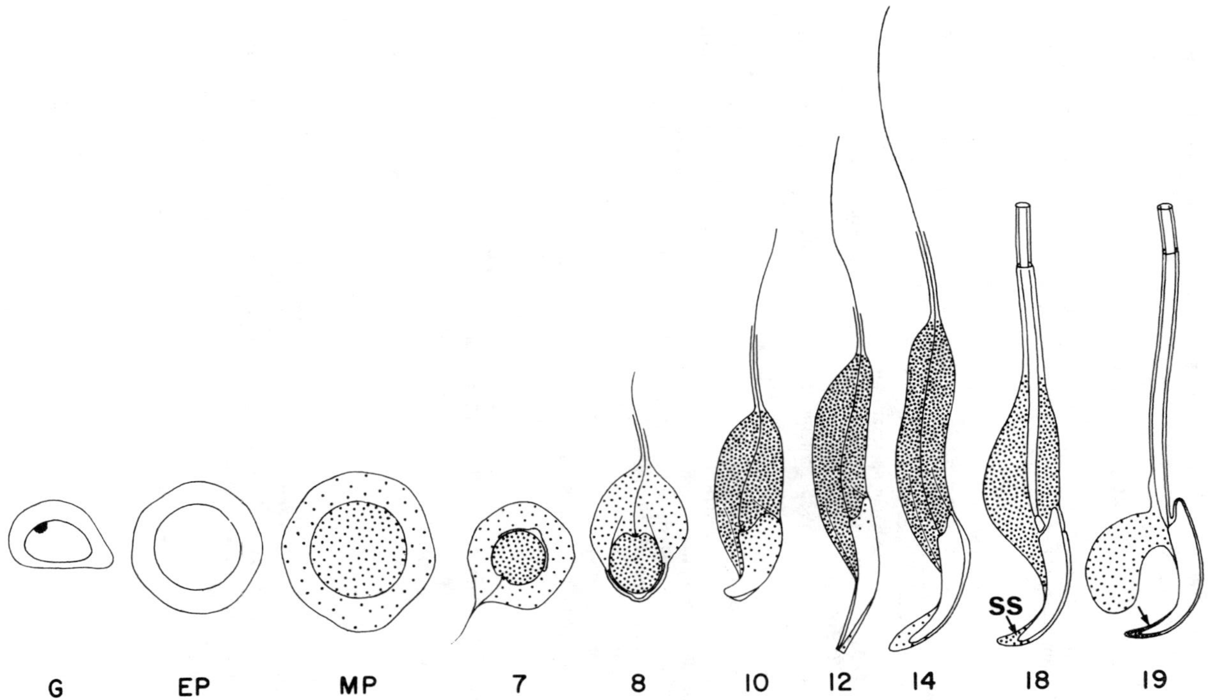

FIGURE 31. Diagrammatical summary of the reactivity (as indicated by the stippling) of rat spermatogenic cells to anti-perforatorial antibodies. The reactivity to the antibodies first appears in both the nuclei and cytoplasm of mid-pachytene spermatocytes (MP), becomes intense in both compartments in round spermatids (steps 1–7), and reaches a peak in the nuclei of step 8 spermatids. Up to this point of spermatogenesis the reactivity is more intense in the nuclei of spermatocytes and round spermatids than in the cytoplasm. During nuclear condensation of the spermatid, as depicted on the diagram by step 10 and 12 spermatids, the reactivity appears to be displaced from the nucleus to the cytoplasm. Thereafter the reactivity is restricted to the elongated spermatid's cytoplasm and the subacrosomal space (SS). In step 19 of spermiogenesis the reactivity becomes most intense around the apical part of the spermatid nuclei (arrow) over the condensed perforatorium. **Labels**: G, spermatogonia; EP, early pachytene spermatocytes; MP, mid-pachytene spermatocytes; 7–19, each number indicates the step of spermiogenesis.

appear to be concentrated in the nuclei of pachytene spermatocytes and round spermatids until their displacement into the cytoplasm during nuclear condensation. Both forms of localization suggest a storage role for these proteins uniquely adapted by the spermatid to regulate the assemblies of the respective cytoskeletal elements.

REFERENCES

1. Calvin, H. I. & J. M. Bedford. 1971. Formation of disulfide bonds in the nucleus and accessory structures of mammalian spermatozoa during maturation in the epididymis. J. Reprod. Fertil. **13**(Suppl.): 65–75.
2. Calvin, H. I. 1976. Isolation and subfractionation of mammalian sperm heads and tails. *In* Methods of Cell Biology. D. M. Prescott, Ed. **13**: 85–104. Academic Press. New York.
3. Olson, G. E., D. W. Hamilton & D. W. Fawcett. 1976a. Isolation and characterization of the perforatorium of rat spermatozoa. J. Reprod. Fertil. **47**: 1–9.
4. Olson, G. E., D. W. Hamilton & D. W. Fawcett. 1976b. Isolation and characterization of the fibrous sheath of rat epididymal spermatozoa. Biol. Reprod. **14**: 517–530.
5. Olson, G. E. & D. W. Sammons. 1980. Structural chemistry of outer dense fibers of rat sperm. Biol. Reprod. **22**: 319–332.
6. Pruslin, F. H. & T. C. Rodman. 1985. Proteins of demembraned mouse sperm heads. J. Biol. Chem. **260**: 5654–5659.
7. Vera, J. C., M. Brito, T. Zavic & L. O. Burzio. 1984. Polypeptide composition of rat sperm outer dense fibers. J. Biol. Chem. **259**: 5970–5977.
8. Brito, M., J. Figueroa, E. U. Maldonado, J. C. Vera & L. O. Burzio. 1989. The major component of rat sperm fibrous sheath is a phosphoprotein. Gamete Res. **22**: 205–218.
9. Oko, R. 1988. Comparative analysis of proteins from fibrous sheath and outer dense fibers of rat spermatozoa. Biol. Reprod. **39**: 169–182.
10. Oko, R. & Y. Clermont. 1988. Isolation, structure and protein composition of the perforatorium of rat spermatozoa. Biol. Reprod. **39**: 673–687.
11. Longo, F. J., G. Krohne & W. W. Franke. 1987. Basic proteins of the perinuclear theca of mammalian spermatozoa and spermatids: A novel class of cytoskeletal elements. J. Cell Biol. **105**: 1105–1120.
12. Eddy, E. M., D. A. O'Brien & J. M. Benziger. 1987. Intermediate filament-like protein in the mouse sperm flagellum. J. Cell Biol. 168a (Abstr.).
13. Franke, W. W., C. Grund & E. Schmid. 1979. Intermediate-sized filaments present in Sertoli cells are of the vimentin type. Eur. J. Cell Biol. **19**: 269–275.
14. Kierszenbaum, A. L., J. A. Crowell, R. B. Shabanowitz, E. C. Smith, W. A. Spruill & L. A. Tres. 1986. A monoclonal antibody recognizes a form of intermediate filament protein in rat Sertoli cells that is not present in seminiferous peritubular cells. Biol Reprod. **35**: 227-238.
15. Fenderson, B. A., K. Toshinori, C. H. Muller, T. F. Lane & E. M. Eddy. 1988. Identification of a protein in the fibrous sheath of the sperm flagellum. Biol. Reprod. **38**: 345.-357.
16. O'Brien, D. A. & A. R. Bellve. 1980. Protein constituents of the mouse spermatozoon. II Temporal synthesis during spermatogenesis. Dev. Biol. **75**: 405–418.
17. Oko, R. & Y. Clermont. 1989. Light microscopic immunocytochemical study of fibrous sheath and outer dense fiber formation in the rat spermatid. Anat. Rec. **225**: 46–55.
18. Clermont, Y., R. Oko & L. Hermo. 1991. Immunocytochemical localization of proteins utilized in the formation of outer dense fibers and fibrous sheath in rat spermatids: An electron microscopic study. Anat. Rec. **227**: 447–457.
19. Oko, R., L. Moussakova & Y. Clermont. 1990. Regional differences in composition of the perforatorium and of the outer periacrosomal layer of rat spermatozoa as revealed by immunocytochemistry. Am J. Anat. **188**: 64–73.
20. Oko, R. & Y. Clermont. 1991. Origin and distribution of perforatorial proteins during spermatogenesis of the rat: An immunocytochemical study. Anat. Rec. **230**: 489–501.
21. Fawcett, D. W. 1970. A comparative view of sperm ultrastructure. Biol. Reprod. [Suppl. 2]: 90–127.

22. LALLI, M. F. & Y. CLERMONT. 1981. Structural changes of the head components of the rat spermatid during late spermiogenesis. Am. J. Anat. **160:** 419–434.
23. COURTENS, J. L., M. COUROT & J. E. FLÉCHON. 1976. The perinuclear substance of boar, bull, ram and rabbit spermatozoa. J. Ultrastruct. Res. **57:** 54–64.
24. CALVIN, H. I. 1979. Electrophoretic evidence for the identity of the major zinc-binding polypeptides in the rat sperm tail. Biol. Reprod. **21:** 873–882.
25. TALIAN, J. C., J. B. OLMSTED & R. D. GOLDMAN. 1983. A rapid procedure for preparing fluorescein-labeled specific antibodies from whole antiserum: Its use in analysing cytoskeletal architecture. J. Cell Biol. **97:** 1277–1282.
26. FAWCETT, D. W. 1975. The mammalian spermatozoon. Dev. Biol. **44:** 394–436.
27. MONESI, V. 1965. Synthetic activity during spermatogenesis in the mouse. RNA and protein synthesis. Exp. Cell Res. **39:** 197–224.
28. MONESI, V. 1971. Chromosome activities during meiosis and spermiogenesis. J. Reprod. Fertil. **13**(Suppl.): 1–14.
29. MONESI, V., R. GEREMIA, A. D'AGOSTINO & C. BOITONI. 1978. Biochemistry of male germ cell differentiation in mammals: RNA synthesis in meiotic and postmeiotic cells. Curr. Top Dev. Biol. **12:** 11–36.
30. HECHT, N. B. 1987. Gene expression during spermiogenesis. Ann. N. Y. Acad. Sci. **513:** 90–101.

Intermediate Filament–like Proteins in the Fibrous Sheath of the Mouse Sperm Flagellum

E. M. EDDY,[a,d] D. A. O'BRIEN,[b]
B. A. FENDERSON,[c] AND J. E. WELCH[a]

[a] *Gamete Biology Section*
Laboratory of Reproductive and Developmental Toxicology
National Institute of Environmental Health Sciences
National Institutes of Health
P.O. Box 12233
Research Triangle Park, North Carolina 27709

[b] *Laboratories for Reproductive Biology and*
Departments of Pediatrics and Cell Biology and Anatomy
University of North Carolina at Chapel Hill
Chapel Hill, North Carolina 27995–7500

[c] *Department of Pathology*
Jefferson Medical College
Thomas Jefferson University
Philadelphia, Pennsylvania 19107

INTRODUCTION

During the process of spermatogenesis, germ cells progress through three phases of development. The first is the stem cell phase in which spermatogonial cells divide mitotically, the second is the meiotic phase of primary and secondary spermatocyte development, and the third is the post-meiotic phase when spermatids remodel into spermatozoa. The cells resulting from this process are highly differentiated in structure and function.[1] The unusual structural features of sperm include a mosaic plasma membrane, an acrosome containing several hydrolytic enzymes, a spatulate- or falciform-shaped head containing a highly condensed nucleus, a helical assembly of mitochondria in the midpiece, and an elaborately constructed flagellum. Protein isoforms specific to germ cells are commonly associated with these features. Such proteins are frequently the products of genes actively transcribed only in spermatogenic cells and/or expressed in a stage-specific manner during male germ cell development.[2]

The unusual shape of mammalian spermatozoa reflects the presence of a complex set of cytoskeletal structures in the head and flagellum.[1] They include subacrosomal, postacrosomal, and para-acrosomal cytoskeletal structures in the sperm head and outer dense fibers and the fibrous sheath in the flagellum. These structures have morpho-

[d] Author to whom correspondence should be addressed.

logical, biochemical, physical and immunological features suggesting that they contain intermediate filament proteins. Although we are beginning to learn about some of the proteins present in these structures, it has not been determined if they are encoded by genes of the intermediate filament family or are the products of genes unique to spermatogenic cells.

We have begun to characterize the composition of sperm cytoskeletal structures by examining the nature of proteins in the fibrous sheath. The fibrous sheath extends throughout the principal piece of the flagellum, where it immediately underlies the plasma membrane and surrounds the outer dense fibers and axoneme.[1] It consists of two longitudinal dense columns connected by circumferential ribs and is synthesized and assembled throughout most of spermiogenesis.[3] The fibrous sheath provides form and rigidity to the flagellum and probably determines the shape of the flagellar beat.[4] Infertility can occur in humans and mice with spermatozoa having defective fibrous sheaths.[5,6]

The fibrous sheath was suggested to be keratin-like in composition because of its disulfide content and resistance to solubilization.[7] Initial biochemical studies identified a protein with an apparent molecular weight (M_r) of 80,000 as the main component in the fibrous sheath of rat sperm.[8,9] More recent studies reported three major fibrous sheath proteins of M_r 75,000–80,000, 24,000–27,000 and 11,000–14,000, with the largest and most abundant protein being phosphorylated.[10,11] Peptide mapping indicated that the two larger proteins were unrelated to outer dense fiber proteins, but compositional data suggested that the small protein was shared by the two structures.[11] Studies with antisera also suggested that the small protein is present in both structures and that common epitopes are present in several proteins of the outer dense fibers and fibrous sheath.[10] We previously demonstrated that a monoclonal antibody recognizes fibrous sheath proteins of M_r 67,000 in mouse, M_r 65,500 in rat, and M_r 66,000 in the hamster.[12] The protein was detected in late spermatids of the mouse by immunohistochemical procedures, but not in brain, kidney, liver or thymus. We have further examined the nature of the fibrous sheath and its proteins in the present study. Although some investigators have reported that sperm contain intermediate filament proteins,[13–15] others have been unable to identify these proteins in spermatogenic cells or sperm.[16–18] The results of the present study indicate that the fibrous sheath contains proteins that are immunologically related to intermediate filament proteins, but have different molecular weights compared to previously reported members of this protein family. We hypothesize that these proteins are products of intermediate filament genes that are expressed only during male germ cell development.

METHODS AND MATERIALS

Cell Preparation

Spermatogenic cells were obtained from day 17 prepuberal or adult CD-1 mice from the NIEHS breeding colony. Testes were disaggregated enzymatically and spermatogenic cells isolated from seminiferous epithelial cell suspensions by unit gravity sedimentation, using procedures described previously.[19–21] Cells were washed twice in enriched Krebs-Ringer buffer solution[19] and used immediately or stored at −70°C.

Sperm were isolated from the cauda epididymides of CD-1 mice or Wistar rats (Charles River Labs, Raleigh, NC) in Dulbecco's phosphate buffered saline (DPBS) on ice and washed three times by centrifugation for 5 min at 650 × g. Cytocentrifuge slides were prepared by centrifugation (5 min at 160 × g) of 1 × 10^4 sperm in 0.2 ml of DPBS onto glass slides in a cytocentrifuge (Shandon Southern Products, Cheshire, UK), and were air dried and stored at 4°C.

3T3 cells and NOR-10 cells were obtained from the American Type Culture Collection (Rockville, MD) and maintained as recommended. For indirect immunofluorescence (IIF) studies, 3T3 and NOR-10 cells grown on Labtek tissue culture/chamber slides (Miles Laboratories, Inc., Naperville, IL) were fixed for 5 min at room temperature in DPBS (pH 7.6) containing 3% formaldehyde (freshly prepared from paraformaldehyde) and 2% sucrose, washed three times with ice cold DPBS, then treated for 2 min on ice with permeabilizing buffer (0.2% Triton X-100, 300 mM sucrose, 3 mM MgCl, 50 mM NaCl, and 2 mM PMSF in 20 mM HEPES, pH 7.4). To prepare cytoskeletons for gel electrophoresis, 3T3 and NOR-10 cells were grown on 100 mm tissue culture dishes, treated for 15 min with permeabilizing buffer and removed from the dishes with a rubber policeman. Cytoskeletons were washed three times by centrifugation at 1200 × g for 10 min in 20 mM Tris hydrochloride, pH 7.4, and prepared for gel electrophoresis as described below.

Cytocentrifuge slides of sperm were prepared for IIF in the same manner as 3T3 and NOR-10 cells or by soaking for 2 h in each of the solutions used for isolating fibrous sheaths.[12]

Enzyme Immunoassay

Enzyme-dissociated seminiferous epithelial cells (1 × 10^7/ml) were solubilized for enzyme-linked immunosorbent assay (ELISA) with freshly prepared extraction buffer (EB) containing 0.05% cetyltrimethylammonium bromide (CTAB), 1 mM ethylene diamine-tetraacetic acid (EDTA), 1 mM ethylene glycol-bis(β-amino ethyl ether) N,N,N′,N′-tetraacetic acid (EGTA), 0.05 μg/ml pepstatin A, 0.05 μg/ml antipain, 0.5 U/ml aprotinin, 0.2 mM phenylmethylsulfonyl fluoride (PMSF) and 20 mM Tris hydrochloride, pH 8) (Sigma Chemical Co., St. Louis, MO), for 40 min on ice with occasional gentle agitation. The supernatant was collected by centrifugation at 1200 × g for 10 min and centrifuged again at 12,500 × g for 5 min, diluted 10-fold in EB, and dialyzed for 24 h at 4°C against two changes of 100 volumes of EB lacking CTAB. Protein concentrations were determined by the procedure of Lowry *et al.*[22] and fibrous sheath isolation procedures were adapted from those of Olson *et al.*[8] as described previously.[12]

ELISA plates were prepared by adding 100 ng protein per well in 50 μl of coating buffer (25 mM citric acid monohydrate, 50 mM $Na_2HPO_4 \cdot 7H_20$, pH 4.5) and incubating 2 h at room temperature or overnight at 4°C. A competition ELISA was performed with culture supernatants containing monoclonal antibody ATC[12] and synthetic peptides by adding peptide to different dilutions of antibody in 100 μl DPBS. After incubation for 30 min at room temperature, the antibody-peptide mixture was then transferred to wells of an ELISA plate coated with mouse sperm fibrous sheaths. Competing peptides used were polyglycine (50 μg), poly(proline-glycine-proline) (100 μg), and poly-L-proline (100 μg) (Sigma Chemical Co., St. Louis, MO). ELISA assays and monoclonal antibody production were performed as described previously.[12]

Gel Electrophoresis and Immunoblotting

Samples were solubilized in 0.5% sodium dodecyl sulfate (SDS), 40 mM dithiothreitol (DTT), and 0.06% Tris hydrochloride (pH 6.8) for 20 min at 50°C. Proteins were separated electrophoretically under denaturing conditions on uniform 10% or continuous gradient 7 to 12% polyacrylamide one-dimensional gels (1D-gels), using the Laemmli[23] discontinuous SDS buffer system. For two-dimensional polyacrylamide gel electrophoresis (2D-gels), proteins were solubilized in 9.5% urea, 2% Nonidet P-40 and 40 mM DTT, and separated in the first dimension by isoelectric focusing (IEF) on 3.6% polyacrylamide tube gels containing pH 3 to 10 Ampholines (LKB Pharmacia Biotechnology Inc., Piscataway, NJ), according to the procedures of Duncan and Hershey.[24] In some studies, proteins were separated in the first dimension by non-equilibrium polyacrylamide gel electrophoresis (NEPHGE) as described.[25] The second dimension was run on 7 to 12% continuous gradient polyacrylamide slab gels, according to the procedure recommended by O'Farrell.[26] Proteins were stained with Coomassie blue or the silver procedure of Wray *et al.*[27] or unstained gels were transferred electrophoretically to nitrocellulose sheets and immunostained as previously described.[28]

Indirect Immunofluorescence

Monoclonal antibodies used for IIF and immunoblot studies were against **vimentin** (Labsystems Oy, Helsinki, Finland; EAB 903, Enzo Biochem, Inc., New York, NY; VIM 13.1, Sigma Chemical Co., St. Louis, MO; V9, Boehringer Mannheim Biochemica, Indianapolis, IN; Amersham Corp., Arlington Heights, IL), **desmin** (Labsystems Oy, Helsinki, Finland; DE-U-10, Sigma Chemical Co., St. Louis, MO; DE-B-5, ICN ImmunoBiologicals, Lisle, IL; Amersham Corp., Arlington Heights, IL), **cytokeratin** (AE1/AE3, Hybritech Inc., San Diego, CA; EAB 902, EAB 903, and EAB 904, Enzo Biochem, Inc., New York, NY; Amersham Corp., Arlington Heights, IL), **glial fibrillary acidic protein** (EAB 906, Enzyo Biochem, Inc., New York, NY; Amersham Corp., Arlington Heights, IL), **neurofilament 68kD polypeptide** (Amersham, Arlington Heights, IL), as well as against all classes of intermediate filaments or **panfilament** (TIB 131, American Type Culture Collection, Rockville, MD; EAB 905, Enzo Biochem, Inc., New York, NY). IIF was performed as described previously.[12]

RESULTS

Characterization of Fibrous Sheath Proteins

Fibrous sheaths isolated from mouse and rat sperm showed similar protein patterns on 1D-gels stained with Coomassie blue (FIG. 1). In the mouse, the main proteins had apparent molecular weights (M_r) of 112,000, 78,000, 67,000, 63,000, 36,000 and 24,000 (FIG. 1, lane 2). In the rat, the main proteins had M_r of 115,000, 80,000, 65,500, 63,000, 35,000, 29,000 and 24,000 (FIG. 1, lane 3). These values were determined by averaging the results of laser densitometric scans on three gels. Furthermore, these scans indicated that in the mouse, the protein of M_r 78,000 was ~40% and the pro-

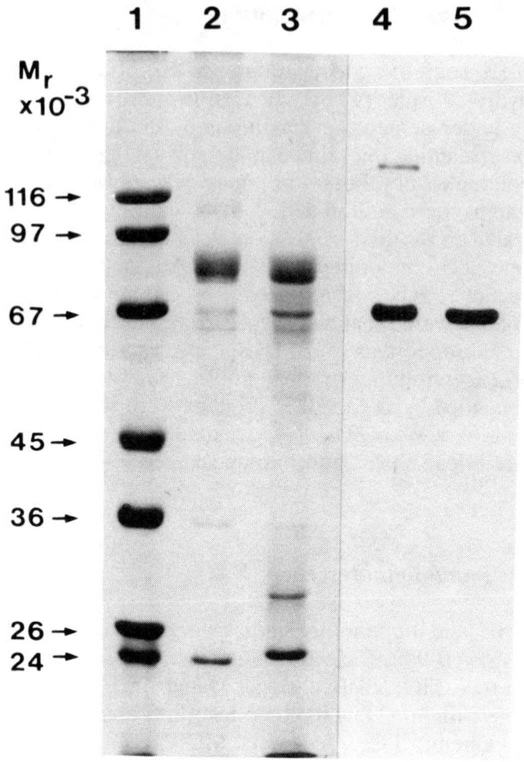

FIGURE 1. One dimensional PAGE and immunoblot characterization of fibrous sheaths isolated from mouse and rat sperm. Lanes 2 and 4 contain mouse fibrous sheaths, lanes 3 and 5 contain rat fibrous sheaths, and lane 1 contains molecular weight standards. Lanes 1–3 were stained with Coomassie blue and lanes 4 and 5 were immunostained with monoclonal antibody ATC. Isolated mouse fibrous sheaths (*lane 2*) contain proteins of M_r 112,000, 78,000, 67,000, 63,000 and 24,000. Isolated rat fibrous sheaths (*lane 3*) contain proteins of M_r 115,000, 80,000, 65,500, 63,000, 35,000, 29,000 and 24,000. Antibody ATC recognized a M_r 67,000 protein in mouse fibrous sheath (*lane 4*) and a M_r 65,000 protein in rat fibrous sheath (*lane 5*). A M_r 135,000 protein sometimes seen in mouse fibrous sheath (*lane 4*) may be a dimer of the M_r 67,000 protein.

tein of M_r 67,000 was ~16% of the total protein in the isolated fibrous sheath. In the rat, the protein of M_r 80,000 was ~35% and the protein of M_r 65,500 was ~12% of the total protein. The mouse fibrous sheath did not contain a protein comparable to the protein of M_r 29,000 in the rat. Although the isolated fibrous sheath preparations appeared homogeneous by light microscopy, we cannot exclude the possibility that some of the proteins detected may have come from other sperm components. On immunoblots prepared from the same samples, monoclonal antibody ATC recognized a protein of M_r 67,000 in mouse fibrous sheath (FIG. 1, lane 4) and of M_r 65,500 in rat fibrous sheath (FIG. 1, lane 5). In addition, a protein of M_r 135,000 was seen in some preparations of mouse fibrous sheath (FIG. 1, lane 4), which may be a dimer of the protein of M_r 67,000.

Fibrous sheaths isolated from mouse and rat sperm were also examined on 2D-gels. The major fibrous sheath proteins migrated as multiple charge forms or with a broad isoelectric point (pI) and/or a broad M_r range on both IEF and NEPHGE 2D-gels (FIGS. 2 and 3). The abundant mouse protein of M_r 78,000 (FIG. 2,A and C) and rat protein of M_r 80,000 (FIG. 3,A and C) were diffuse on IEF and NEPHGE 2D-gels. These proteins and the mouse protein of M_r 67,000 and rat protein of M_r 65,000 focused to the basic pI range on IEF gels, while the smaller proteins generally focused to neutral or acidic pI ranges on IEF gels. On immunoblots of 2D-gels stained with monoclonal antibody ATC, the mouse protein of M_r 67,000 had multiple charge

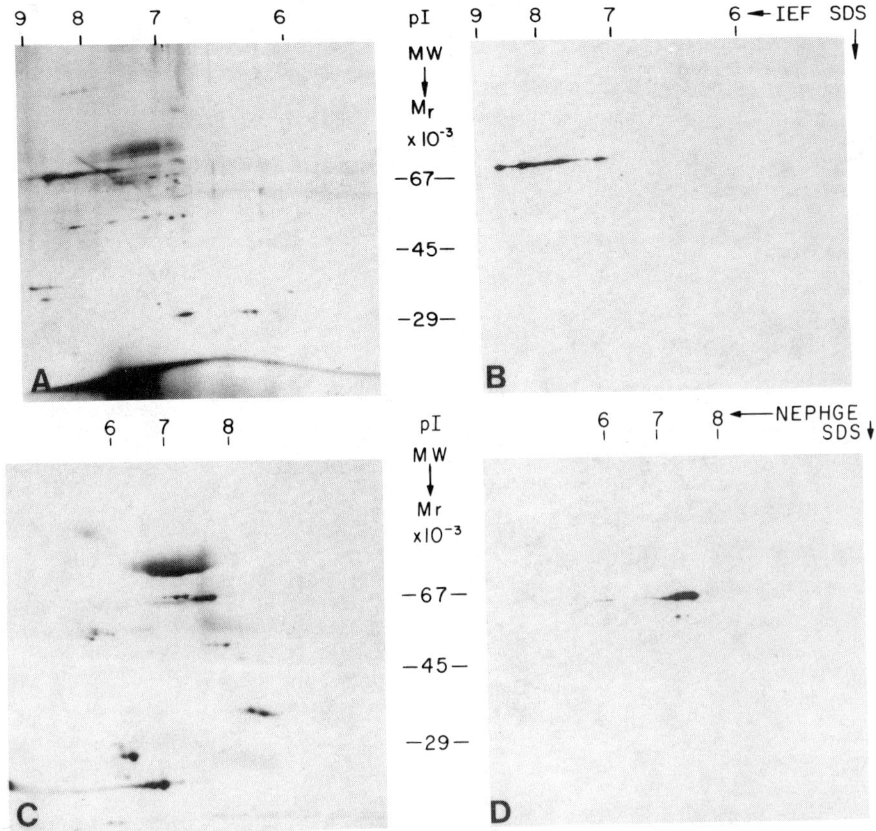

FIGURE 2. Two dimensional PAGE and immunoblot characterization of fibrous sheaths isolated from mouse sperm. **A** and **B** are samples subjected to IEF in the first dimension and 7–12% linear gradient PAGE in the second dimension. Multiple components are silver stained (**A**), but antibody ATC recognizes a protein of M_r 67,000 and pI 7.9–8.7 on the immunoblot (**B**). **C** and **D** are samples subjected to NEPHGE in the first dimension and 7–12% linear gradient PAGE in the second dimension. Multiple components are silver stained (**C**), but antibody ATC recognizes a protein of M_r 67,000 and pI 6.8–7.7 on the immunoblot (**D**).

forms of pI 7.9 to 8.7 on IEF gels and 6.8 to 7.7 on NEPHGE gels (FIG. 2,B and D), while the rat protein of M_r 65,500 had charge forms of pI 7.8 to 8.8 on IEF gels and 7.2 to 7.8 on NEPHGE gels (FIG. 3,B and D). Minor components of lower M_r were immunostained on blots of NEPHGE gels of both mouse (FIG. 2D) and rat (FIG. 3D) fibrous sheaths.

Developmental Appearance of Fibrous Sheath Proteins

The postnatal appearance of the protein recognized by antibody ATC was examined by ELISA on detergent extracts of mouse seminiferous epithelial cells. Immuno-

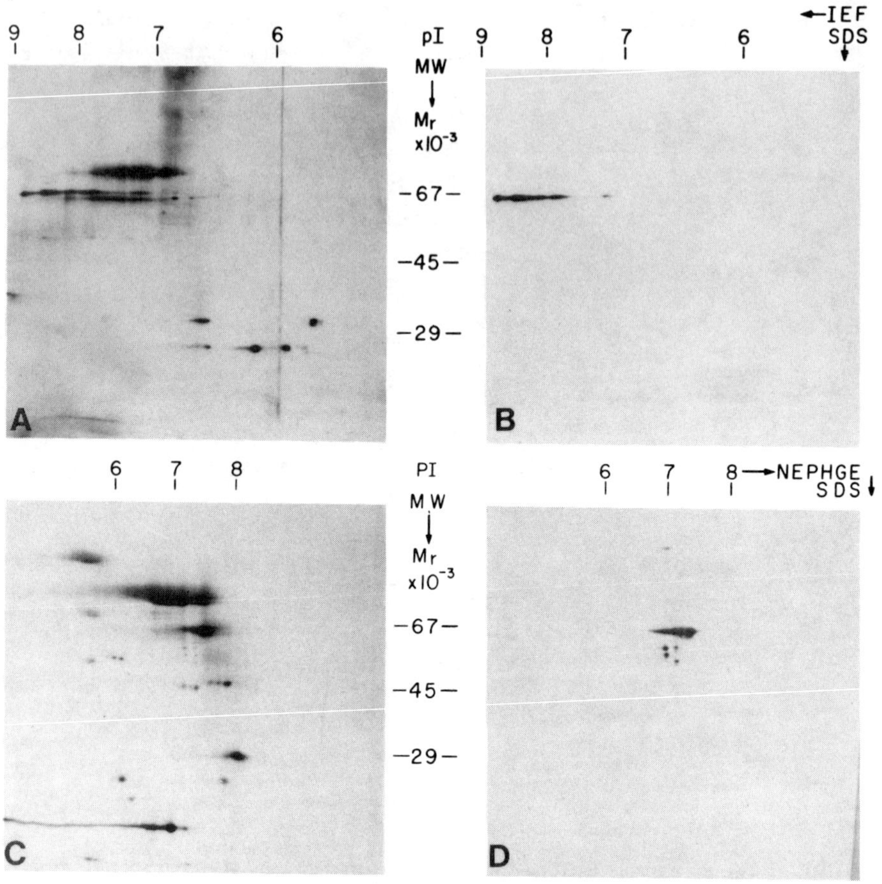

FIGURE 3. Two dimensional PAGE of fibrous sheaths isolated from rat sperm. **A** and **B** are samples subjected to IEF in the first dimension and 7–12% linear gradient PAGE in the second dimension. Multiple components are silver stained (**A**), but antibody ATC recognizes a protein of M_r 65,500 and pI 7.8–8.8 on the immunoblot (**B**). **C** and **D** are samples subjected to NEPHGE in the first dimension and 7–12% linear gradient PAGE in the second dimension. Multiple components are silver stained (**C**), but antibody ATC recognizes a protein of M_r 65,000 and pI 7.2–7.8 on the immunoblot (**D**).

reactivity increased between postnatal days 16 and 18 (when mid-pachytene spermatocytes first appear)[19] and again between postnatal days 20 and 22 (when round spermatids first appear)[19] (FIG. 4). These findings were unexpected because earlier immunohistochemical studies had indicated that the antigen first appeared during the latter part of the postmeiotic phase of spermiogenesis, when spermatids were being remodeled into spermatozoa.[12]

To characterize further the developmental appearance of the fibrous sheath protein recognized by antibody ATC, immunoblotting studies were performed on extracts of isolated germ cells. Preleptotene spermatocytes, a mixture of leptotene and zygotene

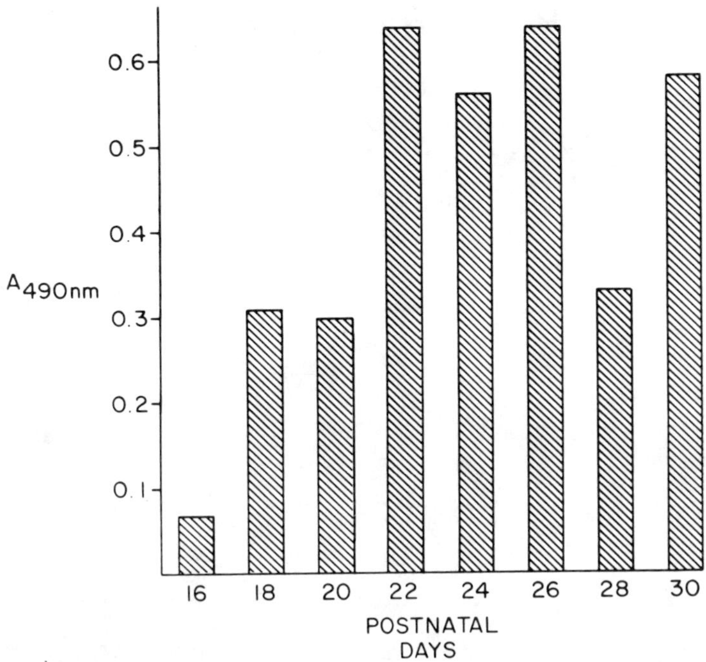

FIGURE 4. Developmental appearance of antigen detected by ELISA with antibody ATC on extracts of seminiferous epithelial cells from mice of different postnatal ages. An increase in immunoreactivity occurs between days 16 and 18, and again between days 20 and 22.

spermatocytes, and pachytene spermatocytes were isolated by unit gravity sedimentation from enzymatically dissociated testes of postnatal day 17 mice. Pachytene spermatocytes, round spermatids, and a mixture of condensing spermatids and residual bodies were isolated in the same manner from adult mouse testes. Extracts of these cells were then examined on immunoblots of 1D-gels. The fibrous sheath protein of M_r 67,000 was recognized by antibody ATC in round and condensing spermatids (FIG. 5). In addition, a protein of M_r 78,000 was recognized in leptotene and zygotene spermatocytes, pachytene spermatocytes and round spermatids (FIG. 5). Some preparations of pachytene spermatocytes isolated from day 17 mice contained minor proteins of M_r 67,000 and 63,000 recognized by antibody ATC (FIG. 5). These usually were not seen in pachytene spermatocytes from adults.

Cytoskeletal Characteristics of Fibrous Sheath Proteins

The possible relationship between fibrous sheath proteins and intermediate filament proteins was examined because of the cytoskeletal nature of the fibrous sheath and suggestions by other investigators that sperm contain intermediate filament proteins.[13-15] In addition, the mouse protein of M_r 67,000 and the rat protein of M_r 65,500 are similar in size, pI and physical characteristics to members of the type II basic

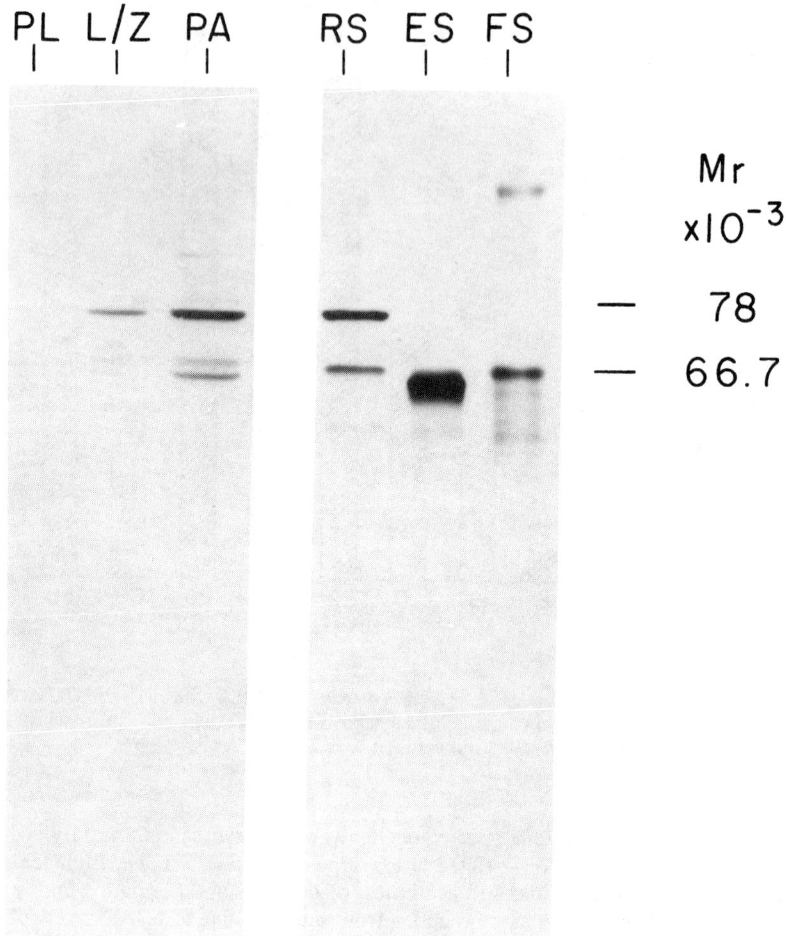

FIGURE 5. Immunoblots of extracts of germ cells from postnatal day 17 and adult mice separated by unit gravity sedimentation. Spermatocytes are from day 17 and spermatids and residual bodies are from adult mice. Antibody ATC reacts with a M_r 78,000 protein in a mixture of leptotene and zygotene primary spermatocytes (L/Z), pachytene spermatocytes (PA), and round spermatids (RS), but not in preleptotene (PL) spermatocytes. It also reacts with a M_r 67,000 protein in round spermatids (RS), and in fibrous sheath (FS). Some preparations of pachytene spermatocytes from day 17 mice (PA) contain minor amounts of a M_r 67,000 protein recognized by antibody ATC, but this was usually not seen in pachytene spermatocytes from adult mice.

keratin family.[29] Monoclonal antibodies to intermediate filament proteins were tested for immunoreactivity with mouse and rat fibrous sheaths by IIF on isolated fibrous sheaths. These included antibodies to vimentin, desmin, cytokeratin, glial fibrillary acidic protein and neurofilament 68 kD polypeptide, and two panfilament antibodies reported to recognize all classes of intermediate filaments. Of the 19 antibodies tested, a vimentin antibody (VIM 13.2) and a cytokeratin antibody (EAB 903) reacted weakly and a panfilament antibody (EAB 905) reacted strongly with fibrous sheaths by IIF

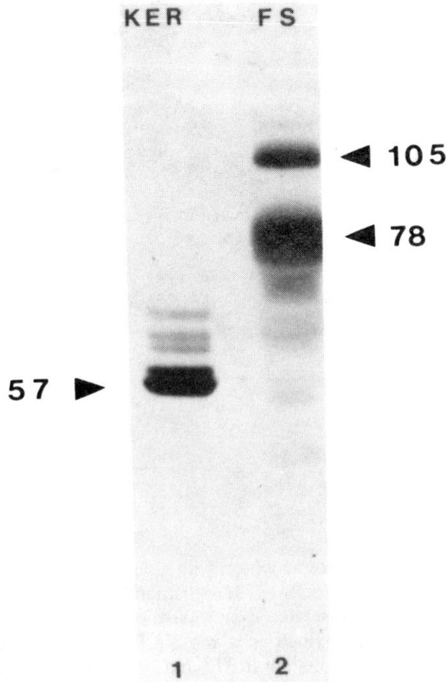

FIGURE 6. Immunoblot with panfilament monoclonal antibody EAB 905 on a cytoskeletal extract from skin of newborn mice (KER) and on fibrous sheaths (FS) isolated from mouse sperm. The major protein recognized in skin is M_r 57,000 and those in the fibrous sheath are M_r 105,000 and 78,000.

(data not shown). When these antibodies were used on immunoblots of mouse fibrous sheath proteins, only EAB 905 showed reactivity. EAB 905 recognized several fibrous sheath proteins, including the protein of M_r 78,000 but not the protein of M_r 67,000 protein (FIG. 6). This antibody also recognized proteins in skin isolated from newborn mice (FIG. 6). However, the M_r of proteins recognized by EAB 905 in skin were not the same as those recognized in the fibrous sheath. The reactivity of the antibodies was verified by IIF on permeabilized mouse 3T3 and NOR-10 cells and on sections of mouse testis, skin and brain. Although the antibodies reacted with various somatic cell types by IIF, they did not react with germ cells.

Additional monoclonal antibodies were generated to mouse fibrous sheath proteins and used on immunoblots of cytoskeletons isolated from 3T3 and NOR-10 cells and of mouse fibrous sheath. Although several of these antibodies recognized proteins in 3T3 and NOR-10 cytoskeletons and in the fibrous sheath, the proteins recognized in somatic cells were of different M_r than those from germ cells (FIG. 7). Most commonly recognized in the fibrous sheath were proteins of M_r 105,000 and 78,000, while proteins of M_r 58,000 and 42,000 were frequently recognized in the somatic cell cytoskeletal preparations.

Identification of the ATC Epitope

The nature of the amino acid sequence recognized by monoclonal antibody ATC was determined by competitive ELISA with synthetic peptides. The antibody reactivity was not reduced by polyglycine, was slightly reduced by poly(proline-glycine-proline),

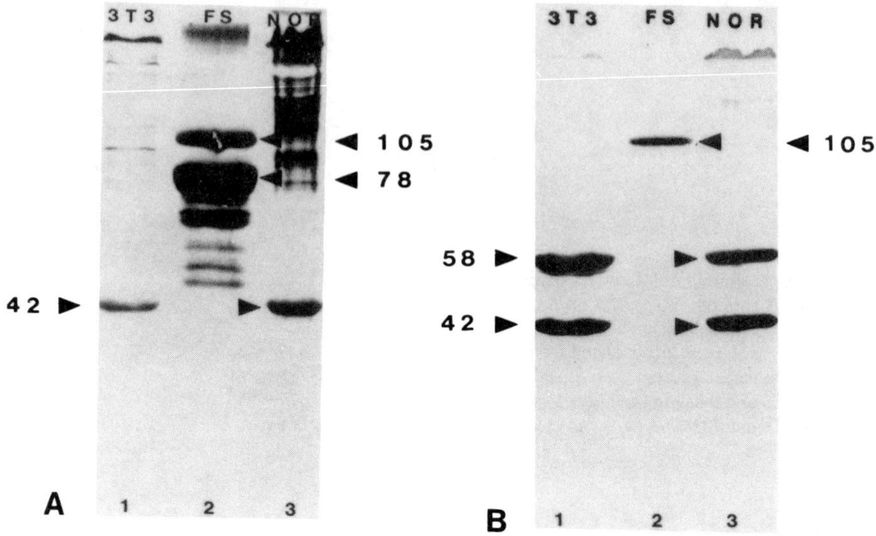

FIGURE 7. Immunoblots with monoclonal antibodies 5A8 and AG13 on cytoskeletal extracts of mouse fibroblast 3T3 cells (3T3) and smooth muscle NOR–10 cells (NOR) grown in culture and on fibrous sheaths (FS) isolated from mouse sperm. Antibody 5A8 (**A**) recognizes a M_r 42,000 protein present in 3T3 and NOR-10 cells and not in fibrous sheath, and M_r 105,000 and 78,000 proteins present in fibrous sheath but not in 3T3 and NOR-10 cells. Antibody AG13 (**B**) recognizes M_r 58,000 and 42,000 proteins only in 3T3 and NOR-10 cells and a M_r 105,000 protein only in fibrous sheath.

and was eliminated by poly-L-proline (FIG. 8). This indicated that the epitope recognized by antibody ATC consisted largely or entirely of a polyproline amino acid sequence.

DISCUSSION

Characteristics of Fibrous Sheath Proteins

Fibrous sheaths isolated from mouse and rat sperm had similar protein patterns on 1D-gels and on IEF and NEPHGE 2D-gels. It should be emphasized that the proteins identified were those which withstood solubilization during rigorous isolation procedures and that important fibrous sheath proteins may be lost prior to gel electrophoresis. The larger proteins migrated with multiple charge forms and/or broad M_r in the basic pI range on IEF gels. In contrast, the smaller proteins showed less diversity in charge and M_r and migrated to neutral or basic pI regions on IEF gels. These studies confirmed that the most abundant protein in the rat fibrous sheath is approximately M_r 80,000.[8–11] In addition, a protein of M_r 78,000 was the most abundant component in the mouse fibrous sheath. The migration of these proteins as diffuse spots on IEF gels indicated heterogeneity of charge and mass, probably due to post-translational modifications. Although the NEPHGE gel system was used in an attempt to better resolve these basic proteins, they remained diffuse even under these sepa-

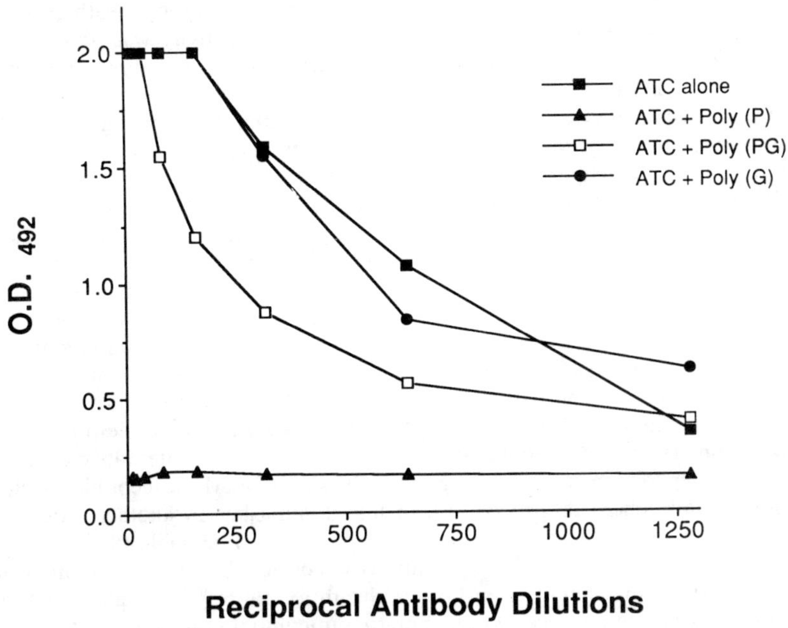

FIGURE 8. Identification of the epitope recognized by monoclonal antibody ATC with a competitive ELISA. Different dilutions of antibody ATC were incubated with the synthetic peptides polyglycine (Poly(G)), poly(proline-glycine-proline) (Poly(PG)), or poly-L-proline (Poly(P)) and then added to an ELISA plate contained fibrous sheaths isolated from mouse sperm. Antibody reactivity was not reduced by polyglycine, slightly reduced by poly(proline-glycine-proline), and eliminated by poly-L-proline.

ration conditions. Previous studies indicated that the protein of M_r 80,000 in rat fibrous sheath contained approximately 3 mol of phosphoserine per mol of polypeptide (Brito *et al.*[11]), which could significantly affect the migration of the protein on 2D-gels.

The mouse protein of M_r 67,000 and the rat protein of M_r 65,500 were recognized by monoclonal antibody ATC on immunoblots of isolated fibrous sheaths. These proteins also showed similar patterns of migration on IEF and NEPHGE 2D-gels, suggesting they are similar proteins. They appeared to be minor components on Coomassie blue stained 1D-gels, but were major proteins on silver-stained IEF and NEPHGE 2D-gels. Although hamster sperm fibrous sheaths contained a protein of M_r 66,000 recognized by antibody ATC, no reactivity was seen with fibrous sheaths of rabbit, guinea pig or human sperm.[12] However, a comparable protein could be present in these species, but lacking the poly-L-proline epitope recognized by antibody ATC.

Developmental Appearance of Fibrous Sheath Proteins

Previous immunohistochemical studies indicated that the protein recognized by antibody ATC appeared late during mouse spermatogenesis. The antigen was first detected in the cytoplasm of step 13 spermatids and in the fibrous sheath of step 14–16 spermatids.[12] However, in the present study immunoreactivity was first detected by ELISA during postnatal development between days 16 and 18 and increased between days 20 and 22. The first period corresponds approximately to the appearance of mid-pachytene spermatocytes and the second period to the development of round spermatids in the initial wave of spermatogenesis.[19] The developmental appearance of the antigen during spermatogenesis was examined further by immunoblotting studies with isolated germ cells. Antibody ATC recognized a protein of M_r 67,000 in round spermatids and in a mixed population of condensing spermatids and residual bodies. The antibody also recognized a protein of M_r 78,000 in populations of leptotene and zygotene spermatocytes, pachytene spermatocytes, and round spermatids.

Why were the antigens of M_r 78,000 and 67,000 detected on immunoblots of spermatocytes and round spermatids not recognized in these cells by immunohistochemistry? We speculate that the proteins are present as relatively soluble monomers until late in spermiogenesis, but associate into insoluble oligomers as assembly of the fibrous sheath begins in step 13 condensing spermatids, allowing the protein of M_r 67,000 to be retained during processing for immunohistochemistry. Alternative explanations are that the epitope in earlier stage germ cells is particularly susceptible to alteration by immunohistochemical procedures, or that it is masked by another protein *in situ* that is removed during processing of cell extracts for immunoblotting. It remains to be determined if any of these explanations is correct, but our results indicate that immunohistochemical studies on fibrous sheath formation[30-32] should be interpreted with caution in the absence of corroborative immunoblotting data.

What is the relationship of the protein of M_r 78,000 in spermatocytes and spermatids to the protein of M_r 67,000 in spermatids and the fibrous sheath? One hypothesis is that the protein of M_r 78,000 is a precursor which is processed to produce the protein of M_r 67,000 during round spermatid development. A second hypothesis is that these are separate proteins produced at different times during spermatogenesis. Consistent with the second hypothesis is the observation that a protein of M_r 78,000 is a major component of the fibrous sheath. However, antibody ATC does not recognize the protein of M_r 78,000 in condensing spermatids and the fibrous sheath. This might be due to posttranslational changes in the protein affecting the epitope, but additional studies will be needed to clarify the relationship between these two proteins.

Relationship of Fibrous Sheath and Intermediate Filament Proteins

Previous studies have indicated that different sperm head and flagellar cytoskeletal structures share proteins or contain related proteins. This suggests that the sperm cytoskeleton may be constructed from a family of related proteins. The perforatorium is the well-developed subacrosomal cytoskeleton in rat sperm and has been shown to contain proteins of M_r 43,000, 35,000, 33,000, 16,000, 13,400 and 13,000.[9,33,34] An antiserum to the protein of M_r 16,000 reacted with the outer dense fibers and fibrous sheath of rat sperm.[33] The postacrosomal cytoskeleton (posterior calyx) of bull and rat sperm was shown to contain a basic protein of M_r 60,000 (calicin).[35] An antibody to calicin reacted with a protein of the same size in the head of sperm of several other mammals, but the protein was not always in the postacrosomal cytoskeleton.[36] Another study found that antisera prepared to either outer dense fibers or fibrous sheaths of rat sperm recognized a major protein of M_r 14,000 present in both structures.[10]

The same amino terminal residue (proline) and quite similar amino acid composition was found for M_r 11,500 proteins present in rat outer dense fibers and fibrous sheath.[11] This may be the same protein as the M_r 14,000 protein described by Oko.[10] Furthermore, affinity-purified antibodies to the outer dense fiber protein of M_r 14,400 reacted with proteins of M_r 63,000, 57,000, 27,500 and 14,400 in the fibrous sheath.[11]

Previous investigators have suggested that different sperm cytoskeletal structures contain intermediate filament proteins. Sperm cytoskeletal structures and keratin have similarities in their relative insolubility in detergents and chaotropic agents,[37] content of zinc-thiol complexes,[38,39] infrared spectra,[40] amino acid composition[40] and filamentous and periodic substructures.[41] Further evidence for similarities between sperm cytoskeletal and intermediate filament proteins has come from studies using antibodies to intermediate filament proteins. An antibody to vimentin reacted with a protein of M_r 58,000 in the equatorial segment of human sperm.[13] In addition, a monoclonal and a polyclonal antibody to vimentin reacted weakly with the flagellum of late spermatids in frozen section of rat testis and with a protein of M_r 58,000 extracted from epididymal sperm.[15] Furthermore, two monoclonal antibodies to human sperm reacted with vimentin from skin and with a keratin-like protein in the acrosomal cap of human sperm.[14] However, several other studies failed to identify intermediate filament proteins in male germ cells.[16–18]

The present study used two approaches to examine the possible relationship between intermediate filament proteins and cytoskeletal proteins present in male germ cells. One was to use a group of commercially available monoclonal antibodies to intermediate filament proteins in IIF and immunoblot assays on mouse sperm fibrous sheaths. These antibodies were to keratin, cytokeratin, vimentin, desmin, neurofilament protein, glial fibrillary acidic protein, or to all classes of intermediate filament proteins (panfilament antibodies). Although three antibodies reacted with fibrous sheath by IIF, only one (panfilament antibody EAB 905) showed reactivity on immunoblots. It recognized several proteins in mouse fibrous sheath, including the protein of M_r 78,000, and several proteins in skin and cytoskeletal proteins from 3T3 and NOR-10 cells. This indicates that fibrous sheath and somatic cell intermediate filament proteins share a common epitope. However, the M_r of proteins recognized in mouse somatic cells were different from those in fibrous sheath, indicating that different proteins were recognized. Because the other commercially available monoclonal antibodies did not recognize mouse fibrous sheath, but did react with somatic cell cytoskeletal proteins, these data argue that it is unlikely that the fibrous sheath contains conventional intermediate filament proteins.

The second approach to comparing sperm cytoskeleton and intermediate filament proteins was to produce monoclonal antibodies to the fibrous sheath and to use those antibodies on immunoblots of 3T3 and NOR-10 cytoskeletons and fibrous sheath. Several of the antibodies recognized proteins in both somatic cell cytoskeletons and fibrous sheath. However, in all cases the proteins were of different M_r in the somatic and germ cell cytoskeletons. This suggests that while fibrous sheath proteins have epitopes in common with those of intermediate filament proteins, the fibrous sheath proteins are not the same as intermediate filament proteins of somatic cells. This is likely to be the basis for why antibodies to intermediate filament proteins reacted with sperm in some studies,[13–15] while this was not observed in other studies.[16–18]

These results have led us to hypothesize that at least some sperm cytoskeletal proteins are products of genes related to the intermediate filament gene family[29] which are expressed only during male germ cell development. Several recent studies have begun to characterize proteins of the sperm cytoskeleton and it is likely that the genes for some of these proteins will be cloned in the near future. It is this approach that has the greatest likelihood of determining the nature of the proteins contained within sperm cytoskeletal components.

REFERENCES

1. Eddy, E. M. 1988. The spermatozoon. *In* The Physiology of Reproduction. E. Knobil & J. Neill, Eds.: 27–68. Raven Press, Ltd. New York.
2. Eddy, E. M., D. A. O'Brien & J. E. Welch. 1991. Mammalian sperm development *in vivo* and *in vitro*. *In* Elements of Mammalian Fertilization. P. M. Wassarman, Ed. Vol. **1:** 1–28. CRC Press. Boca Raton, FL.
3. Irons, M. J. & Y. Clermont. 1982. Kinetics of fibrous sheath formation in the rat spermatid. Am. J. Anat. **165:** 121–130.
4. Phillips, D. M. 1972. Comparative analysis of mammalian sperm motility. J. Cell Biol. **53:** 561–573.
5. Escalier, D. & C. Serres. 1985. Aberrant distribution of the peri-axonemal structures in the human spermatozoon: Possible role of the axoneme in the spatial organization of the flagellar components. Biol. Cell **53:** 239–250.
6. Handel, M. A. Genetic control of spermatogenesis in mice. *In* Spermatogenesis: Genetic Aspects Results and Problems in Cell Differentiation. W. Henning, Ed. Vol. **15:** 1–62. Springer-Verlag. Berlin-Heidelberg.
7. Bedford, J. M. & H. I. Calvin. 1974. Changes in -S-S- linked structures of the sperm tail during epididymal maturation, with comparative observations in sub-mammalian species. J. Exp. Zool. **187:** 181–204.
8. Olson, G. E., D. W. Hamilton & D. W. Fawcett. 1976. Isolation and characterization of the fibrous sheath of rat epididymal spermatozoa. Biol. Reprod. **14:** 517–530.
9. Olson, G. E. 1979. Isolation of the fibrous sheath and perforatorium of rat spermatozoa. *In* The Spermatozoon. D. W. Fawcett & J. M. Bedford, Eds.: 395–400. Urban & Schwarzenberg, Inc. Baltimore-Munich.
10. Oko, R. 1988. Comparative analysis of proteins from the fibrous sheath and outer dense fibers of rat spermatozoa. Biol. Reprod. **39:** 168–182.
11. Brito, M., J. Figueroa, E. U. Maldonado, J. C. Vera & L. O. Burzio. 1989. The major component of the rat sperm fibrous sheath is a phosphoprotein. Gamete Res. **22:** 205–217.
12. Fenderson, B. A., K. Toshimori, C. H. Muller, T. F. Lane & E. M. Eddy. 1988. Identification of a protein in the fibrous sheath of the sperm flagellum. Biol. Reprod. **38:** 345–357.
13. Virtanen, I., R. A. Badley, R. Paasivuo & V.-P. Lehto. 1984. Distinct cytoskeletal domains revealed in sperm cells. J. Cell Biol. **99:** 1083–1091.
14. Ochs, D., D. P. Wolf & R. L. Ochs. 1986. Intermediate filament proteins in human sperm heads. Exp. Cell Res. **167:** 495–504.
15. Mali, P., I. Virtanen & M. Parvinen. 1987. Vimentin expression in spermatogenic and Sertoli cells is stage-related in rat seminiferous epithelium. Andrologia **19:** 644–653.
16. Franke, W. W., C. Grund & E. Schmid. 1979. Intermediate filament-sized filaments present in Sertoli cells are of vimentin type. Eur. J. Cell Biol. **19:** 269–275.
17. Puchtler, H., B. P. Barton, F. S. Waldrop, S. N. Meloan & J. L. Hobbs. 1985. A comparative study of myosins and prekeratin in epithelial cells of methacarn-fixed tissues. Histochemistry **82:** 403–409.
18. Aumüller, G., M. Steinbruck, W. Krause & H.-J. Wagner. 1988. Distribution of vimentin-type intermediate filaments in Sertoli cells of the human testis, normal and pathologic. Anat. Embryol. **178:** 129–136.
19. Bellvé, A. R., J. C. Cavicchia, C. F. Millette, D. A. O'Brien, Y. M. Bhatnagar & M. Dym. 1977. Spermatogenic cells of the prepuberal mouse. Isolation and morphological characterization. J. Cell Biol. **74:** 68–85.
20. Bellvé, A. R., C. F. Millette, Y. M. Bhatnagar & D. A. O'Brien. 1977. Dissociation of the mouse testis and characterization of isolated spermatogenic cells. J. Histochem. Cytochem. **25:** 480–494.

21. O'BRIEN, D. A. 1987. Stage-specific protein synthesis by isolated spermatogenic cells throughout meiosis and early spermiogenesis in the mouse. Biol. Reprod. **37:** 147–157.
22. LOWRY, O. H., N. J. ROSEBROUGH, A. L. FARR & R. J. RANDALL. 1951. Protein measurement with the folin phenol reagent. J. Biol. Chem. **193:** 265–275.
23. LAEMMLI, U. K. 1970. Cleavage of structural proteins during the assembly of the head of bacteriophage T4. Nature **277:** 680–685.
24. DUNCAN, R. & J. W. B. HERSHEY. 1984. Evaluation of isoelectric focusing running conditions during two-dimensional isoelectric focusing/sodium dodecyl sulfate-polyacrylamide gel electrophoresis: Variations of gel patterns with changing conditions and optimized isoelectric focusing conditions. Anal. Biochem. **138:** 144–155.
25. O'FARRELL, P. Z., H. M. GOODMAN & P. H. O'FARRELL. 1977. High resolution two-dimensional electrophoresis of basic as well as acidic proteins. Cell **12:** 1133–1142.
26. O'FARRELL, P. H. 1975. High resolution two-dimensional electrophoresis of proteins. J. Biol. Chem. **250:** 4007–4021.
27. WRAY, W., T. BOULIKAS, V. P. WRAY & R. HANCOCK. 1981. Silver staining of proteins in polyacrylamide gels. Anal. Biochem. **118:** 197–203.
28. ALLEN, R. L., D. A. O'BRIEN, C. C. JONES, D. L. ROCKETT & E. M. EDDY. 1988. Expression of heat shock proteins by isolated mouse spermatogenic cells. Mol. Cell. Biol. **8:** 3260–3266.
29. STEINERT, P. M. & D. R. ROOP. 1988. Molecular and cellular biology of intermediate filaments. Ann. Rev. Biochem. **57:** 593–625.
30. SAKAI, Y., Y.-I. KOYAMA, H. FUJIMOTO, T. NAKAMOTO & S. YAMASHINA. 1986. Immunocytochemical study of fibrous sheath formation in mouse spermiogenesis using a monoclonal antibody. Anat. Rec. **215:** 119–126.
31. OKO, R. & Y. CLERMONT. 1989. Light microscopic immunocytochemical study of fibrous sheath and outer dense fiber formation in the rat spermatid. Anat. Rec. **225:** 46–55.
32. CLERMONT, Y., R. OKO & L. HERMO. 1990. Immunocytochemical localization of proteins utilized in the formation of outer dense fibers and fibrous sheath in rat spermatids: An electron microscope study. Anat. Rec. **227:** 447–457.
33. OKO, R. & Y. CLERMONT. 1988. Isolation, structure and protein composition of the perforatorium of rat spermaozoa. Biol. Reprod. **39:** 673–687.
34. OLSON, G. E., D. W. HAMILTON & D. W. FAWCETT. 1976. Isolation and characterization of the perforatorium of rat spermaozoa. J. Reprod. Fertil. **47:** 293–297.
35. LONGO, F. J., G. KROHNE & W. W. FRANKE. 1987. Basic proteins of the perinuclear theca of mammalian spermatozoa and spermatids: A novel class of cytoskeletal elements. J. Cell Biol. **105:** 1105–1120.
36. PARANKO, J., F. LONGO, J. POTTS, G. KROHNE & W. W. FRANKE. 1988. Widespread occurrence of calicin, a basic cytoskeletal protein of sperm cells, in diverse mammalian species. Differentiation **38:** 21–27.
37. CALVIN, H. I. & J. M. BEDFORD. 1971. Formation of disulphide bonds in the nucleus and accessory structures of mammalian spermatozoa during maturation in the epididymis. J. Reprod. Fertil. **13**(Suppl.): 65–75.
38. CALVIN, H. I. & G. BLEAU. 1974. Zinc-thiol complexes in keratin-like structures of rat spermatozoa. Exp. Cell Res. **86:** 280–284.
39. CALVIN, H. I. 1975. Keratinoid proteins in the heads and tails of mammalian spermatozoa. *In* Biology of the Male Gamete. J. G. Duckett & P. A. Racy, Eds.: 257–273. Academic Press. London.
40. BACCETTI, B., V. PALLINI & A. G. BURRINI. 1976. The accessory fibers of the sperm tail. III. High-sulphur and low-sulphur components in mammals and cephalopods. J. Ultrastruct. Res. **57:** 289–308.
41. OLSON, G. E., V. P. WINFREY & S. P. FLAHERTY. 1987. Cytoskeletal assemblies of mammalian spermatozoa. Ann. N. Y. Acad. Sci. **513:** 222–246.

Structure-Function Relationships in the Sperm Acrosome[a]

GARY E. OLSON AND VIRGINIA WINFREY

Department of Cell Biology
School of Medicine
Vanderbilt University
Nashville, Tennessee 37232

INTRODUCTION

The polarized mammalian spermatozoon is constructed from a limited set of intracellular organelles which are sequestered to specific domains. The striking species differences in the size and shape of spermatozoa results from differences in the size and shape of this common set of organelles and not from differences in their distribution, which is consistent between species.[1] Based on anatomical and physiological criteria the major subdivisions of the spermatozoon are the acrosomal and postacrosomal domains of the head and the midpiece and principal piece domains of the flagellum. These domains differ in their assemblage of organelles, in the composition and structure of the overlying plasma membrane and in their function in fertilization events.[1-6]

The acrosomal segment comprises the anterior one-half to two-thirds of the sperm head and it functions in sperm-egg binding, penetration of the egg investments, and ultimately fusion with the egg plasma membrane.[1-6] Proceeding inward the major components of this segment include the plasma membrane, the underlying membrane-bounded acrosome, a layer of electron dense perinuclear material and, innermost, the condensed nucleus. The acrosome contains a variety of hydolases which are thought to facilitate sperm penetration of the egg investments[7] and it is made up of three major subdivisions termed the apical segment, the principal segment, and, distally, the equatorial segment. The limiting membrane of the acrosome consists of two major subregions: the outer acrosomal membrane immediately underlies the plasma membrane while the inner acrosomal membrane faces the nucleus and is in apposition with the perinuclear electron dense material. The subdomains of the inner and outer acrosomal membranes corresponding to the three acrosomal segments exhibit different functions. During fertilization the outer acrosomal membrane of the apical and principal segments participates in the membrane fusion events of the acrosome reaction, forming in conjunction with the adjacent plasma membrane, a fenestrated hybrid membrane complex which permits release of the acrosomal contents. In contrast, the inner acrosomal membrane becomes the plasma membrane-equivalent of acrosome reacted spermatozoa; in some species, this membrane is believed to function in the primary binding of spermatozoa to the zona pellucida or in maintenance of sperm-zona interactions

[a] This work was supported by NIH Grant HD20419 and Center Grant NIH HD05797.

during sperm penetration, and, although controversial, some investigators have suggested that this membrane retains bound acrosomal enzymes important in the penetration process. The equatorial segment is the most poorly understood of the acrosomal segments. The equatorial segment appears unusually stable and, morphologically, it is relatively unchanged during the acrosome reaction and egg penetration. The plasma membrane overlying the equatorial segment is thought to represent the initial site of fusion of the sperm and egg plasma membranes so that this segment could play crucial, although at present poorly understood, functions in the fertilization process.[2,5,8]

Little is known of the molecular mechanisms by which the different acrosomal membrane domains perform their specific functions. Structural studies have revealed a number of unique features of the different acrosomal membrane domains.[1,3,4,10] For example, freeze-fracture analyses have revealed ordered intramembranous particle arrays in the outer acrosomal membrane of the apical and principal segments of several mammalian species. In some species, specific cytoskeletal elements have been shown to mediate the interaction of the plasma membrane with specific subregions of the outer acrosomal membrane of the apical segment,[11-13] while the molecular composition of these assemblages is unknown, they may affect the patterns of membrane fusions noted during an acrosome reaction. A characteristic feature of the outer acrosomal membrane of the apical and principal segment is the presence of a layer of electron-dense material on the luminal membrane surface[14,15]; this layer, termed the acrosomal lamina, may be structurally and functionally analogous to the plasma membrane-skeleton of somatic cells, and could play a pivotal role in the regulation of the dynamic properties of this membrane domain in the membrane fusion events of the acrosome reaction.[13] The inner acrosomal membrane of the principal segment also displays a regular pattern in freeze-fracture replicas which is distinctive from the outer acrosomal membrane thereby suggesting their compositional differences.[4,10] Unique membrane differentiations have been noted in the equatorial segment region. In this segment the outer and inner acrosomal membranes are in close proximity and run parallel to one another; this relationship is maintained by a set of bridges joining the luminal surfaces of these two membrane domains.[8,16,17] These bridges are arrayed in a paracrystalline fashion and freeze-fracture analyses of these membranes shows a paracrystalline pattern within the membrane interior which may reflect the distribution of these bridging elements. The molecular composition of these elements has not yet been identified.

The acrosomal interior contains a variety of hydrolytic enzymes with hyaluronidase and acrosin representing the major enzymatic constituents.[7] In various species, heterogeneity of the acrosomal matrix is noted by electron microscopic analysis. In the guinea pig a specific hydrolase, dipeptidyl peptidase II, has been demonstrated to reside within a specific intraacrosomal compartment of characteristic morphology.[18] How this partitioning of constituents is regulated is poorly understood, but a sequestered localization of various components could provide a mechanism for regulating their temporal release during the acrosome reaction.

We have employed structural, biochemical and immunological approaches to examine both the different domains of the inner and outer acrosomal membrane and the acrosomal matrix in an effort to identify structural and biochemical features pertinent to their specific functions. In this manuscript we present data obtained primarily from hamster spermatozoa and discuss the findings with respect to the function of the acrosome in fertilization events.

METHODS

Sperm Preparation

Mature male golden hamsters were lethally anesthetized with Nembutal or asphyxiated with CO_2. Sperm were obtained from the cauda epididymides either by mincing the tubule in warm physiological saline or by luminal perfusion of saline solution. Sperm pellets were obtained by gentle centrifugation of the suspensions at $400 \times g$ for 5 minutes. These pellets were employed for various extraction regimens and isolation protocols.

Isolation of Sperm Fractions

An acrosomal lamina-acrosomal matrix (ALM) fraction was isolated from the apical and principal segments of the acrosomal domain of hamster spermatozoa by a previously published procedure.[19] Acrosomal caps were released by extraction in buffer containing Triton X-100 and the released acrosomal components were then separated from the spermatozoa by centrifugation onto Percoll density gradients.

To investigate the structural and biochemical properties of the inner acrosomal membrane of the principal segment and the acrosomal membranes of the equatorial segment, a purified fraction of hamster sperm heads was isolated from a sonicated suspension by centrifugation onto discontinuous sucrose gradients composed of steps of 60%, 70% and 75% sucrose. The resultant pellet was highly enriched for sperm heads which retained the acrosomal membranes of the equatorial segment and the inner acrosomal membrane over the principal segment.

Microscopic Techniques

Light microscopic immunohistochemistry was performed as previously described.[12] Spermatozoa and sperm fractions were allowed to adhere to Poly-L-lysine–coated coverslips. They were rinsed in buffer, fixed with $-20°$ acetone or a solution of 4% formaldehyde, 0.1% Triton X-100 and 0.1M phosphate buffer and then blocked with phosphate-buffered saline containing normal, nonimmune, serum. Cells were then exposed to primary antiserum against specific acrosomal components, washed in buffer, incubated in FITC- or Texas Red-conjugated secondary antibody, washed and then examined by epifluorescence. Specificity was assessed utilizing preimmune control antiserum. To demonstrate lectin binding sites, fractionated sperm were exposed to FITC-conjugated lectins and observed by fluorescence microscopy.

Electron microscopic histochemistry employed pre-embedding labeling protocols. Sperm fractions were exposed to primary antibodies followed by gold-labeled secondary antibodies. For identification of lectin-binding sites, sperm fractions were exposed to biotinylated lectins followed by streptavidin-10 nm gold conjugates. For all labeling protocols, sperm were washed at least three times between successive treatments. The final sperm pellets were fixed with 4% glutaraldehyde, postfixed in 1% OsO_4, and embedded in epoxy resin for thin sectioning.

RESULTS

Structural Characterization of the Outer Acrosomal Membrane and Acrosomal Matrix

The hamster acrosome forms a caplike structure applied over the dorsal and lateral but not the ventral surface of the hook-shaped head. The apical and principal segments of the acrosome of intact hamster spermatozoa contain an electron dense matrix which in conventionally fixed specimens (FIG. 1), generally appears homogeneous, although in some cases regions of differing electron density are noted. Along the ventral surface of the acrosome a parallel array of filaments, following the long axis of the head, forms a cytoskeletal complex adherent to a specific subregion of the outer acrosomal membrane (FIG. 1).[11,12]

Distinct differentiations of the outer acrosomal membrane and the acrosomal matrix are evident in cells disrupted by brief Triton X-100 extraction (FIGS. 2–4), frequently these treatments result in detachment of the acrosomal cap. The outer acrosomal membrane of the apical and principal segment possesses a prominent layer of electron dense material on its luminal surface (FIG. 2); this complex, termed the acrosomal lamina, has been isolated from bovine sperm acrosomes[14] and shown in guinea pig sperm to comprise a paracrystalline lattice of filamentous elements.[15] Whether the acrosomal lamina comprises a filamentous network in hamster spermatozoa remains to be determined. Although Triton extraction solubilized the trilaminar component of the outer acrosomal membrane, the acrosomal lamina remained intact and adherent to a solubilization-resistant acrosomal matrix complex (FIG. 4).

Two structurally different domains are noted in the stable acrosomal matrix and each is restricted to a specific intra-acrosomal location (FIG. 2). The more electron-dense domain, termed M_2, which is located ventrally, is contiguous with the second domain, termed M_1, which is less electron dense and extends over the lateral to the dorsal surface of the acrosome (FIGS. 2 and 4). Since the acrosome is bilaterally symmetric, cross sections reveal two electron-dense ovoid-shaped plaques of M_2 matrix positioned along the ventral acrosomal surface (FIG. 2). Frequently the M_1 matrix domain is discontinuous at the dorsal apex of the acrosome (FIG. 2). Both of the matrix domains have a granular texture in thin sections with M_1 having a looser, more coarse, appearance. In whole mount preparations of Triton-extracted spermatozoa the two matrix domains can be distinguished; both have a somewhat fibrous appearance but M_1 has a more porous appearing meshwork (FIG. 5).

Triton-extracted sperm suspensions were centrifuged on Percoll density gradients to separate spermatozoa from the insoluble acrosomal components. A highly purified fraction was obtained which contained both matrix components, M_1 and M_2, and the acrosomal lamina (FIG. 6). The matrix remained adherent to the acrosomal lamina (FIGS. 4 and 6).

SDS-PAGE was utilized to identify the major polypeptide constituents of the acrosomal matrix-acrosomal lamina (ALM) fraction. A spectrum of polypeptides was noted by Coomassie Blue staining. Minor components included a diffuse band of M_r 64,000–62,000, a doublet band of M_r 56,000, a faint complex of M_r 43,000–50,000 and a band of M_r 35,000. Major components included a doublet band of M_r 29,000 and 27,000 and a band of M_r 22,000; a group of evenly spaced minor bands was present

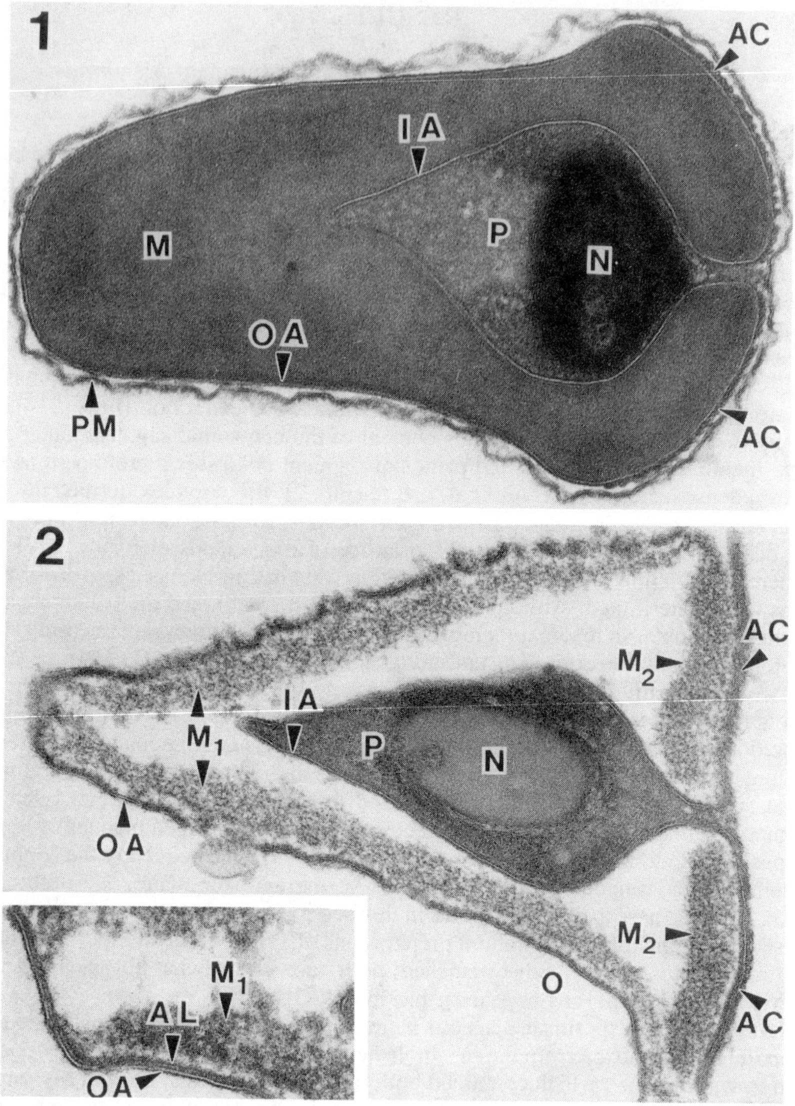

FIGURE 1. Cross section through the anterior end of the acrosomal segment of a hamster spermatozoon, the ventral surface is oriented toward the right side of the plate. The nucleus (n) is surrounded by a prominent accumulation of perinuclear material (p) and it in turn is surrounded by an adherent inner acrosomal membrane (ia). The matrix (m) of the acrosome is homogenous and within the confines of the outer acrosomal membrane (oa). Along the ventral surface of the acrosome the outer acrosomal membrane is adherent to a network of filaments termed the acrosomal cytoskeleton (ac). The acrosome is surrounded by the plasma membrane (pm).

FIGURE 2. Cross section through the acrosomal segment of a sperm disrupted by exposure to 0.01% Triton for 1 minute. The plasma membrane is absent but the outer acrosomal membrane (oa) remains. Note that much of the acrosomal matrix is lost but that a well-defined layer of matrix material re-

between these major bands (FIG. 7). Both of the major bands exhibited a negative image on silver-stained SDS-PAGE gels while all other bands stained darkly. These two major polypeptides exhibit common peptide fragments after digestion with V8 protease, suggesting that they are structurally related (not shown). In addition a monoclonal antibody was prepared against the ALM fraction which recognized both the M_r 29,000/27,000 and 22,000 polypeptides as well as the array of minor polypeptides located between these two components on SDS-PAGE gels; the antibody displayed no reactivity against the higher molecular weight polypeptides of the ALM complex. This result further confirms the presence of structural similarity between this complex of polypeptides.

Immunostaining of permeabilized spermatozoa with the anti-29-22 monoclonal antibody revealed intense staining of the acrosomal cap, but the inner acrosomal membrane and equatorial segment were negative as were all other sperm components (FIG. 8). Thus these polypeptides are restricted to the apical and principal segments of the acrosome.

The distribution of the acrosomal matrix constituents was compared to that of proacrosin/acrosin. A monospecific antibody that specifically interacts with guinea pig testicular and epididymal sperm proacrosin[20] was employed to immunostain permeabilized cauda epididymal hamster spermatozoa. The staining pattern was specific for the acrosomal cap but no staining of the inner acrosomal membrane or equatorial segment was noted (FIG. 9). Hamster proacrosin/acrosin has been previously shown by SDS-PAGE to be a complex of four major bands in the molecular weight range M_r 43,000–50,000 range;[17,21] moreover, although protease activity is present in the isolated ALM fraction, much of the activity can be extracted by conditions that do not solubilize the M_r 29,000, 27,000 or 22,000 matrix polypeptides.[17] These data indicate that the anti-matrix and anti-proacrosin antibodies are recognizing distinct constituents that co-localize to the same acrosomal domain.

Equatorial Segment

The equatorial segment represents the posterior-most segment of the acrosome and it is characterized by the relatively close positioning and parallel arrangement of the inner and outer acrosomal membranes (FIGS. 10 and 11). Previous work has demonstrated that these two membranes are linked together by bridging elements located within the interior of the acrosome,[8,16,17] but their molecular composition remains to be identified. In the equatorial segment the inner acrosomal membrane is associated with a discontinuous layer of perinuclear electron dense material and at the zone of transition between the inner and outer acrosomal membrane, the equatorial segment attaches to the leading edge of the postacrosomal sheath (FIGS. 4 and 10). Thus the equatorial segment membranes appear firmly adherent to other nuclear struc-

---

mains associated with the outer acrosomal membrane. The matrix contains two distinct domains, M_1, which extends over the dorsal and lateral surface of the acrosome and a contiguous, more electron-dense domain, M_2 which is located ventrally and adjacent to the subdomain of the outer acrosomal membrane associated with the acrosomal cytoskeleton (ac). Note that the inner acrosomal membrane (ia) is not associated with the matrix but remains apposed to the perinuclear material (p). The inset shows a higher magnification view of the outer acrosomal membrane and the well-defined acrosomal lamina (al) which coats its luminal surface.

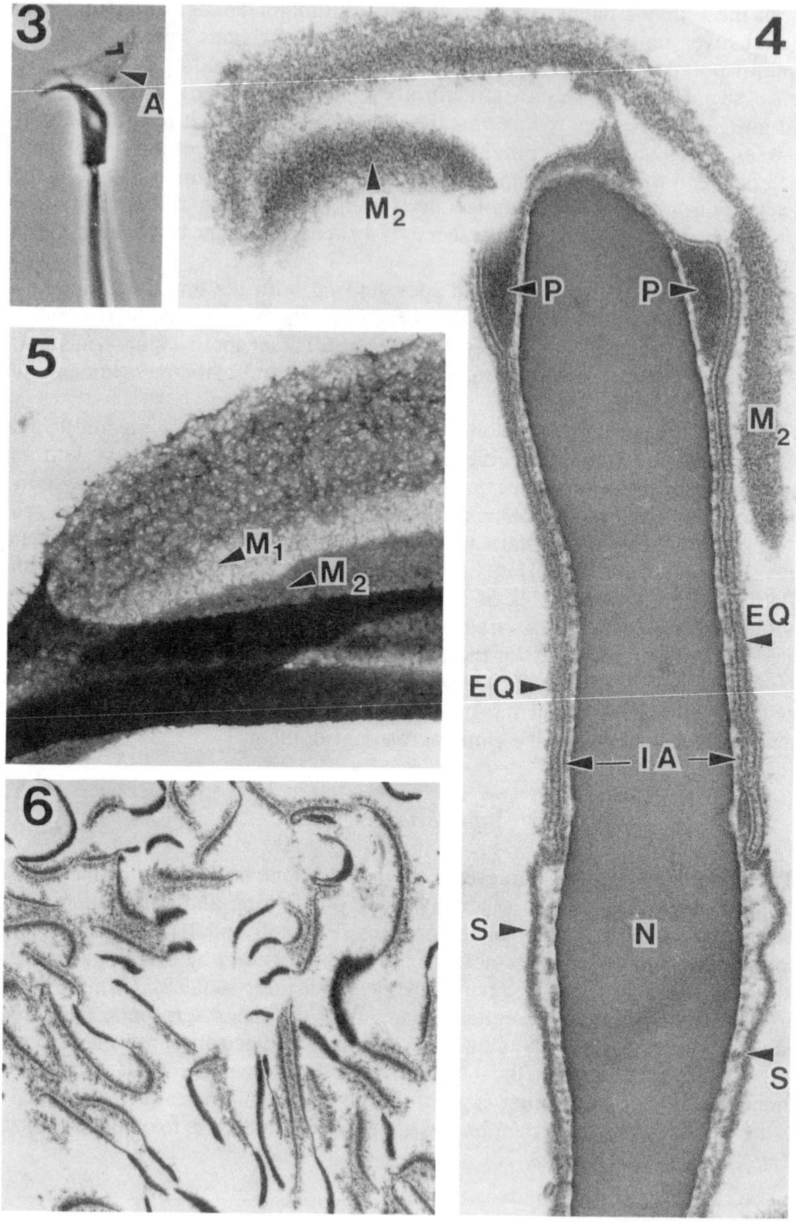

FIGURE 3. Phase contrast photomicrograph of a Triton-extracted spermatozoon showing the detachment of the acrosome (a) from the underlying nucleus.

FIGURE 4. Electron micrograph of a Triton-extracted spermatozoon. Note the acrosomal lamina-acrosomal matrix complex detaching from the sperm head. Also on the sperm head note the periodic bridges within the equatorial segment region (eq). A bulge of perinuclear material (p) underlies the

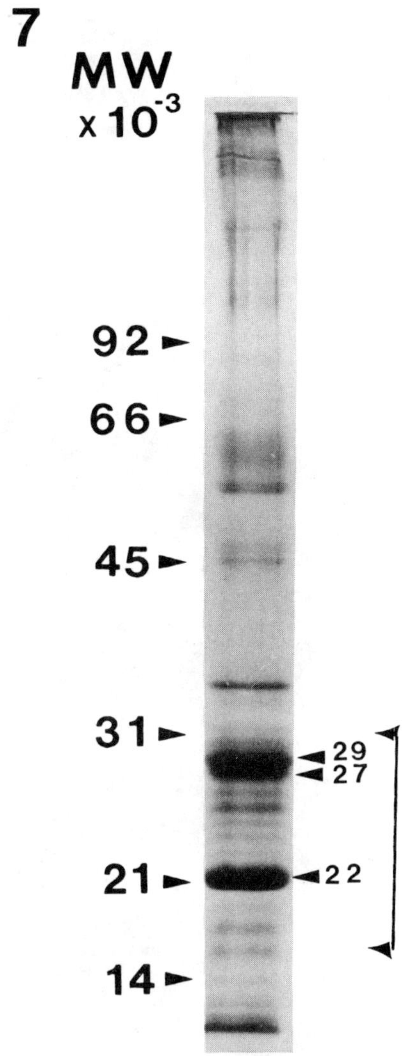

FIGURE 7. Coomassie blue–stained SDS-PAGE gel showing the polypeptide composition of the purified ALM fraction. Note the prominent doublet of polypeptides of M_r 29,000 and 27,000 and the other major component of M_r 22,000. A cluster of evenly spaced minor components is associated with these major bands and all of the bands within the brackets are recognized by the monoclonal antibody employed in FIGURE 8.

---

anterior edge of the equatorial segment. At the posterior margin of the equatorial segment the acrosomal membrane is attached to the postacrosomal sheath (s).

FIGURE 5. Whole mount preparation of the Triton-extracted acrosomal matrix. Note the fibrous substructure of the different matrix domains.

FIGURE 6. Electron micrograph showing a purified fraction of acrosomal lamina-acrosomal matrix complexes isolated from a suspension of Triton-extracted spermatozoa.

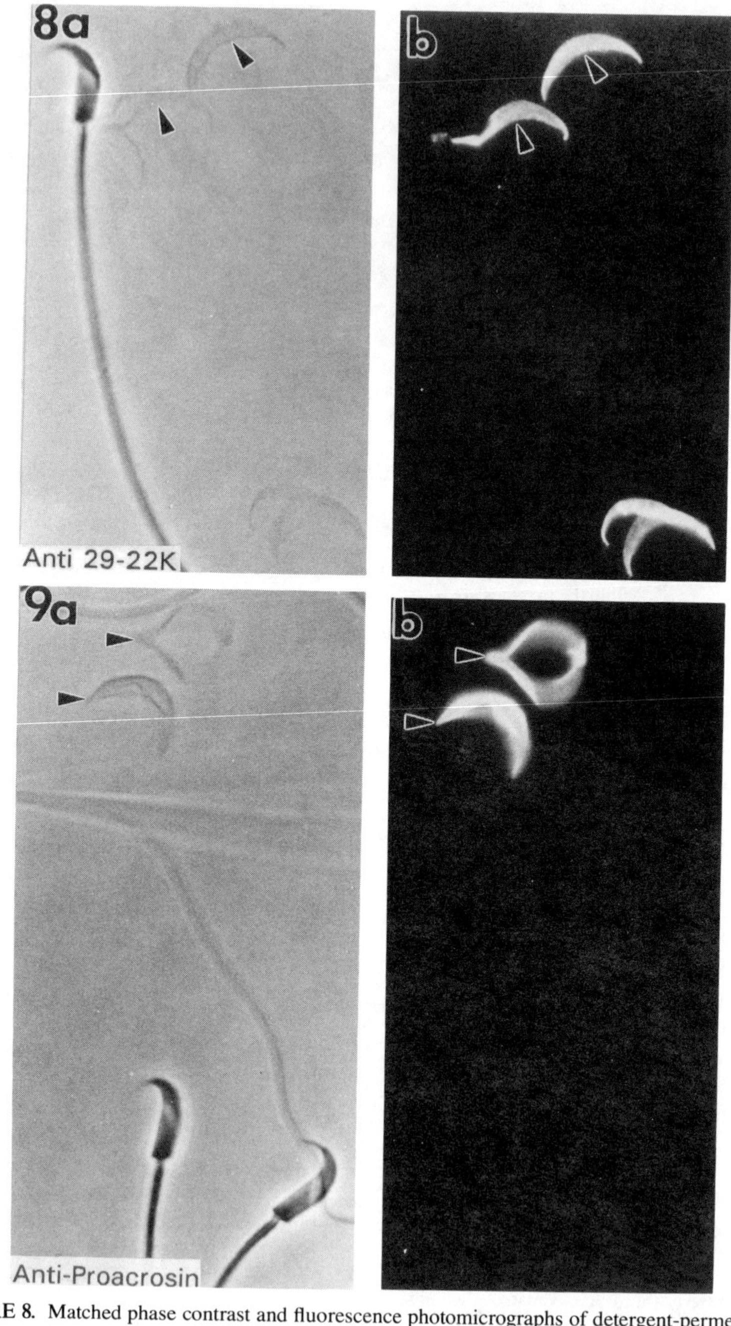

FIGURE 8. Matched phase contrast and fluorescence photomicrographs of detergent-permeabilized spermatozoa stained with monoclonal antibody specific to polypeptides within the brackets of FIGURE 7. The antibody reacts exclusively with the detached acrosomal caps (*arrowheads*) and not with any other sperm component.

tures. A distinctive specialization of the anterior margin of the hamster equatorial segment is the presence of a prominent subacrosomal accumulation of perinuclear material, this accumulation is thickest at the dorsal edge of the sperm head[2] and the inner acrosomal membrane is closely apposed to this material (FIGS. 4, 10, and 11).

A purified sperm head fraction was isolated from a suspension of sonicated spermatozoa. The only components of the acrosome that remained associated with the heads was a continuous inner acrosomal membrane over the principal segment and the acrosomal membranes of the equatorial segment (FIG. 10). The outer acrosomal membrane terminated at the anterior margin of the equatorial segment (FIGS. 10 and 11). Regularly spaced bridging elements were noted within the interior of the equatorial segment (FIG. 11). In tangential sections these elements appear arrayed as a paracrystalline lattice. Triton X-100 extraction of the sperm heads solubilized the outer acrosomal membrane, but a recognizable inner acrosomal membrane remained associated with the underlying perinuclear material (FIG. 12). The bridging elements also remained associated with the inner acrosomal membrane-perinuclear material complex and the individual bridging elements appeared to be asymmetric in shape, terminating in a globular shaped structure (FIG. 12). Subsequent extraction of the heads in a solution of elevated ionic strength or pH released most of the structural elements of the equatorial segment, although the accumulation of perinuclear material at the principal segment-equatorial segment junction remained intact (FIG. 13).

Isolated sperm heads were exposed to a variety of FITC-lectins in order to identify glycosylated domains of the inner acrosomal membrane and equatorial segment. Isolated heads displayed a characteristic wheat germ agglutinin (WGA)–binding pattern. The anterior tip of the spermatozoon stained intensely while the remainder of the surface of the principal segment appeared negative. A positive stripe of fluorescence extending from the dorsal to the lateral surface of the head was noted at the anterior edge of the equatorial segment (FIG. 14). Electron microscopic experiments employing lectin-gold conjugates confirmed that the label was associated with the inner acrosomal membrane (FIG. 15). The remainder of the equatorial segment exhibited variable staining between spermatozoa, most exhibited no or dull fluorescence while others appeared positive (FIG. 14). Pretreatment of heads with Triton X-100 resulted in significant alterations in the fluorescence pattern. The anterior tip of the sperm head remained positive as did the stripe at the anterior edge of the equatorial segment; however, the entire equatorial segment region now exhibited intense fluorescence (FIG. 14). Electron microscopic analyses of Triton-extracted sperm treated with lectin-gold conjugates demonstrates that at the anterior tip of the sperm the gold binds to what is apparently residual inner acrosomal membrane associated with the underlying perinuclear material (FIG. 16) and in the equatorial segment the lectin binds to the bridging elements which remain associated with the inner acrosomal membrane (FIG. 17).

Triton-treated sperm heads were subjected to extraction regimens of varying pH and salt concentrations in an effort to release the equatorial segment WGA-binding components. Extraction of the heads with 25 mM TAPS, pH 8.5 containing 0.2M KCL, 2 mg/ml dithiothreitol and protease inhibitors prior to exposure to FITC-WGA resulted in a dramatic decrease of fluorescence of the equatorial segment (FIG. 14). However, the extracted sperm retained intense fluorescence both at the tip of the head

FIGURE 9. Matched phase contrast and fluorescence photomicrographs of detergent-permeabilized spermatozoa stained with monospecific antibody to guinea pig proacrosin. Specific and exclusive staining of the detached acrosomal complexes is seen.

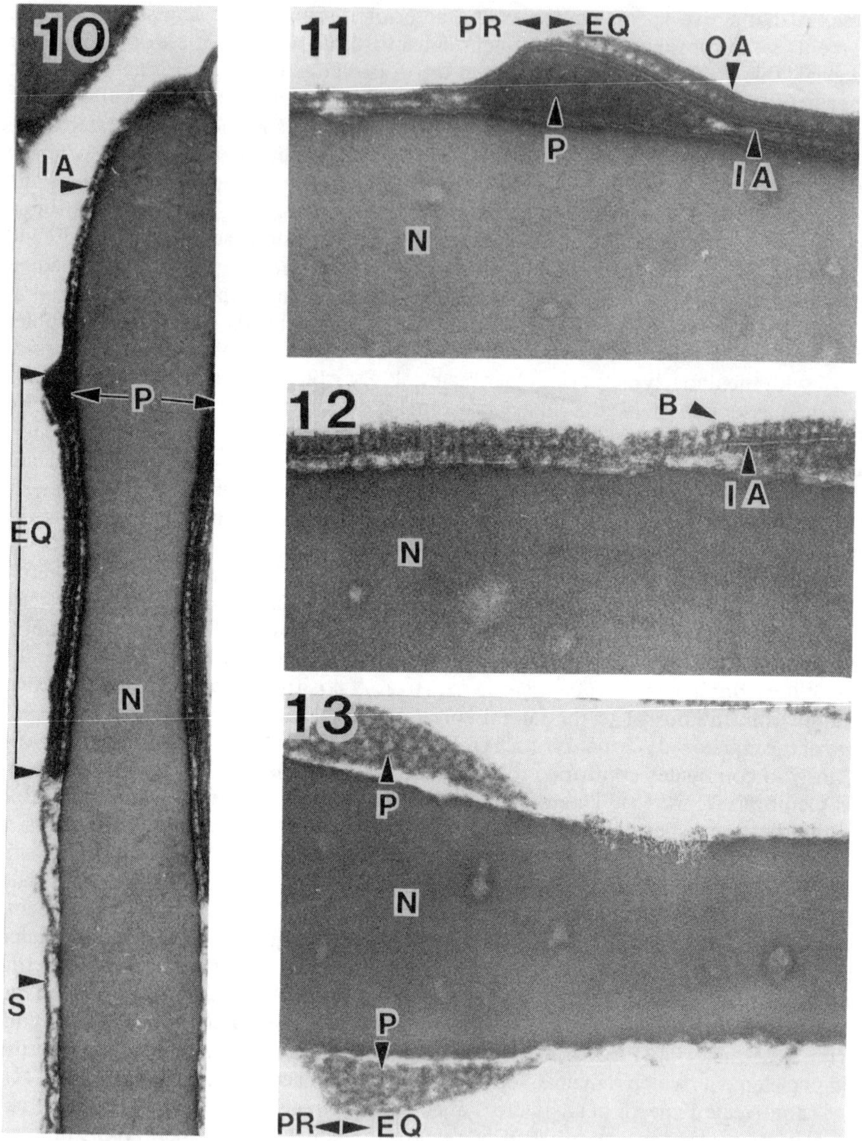

FIGURE 10. Electron micrograph of isolated sperm head. In the equatorial segment region (eq) both the inner and outer acrosomal membranes are present while in the principal segment only the inner acrosomal membrane (ia) remains. The postacrosomal sheath (s) is adherent to the posterior margin of the equatorial segment while a prominent accumulation of perinuclear material (p) is associated with the anterior border of the equatorial segment.

FIGURE 11. High power view of the principal segment (pr)-equatorial segment (eq) junction of an isolated head. Note both the outer (oa) and inner (ia) acrosomal membranes of the equatorial segment and the periodic bridging elements joining between them. In the principal segment the inner acrosomal membrane remains intact.

and at the stripe at the equatorial segment-principal segment border (FIG. 14). This supports the electron microscopic analysis of the extracted heads revealing loss of the bridging elements of the equatorial segment (FIG. 13); the perforatorium as well as the accumulation of perinuclear material at the junction of the equatorial and principal segments were not solubilized by this treatment.

SDS-PAGE analysis of the pellet and the supernatant fluid fractions at specific steps of the extraction procedure revealed that Triton X-100 and high salt extractions each released a specific subset of polypeptides from the sperm head. Western blots of the fractions stained for glycoproteins with WGA and RCA, revealed that the high salt extraction specifically released a major band of M_r 40,000 as well as several minor bands which were WGA-binding components. Under all extraction conditions examined, loss of lectin binding over the bulk of the equatorial segment correlated with solubilization of the M_r 40,000 component. The M_r 40,000 band was absent in the pellet fraction of the high salt–extracted heads suggesting that the extraction resistant WGA-binding components at the tip of the head and at the equatorial segment-principal segment represent different glycoproteins; several lectin-binding glycoproteins remained in the residual head fraction (FIG. 18). These data suggest that specific glycoproteins of the inner acrosomal membrane of the principal segment and equatorial segment are anchored to underlying structural elements and that different constituents vary in the firmness of their association to the underlying structures. The observations that the WGA-binding constituents of the tip of the sperm and at the equatorial-principal segment junction are the most resistant to extraction suggests that they are firmly anchored to the underlying perinuclear material.

DISCUSSION

The acrosomal segment of the spermatozoon performs a number of distinctive functions during fertilization with respect to the binding and penetration of the egg investments and ultimately in the fusion with the egg plasma membrane. A set of distinctive structural assemblies, with limited and specific distributions within the acrosomal segment, have been identified which may play functionally important roles in the membrane fusion processes, in the organization of acrosomal hydrolases, and in the maintenance and/or generation of functionally distinct acrosomal membrane domains. Assemblies included in this set which have been discussed in the present paper include: first, cytoskeletal elements restricted to the apical and principal segments which are interposed between the plasma membrane and outer acrosomal membrane and associate with specific subdomains of these membranes; second, the acrosomal lamina which is a membrane-skeleton like complex adherent to the luminal surface of the

---

FIGURE 12. View of the equatorial segment of a Triton-extracted sperm head. The outer acrosomal membrane is mostly solubilized but the inner acrosomal membrane (ia) remains intact. Note the regularly spaced bridging elements (b) which remain associated with the inner acrosomal membrane.

FIGURE 13. Electron micrograph of the principal segment (pr)-equatorial segment (eq) junction of a sperm head which, after initial Triton treatment, was extracted with 25 mM TAPS, pH 8.5 containing 0.2M KCL, 2 mg/ml dithiothreitol and protease inhibitors. Most elements of the equatorial segment are absent while the prominent accumulations of perinuclear electron dense material (p) at the anterior margin of the equatorial segment remain associated with the nucleus (n).

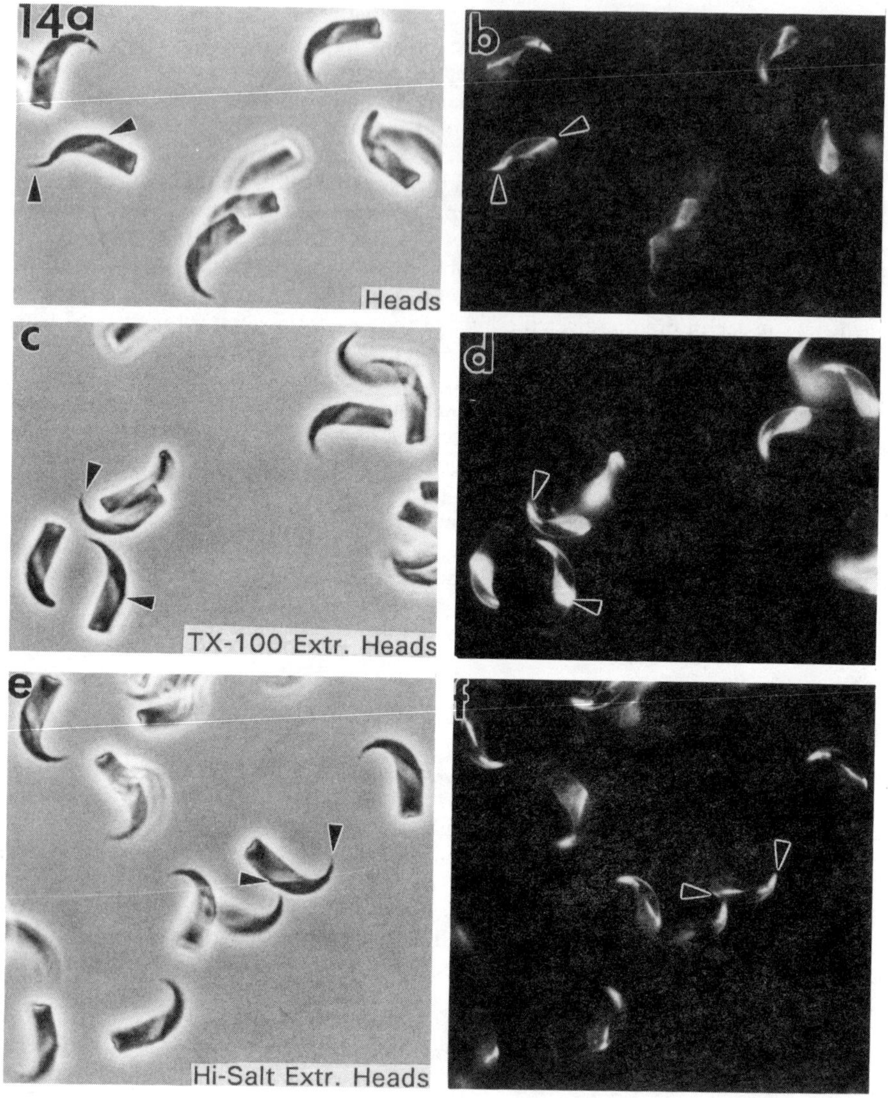

FIGURE 14. Matched phase contrast (**a**,**c**,**e**) and fluorescence (**b**,**d**,**f**) of sperm heads which were labeled with FITC-WGA after extraction. Panels **a** and **b** show freshly isolated heads; panels **c** and **d** show heads extracted with Triton X-100; and panels **e** and **f** show heads subjected to sequential Triton extraction followed by extraction at elevated pH ionic strength. Note the prominent staining of the equatorial segment after Triton extraction (**d**) and its lack of fluorescence after high salt extraction (**f**).

FIGURE 15. Cross section through the anterior end of an isolated sperm head labeled to demonstrate WGA binding sites. Note the extensive binding to the inner acrosomal membrane which is associated with the underlying perforatorium (p).

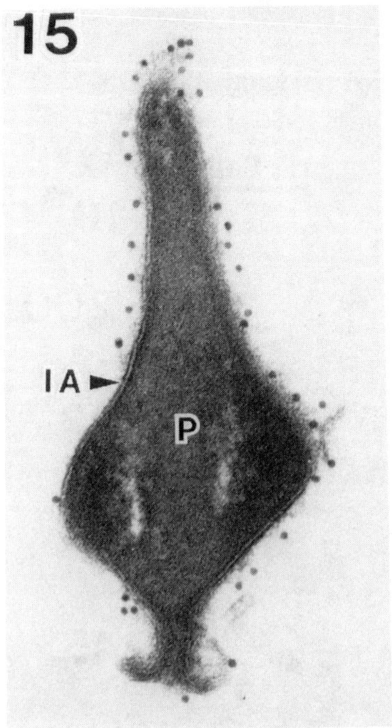

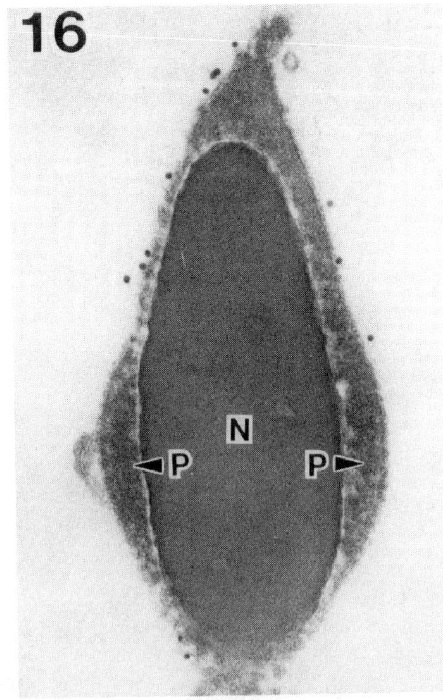

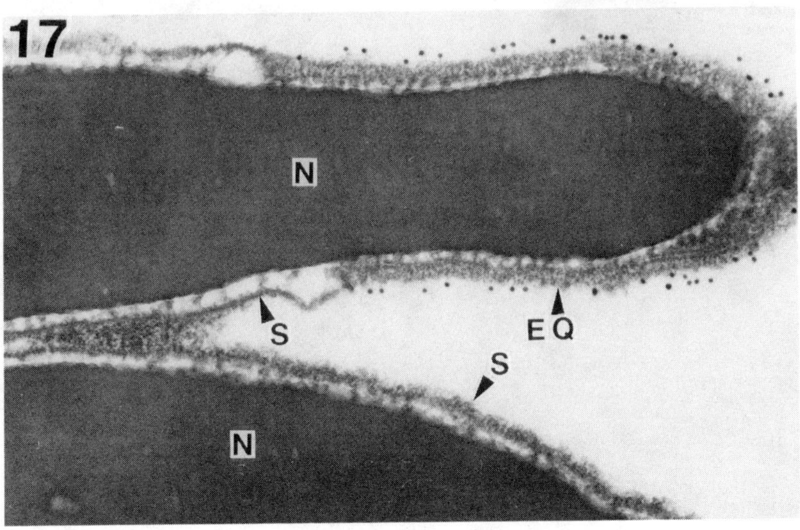

FIGURE 16. Cross section through anterior end of an isolated sperm head which was extracted with Triton X-100 prior to labeling with WGA. Note the gold particles overlying the perinuclear material (p).

FIGURE 17. Section showing the junction of the postacrosomal and equatorial segment of a sperm head which was extracted with Triton and then prepared for localization of WGA-binding components. Note the extensive binding to the bridges of the equatorial segment (eq) but not to the postacrosomal sheath (s).

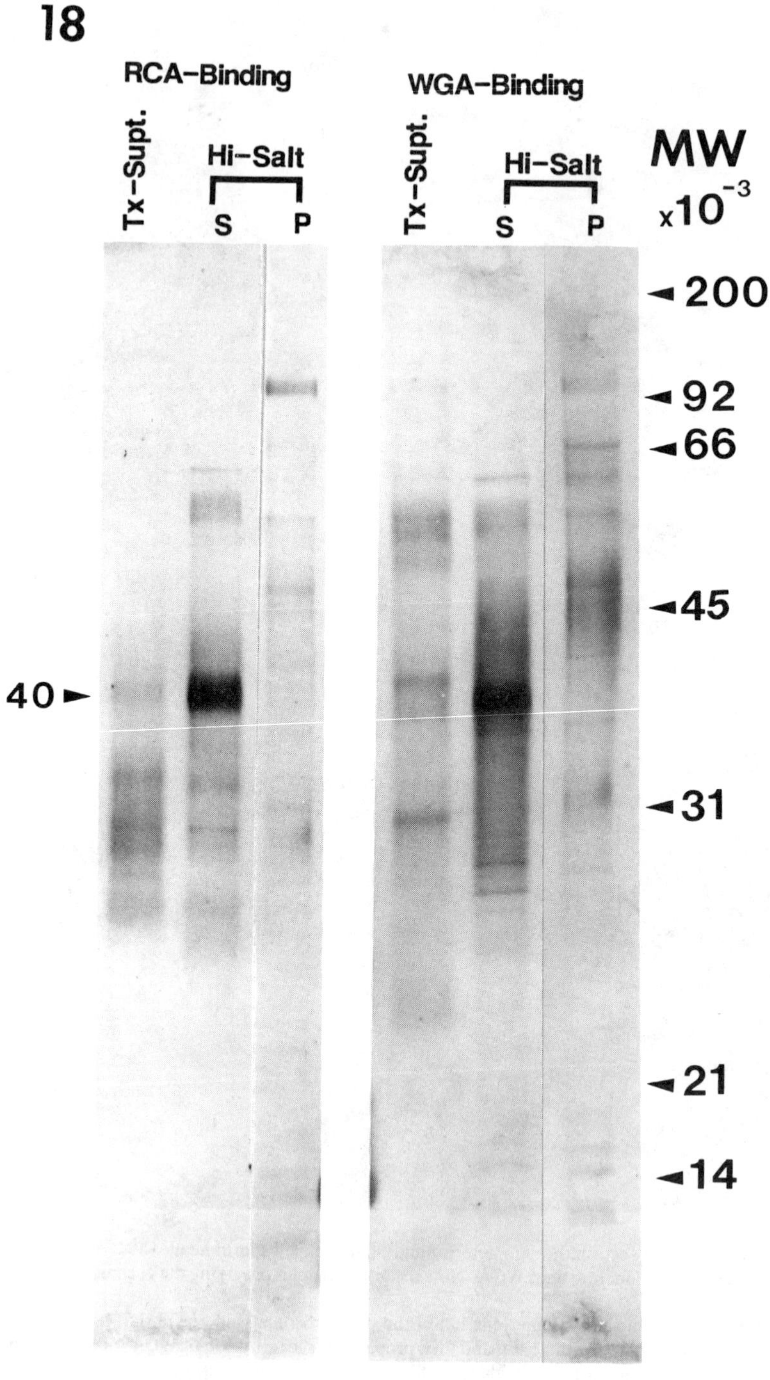
18
RCA-Binding
WGA-Binding
Tx-Supt.
Hi-Salt
S
P
Tx-Supt.
Hi-Salt
S
P
MW
x10^{-3}
200
92
66
45
40
31
21
14

outer acrosomal membrane of the apical and principal segments; third, a paracrystalline network of membrane-associated bridging elements within the equatorial segment; fourth, specific matrix structures within the apical and principal segments; and fifth the subacrosomal perinuclear substance which displays regional differences in its structure and is associated with the inner acrosomal membrane.

A variety of hydrolases are sequestered within the acrosome and during the acrosome reaction these are released and the acrosomal matrix, for the most part is dispersed, although matrix remnants have been noted to remain associated with the shed hybrid membrane complex. In the hamster we have identified a detergent-insoluble matrix complex comprised of several polypeptides and two major polypeptides of M_r 29,000/27,000 and 22,000. Whether these are related to other acrosomal constituents identified in other studies such as acrogranin a polypeptide of M_r 67,000 in the guinea pig,[23] acrosomal antigen SP-10 of the human which is a complex of polypeptides between M_r 18,000–34,000[24] or another constituent recently identified in the hamster acrosome[25] remains to be elucidated. The co-localization of proacrosin/acrosin with the insoluble matrix of hamster spermatozoa suggests that this complex could play a role in sequestering hydrolases to specific domains within the acrosome interior and further could function in effecting a controlled rate of release of soluble acrosin during the acrosome reaction. Whether complexes such as this could act to sequester other proteases such as dipeptidyl peptidase II which has been shown to clearly reside in a morphologically distinct compartment of the guinea pig acrosome[18] remains to be established. It is an attractive hypothesis, however, that an acrosomal infrastructure made up of spatially segregated distinct matrix components could interact with and define the distribution of selected hydrolases.

How the different domains of the acrosomal membrane are generated and maintained is poorly understood, but the observations of the present study suggest potential mechanisms relevant to the outer acrosomal membrane of the apical and principal segments, to the inner acrosomal membrane and both the inner and outer membrane of the equatorial segment. Ultrastructural studies of several species have demonstrated that the outer acrosomal membrane of the apical and principal segment possesses a distinct coating of electron dense material on its luminal surface.[11,13–15,19] This complex, termed the acrosomal lamina, has been isolated and shown to be a sheet-like complex; it may be analogous to the well-characterized "membrane-skeleton" of the plasma membrane of somatic cells or to the nuclear lamina, which is a network of intermediate sized filaments associated with the inner nuclear membrane. The acrosomal lamina of guinea pig sperm is a two-dimensional lattice of filaments;[13,15] whether the acrosomal lamina is a filamentous network in other species remains to be determined. Freeze-fracture analysis of guinea pig spermatozoa have shown that the intramembranous particles of the outer acrosomal membrane are arranged into a two dimensional lattice,[1,4,9] and it is tempting to speculate that interaction of the lamina with the integral proteins facilitates this arrangement. Another potential function of the

---

FIGURE 18. Western blot showing RCA-binding (*left lanes*) and WGA-binding polypeptides. Sperm heads were extracted with Triton and centrifuged; the supernatant (TX-supt.) is the first lane of each set. The pelleted nuclei were then extracted with high salt and centrifuged to prepare a supernatant fluid (s) and pellet (p) fraction. Each lane represents extract from an equivalent number of heads. Note that the supernatant of the high salt fraction had a prominent lectin-binding band of M_r 40,000 which is not present in the corresponding pellet (p) fraction.

acrosomal lamina is participation in the membrane fusion events of the acrosome reaction. Supporting this idea is data from guinea pig sperm where it has been demonstrated that the pattern of membrane fusions in acrosome reacting sperm is related to the arrangement of filaments of the acrosomal lamina.[13,26] It is suggested that this membrane-associated assembly may play important roles both in the maintenance of the outer acrosomal membrane domain and in the membrane fusion events of the acrosome reaction.

The molecular composition of the inner acrosomal membrane of the principal segment and of the acrosomal membranes of the equatorial segment has not been well established. In this present study we demonstrate that specific glycoconjugates associated with specific subregions of the inner acrosomal membrane are resistant to extraction with detergents. This suggests these membrane components may be linked to submembranous structures. Two segments of the inner acrosomal membrane which are most resistant to release of the glycoconjugates include the apical tip of the inner acrosomal membrane, where the membrane is associated with a specialization of underlying perinuclear material termed the perforatorium, and the junction of the principal and equatorial segments; where there is also a prominent accumulation of perinuclear material. While the perforatorium has been generally considered to be a rigid structural element playing a role in maintenance of head shape,[27,28] the data presented here suggest that it could have a direct role in the generation and maintenance of biochemically distinct subdomains of the inner acrosomal membrane. Similarly, the paracrystalline lattice of bridging elements associated with the inner acrosomal membrane of the equatorial segment resists solubilization by detergent and they appear to be associated with a looser network of underlying perinuclear material. Regional variations in the composition of the perinuclear material of the acrosomal segment could provide a biochemical basis for segregating specific inner acrosomal membrane proteins to selected subdomains.

ACKOWLEDGMENTS

We thank Drs. Ken Tung and Dan Hardy for providing a monospecific antiserum to guinea pig proacrosin.

REFERENCES

1. FAWCETT, D. W. 1975. Dev. Biol. **44:** 394–436.
2. YANAGIMACHI, R. 1988. *In* The Physiology of Reproduction. E. Knobil and J. D. Neil, Eds. **1:** 135–186. Raven Press. New York.
3. EDDY, E. M. 1988. *In* The Physiology of Reproduction. E. Knobil and J. D. Neil, Eds. **1:** 27–68. Raven Press. New York.
4. BEARER, E. L. & D. S. FRIEND. 1990. J. Electron Micros. Tech. **16:** 281–297.
5. OUARA, C. & K. TOSHIMORI. 1990. Int. Rev. Cytol. **122:** 105–151.
6. WASSARMAN, P. 1987. Science **235:** 553–560.
7. MEIZEL, S. 1984. Biol. Rev. **59:** 125–157.
8. BEDFORD, J. M., H. D. M. MOORE & L. E. FRANKLIN. 1979. Exp. Cell Res. **119:** 119–126.
9. FRIEND, D. S. & D. W. FAWCETT. 1974. J. Cell Biol. **63:** 641–664.
10. HOLT, W. V. 1984. Int. Rev. Cytol. **87:** 159–194.
11. OLSON, G. E. & V. P. WINFREY. 1985. J. Ultrastruct. Res. **92:** 167–179.
12. OLSON, G. E., V. P. WINFREY & S. P. FLAHERTY. 1987. Ann. N.Y. Acad. Sci. **513:** 222–246.

13. Flaherty, S. P. & G. E. Olson. 1988. Anat. Rec. **220:** 267–280.
14. Olson, G. E., V. P. Winfrey, D. L. Garbers & T. D. Noland. 1985. Biol. Reprod. **33:** 761–779.
15. Olson, G. E., V. P. Winfrey, M. A. Winer & G. R. Davenport. 1987. Gamete Res. **17:** 77–94.
16. Russell, L., R. N. Peterson & M. Freund. 1980. Anat. Rec. **198:** 449–459.
17. Olson, G. E. & V. P. Winfrey. 1985. J. Ultrastruc. Res. **90:** 9–25.
18. Talbot, P. & G. DiCarlantonio. 1985. J. Histochem. Cytochem. **33:** 1169–1172.
19. Olson, G. E., V. P. Winfrey & G. R. Davenport. 1988. Biol. Reprod. **39:** 1145–1158.
20. Hardy, D. M., G. C. Wild & K. S. K. Tung. 1987. Biol. Reprod. **37:** 189–199.
21. Siegel, M. S., D. S. Bechtold, J. L. Willand & K. L. Polakoski, 1987. Biol. Reprod. **35:** 485–491.
22. Yanagimachi, R. & Y. D. Noda. 1970. Am. J. Anat. **128:** 367–388.
23. Anakwe, O. O. & G. L. Gerton. 1990. Biol. Reprod. **42:** 317–328.
24. Herr, J. C., R. M. Wright, E. John, J. Foster, T. Kays & C. J. Flickinger. 1990. Biol. Reprod. **42:** 377–382.
25. Longo, F. J., S. Cook & R. Baillie. 1990. Biol. Reprod. **42:** 553–562.
26. Flaherty, S. P. & G. E. Olson. 1991. Anat. Rec. **229:** 186–194.
27. Oko, R. & Y. Clermont. 1988. Biol. Reprod. **39:** 673–687.
28. Oko, R., L. Moussakova & Y. Clermont. 1990. Am. J. Anat. **188:** 64–73.

Endocytosis of Human Sex Steroid-binding Protein in Monkey Germ Cells

ANNE GERARD,[a,c] AMINA EN NYA,[a]
MONIQUE EGLOFF,[b] MAURICETTE DOMINGO,[b]
HERVÉ DEGRELLE,[b] AND HUBERT GERARD[a]

[a] *Laboratoire d'Histologie-Embryologie II*
Faculté de Médecine de Nancy I
9, Avenue de la forêt de Haye, BP 184
54505 Vandoeuvre les Nancy Cedex, France

[b] *Laboratoire de Biochimie Endocrinienne*
Faculté de Médecine de Paris VI
45, rue des Saints-Pères
75270 Paris Cedex 06, France

INTRODUCTION

During the past decade, it has become increasingly clear that steroid-binding proteins such as androgen-binding protein (ABP) and sex steroid–binding protein (SBP) could act as transmembrane carriers for the transport of steroid hormones from extracellular milieu into intracellular compartments.[1-6] Sperm are known to bind steroids.[7-10] Binding sites for 17β estradiol, progesterone and testosterone have been detected on the midpiece of human spermatozoa.[11] But, as stressed by Frankel in 1989,[10] the nature of the molecule responsible for the binding of androgens in sperm cells is uncertain, one of their hypothesis being that ABP could be adsorbed on sperm, thus accounting for the specific androgen binding activity observed in their study on rat sperm cells.

In the rabbit in fact, using immunocytochemistry, the presence of SBP, which is equally able to bind testosterone, has been identified in ejaculated spermatozoa at the junction of the head and midpiece and, occasionally, along the head, supporting the finding of steroid binding sites on sperm cells and suggesting a possible role of SBP as a steroid carrier protein across the plasma membrane of these cells.[12] This raises, however, the question of the origin of the SBP detected in mature sperm cells since 1) differentiated post-meiotic sperm cannot be held to be able to synthesize SBP or ABP and such a synthesis has not been reported in the literature, and 2) no SBP or only trace amounts have been found in seminal fluid to be taken up by sperm cells,[13] which, in addition, are not known to contain specific endocytic structures. Taken all together, this suggests that the SBP molecules detected in rabbit spermatozoa could have been either internalized or synthesized at some earlier stage in their development.

[c] Author to whom correspondence and reprint requests should be addressed.

The present study was undertaken to test in a primate model the ability of germ cells to internalize labeled human sex steroid-binding protein. The labeling of the pure protein was obtained either by conjugating with colloidal gold particles, or by coupling to $[^3H]\Delta_6$-testosterone using photoaffinity treatment, as already described.[6] Uptake experiments were analyzed by transmission electron microscopy, directly for gold conjugated protein and after autoradiography processing for the radiolabeled protein.

MATERIALS AND METHODS

Chemicals

$[1,2\text{-}^3H]17\beta$-hydroxy-4,6-androstadien-3-one ($[^3H]\Delta_6$-testosterone; 48 Ci/mmol) was obtained from New England Nuclear Corp. (Boston, MA). All other chemicals used were of analytical reagent grade and obtained from Merck (Darmstadt).

Animals and Cell Preparation

Two adult, healthy, laboratory-born monkeys (*Macaca fascicularis*) were studied. They were housed in individual cages under photoperiod in Paris and laboratory conditions described elsewhere.[14]

Isolation of Germ Cells

Testes were dissected free from surrounding fat and connective tissue and minced with scissors. Under a stereomicroscope, the seminiferous tubules were gently unraveled with forceps in RPMI 1640 medium (pH 7, Sigma) in order to eliminate all the interstitial tissue. Germ cells were isolated using mechanical means (a glass homogenizer, Potter n° 10, VSC, Paris), then washed with RPMI medium, filtered through cotton wool in order to trap testicular sperm and cellular debris, then recovered by centrifuging at 1000 $\times$ *g* for 5 minutes. Pellets were resuspended in fresh culture medium and cell viability, assessed by trypan blue (Sigma) exclusion test, was greater than 95%. Cells were counted under phase contrast microscope, the suspension was adjusted to 4 $\times$ 10^7 cells/ml and divided into 100 μl aliquots. Each of these groups was further exposed to one of the labeled proteins.

Smears were prepared with excess cell suspension and stained in order to quantify the germ cells in particular respect to their maturation steps and the level of contamination with Leydig and Sertoli cells and fragments.

Collection of Epididymal Spermatozoa

Epididymal sperm cells were obtained from the caput epididymides by making multiple slits with a razor blade and gently squeezing out the content into a tube containing 2 ml RPMI culture medium. Sperm cells were washed, centrifuged at 1000 $\times$ *g* for 5 min, resuspended in fresh culture medium and adjusted to a final concentration of 4 $\times$ 10^7 cells/ml and divided into 100 μl aliquots to be used for the uptake study.

Purification of Human SBP

The sex steroid-binding protein was purified from human late-pregnancy serum using a modification of the method previously described.[15] Four steps were performed including ammonium sulfate precipitation, carboxymethyl cellulose chromatography, DEAE cellulose chromatography and gel filtration. Purity of hSBP was checked by polyacrylamide gel electrophoresis, both under nondenaturing conditions and in the presence of sodium dodecyl sulfate (SDS-PAGE), and by immunoelectrophoresis against antiserum to whole human serum. The concentrations of solutions of purified hSBP were determined spectrophotometrically, using the absorbance coefficient value 1.14 $\times$ 10^5/mol per cm-1 at 280 nm and a M_r of 93,400.[16] Quantitative estimation of hSBP was also performed by electroimmunoassay using a polyclonal rabbit anti-SBP serum.

Colloidal Gold Coupling to Pure hSBP

Colloidal gold particles were prepared according to Frens[17] and the monodisperse colloidal sol was checked at the electron microscope level as having an average size of 18 nm in diameter. Conjugation of colloidal gold to hSBP was performed after first determining minimal concentration of protein needed to stabilize the gold colloid: 150 µg of freshly dialyzed hSBP were diluted to 500 µg with double-distilled water and 5 ml of colloidal gold solution was added in a fast jet. After 5 min, the solution was centrifuged at 250 $\times$ *g* for 20 min at 4°C to remove the large gold aggregates. To eliminate the unbound hSBP, the preparation was washed twice in phosphate-buffered saline (PBS pH 7.4) using ultracentrifugation at 13,000 $\times$ *g* for 30 min. The supernatant was eliminated and the pellet was resuspended in PBS containing 0.2 mg/ml of polyclonal rabbit anti hSBP serum and was found to be 30 µg of protein per ml of buffer. Just before use, this solution was again centrifuged at 250 $\times$ *g* for 20 min and filtered through a 0.2 µm millipore filter. Quantitative estimation of gold-hSBP was performed by electroimmunoassay using a polyclonal rabbit anti-SBP serum by comparison with the migration of known quantities of pure SBP (FIG. 1).

Covalent Coupling of [^{3}H]-Δ_6 Testosterone to Pure hSBP

hSBP (30 µg) was incubated overnight at 4°C with 20 nM [^{3}H]Δ_6-testosterone and then photolyzed in a reactor using a 450 Watt quartz jacketed mercury lamp. A Pyrex filter was used to prevent the transmission of light of wavelengths less than 300 nm. The hSBP was irradiated during four periods of 15 min, separated by periods of 10 min to avoid overheating.[6] SDS-polyacrylamide slab gel electrophoresis was performed with labeled hSBP, and the radioactive component was visualized by fluorography. The concentration of labeled hSBP was estimated to 2 µg/ml and 400,000 cpm.

Experimental Protocols for Studies of Endocytosis

Gold-labeled Protein

Sixty nanograms of hSBP-gold complex were added to each 100 µl aliquot of cell suspension containing 4 $\times$ 10^6 cells. Cells were further incubated for 2, 5, 15, and

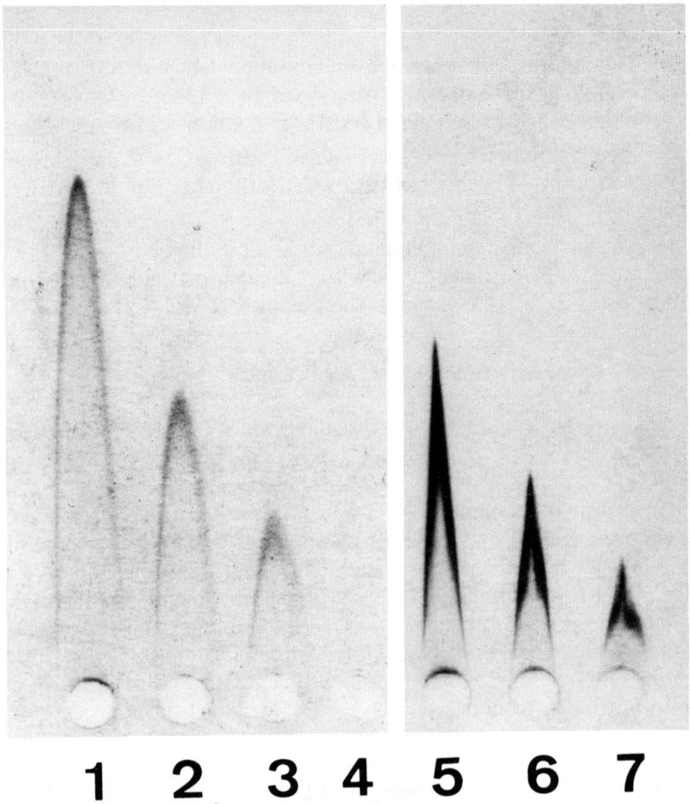

FIGURE 1. Rocketline immunoelectrophoresis against a polyclonal rabbit antihuman SBP serum. Standards (wells 1–3): **1** = undiluted (14 μg/ml), **2** = half-diluted (7 μg/ml), and **3** = quarter-diluted (3.5 μg/ml). hSBP-gold complex (wells 5–7): **5** = undiluted sample, **6–7** = half- and quarter-diluted; 5 μl in each well.

60 min in a shaking water bath at 34°C and then washed extensively in cooled RPMI before electron microscopy processing.

Radiolabeled Protein

Fifty microliters of buffer containing hSBP [^{3}H]Δ_6-testosterone (20,000 cpm) was added to each 100 μl aliquot of cell suspension containing 4 × 10^6 cells. Cells were further incubated for 2, 5, 15, and 60 min in a shaking water bath at 34°C and then washed extensively in cooled RPMI before electron microscope autoradiography processing.

In addition, 100 μl RPMI containing 4 × 10^6 epididymal spermatozoa were exposed to 50 μl radiolabeled hSBP (20,000 cpm) for 15 min at 34°C.

Inhibition Procedures

- To determine nonspecific binding excess unlabeled pure hSBP (1200 ng/30 μl) was added to germ cells or epididymal spermatozoa suspensions for 10 min before the gold-labeled or radiolabeled hSBP for another 15 min.
- The effect of calcium ions on the uptake of hSBP-gold was studied by incubating the cells in 100 μl PBS containing EDTA (400 μM), for 10 min before adding labeled hSBP (60 ng) for 15 min.
- To prevent endocytosis and enhance surface binding, the cell temperature was equilibrated at 4°C during the whole incubation with hSBP-gold complex (60 ng) or hSBP-[^{3}H]Δ_6-testosterone complex (66 ng/100 μl, 20,000 cpm) for 60 min.

Each of the above experiments was performed in triplicate.

Electron Microscopy

After completion of incubation, cells were washed twice in cooled culture medium before being fixed for 90 min in 2.5% glutaraldehyde/0.1 M cacodylate buffer, pH 7.4 at 4°C, and for 60 min in 5% glutaraldehyde in the same buffer. The samples were washed three times with the cacodylate buffer and postfixed in 1% osmium tetroxide at room temperature for one hour, washed in the buffer, and dehydrated in graded ethanols and embedded in Epon 812. Thin sections (80 nm thick) were stained with uranyl acetate and lead citrate and examined in a CM12 Philips electron microscope equipped with a LaB6 cathode.

Autoradiographic Method

Eighty nanometer sections were prepared for ultrastructural autoradiography using Ilford L4 nuclear emulsion, as already described.[3] The autoradiographs were developed with the Microdol-X Kodak developer to obtain filamentous grains 3 months after exposure at 4°C and examined on a CM12 Philips electron microscope.

Significance of the Labeling

hSBP-Gold

To detect the gold particles, examinations were performed at a minimum magnification of ×25,000. The surface binding and the uptake of protein-gold conjugates in the different organelles was determined by counting the incidence of at least 100 gold particles in the different organelles.

Radiolabeled hSBP

The silver grain distribution was analyzed at magnifications of ×6000 and ×8000. A cell was considered labeled as soon as at least one silver grain was located over it. The cell labeling according to maturation stage was determined by counting the incidence of at least 300 silver grains at either stage. The determination, at each maturation stage, of the labeled versus total cell number was restricted to 15 min, incubation at 34°C. The background grains were extremely few, calculated from silver grains counted over celloidin in random fields at some distance from the cells.

The labeling of different cellular organelles was analyzed by counting the incidence of at least 100 silver grains located over the organelles or within one half distance (HD) of them as previously described.[3,4,6] The HD used here was 145 nm, according to the emulsion thickness and the radioelement (tritium) used.[18]

Morphometric Analysis

The diameter of the germ cells, nuclei, endocytic organelles (coated pits and vesicles, early and late endosomes, multivesicular bodies, prelysosomes), as well as all distances between silver grains and the proximal organelles, were measured with the Philips computer measuring software integrated into the microscope.

RESULTS

Germ Cell Suspensions

Germ cell populations examined at light microscope level on smears contained a few spermatogonia (5.5 ± 0.59%), primary and secondary spermatocytes (34 ± 2.66%), round spermatids (25 ± 0.54%), elongated spermatids (21 ± 0.34%), residual bodies (10 ± 2.7%), spermatozoa (3 ± 0.8%), and a few identifiable Sertoli cell processes and migrating cells (2 ± 1.5%). At the electron microscope level, the different cell types were defined according to their known morphological characteristics.

Fine Structure of the Endocytic Apparatus in Monkey Germ Cells during Spermatogenesis

All the different germ cell types including spermatogonia and premeiotic spermatocytes as well as meiotic, postmeiotic and differentiated testicular spermatozoa, revealed the presence of indentations on their plasma membrane, showing a dense "fuzzy coat" on the cytoplasmic surface of the membrane (FIGS. 2–6). Their size was 95 ± 22 nm in diameter as the regular clathrin-coated pits. Internalized coated vesicles of 105 ± 12 nm in diameter were also seen in the peripheral cytoplasm in all spermatogenic cell types (FIGS. 3 & 4).

The mean number of these peripheral coated structures was of 3.7 ± 1.6 in spermatogonia sections, 4.3 ± 1.2 in spermatocytes I sections, 2.0 ± 0.6 in round spermatid sections and 3.5 ± 2.1 in elongated spermatid sections. Frequently, two coated structures appeared very near to each other (FIGS. 2–4). In maturation phase spermatids, the coated structures were seen along the head, in the midpiece and the neck region. In differentiated testicular spermatozoa and caput epididymal spermatozoa, coated structures were only observed in the midpiece cytoplasm (FIG. 5).

The disappearance of coated pits and subsequent coated vesicles surged after EDTA treatment. This induced the formation of large mats of coating material adherent to

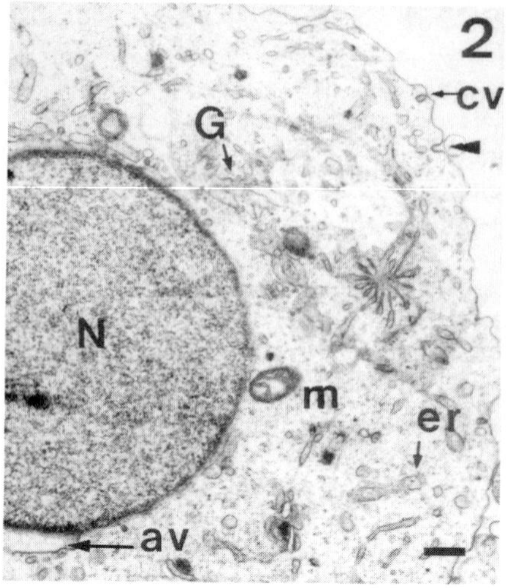
2
cv
G
N
m
er
av

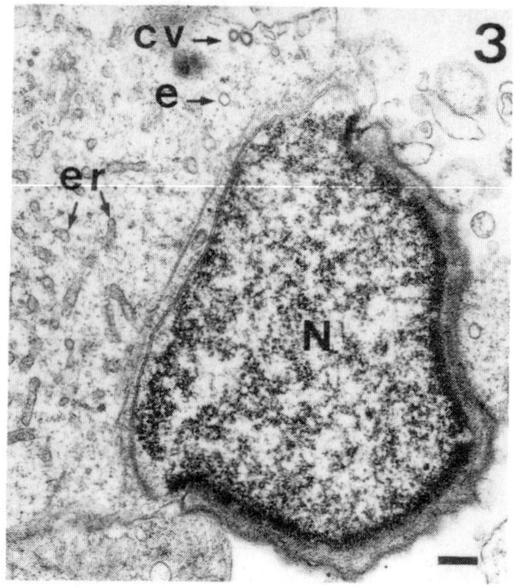
3
cv
e
er
N

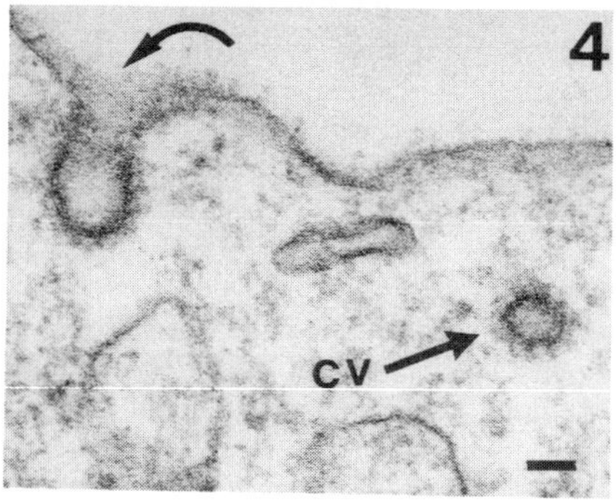
4
cv

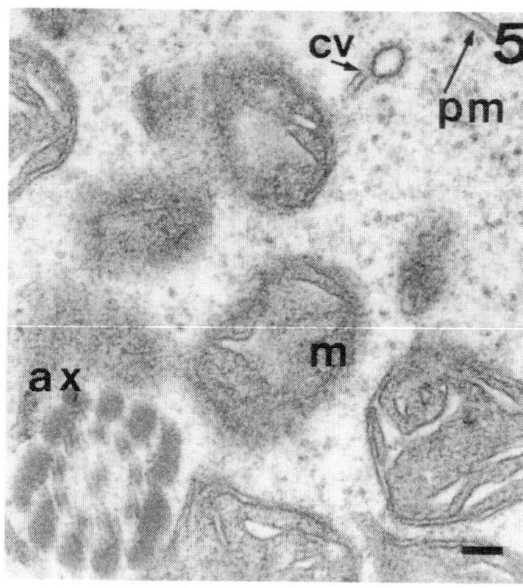
5
cv
pm
m
ax

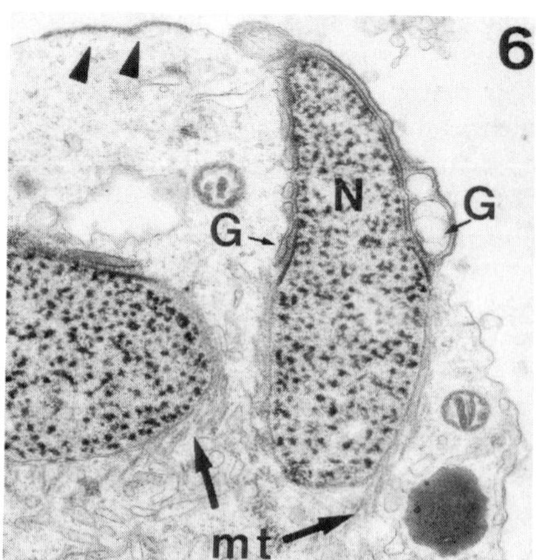
6
N
G
G
mt

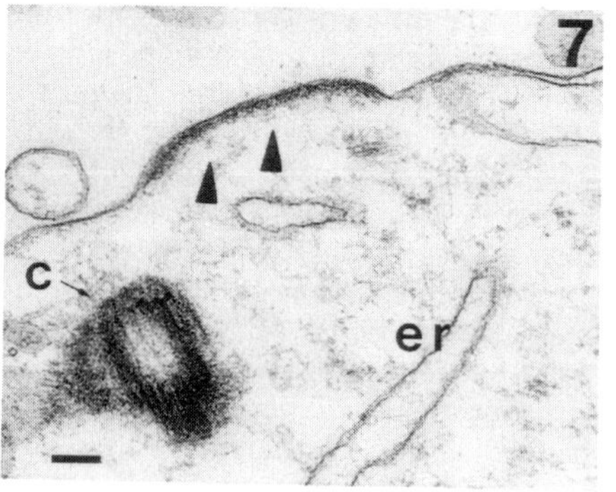
7
c
er

the endodomain of the plasma membrane, abnormal in shape (FIGS. 6 & 7). The cell membranes were not able to bud into internalized vesicles. This yields evidence of a mechanism highly sensitive to the lowering of the calcium concentration.

Some fusion-pictures of coated vesicles with early large multivesicular uncoated endosomes (1500 to 2300 nm in diameter) were encountered in the peripheral cytoplasm (FIG. 12) of spermatids. Small uncoated endocytic vesicles of 160 to 250 nm in diameter were observed in all spermatogenic cells, and more frequently in developing spermatids (acrosome phase), in the postacrosomal cytoplasm. In late spermatogenetic cells and in the residual bodies, late multivesicular endosomes (1500 ± 3200 nm in diameter) revealed a "mature" aspect including the appearance of dense heterogenous pre-lysosomal structures; they were mainly located in the infranuclear cytoplasm that will be detached from the mature spermatids. A well-developed Golgi apparatus was observed through its morphological changes during the spermiogenic events.

Pathways of Endocytosis of the Labeled Proteins

Endocytosis of both tracers, gold-hSBP complex and $[^3H]\Delta_6$-testosterone-hSBP complex occurred in germ cells lineage from spermatogenesis onset to epididymal maturation and was significantly decreased by incubation of the cells with excess unbound protein indicating that the mechanism of uptake could be receptor-mediated.

Gold-hSBP Complex

Most of the preparations showed the majority of markers to be dispersed as single particles. Approximately 20% of the particles were arranged in clusters of 2 to 5 particles especially when located at the cell surface.

FIGURES 2–5. Mechanically isolated, drug untreated monkey germ cells. **2.** Golgi phase spermatid. The plasma membrane presents numerous indentations, some are coated on their cytoplasmic face (*arrowhead*). One coated vesicle (CV) is pinching off the plasma membrane. Mitochondria (m) are grouped around the nucleus (N); av = acrosomal vesicle; G = Golgi; er = endoplasmic reticulum. bar = 0.5 μm. **3.** Acrosome phase spermatid. The peripheral infranuclear cytoplasm revealed the presence of two adjacent internalized coated vesicles of around 100 nm in diameter. N = nucleus; er = endoplasmic reticulum; e = endosome. bar = 0.34 μm. **4.** High magnification of a coated pit (*arrow*) and of a coated vesicle (CV) located at the periphery of a premeiotic spermatocyte (16 μm in diameter). These organelles display ultrastructural features and size of clathrin-coated structures described in other cell systems. bar = 0.06 μm. **5.** Midpiece of a testicular spermatozoa. In the cytoplasm surrounding the axoneme (Ax) and the mitochondrial sheath (m) a clathrin-like coated vesicle (100 nm in diameter) is visible; pm = plasma membrane. bar = 0.09 μm.

FIGURES 6 & 7. Mechanically isolated monkey germ cells treated with EDTA (400 μM/μl). **6.** Elongating spermatids following EDTA treatment. Coated pit invaginations and coated vesicles are no longer present at the cell surface. Conversely, cells were observed bearing an abnormal coating adherent material on the endodomain of their membrane (*arrowheads*). The periacrosomal Golgi saccules (G) exhibit a modified, dilated volume. N = condensing nucleus; mt = microtubules. bar = 0.53 μm. **7.** High magnification of an abnormally shaped and sized coated membrane in a premeiotic spermatocyte after EDTA treatment. Coat proteins were only assembled at the cell surface forming a protrusion of 950 nm length. A centriole (c) is present in the peripheral cytoplasm of this cell. er = endoplasmic reticulum. bar = 0.13 μm.

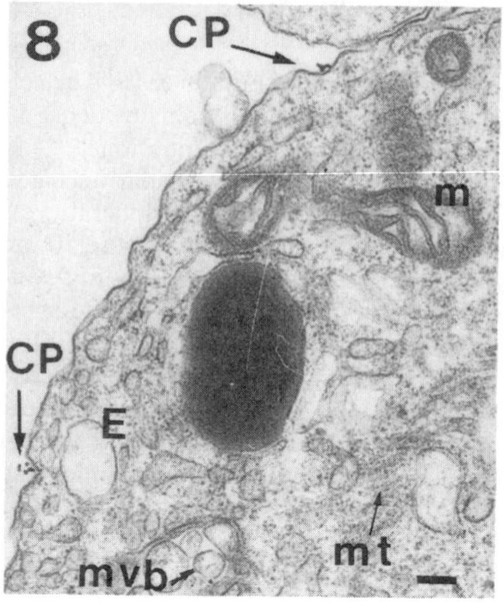
8
CP
m
CP
E
mt
mvb

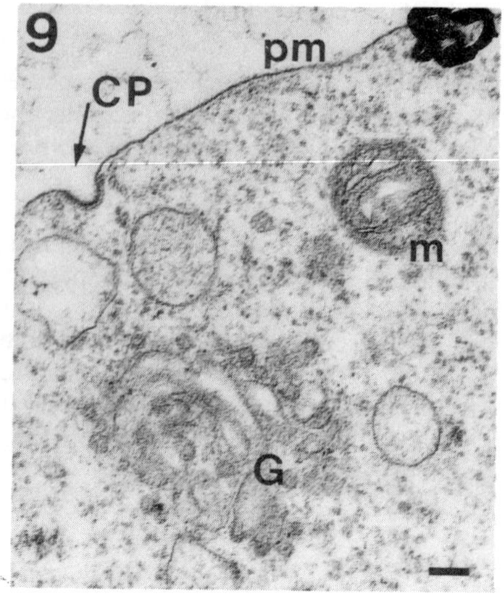
9
pm
CP
m
G

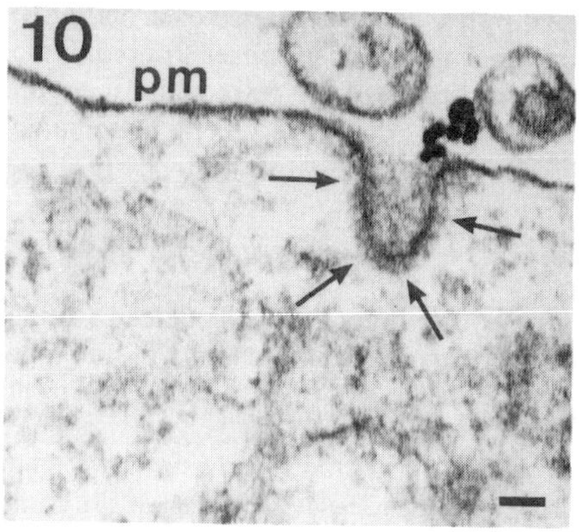
10
pm

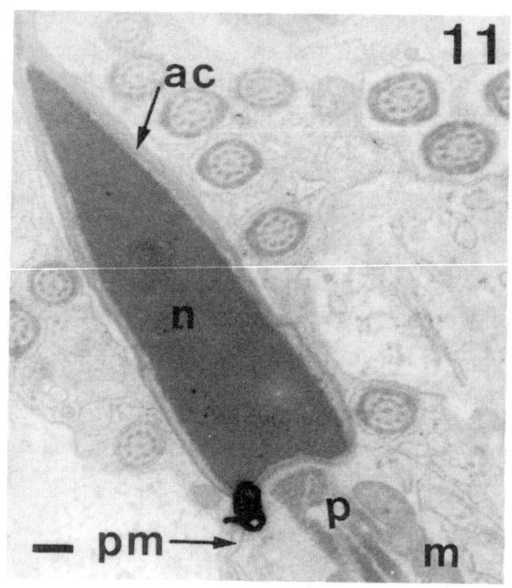
11
ac
n
p
pm
m

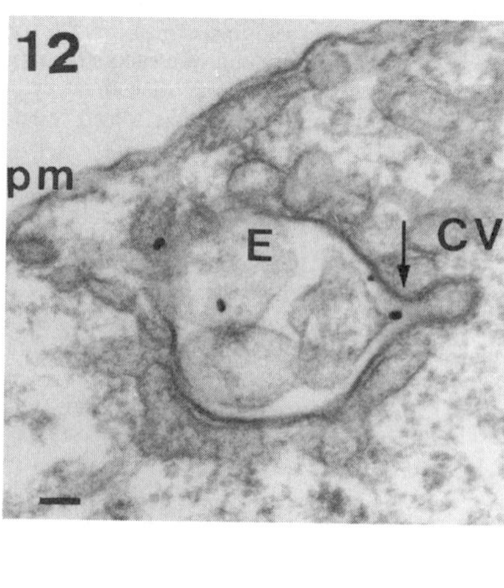
12
pm
E
CV

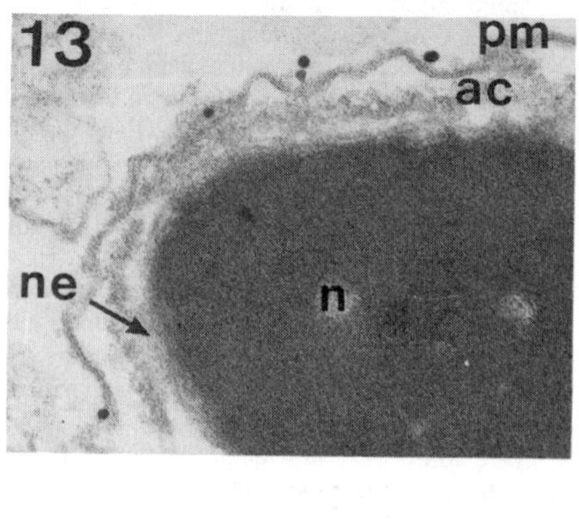
13
pm
ac
ne
n

The gold particles were found in all different types of Macaca germ cells, in pre- and postmeiotic cells, either attached to the plasma membrane or internalized within cytoplasmic organelles. The labeled ligand was initially bound to the plasma membrane predominantly in coated pits (FIGS. 8 & 10). Lowering the incubation temperature to 4°C for 60 min enhanced the plasma membrane bindings (FIG. 13).

At all experimental times, gold particles were seen internalized in coated vesicles, in peripheral uncoated endosomes (FIG. 12), in more internal late endosomes corresponding to multivesicular bodies (1336 ± 43 μm). In late spermatogenic cells, in late cytoplasts and residual bodies, gold particles were accumulated in prelysosomes (FIG. 17). Within the endocytic apparatus, gold particles were seen mainly attached, or close to the internal surface of the delimiting membrane.

No gold particle was observed over the nuclear area of the late spermatids or testicular or epididymal spermatozoa. On the contrary, in spermatogonia, spermatocytes and early spermatids, gold particles were detected bound to the nuclear envelope and/or the lamina and over nuclear area (FIGS. 14–16).

Except for the prelysosomal and nuclear localizations which were never observed before 15 min, our results did not show significant time-related differences in the labeling of the various organelles.

The higher labeling score (number of gold particles in one defined organelle) was recorded in the prelysosomes found in residual bodies (up to 30 grains per prelysosomal section at 60 min).

The incubation with excess unlabeled hSBP before gold-hSBP prevented the binding and internalization of the labeled ligand in most cell types and markedly decreased the number of labeled cells.

FIGURES 8, 10, 12, & 13. Mechanically isolated monkey germ cells treated with human SBP-gold (60 ng/100 μl). **8.** Representative examples of surface compartments with gold particles preferentially associated with coated pits (CP) in acrosome-phase spermatid following the incubation with gold-hSBP complex for 2 min at 34°C. An early uncoated endosome (E) and a multivesicular body (mvb) are visible in the peripheral cytoplasm as well as mitochondria (m). mt = microtubules of the manchette. bar = 0.26 μm. **10.** High magnification of gold particles bound to a clathrin-like coated pit (85 nm in diameter) in a primary spermatocyte 5 min after incubation with gold-hSBP complex. The arrows denote the typical architectural features of the cytoskeleton proteins on the cytoplasmic face of this pit. pm = plasma membrane. bar = 0.05 μm. **12.** Intracellular localization of the protein-gold complex in an acrosome phase spermatid 15 min after incubation at 34°C. In the peripheral cytoplasm, an obvious coated vesicle (CV) delivers its cargo (gold particle) by membrane-fusion with a multivesicular early uncoated endosome (E). The arrow denotes a gold particle leaving the coated vesicle and entering the uncoated endosomal structure. pm = plasma membrane. bar = 0.09 μm. **13.** Head of a late spermatid after incubation with gold-hSBP complex at 4°C for 60 min. Only surface labeling is observed. Gold particles are bound to numerous pits visible on the plasma membrane (pm). ac = acrosome; n = nucleus; ne = nuclear envelope. bar = 0.07 μm.

FIGURES 9 & 11. Mechanically isolated monkey germ cells treated with [^{3}H]Δ_6-testosterone-hSBP (66 ng/100μl, 20,000 cpm); ultra-thin sections were coated with Ilford L4 nuclear emulsion and treated with Microdol-X developer after three months exposure at 4°C). **9.** Silver grains are overlying the plasma membrane (pm) of a premeiotic spermatocyte after 2 min incubation at 34°C. One of the obvious clathrin-like coated pits (CP) of 98 nm diameter is present on this cell surface. m = mitochondria; G = Golgi complex. bar = 0.15 μm. **11.** Spermatozoa from the caput epididymis. Silver grains are localized at the junction of the head and the midpiece 15 min following the incubation with [^{3}H]Δ_6-testosterone-hSBP complex at 34°C. The grains overlay the plasma membrane (pm). Numerous unlabeled tails are seen in cluster. n = nucleus; ac = acrosome. Ax = axoneme; m = mitochondrial sheath; p = proximal centriole. bar = 0.4 μm.

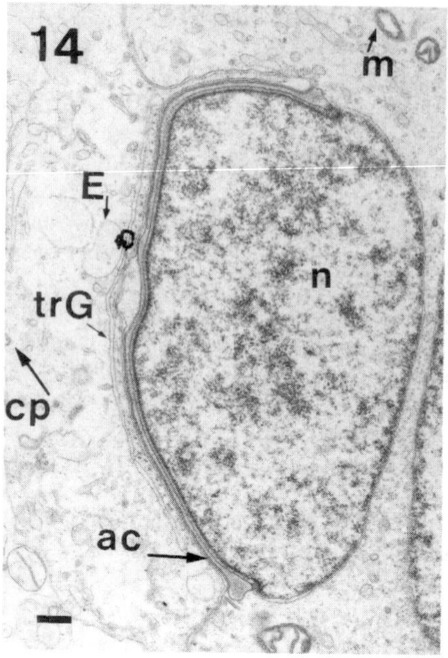
14
m
E
n
trG
cp
ac

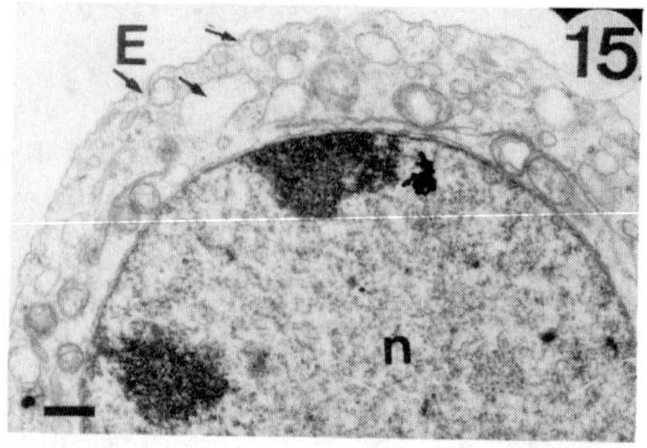
15
E
n

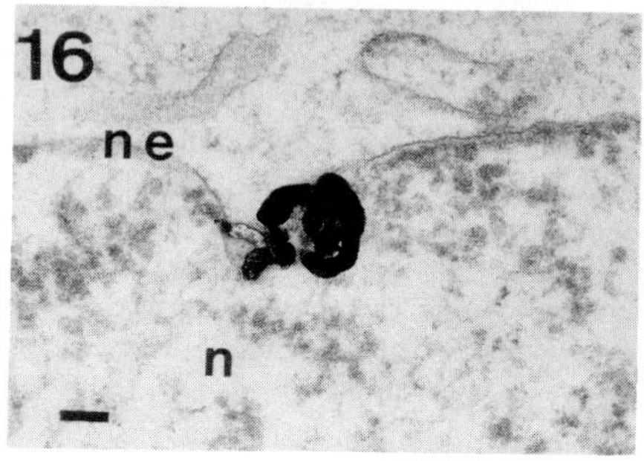
16
ne
n

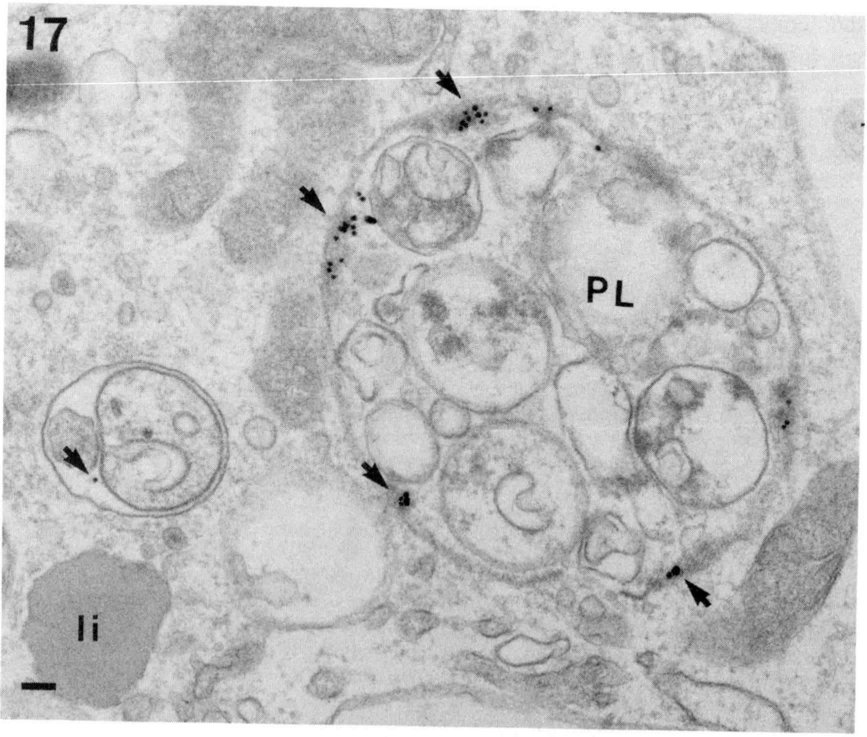
17
PL
li

The incubation with EDTA before gold-hSBP decreased the label of germ cells. In addition, numerous cells exhibited highly modified coated structures as already mentioned.

Radiolabeled hSBP-Steroid Complex

The behavior of [^{3}H]Δ_6-testosterone-hSBP was qualitatively similar to that observed with gold-hSBP, both at the cell surface and intracellularly.

At all maturation stages, silver grains were seen in association with the plasma membrane, overlying coated pits (FIG. 9) and subsequently internalized into endocytic vesicles and multivesicular bodies. In these endocytic related structures, the radiolabeled complex was markedly associated with the membrane component although the large size of the silver grains was somewhat masking the radioactive source, thus rendering the localization less evident than shown using gold-hSBP complex. Statistical analysis did not show significant differences in the silver grain counts according to time within the different parts of the endocytic apparatus whatever the cell type. In spermatogonia and spermatocytes, evidence was also obtained that the nucleus was labeled at 15 and 60 min (FIGS. 15 & 16). Some grains were also detected in Golgi saccules during the acrosome formation (FIG. 14).

When labeled, one organelle was usually associated with only one cluster of silver grains, except the prelysosomal multivesicular bodies present in the residual bodies, which were often associated with several clusters, suggesting a final accumulation step, and the nuclei of the spermatogonia and spermatocytes which shared up to 4 clusters.

As shown in TABLE 1, the labeled cells versus total cells ratio was negatively correlated to the maturation steps of the germinal lineage ($r = 0.942$), more than 50% of the spermatogonia and less than 6% of the epididymal spermatozoa being labeled.

Lowering the incubation temperature to 4°C for 60 min inhibited intracellular labeling.

FIGURES 14, 15, & 16. Intracellular localization of radiolabeled hSBP in mechanically isolated monkey germ cells treated with [^{3}H]Δ_6-testosterone-hSBP (66 ng/100 µl, 20,000 cpm); ultra-thin sections were coated with Ilford L4 nuclear emulsion and treated with Microdol-X developer after three months exposure at 4°C). **14.** Intracytoplasmic localization of silver grains in elongating spermatid following incubation for 30 min. The radioactive source is located on the peripheral membrane of a late endosome (E) which is in close association with trans sacculotubular elements (trG) of the Golgi apparatus; ac = acrosome; n = nucleus; m = mitochondria. A clathrin-like coated pit is denoted at the cell surface (*arrow*). bar = 0.47 µm. **15.** Intranuclear localization of silver grains in a type B spermatogonia 15 min after incubation with [^{3}H]Δ_6-testosterone-hSBP complex. The plasma membrane (pm) of this cell-type presents numerous indentions on the cell surface. In the cytoplasm, endocytic vesicles (E) of different size are visible. bar = 0.49 µm. **16.** Labeling of the nuclear envelope (ne) in a premeiotic spermatocyte 15 min after incubation with [^{3}H]Δ_6-testosterone-hSBP complex. n = nucleus. bar = 0.12 µm.

FIGURE 17. Intracellular localization of gold particles in mechanically isolated monkey germ cells treated with hSBP-gold (60 ng/100 µl) at 34°C. Gold particles (*arrows*) are accumulated in a residual body within a prelysosomal multivesicular structure (PL, 1440 nm in diameter) 60 min after the incubation with the gold-hSBP complex. The gold particles are notably attached to the peripheral membrane of this late endocytic organelle; one particle is also visible in smaller multivesicular structure. li = lipid; m = mitochondria. bar = 0.11 µm.

TABLE 1. Relative Labeling of the Different Germ Cells of *Macaca fascicularis* following Incubation in the Presence of the $[^3H]\Delta_6$-Testosterone-hSBP Complex at 34°C for 15 Minutes with or without Inhibiting Pretreatment

Cell Types	Radiolabeled hSBP	Unlabeled hSBP Pretreatment	EDTA Pretreatment
Spermatogonia	**56.4 ± 5.8**	5.3 ± 2.63 (a)	29.3 ± 7.08 (a)
Spermatocytes	**43.3 ± 8.89 (NS)**	4.4 ± 1.67 (b)	30 ± 4.18 (b)
Round spermatids	**32.6 ± 3.9 (B)**	4.6 ± 2.19 (a)	22.7 ± 5.69 (b)
Elongated spermatids	**34.12 ± 2.67 (NS)**	3.4 ± 1.67 (a)	19 ± 6.89 (a)
Testicular spermatozoa	**16.02 ± 5.68 (A)**	3.6 ± 2.7 (a)	8.6 ± 3.91 (b)
Epididymal spermatozoa	**5.9 ± 1.5 (A)**	0.8 ± 0.8 (a)	1.4 ± 1.14 (a)

A cell was considered labeled as soon as at least one silver grain was over it. Values (means ± SD from 3 scores for each experimental condition) are percentages of the number of labeled per total cells observed for each category. A significant negative correlation was found between the number of labeled cells and the steps of maturation. The linear regression correlation coefficient was calculated ($r = 0.942$) followed by a F test for the statistical assessment of differences between the different cell types ($F = 213.45$; significant, $p < 0.0001$).

Pretreatment with excess unlabeled hSBP significantly decreased the labeling level as did EDTA pretreatment. Values were statistically compared using a Student's *t* test. a = significant, $p < 0.001$; b = significant, $p < 0.05$.

Significant differences were estimated between the different germ cell categories using a Student's *t* test. **A** = significant, $p < 0.001$; **B** = significant, $p < 0.05$; **NS** = not significant.

Pretreatment with excess unlabeled hSBP significantly decreased the labeling level as also did EDTA pretreatment (TABLE 1).

DISCUSSION

Since the demonstration by Steinberger[19] that rat germ cells expressed binding sites for rat ABP and since the detection by David[12] of immunoreactive sites to anti-rabbit SBP antibodies in the midpiece of the rabbit spermatozoa it became of interest to study the possible interactions between sex steroid-binding proteins in general and the germ cell lineage.

Our *in vitro* study clearly showed that purified hSBP, either $[^3H]\Delta_6$-testosterone-photoaffinity labeled or colloidal gold labeled, not only bound to macaca germ cell plasma membrane when infused in the culture medium but, moreover, was rapidly internalized through coated pits and coated vesicles which are highly specialized structures of endocytosis. Germ cells have been occasionally shown to be able to exert fluid and/or adsorptive endocytosis through uncoated non-specific vesicles[20-24] and recently transferrin was demonstrated to enter rat spermatogonia, spermatocytes and young spermatids,[25] but, to our knowledge, it is the first report of the existence of coated structures in germ cells. This finding could be of wider significance since such structures are also present in rat germ cells and in rabbit germ cells (manuscript in preparation).

Coated membranes play a central role in endocytosis.[26,27] Observations on various tissues have confirmed that endocytosis of macromolecules involves coated pit formation, coated vesicle budding, coat disassembly, and component recycling.[28] Specific receptors in the membrane mediate the uptake of many different macromolecules by concentrating them in coated pits and vesicles.[26,27]

In our *in vitro* conditions, the peglike coated structures shown here are morphologically similar to the clathrin-coated structures well characterized in numerous different cells.[26-29] They also functioned as the clathrin-coated structures could be expected to do, concentrating the labeled ligand at the sites of internalization. The use of colloidal gold as label, in providing unequivocal ultrastructural detection, contrary to the autohistographic method for which the radiation dispersion as well as the masking effect of the oversized silver grains, have to be taken into account, allowed to clearly show that, from the very first step of binding, hSBP is concentrated exclusively within coated structures. Moreover, our results revealed the coincidence between the highest "labeled cells/total cells" ratio and the highest "coated structures/cell section" score, both corresponding to spermatogonia and spermatocytes I. The polymerization of the individual clathrin triskelions into cages, which is responsible for the internalization onset, is highly dependent upon the presence of calcium ions.[30] After lowering the calcium concentration by EDTA pretreatment, germ cells, at any maturation stage, were almost devoid of coated structures. In the same way EDTA pretreatment was found to reduce the "labeled cells/total cells" ratio. Taken together with the fact that labeled hSBP binding is inhibited in the presence of excess unlabeled hSBP, this leads to the conclusion that the binding of hSBP to the germ cell plasma membrane and its subsequent internalization is dependent on clathrin-like coated structures and suggests a receptor-mediated endocytosis. Human sex steroid-binding protein was already demonstrated to interact with plasma membrane of human steroid target tissues[31-37] and to enter the human carcinoma cell line MCF7 after *in vitro* incubation with the pure protein.[1] We have recently provided evidence that the human sex steroid–binding protein was also able to bind the cell surface of the monkey epididymal cells and to enter these cells by specific endocytosis.[6]

Although the finding that hSBP could be internalized into germ cells is consistent with the immunoreactive SBP found previously in the human or monkey testis,[1,38] one cannot exclude that the immunoreactive molecule detected in these earlier studies was in fact ABP, or a closely related molecule, since human SBP and monkey ABP are antigenically related and since rabbit antiserum raised to hSBP cross-reacts with mABP.[39] Furthermore, because of the intimate relation between Sertoli cell lineage and germ cell lineage,[20,40,41] at least above the blood testis barrier, testicular ABP would seem to be a better candidate for an interaction with germ cells than plasma extracted SBP used in the present *in vitro* study. Indeed, Steinberger *et al.*[19] have biochemically demonstrated rABP binding activity in rat pachytene spermatocytes, and, more recently, we have been able to show rat ABP endocytosis within spermatocytes, and round and elongated spermatids.[42] In any case, ABP and SBP of different species and tissue origin share such physicochemical, immunological as well as cDNA sequence similarities,[43-48] that it would not be surprising if they could partly express common cytophysiological behavior. Therefore it can be suggested that, in our *in vitro* experiments, hSBP would have functioned as an alternative tracer for *in situ* ABP behavior, or for the behavior of another not yet defined steroid-binding protein. Binding competition experiments will allow this question to be answered.

It is well-established that spermatogenesis in mammals is totally dependent upon testosterone; however the molecular mechanisms by which androgens act in the testis remain to be elucidated. Moreover, direct or indirect effect of steroids on germ cells has been the matter of controversy[49–51] as well as the presence of androgen receptors in germ cell nuclei.[52,53]

Testosterone is needed for onset of spermatogenesis (spermatogonia level) and for acrosome formation (spermiogenesis). In different species, a high concentration of testosterone has been reported in the zone with spermatogonia as well as an important relationship between androgens and the last step of spermiogenesis.[54,55] However, recent intratesticular testosterone measurements provided no correlation with a specific stage of the spermatogenic cycle.[56]

Keeping *et al.*[57] demonstrated that ABP and SBP exhibited independent modifications during the various stages of sexual development in the Macaca. But the highest level of circulating SBP as well as the testicular ABP is respectively the prepubertal and the pubertal stage which is consistent with a role for these proteins in the process of testicular maturation. Moreover, Sjögren[58] recently showed that, in rat testes, a major increase in ABP-mRNA just precedes the major development of the spermatogenesis at the pubertal stage.

It can therefore be suggested that steroid-binding proteins play a role locally during spermatogenesis either in concentrating steroids at the germ cell surface as deduced from results of others,[59] or in transporting them across the plasma membrane as deduced from our present study. Interestingly, although all spermatogenic monkey germ cells were able to endocytose hSBP, spermatogonia and premeiotic spermatocytes were the more frequently labeled cells, which could reflect an important requirement of steroids for meiosis onset. In addition, specifically at these two stages, the nuclear compartment displayed, from 15 to 60 min, the highest silver grain count. In elongated spermatids nuclei were not labeled any more and after spermiogenesis completion the proportion of labeled cells dramatically decreased as shown on epididymal spermatozoa. Nevertheless, at that step, hSBP internalization was not totally absent but seemed restricted to the mid-piece and postacrosomal region which is consistent with the earlier immunodetection studies.[12]

Another salient feature consisted in the accumulation of both forms of labeled SBP in the multivesicular bodies of the residual bodies. As stressed by Morales,[60] these organelles do not contain hydrolytical lysosomal enzymes and cannot be held as final catabolic structures. Most residual bodies when detached from the mature spermatid are specifically phagocytosed by Sertoli cells.[61] Interestingly, cocultures of residual bodies together with Sertoli cells have been demonstrated to increase the release of ABP in the culture medium.[62] This could be attributed to a stimulating effect of residual bodies on ABP synthesis by Sertoli cells. In view of our findings, the possibility of the recycling of the steroid-binding protein through residual body phagocytosis has also to be considered.

In conclusion, monkey germ cells are equipped with a specialized endocytic apparatus involving clathrin-like coated pits and vesicles which actively internalize hSBP. Although we present morphological evidence for specificity in our *in vitro* model, it cannot be assumed that, within the seminiferous tubule, SBP must be the natural ligand concerned by this receptor-mediated endocytosis. It cannot also be excluded that the physiologic ligand to be internalized could act directly at the germ cell metabolic level apart from serving as steroid transmembrane carrier.

These two important points need further investigation.

SUMMARY

We investigate in this study the hypothesis of human sex steroid–binding protein hSBP internalization into germ cells in a primate model. Human SBP was purified from late-pregnancy serum and labeled either with colloidal gold particles (18 nm) or with $[^3H]\Delta_6$-testosterone by photoaffinity treatment. The germ cells were isolated from sexually mature monkey testis or caput epididymis (*Macaca fascicularis*) by mechanical means and cell suspensions (4×10^6 per 100 μl culture medium) were incubated in presence of hSBP-gold complex (60 ng/100 μl) or hSBP-$[^3H]\Delta_6$-testosterone complex (66 ng/100 μl, 20,000 cpm) for 2, 5, 15, 45, and 60 min. The samples were processed for electron microscopy followed by autoradiographic treatment for the radiolabeled samples.

Localization of the label occurred over the whole germ cell lineage whichever tracer was used. Spermatogonia, spermatocytes, spermatids, testicular and epididymal spermatozoa exhibited specific binding sites over the plasma membrane associated with clathrin-like coated pits and vesicles. At 34°C, intracellular localization of the labeled ligand was found within coated vesicles, in early and late endosomes. In addition, in early spermatogenic cells, labeled ligand was detected in the nuclei and/or associated with the nuclear envelope whereas in late spermatids and residual bodies, the labeling was accumulated in multivesicular, prelysosomal structures. Quantitative analysis of the "labeled cells/total cells" ratio exhibited a negative correlation to the maturation steps, epididymal spermatozoa being the least labeled. The cellular distribution is similar with one or the other protein in the same spermatogenic cells. Unlabeled hSBP treatment prior to labeled hSBP reduced significantly the internalization. Lowering the temperature to 4°C prevented endocytosis and enhanced membrane binding. EDTA pretreatment strongly decreased hSBP internalization and modified the early endocytic steps, namely, the pinching off of the coated vesicles. It is concluded that monkey germ cells are able to internalize the human sex steroid-binding protein through specific endocytic organelles. This endocytosis leads to the labeling of the nuclei in the early spermatogenic cells and of the multivesicular bodies in the late germ cells. This strongly suggests that steroid-binding proteins may be required for spermatogenesis in acting at the germ cell lineage level either by themselves or by serving as steroid transmembrane carriers.

ACKNOWLEDGMENTS

The authors express their gratitude to J. D. Gradeler and J. Poirson for technical assistance, and to Professors M. Gantois, A. Duprez, and F. Plenat for electron microscope and ultramicrotome facilities.

REFERENCES

1. BORDIN, S. & P. H. PETRA. 1980. Immunochemical localization of the sex steroid-binding-protein of plasma in tissues of the adult monkey *Macaca nemestrina*. Proc. Natl. Acad. Sci. USA **77**: 5678–5682.
2. GERARD, A., H. GERARD, G. GRIGNON, J. L. GUEANT, J. KHANFRI, S. FREMONT & J. P. NICOLAS.

1986. Isolation of androgen binding protein from rat testis by HPLC and uptake study of the iodinated molecule by rat epididymis using electron microscope autoradiography. *In* Binding Proteins of Steroid Hormones. M. G. Forest & M. Pugeat, Eds. **149:** 647. John Libbey. London/Paris.
3. GERARD, A., J. KHANFRI, J. L. GUEANT, S. FREMONT & J. P. NICOLAS. 1988a. Electron microscope radioautographic evidence of *in vivo* androgen-binding protein internalization in the rat epididymis principal cells. Endocrinology **122:** 1297–1307.
4. GERARD, H., J. L. GUEANT, A. GERARD, A. EL HARATE, S. FREMONT, J. P. NICOLAS & G. GRIGNON. 1988b. L'endocytose de l'androgen-binding protein (ABP) par les cellules principales de l'épididyme chez le rat. Reprod. Nutr. Dev. **28:** 1257–1266.
5. GERARD, A. , A. EL HARATE, J. L. GUEANT, S. FREMONT, G. GRIGNON & H. GERARD. 1988c. Clues for receptor mediated endocytosis of intraluminal injected ABP in the rat: A TEM radioautographic study. Steroids **52:** 347–349.
6. GERARD, A., M. EGLOFF, H. GERARD, A. EL HARATE, M. DOMINGO, J. L. GUEANT, C. D. DANG & H. DEGRELLE. 1990. Internalization of human sex steroid-binding protein in the monkey epididymis. J. Mol. Endocrinol. **5:** 239–251.
7. ERICSSON, R. I., J. C. CORNETTE & D. A. BUTTALA. 1967. Binding of sex steroids to rabbit sperm. Acta Endocrinol. **56:** 424–432.
8. WEBSTER, R. C. & R. H. FOOTE. 1972. Ouabain effect on bovine spermatozoan mobility and testosterone binding. Proc. Soc. Exp. Biol. Med. **141:** 26–30.
9. KOEHLER, J. K., J. A. BROWN & P. H. PETRA. 1984. Localization of steroid-binding protein in rabbit spermatozoa. Anat. Rec. **208:** 94A (abstract).
10. FRANKEL, A. I., J. C. CHAPMAN & W. W. WRIGHT. 1989. The equivocal presence of nuclear androgen-binding proteins in mammalian spermatids and spermatozoa. J. Steroid Biochem. **33:** 71–79.
11. CHENG, C. Y., B. BOETCHER, R. J. ROSE, D. J. KAY & H. R. TINNENBERG. 1981. The binding of sex steroids to human spermatozoa. An autoradiographic study. Int. J. Androl. **4:** 1–17.
12. DAVID, G. F. X., J. K. KOEHLER, J. A. BROWN, P. H. PETRA & A. G. FARR. 1985. Light and electron microscopic studies on the localization of steroid-binding protein (SBP) in rabbit spermatozoa. Biol. Reprod. **33:** 503–514.
13. MORVAY, J. & A. TRAUB. 1984. Determination of sex hormone-binding globulin in human semen by selective ammonium sulphate precipitation. Andrologia **16:** 299–302.
14. DANG, D. C. 1977. Absence of seasonal variation in the length of the menstrual cycle and the fertility of the crab-eating macaque (*Macaca fascicularis*) raised under natural daylight ratio. Ann. Biol. Anim. Biochem. Reprod. **8:** 1–7.
15. EGLOFF, M., R. VRANCKX, J. TARDIVEL-LACOMBE & H. DEGRELLE. 1981. Immunochemical characterization and quantitation of human sex steroid-binding plasma protein. Steroids **37:** 455–462.
16. PETRA, P. H., S. KUMAR, R. HAYES, L. H. ERICSSON & K. TITANI. 1986a. Molecular organization of the sex steroid-binding protein (SBP) of human plasma. J. Steroid Biochem. **11:** 245–252.
17. FRENS, G. 1973. Controlled nucleation for the regulation of the particle size in monodisperse gold suspension. Nature (Phys. Sci.) **241:** 20–22.
18. SALPETER, M. M., F. A. MCHENRY & E. E. SALPETER. 1978. Resolution in electron microscope autoradiography. IV. Application to analysis of autoradiographs. J. Cell Biol. **76:** 127–130.
19. STEINBERGER, A., R. R. DIGHE & J. DIAZ. 1984. Testicular peptides and their endocrine and paracrine functions. Arch. Biol. Med. Exp. **17:** 267–271.
20. FAWCETT, D. W. 1974. Interactions between Sertoli cells and germ cells. *In* Male Fertility and Sterility. R. E. Mancini & L. Martini, Eds.: 13–36. Academic Press. London.
21. SOARES-PESSOA, J. F. & J. F. DAVID-FERREIRA. 1980. Bidirectional transport of horseradish peroxidase by the rat Sertoli cells. An *in vitro* study. Biol. Cell **39:** 301–304.
22. HINTON, B. T. & D. A. KEEFER. 1983. Evidence for protein absorption from the lumen of the seminiferous tubule and rete of the rat testis. Cell Tissue Res. **230:** 367–375.
23. SEGRETAIN, D. & C. ROUSSEL. 1988. Endocytic origin for periaxonemal vesicles along the flagellum during mouse spermiogenesis. Gam. Res. **21:** 451–463.
24. SEGRETAIN, D. 1989. Endocytosis in spermatids during spermiogenesis of the mouse. Biol. Cell **67:** 289–298.
25. SEGRETAIN, D., M. EGLOFF, C. PINEAU, N. GERARD, M. DOMINGO, B. DEGROSSAS & B. JEGOU.

1990. Endocytose de la transferrine par les cellules germinales de rat. IXe Congress Morphol. Sci. 133 (Abstract).
26. Goldstein, J. L., M. S. Brown, R. G. W. Anderson, D. W. Russel & W. J. Schneider. 1985. Receptor-mediated endocytosis: Concepts emerging from the LDL receptor system. Ann. Rev. Cell Biol. **1:** 1–39.
27. Pearse, B. M. F. & M. S. Bretscher. 1981. Ann. Rev. Biochem. **50:** 85.
28. Pearse, B. M. F. & R. A. Crowther. 1987. Structure and assembly of coated vesicles. Ann. Rev. Biophys. Chem. **16:** 49–68.
29. Goldstein, J. L., R. G. W. Anderson & M. S. Brown. 1979. Coated pits, coated vesicles, and receptor-mediated endocytosis. Nature **279:** 679–685.
30. Irace, G., R. E. Lippoldt, H. Edelhoch & P. K. Nandi. 1982. Properties of clathrin coat structures. Biochemistry **9:** 5764–5769.
31. Tardivel-Lacombe, J., M. Egloff, A. Mazabraud & H. Degrelle. 1984. Immunohistochemical detection of the sex steroid-binding plasma protein in human mammary carcinoma cells. Biochem. Biophys. Res. Commun. **118:** 488–494.
32. Strel'chyonok, O. A., G. V. Avvakumov & L. I. Survilo. 1984. A recognition system for sex hormone-binding protein-estradiol complex in human decidual endometrium plasma membrane. Biochim. Biophys. Acta **802:** 459–466.
33. Hryb, D. J., M. S. Khan & W. Rosner. 1985. Testosterone-estradiol-binding globulin binds to human prostatic cell membranes. Biochem. Biophys. Res. Commun. **128:** 432–440.
34. Hryb, D. J., M. S. Khan, N. A. Romas & R. W. Rosner. 1989. Solubilization and partial characterization of the sex hormone-binding globulin receptor from human prostate. J. Biol. Chem. **264:** 5378–5383.
35. Hryb, D. J., M. S. Khan, N. A. Romas & R. W. Rosner. 1990. The control of the interaction of sex hormone-binding globulin with its receptor by steroid hormones. J. Biol. Chem. **265:** 6048–6054.
36. Rosner, W. 1990. The functions of corticosteroid-binding globulin and sex hormone-binding globulin: recent advances. Endocr. Rev. **11(1):** 80–91.
37. Strel'chyonok, O. A. & G. V. Avvakumov. 1990. Specific steroid-binding glycoproteins of human blood plasma: Novel data on their structure and function. J. Steroid Biochem. **35:** 519–534.
38. Egloff, M., E. Vendrely, J. Tardivel-Lacombe, J. P. Dadoune & H. Degrelle. 1982. Etude immunohistochimique du testicule et de l'épididyme humains à l'aide d'un antiserum monospécifique dirigé contre la proteine plasmatique liant les hormones sexuelles. C. R. Acad. Sci. (Paris) **295:** 107–111.
39. Keeping, H. S., S. J. Winters & P. Troen. 1985. Identification of androgen-binding protein from testis cytosol and Sertoli cell culture medium of the cynomolgus monkey, Macaca fascicularis. Endocrinology **117(4):** 1521–1529.
40. Russel, L. D. 1980. Sertoli-germ cell interrelations: A review. Gamete Res. **3:** 179–202.
41. Ziparo, E., R. Geremia, M. A. Russo & M. Stefanini. 1980. Surface interaction in vitro between Sertoli cells and germ cells of different stages of spermatogenesis. Amer. J. Anat. **159:** 385–388.
42. Gerard, H., A. En Nya, J. L. Gueant, W. Anwar, S. Fremont & A. Gerard. 1989. Regards sur la Biochimie **3:** 9 (Abstract).
43. Petra, P. H., P. C. Namkung, D. F. Senear, D. A. McCrae, K. W. Rousslang, D. C. Teller & J. B. A. Ross. 1986. Molecular characterization of the sex steroid-binding protein (SBP) of plasma. Re-examination of rabbit SBP and comparison with the human, macaque and baboon proteins. J. Steroid Biochem. **25:** 191–200.
44. Joseph, D. R., S. H. Hall & F. S. French. 1987. Rat androgen-binding protein: Evidence for identical subunits and amino acid sequence homology with human sex hormone-binding globulin. Proc. Natl. Acad. Sci. USA. **84:** 4339–4343.
45. Joseph, D. R., S. H. Hall, M. Conti & F. S. French. 1988. The gene structure of rat androgen-binding protein: Identification of potential regulatory deoxyribonucleic acid elements of a follicle-stimulating hormone regulated protein. Mol. Endocrinol. **2:** 3–13.
46. Reventos, J., G. L. Hammond, A. Crozat, D. E. Brooks, G. L. Gunsalus, C. W. Bardin & N. A. Musto. 1988. Hormonal regulation of rat androgen-binding protein (ABP) messenger ribonucleic acid and homology of human testosterone-estradiol-binding globulin and ABP complementary desoxyribonucleic acids. Mol. Endocrinol. **2:** 125–132.

47. HAMMOND, G. L., D. A. UNDERHILL, H. M. RYKSE & C. L. SMITH. 1989. The human sex hormone-binding globulin gene contains exons for androgen-binding protein and two other testicular messengers. Mol. Endocrinol. **3:** 1869–1876.
48. HAMMOND, G. L. 1990. Expression of the SHBG/ABP gene in the human testis: Identification of novel testicular proteins. 6th European Workshop on Molecular and Cellular Endocrinology of the Testis. Mariehamn, 1990 (Abstract book, p2).
49. FRITZ, I. B. 1978. *In* Biochemical actions of hormones. G. Litwack, Ed. **5:** 249. Academic Press. New York.
50. RITZEN, E. M., V. HANSSON & F. S. FRENCH. 1981. The Sertoli cell. *In* The Testis. H. Burger & D. de Kretser, Eds.: 172–194. Raven Press, New York.
51. PARVINEN, M., K. M. VIHKO & J. TOPARI. 1984. Interaction between Sertoli and germinal cells in the testis. *In* Recent progress in Cellular Endocrinology of the Testis. J. M. Saez, M. G. Forest, J. Dazord & J. Bertrand, Eds. **123:** 387–406. John Libbey. London, Paris.
52. GROOTEGOED, J. A., M. J. PETERS, E. MULDER, F. F. G. ROMMERTS & H. J. VAN DER MOLEN. 1977. Absence of nuclear androgen receptor in isolated germinal cells of rat testis. Mol. Cell. Endocrinol. **9:** 159–167.
53. WRIGHT, W. W. & A. I. FRANKEL. 1979. Characterization of the androgen receptor in nuclei of seminiferous tubules of the mature male rat based upon radioimmunoassay of endogenous levels of bound testosterone. Endocrinology **104:** 1580–1587.
54. SOURDAINE, P., D. H. GARNIER & B. JEGOU. 1990. The adult dogfish testis: A model to study stage-dependent changes in steroid levels during spermatogenesis. J. Mol. Endocrinol. **127:** 451–460.
55. OJEIFO, J. S. BYERS & M. DYM. 1988. *In vitro* effects of Sertoli cell secreted proteins on testosterone production by highly purified Leydig cells. Biol. Reprod. **38(1):** 185.
56. BARTLETT, J. M. S., G. F. WEINBAUER & E. NIESCHLAG. 1989. Quantitative analysis of germ cell numbers and relation to intratesticular testosterone following vitamin A-induced synchronization of spermatogenesis in the rat. J. Endocrinol. **123:** 403–412.
57. KEEPING, H. S., S. J. WINTERS & P. TROEN. 1987. Age-dependent differences in testicular and epididymal androgen-binding protein in the cynomolgus monkey, *Macaca fascicularis.* Ann. N. Y. Acad. Sci. **513:** 455–457.
58. KEEPING, H. S., S. J. WINTERS, B. ATTARDI & P. TROEN. 1990. Developmental changes in testicular inhibin and androgen-binding protein during sexual maturation in the cynomolgus monkey, *Macaca fascicularis*. Endocrinology **126(6):** 2858–2867.
59. SJÖGREN, D., B. OLLARS, M. RITZEN & L. HÄGENAS. 1990. Ontogeny of mRNA for testicular androgen-binding protein and cellular retinol-binding protein in the rat. 6th European Workshop on Molecular and Cellular Endocrinology of the Testis, Mariehamn, 1990 (Abstract book, F7).
60. CAMPO, S., E. PELLIZARI, S. CIGORRAGA, C. MONTEAGUDO, G. NICOLAU & M. A. RIVAROLA. 1982. Androgen-binding to subcellular particles of rat testis. J. Steroid Biochem. **17:** 165–173.
61. MORALES, C. & Y. CLERMONT. 1990. Endocytosis in Sertoli cells. IXe Congress Morphol. Sci. Nancy (Abstract).
62. CLERMONT, Y., C. MORALES & L. HERMO. 1987. Endocytic activities of Sertoli cells in the rat. Ann. N. Y. Acad. Sci. **513:** 1–15.
63. LE MAGUERESSE, B., F. LE GAC, M. LOIR & B. JEGOU. 1986. Stimulation of rat Sertoli cell secretory activity *in vitro* by germ cells and residual bodies. J. Reprod. Fertil. **77:** 489–498.

First Expression of Protamine Message in Trout Testis[a]

NADINE A. SENIUK[b,d] AND WILLIAM G. TATTON[b,c]

[b] *Centre for Research in Neurodegenerative Diseases*
[c] *Department of Physiology*
University of Toronto
Toronto, Ontario, Canada M5S 1A8

PAUL D. CANNON, ANTHONY T. GARBER,
AND GORDON H. DIXON

Department of Medical Biochemistry
University of Calgary
Calgary, Alberta, Canada T2N 4N1

INTRODUCTION

The protamines, a unique set of sperm-specific nuclear proteins, are synthesized in the testis during the terminal stage of spermatogenesis. Primordial stem cells undergo repeated mitotic divisions to create a pool of spermatogonial cells which then become committed to meiosis as spermatogonia and subsequently as primary spermatocytes. Two meiotic divisions follow, giving rise to secondary spermatocytes and then spermatids.[1,2] The mRNA for protamine is translated in spermatids which then undergo nuclear condensation, loss of their cytoplasm and the development of a flagellum to become spermatozoa.

Earlier studies of rainbow trout spermatogenesis sought to determine whether protamine messenger RNA (mRNA) is synthesized immediately prior to its translation, or whether protamine synthesis depends upon utilization of pre-existing mRNA templates. Separation of different trout testis cell types by gravity sedimentation with subsequent solution hybridization of the RNA extracts from each cell population with ^{3}H-DNA probes[3] complementary to protamine mRNA,[4] indicated that protamine message sequences could be detected in the cell sap of primary spermatocytes. It was proposed therefore that these protamine mRNAs were later bound to polysomes at the spermatid stage[5] in a translationally active state[6] so that protamine synthesis could begin. Protamine polypeptides do not accumulate in the cell cytoplasm but are monophosphorylated[2] and transported into the spermatid nucleus.[7]

In contrast to the studies in rainbow trout, subsequent investigations of protamine

[a] The research upon which this paper is based was supported by a Medical Research Council of Canada grant numbers MA5218 and MT6078. P. D. C. and A. T. G. were supported by the Alberta Heritage Foundation for Medical Research.

[d] Address correspondence to Dr. Seniuk at the Centre for Research in Neurodegenerative Diseases, Tanz Building, 6 Queen's Park Cr. W., University of Toronto, Toronto, Ontario, Canada M5S 1A8.

transcription during spermatogenesis of mouse,[8] rat,[9] and rooster[10] have detected protamine mRNAs only in post-meiotic cell-types, that is spermatids. These findings may reflect a real difference in the timing of protamine mRNA expression in trout as opposed to other species but could also be due to differences in the results of the sedimentation separation. Cross contamination with cells from adjacent sedimentation velocity peaks can occur. Hence, it would be valuable to use *in situ* hybridization to examine the cytoplasm of different intact testis cells for protamine mRNA. Yet, given the small size of the terminal spermatogenic cells (*i.e.*, spermatocytes and spermatids are four to five microns in diameter with a rim of cytoplasm about one to one and one-half microns wide), the resolution at the light microscope level of ^{35}S- or ^{32}P-labeled hybridization probes was considered unlikely to unequivocally localize protamine mRNA to a specific cell type given the degree of grain scatter. Alternately, hybridization studies at the electron microscope level, although providing for adequate resolution, make it difficult to scan large volumes of testis for possible variations in protamine mRNA expression. We therefore chose an *in situ* hybridization method employing biotin-UTP–labeled RNA probes suitable to detect protamine RNA within small subcellular volumes at the light microscope level. The *in situ* hybridizations detected protamine mRNA in the cytoplasm of spermatids but not in spermatogonia or spermatocytes.

METHODS

Immature rainbow trout were purchased from Allen's Trout Farm Inc., Calgary, Alberta and housed in 200 liter self-cleaning aquaria kept at 10–12°C. In order to induce spermatogenesis, the trout were injected with pituitary gonadotropin as previously described,[4] accelerating the process of spermatogenesis from the normal 9 months to 10–12 weeks.[11] Fish were culled at various times after completion of the injection schedule (n = 12) and anesthetized in a solution of tricaine methane sulfonate (MS 222, 50 mg/liter). A cannula was inserted into the ascending aorta via the heart, the right atrium was cut and the animal was perfused with 100 ml of a mixture of saline and MS 222, followed by approximately 600 ml of fixative (4% (w/v) paraformaldehyde in 0.1M phosphate buffer (pH 7.2) with 0.02% (v/v) diethylpyrocarbonate (DEPC)). The testes were removed and placed in fixative for approximately 1–4 hours. The testes were then blocked into various sized pieces and placed overnight in two changes of 0.1M phosphate buffer, pH 7.2, 3% (w/v) polyethylene glycol. The tissue pieces were then frozen in 2-methylbutane and stored in a −70°C freezer until ready to be sectioned. Serial sections (5–8 μm) were cut on a Reichert-Jung Frigocut microtome, thaw-mounted on gel coated slides, freeze-dried, and stored in air-tight containers at −20°C.

A 180 base-pair Nar I-Mae III fragment, containing a significant portion of the translated region of the trout protamine gene TP101,[12] was excised from the plasmid pJP22, rendered blunt-ended and subcloned into the Sma I site of the vector Bluescript KS (+) (Stratagene). The orientation of the inserts was determined, and clones with the opposite orientations were each cut with Bam HI and transcribed using T3 RNA polymerase to generate antisense (complementary to the mRNA) and sense (identical to the message) riboprobes. Transcriptions were performed for one hour at 37°C in the reaction buffer recommended by the enzyme manufacturer (Stratagene). Each reaction contained 1 μg linearized template, 20 units RNA guard (Pharmacia), 40 units

T3 RNA polymerase (Stratagene), 1 mM biotin-(11)-UTP (Enzo Biochemicals Inc.), 0.4 mM ATP, CTP and GTP, and a small amount of ^{32}P-GTP included to allow quantitation of the amount of RNA synthesized. The DNA template was removed by digestion with DNAse I, and the riboprobe purified by gel filtration on Sephadex G-50.

Slide-mounted sections were post-fixed for 10 minutes in cold fixative (described above). The slides were then rinsed with 0.1 M phosphate buffered saline (PBS, Na-monobasic,Na-dibasic,0.9% NaCl), followed by 2x SSC (0.3M sodium chloride, 30 mM sodium citrate) and then incubated for 30 minutes in a 0.1M glycine/0.1M Tris buffer, pH 7.0. Sections were permeabilized with proteinase K (1 μg/ml) for 2 minutes to aid probe access to cellular RNA. Sections were held in ice-cold 0.1M PBS for 15 minutes to inactivate the enzyme. After a brief rinse in 2x SSC, the sections were taken through a series of graded alcohols containing 0.3M sodium acetate to promote RNA retention and left to air dry. Sections were hybridized at 45°C for 4 hours at an antisense riboprobe concentration of 1000 ng/ml in a buffer containing 50% (v/v) formamide, 10 mM dithiothreitol, 10% dextran sulfate and 0.02% (w/v) each of bovine serum albumin, Ficoll 400, polyvinylpyrolidone. Sections were covered with a parafilm "coverslip" and slides were kept in a humid chamber for the duration of the hybridization. Slides were dipped briefly in 2x SSC to remove the "coverslips." This was followed by a series of washes (2x SSC/20% formamide, 5 min; 2x SSC/10% formamide, 20 min; 2x SSC/5% formamide, 5 min, @ 40°C; 2x SSC, 5 min, @ 21°C) to remove unbound riboprobe. After a rinse in 0.1M PBS the sections were incubated with avidin-conjugated HRP for 30 minutes (Elite Kit, Vector Labs) and reacted with a 0.05% solution of DAB in a 0.01% solution of hydrogen peroxide to chromogenically localize the sites of biotin-UTP–labeled probe hybridization. The corresponding sense probe was used as a control for non-specific hybridization.

All sections were counterstained with the DNA-specific stain 4,6-diamidino-2-phenylindole (DAPI; Boehringer Mannheim) and observed under oil immersion fluorescence microscopy (excitation wavelength 340–380 nm with a beam splitting wavelength of 400 nm and a viewing suppression low pass filter wavelength of 430 nm) at 1000× on a Leitz Orthoplan microscope. A number of representative sections were also stained with thionin in order to compare their light morphology to that in previous reports[13] and to examine the same sections under fluorescence microscopy for DAPI in order to develop criteria for identifying the different germ cell–derived phenotypes in the testis according to the size and staining pattern of their DAPI-labeled nuclei. The thionin stained sections were also used to measure the diameter of the cytoplasmic annuli of the different cell types.

The 1000× brightfield and transmission images from the testicular sections were digitized from the Orthoplan microscope using an IBM 386 computer via a Javelin MOS solid state video camera and a Correco frame-grabber (see ref. 14 for details). A fluorescent image for the DAPI-labeled nuclei and the exactly corresponding brightfield image for the DAB-reacted cytoplasm for the same region of a testicular section were stored in the computer hard disc as 512 by 512 images. The system allowed a value in range of 0–127 to be assigned to each pixel. The two images were then overlaid using an alternating flicker method to insure that the DAPI-labeled nuclei of cells showing a DAB reaction in their cytoplasm were correctly aligned so that the nuclei were exactly centrally placed in the DAB-reacted cytoplasmic annulus. DAPI-labeled nuclei were selected randomly using a grid selection method[14] from regions containing "spermatid nests" or relatively high concentrations of nuclei identified as spermatogonia or spermatocytes (see below). A mouse-controlled tracing system allowed each selected cell's nuclear outline to be traced onto the computer image for the brightfield image. A standard diameter of 1.0 μm from the outer border of each selected nucleus was taken to provide a standard annular outline for the cell's cytoplasm. The standard annular diameter was taken to ensure that the optical density (OD) measurements were taken for the cytoplasmic annulus surrounding each identified nucleus and did not extend into the cytoplasmic domains of nearby cells (see justification in results below).

The OD per unit area was measured within each perinuclear annulus and was subtracted from the mean background OD taken from a cell free area on the same section to provide an estimate of the cytoplasmic OD per unit area surrounding each selected nucleus. The cytoplasmic OD for 5–10 spermatid nuclei and a similar number of spermatogonia or spermatocyte nuclei were measured from each randomly selected section. On most sections approximately even numbers of spermatogonia and spermatocyte nuclei were selected even though the number of spermatogonia outnumbered the number of spermatocytes by 4–5:1 on most sections that were measured. The mean value for the spermatogonia/spermatocyte population for each section was used to normalize each value so as to avoid any variation that might result from variable exposure to the hybridization and peroxidase solutions. The normalized values were pooled for 100 nuclei identified as spermatids and 200 nuclei identified as either spermatogonia or spermatocytes for both the sense (taken for 17 different sections) and antisense (taken for 22 different sections) riboprobe hybridizations pooled from three different testes. Hence, the distributions for normalized values provided an estimate of the density of hybridization for the antisense riboprobes relative to the sense riboprobes for each cell type and for the spermatid population relative to spermatogonia or spermatocyte populations.

RESULTS

The nuclear diameters and characteristics of the different cell types examined with thionin stain corresponded well with those previously reported for the trout testis following treatment with gonadotrophin.[13] Within 10 to 12 weeks of the gonadotrophin injections, we found that the testis transiently contained all cell types. During this brief period, the testis contained isolated islands or "nests" comprised largely of spermatids surrounded by smaller numbers of spermatocytes and spermatogonia while nearby lobules contained only the primordial cells, spermatogonia or spermatocytes. At times shorter than 10 weeks, spermatids were not evident in the sections while at 12 or more weeks the testicular sections were dominated by sheets of mature sperm cells and some spermatids with few, if any, spermatocytes or spermatogonia.

Using criteria for identifying the different cell types reported by Drance and his colleagues,[13] cells with nuclei exceeding 4.5 μm in diameter appeared to correspond to primordial germ cells (4.8–5.7 μm) or Sertoli cells (7.3–16.6 μm). Nuclei in both cell types were often oblong in shape. Nuclei for cells corresponding to primary and secondary spermatogonia ranged from 3.5–4.4 μm in diameter, were round in shape and showed a reticulated thionin staining pattern. Spermatocytes (primary and secondary) displayed nuclear diameters of 2.7–3.8 μm. Their nuclei were round and showed a condensed, almost uniform, pattern of thionin staining in contrast to the reticulated pattern of the spermatogonia. Spermatid nuclei were even more highly condensed with uniform thionin staining and small nuclear diameters ranging from 2.0–2.3 μm.

Similar to previous reports,[13] the cytoplasmic annulus surrounding the spermatid nucleus was only 1.0–1.2 μm in diameter, smaller than the 1.3–1.5 μm for the spermatocytes and 1.4–1.7 μm for the spermatogonia. Hence there was a progressive reduction in both nuclear and cytoplasmic volumes with the meiotic divisions from spermatogonia to spermatocytes and then from spermatocytes to spermatids. In the optical density measurements reported below, we restricted the computer image measurements to a uniform diameter extending 1.0 μm from the nuclear borders for spermatogonia, spermatocytes and spermatids. This ensured that the measurements reflected the optical density of the cytoplasm for the nuclei in the center of the annulus since the spermatid cytoplasmic diameters were smaller than those of the other two cell populations.

The DAPI-labeling of the nuclei revealed characteristic patterns of blue fluorescence for each of the three major cell populations as illustrated in FIGURE 1. FIGURE 1a shows a low power fluorescent photomicrograph of a DAPI-labeled testicular section after 11 weeks of gonadotrophin injection which illustrates a nest of spermatid nuclei marked by the arrow and surrounded by a variety of other cell types including primordial cells, spermatogonia and spermatocytes. A second smaller group of seven or eight spermatid nuclei are evident in the photomicrograph just below and to the right of the larger nest (at about 4 o'clock from the center of the larger nest).

FIGURE 1b shows an intermediate power fluorescent photomicrograph of a group of spermatids (one is marked by an arrow) surrounded by the larger nuclei of more primitive sperm cell precursors as well as fibroblasts and other stromal cells. Several spermatocyte nuclei are evident to the right of the spermatid group. The high power photomicrographs in FIGURES 1c and 1d illustrate the typical DAPI fluorescent labeling patterns found for spermatid nuclei as compared to spermatocyte and spermatogonia nuclei. As well as having a smaller nuclear size, spermatid nuclei had a markedly condensed, uniform pattern of DAPI-labeling (an example is marked by an arrow in FIG. 1c). The nuclei frequently showed a characteristic narrow depression or "crack" in the fluorescence at one pole which appears to correspond to a region in which flagellar components are first being assembled in trout spermatids as viewed with the electron microscope (J.B. Rattner, personal communication).

The larger spermatocyte nuclei were similarly condensed in DAPI-labeling but contained irregular unlabeled areas of DAPI fluorescence that were sometimes almost circular and appeared as holes or "punched out" regions. An example is labeled by an arrow at the lower left of FIGURE 1d with other spermatocyte nuclei above and to the right of the labeled nucleus in 1d and in the upper and right portions of FIGURE 1c. The even larger spermatogonia nuclei showed an irregular or bubbly pattern of DAPI-labeling so that there were numerous circular regions of intense labeling separated by regions of little or no labeling throughout the nuclei (an example of a nucleus meeting the criteria for primary spermatogonia is marked by an arrow in the upper right portion of FIGURE 1d). With experience, we were able to use nuclear size and shape together with DAPI-labeling pattern to distinguish spermatids from spermatogonia and spermatocytes with fluorescence microscopy.

The *in situ* hybridizations for the antisense protamine riboprobes using the DAB chromogen showed localized groups of labeled annular shapes corresponding to the spermatid nests. The brown pigment from the peroxidase reaction in these annular shapes appeared to correspond to the spermatid cytoplasm. FIGURE 1e shows three localized regions of peroxidase reaction product in a low power photomicrograph for an antisense hybridization. Note that there is no detectable peroxidase reaction outside

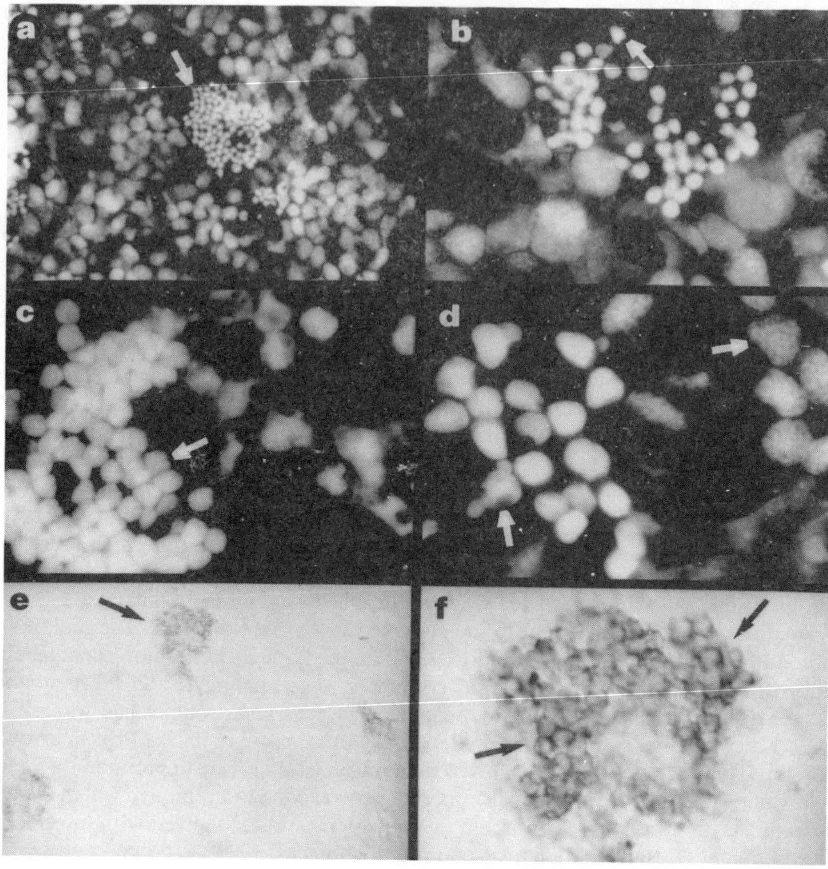

FIGURE 1. Fluorescence and brightfield photomicrographs for sections of trout testis stained with DAPI and hybridized with an antisense protamine riboprobe. Panels **a–d** are fluorescence photomicrographs showing the characteristic DAPI labeling of spermatogonia, spermatocyte, and spermatid nuclei. Panels **e** and **f** show the distribution of the peroxidase reaction for the antisense protamine riboprobe viewed under brightfield microscopy. See text for further details.

of the three localized regions. FIGURE 1f shows a higher power photomicrograph of the upper localized region of peroxidase reaction in FIGURE 1e marked by the arrow. Even though only a proportion of the cells are in focus at high power in the 5 μm thick section, the annular shapes of the individual areas of peroxidase reaction are clearly visible, particularly in the cells that are in focus (several examples of in focus cells are marked by arrows). The annular shapes consistently were 4.0–4.4 μm in diameter with a central zone, 2.0–2.3 μm in diameter, free of peroxidase reaction.

The photomicrograph of FIGURE 2 is included to show that the peroxidase-reactive annuli in the antisense hybridizations only surrounded those nuclei identified as belonging to spermatids. FIGURE 2a shows the DAPI fluorescent nuclei of a spermatid nest surrounded by the nuclei of a variety of other cell types including spermatogonia

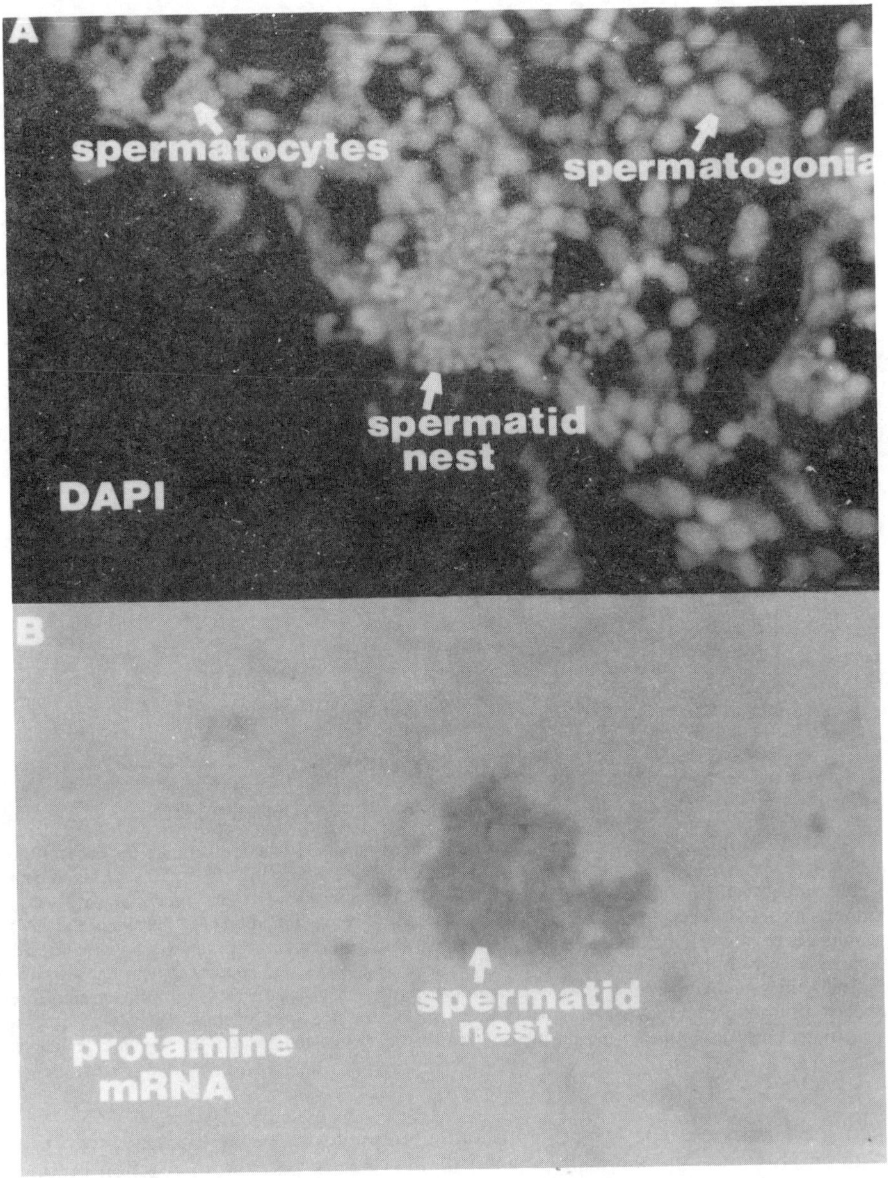

FIGURE 2. Section of immature trout testis. Panel **a**: DAPI staining of testis cell nuclei under UV fluorescence. Panel **b**: Identical region of the same section under brightfield illumination showing the distribution of the brown peroxidase reaction for protamine antisense riboprobe hybridization. Note the annular areas of brown product from the peroxidase reaction are limited to the area surrounding nuclei characteristic of spermatids.

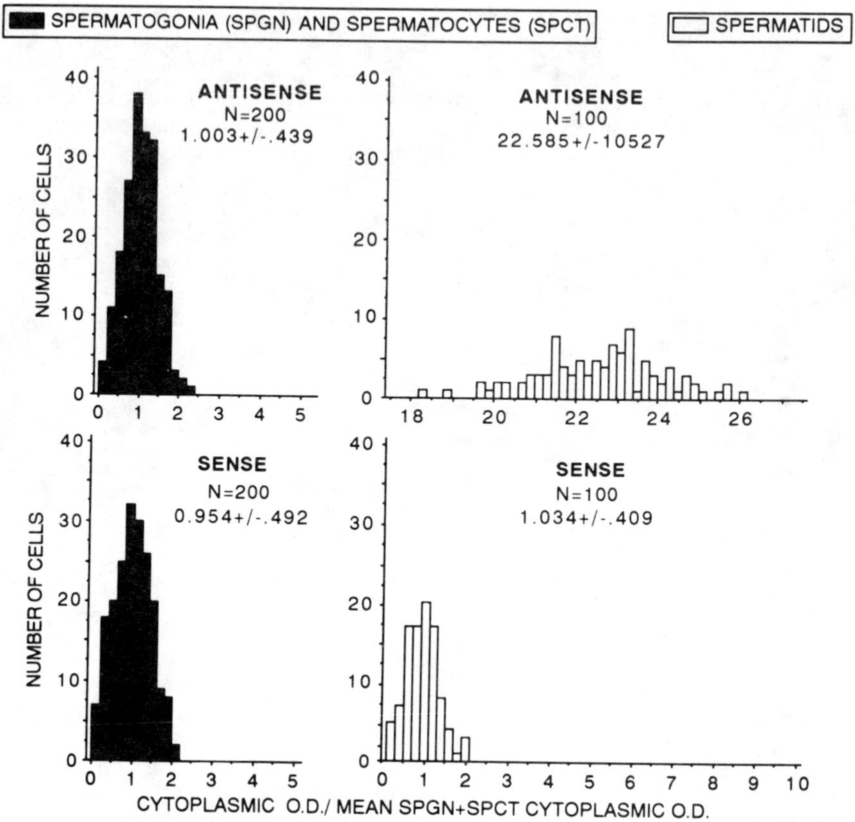

FIGURE 3. Normalized densitometry measurements of the DAB reaction product for each of the cell types hybridized to either a sense or antisense protamine riboprobe. There was no significant difference between the relative optical density of the spermatogonia (SPGN) and spermatocyte (SPCT) cytoplasm ($p < .01$) when hybridized with the protamine antisense riboprobe. The density of the DAB chromogen reaction product for hybridization with the antisense protamine probe was on average 22.5 times as dense in the spermatids as compared to spermatogonia and spermatocytes. Sense probe hybridizations for all three cell types gave values that were not significantly different from the antisense probe hybridizations for the spermatogonia and spermatocytes. See text for details of the normalization procedure. The values adjacent to each distribution are the normalized mean ± the standard deviation.

and spermatocytes. The brightfield photomicrograph of exactly the same region in FIGURE 2b shows an identically shaped region of dark peroxidase reaction product corresponding to the spermatid nest in FIGURE 2a. The annular shapes of the brown peroxidase reaction are clearly evident in FIGURE 2b and can be superimposed upon annular regions surrounding the nuclei identified as spermatids in FIGURE 2a. Sense riboprobe hybridizations used as negative controls revealed no brown reaction products in any cell type.

Normalized densitometry measurements of the DAB reaction product for each of the cell types are shown in FIGURE 3. The number of cells is displayed on the ordinates while relative density per unit area of cytoplasm is displayed along the abscissa. There was no significant difference between the relative OD per unit area for the spermatogonia (SPGN) and spermatocyte (SPCT) cytoplasms ($p < .01$) when hybridized with the protamine antisense or sense riboprobe. The density of the DAB chromogen reaction product for hybridization with the antisense protamine probe was on an average 22.5 times as dense in the spermatid cytoplasm as compared to the other two cell types and ranged from about 18 times to 26 times as dense (note the abscissa scale for the antisense distribution for the spermatids extends from 17–27). There was no difference in the optical densities for the spermatid sense riboprobe hybridizations from the sense hybridizations for the spermatogonia and spermatocytes. Given the absence of any detectable brown color in the spermatogonia or spermatocyte cytoplasm with the antisense probes and the fact that we have obtained similar OD values for unstained and unhybridized sections of the trout testis, the OD values for their cytoplasm represent attenuation of the transmitted light by the unstained tissue without any contribution from the hybridization of the biotinylated probes.

DISCUSSION

In situ hybridization with biotinylated riboprobes offers distinct advantages over solution hybridization in terms of speed of the procedure, resolution and a significant reduction in the number of cells required as starting material. RNA probes are single stranded and cannot reanneal during hybridization as compared to the more routinely used double-stranded cDNA probes; hence, the amount of probe available for hybridization is increased. RNA-RNA hybrids are also more stable than DNA-RNA hybrids[15] permitting higher stringency washing and improved signal-to-noise ratios. Most importantly, this *in situ* hybridization method can provide information on gene expression within individual cells of a heterogeneous population because of the discrete localization of the horseradish peroxidase–chromogenic reaction.

Our results demonstrate that rainbow trout mRNA is detectable only in spermatids using the biotinylated riboprobes. Although these results disagree with those obtained in earlier studies in this system,[3] they are consistent with the results in mouse,[8] rat,[9] and rooster,[10] that showed by other methods that protamine mRNAs are detectable only in post-meiotic cells. It is conceivable that we did not detect protamine message in spermatocytes because the transcript abundance was below the sensitivity limit for biotinylated riboprobes under our conditions of hybridization. At present, we have not yet determined the sensitivity of non-isotopic probe detection on a system where mRNA copy number per cell has been determined as for actin.[16,17] In order to resolve the issue of first appearance of protamine message in trout spermatogenesis, a comparison should be made between the sensitivity limits of an RNase protection assay on a known number of a pure cell population and *in situ* hybridization with the biotinylated probe for an equal number of cells. It remains to be determined whether the relationship between the density of the chromogen reaction is linearly related to the number of mRNA copies per cell. However, relating the number of grain counts to RNA copy number is equally problematic, especially since the efficiency of hybridization must be considered.[18,19]

It is possible that we may have caused some RNA to be lost by permeabilizing the cells with the proteinase K treatment.[17] However, in some of the experiments, we employed proteinase K concentrations that were much lower than recommended for RNA probes, as well as reducing the digestion from thirty minutes as is commonly employed[20] down to two minutes. Alternatively, protamine mRNA may be masked in spermatocytes, although various increased periods of incubation with proteinase K did not produce any increase in signal in these cell types (data not shown). It may also be argued that the protamine riboprobes had limited access to tissue mRNA sites, as compared to the free access to mRNA achieved in solution hybridizations. This difference in accessibility may be a consequence of the attached biotin creating a "stiff" nucleic acid backbone which would hinder permeability. This effect, however, has been reported to be a factor only with probes of length greater than 1500 nucleotides.[17]

In our hands we have found very low background signals with the HRP-avidin/DAB chromogenic detection of the biotin-RNA hybridizations. Our signal to noise ratio was of the order 40–80:1. This compares most favorably to values of 70:1 for isotopically labeled cDNA probes and is at least four times better than the 20:1 ratio reported for biotin-cDNA probes using a rhodamine-rabbit IgG conjugate detection system or the 15:1 ratio reported for ^{125}I-avidin.[17] It was previously determined by Reis and his colleagues[21] that with a hydrogen peroxide concentration in excess of 0.003% and at least a 0.05% solution of DAB the peroxidase reaction followed a linear time course up to six minutes, background staining being minimal over this time. All peroxide/chromogen incubations in this study were terminated after five minutes.

The average increase in optical density of 22.5 times for the antisense hybridizations in the spermatids compared to the spermatogonia and spermatocytes could be considered to reflect the condensation in the cell cytoplasm that accompanies the meiotic progression from spermatocyte to spermatid. By our calculations, the cytoplasmic volume of an average secondary spermatocyte is 84.2 μm^3 while that of an average spermatid is 74.5 μm^3 (using the nuclear and cell diameters reported previously[13] for thin plastic sections and assuming the nuclei and the cells to be spherical in shape). Hence, for a single average cell this represents a cytoplasmic reduction to 87% for the spermatids as compared to spermatocytes. With the further doubling of the total cytoplasmic volume with the meiotic division from secondary spermatocyte to spermatid, the total cytoplasmic volume of the two spermatids would be 174% that of the parent spermatocyte. Hence one would expect the average spermatid would contain about 60% of the protamine mRNA concentration found in the spermatocytes if the mRNA was merely held over after the meiotic division. This is not consistent with the average increase in optical density of 22.5 times we found for the antisense riboprobe hybridization in the spermatids compared to the spermatocytes.

The distribution of protamine antisense hybridization density in spermatid cell cytoplasm, ranging from 18–26 times the optical density for spermatogonia and spermatocytes, suggests that protamine mRNA transcription in spermatids increases to higher levels. This is supported by previous studies which reported that low levels of protamine mRNA transcription occur in early spermatids; the levels of the message steadily increase with the RNA initially sequestered in 11S messenger ribonucleoprotein (mRNP) particles in the cell supernatant in a translationally inactive form.[6] Negligible optical density measurements of protamine antisense hybridization in the other cell populations could be interpreted as an absence of protamine transcription prior to meiosis. The previous finding of low levels of protamine mRNA in spermatocyte total RNA by solution hybridization[3] could conceivably be the result of low level contamination of the separated spermatocyte fraction by spermatids (or aggregates of spermatids). Since such contaminating spermatids individually might be considered to contain protamine mRNA levels up to 22.5 fold higher than the level in secondary spermatocytes seen in the present study (FIG. 3), as little as 3–4% cross-contamination could lead to the previously observed low levels of protamine mRNA in total RNA extracted from the spermatocyte fraction.[3] Until a comparison is made between the sensitivity thresholds of the two methods with respect to protamine mRNA copy number per cell the question of the first appearance of protamine message is still unresolved.

ACKNOWLEDGMENTS

The authors would like to thank Gil Schultz and Kostas Iatrou for helpful discussions and Karl Lederis for unlimited access to his cryotome.

SUMMARY

In situ hybridizations were performed using a biotinylated riboprobe complementary to protamine messenger RNA in order to directly examine the various cell types in the trout testis for the presence of protamine message. Computer-aided optical density measurements were used to provide estimates of transcript abundance for cells identified by their DAPI-labeled nuclei. Optically detectable protamine hybridization occurred only in spermatid cells. These findings are in accord with results obtained in other species which report protamine mRNA only in the post-meiotic spermatid cell; but they are in conflict with a previous study employing solution hybridization which noted that protamine message first appears in the spermatocytes of rainbow trout.

REFERENCES

1. ANGERER, L. M., M. H. STOLER & R. C. ANGERER. 1987. RNA probes: An annotated protocol. *In* In Situ Hybridization: Applications to Neurobiology. K. Valentino, J. Eberwine & J. Barchas, Eds.: 42–71. Oxford University Press. New York
2. DIXON, G. H., J. M. AIKEN, J. M. JANKOWSKI, D. I. MCKENZIE, R. MOIR & J. C. STATES. 1986. Organization and evolution of the protamine genes of salmonid fishes. *In* Chromosomal Proteins and Gene Expression. G. R. Raeck, G. A. Goodwin & P. Puigdomenech, Eds.: 287–314. Plenum Publishing Corp. New York.
3. DRANCE, M. G., M. J. HOLLENBERG, M. SMITH & V. WYLIE. 1976. Can. J. Zool. **54:** 1285–1293.
4. GEDAMU, L., P. L. DAVIES & G. H. DIXON. 1977. Biochemistry **16:** 1383–1391.
5. IATROU, K. & G. H. DIXON. 1977. Cell **10:** 433–441.
6. IATROU, K., A. W. SPIRA & G. H. DIXON. 1978. Devel. Biol. **64:** 82–98.
7. JANKOWSKI, J. M. & G. H. DIXON. 1984. Can. J. Biochem. Cell Biol. **62:** 291–300.
8. KLEENE, K. C., R. J. DISTEL & N. B. HECHT. 1983. Dev. Biol. **98:** 455–464.
9. KLEENE, K. C., R. J. DISTEL & N. B. HECHT. 1984. Dev. Biol. **105:** 71–79.
10. LOUIE, A. J. & G. H. DIXON. 1972. J. Biol. Chem. **247:** 7962–7968.
11. MALI, P., M. SANDBERG, E. VUORIO, P. C. YELICK, N. B. HECHT & M. PARVINEN. 1988. J. Cell Biol. **107:** 407–412.
12. OLIVA, R., J. MEZQUITA, C. MEZQUITA & G. H. DIXON. 1988. Dev. Biol. **125:** 332–340.
13. OLIVA, R. & G. H. DIXON. 1990. J. Mol. Evol. **30:** 333–346.
14. PESCHON, J. J., R. R. BEHRINGER, R. L. BRINSTER & R. D. PALMITER. 1987. Proc. Natl. Acad. Sci. USA **84:** 5316–5319.
15. REIS, D. J., R. H. BENNO, L. W. TUCKER & T. H. JOH. 1982. Quantitative immunocytochemistry of tyrosine hydroxylase in brain. *In* Cytochemical Methods in Neuroanatomy. V. Chan-Palay & S. L. Palay, Eds.: 205–228. Alan R. Liss, Inc. New York.

16. Schmidt, P. J., B. S. Mitchell, M. Smith & H. Tsuyuki. 1965. Gen. Comp. Endocrinol. **5:** 197–206.
17. Schwartz, R. J. & K. N. Rothblum. 1981. Biochemistry **20:** 4122–4129.
18. Sinclair, G. D. & G. H. Dixon. 1982. Biochemistry **21:** 1869–1877.
19. Singer, R. H., J. B. Lawrence & R. N. Rashtchian. 1987. Toward a rapid and sensitive in situ hybridization methodology using isotopic and nonisotopic probes. *In* In Situ Hybridization: Applications to Neurobiology. K. Valentino, J. Eberwine & J. Barchas, Eds.: 71–96. Oxford University Press. New York.
20. Tatton, W. G., M. M. Kwan, M. C. Verrier, N. A. Seniuk & E. Theriault. 1990. Brain Res. **527:** 21–32.
21. Tecott, L. H., J. H. Eberwine, J. D. Barchas & K. L. Valentino. 1987. Methodological considerations on the utilization of in situ hybridization. *In* In Situ Hybridization: Applications to Neurobiology. K. Valentino, J. H. Eberwine & J. Barchas, Eds.: 3–24. Oxford University Press. New York.
22. Trevithick, J. R., C. J. Ingles & G. H. Dixon. 1969. Can. J. Biochem. **47:** 51–60.
23. Wetmur, J. G., W. T. Ruyechan & R. J. Douthart. 1981. Biochemistry **20:** 2999–3002.
24. Young, W. S. 1986. Quantitative in situ hybridization and determination of mRNA content. *In* In Situ Hybridization in Brain. G. R. Uhl, Ed.: 243–248. Plenum Press. New York.

Expression and Processing of the Rooster Protamine mRNA[a]

RAFAEL OLIVA[b,c] AND GORDON H. DIXON[b,d]

[b] *Department of Medical Biochemistry*
Faculty of Medicine, University of Calgary
3330 Hospital Drive N.W.
Calgary, Alberta T2N 4N1, Canada

[c] *Molecular Genetics Research Group*
Department of Physiological Sciences
Faculty of Medicine, University of Barcelona
Barcelona, Spain

INTRODUCTION

Spermatogenesis is a developmentally regulated process which involves marked changes in cell morphology and a dramatic rearrangement in the structure of the chromatin in many species with the formation of a compact sperm nucleus in which the DNA is highly compacted as a complex with protamine.[1-8] The formation of the compacted sperm nucleus is accompanied by a general cessation of transcription.[9] Therefore, spermiogenesis provides an excellent system in which to study the postranscriptional processing of mRNAs in the absence of endogenous transcription in the late stages of spermiogenesis.

In this paper we determine the timing of expression of the chicken protamine gene using *in situ* hybridization. We also characterize the two populations of mRNA expressed at this stage by Northern blot analysis of RNA at different stages of spermatogenesis (using a series of transcriptional unit probes under different stringency conditions), by 3′ S1 mapping and by RNAse H digestion of mRNA-oligo-dT hybrids.

METHODS

White leghorn roosters (5–55 weeks old) were obtained from P. Knievel or A/K. Waddell through the University of Calgary Purchasing services. Reagents and RNA isolation were as described.[10]

In Situ *Hybridizations*

Small fragments (10–50 mm^3) of fresh testis tissue were fixed in Carnoy's fluid (ethanol/chloroform/acetic acid; 6:3:1) for 30 min. The fragments were dehydrated

[a] This work was supported by grants from the Medical Research Council to Gordon H. Dixon and the Alberta Heritage Foundation for Medical Research to Rafael Oliva.

[d] Author to whom correspondence should be addressed.

by dipping in 80% ethanol for 1 h, 95% ethanol 1 h, 100% ethanol 1 h and again 100% ETOH 1 h. The tissue was cleared with xylenes (Fisher) for 1 h, embedded in Paraplast (59°C) for 90 min, poured into molds and let solidify at 4°C overnight. Sections (5 μm) were cut and stretched for 10 sec by floating on a sterile water bath at 92°C layered, on a slide, left to dry-fix for 2 days at 42–45°C, and stored dry at 4°C. The embedding medium was removed by extractions with xylenes (5 min each) followed by 100% ethanol, 95%, 80%, 70%, 40% ethanol and two changes in water. Hybridizations were performed at 42°C overnight in 50% formamide, 5x Denhardt's, 5xSSPE and 250 μg/ml tRNA (120 μl containing 0.2×10^6 cpm of probe). The sections were washed for 5 min twice in 2xSSC at room temperature, twice for 30 min in 2xSSC, at 50°C and twice for 30 min in 0.1xSSC at room temperature. The sections were then dehydrated (70%, 80%, 90%, 95% ethanol, 2 min of each) and air dried. Each slide was dipped in a 1:1 dilution of Kodak NBT nuclear track emulsion in absolute darkness, exposed for 1 week, developed for 2.5 min in Kodak Dektol (No. 123 3113), followed by 30 sec in water, and then fixed for 5 min in Kodak rapid fixer (no. 146 4106), washed three times for 5 min in water and air-dried. They were then stained with hematoxylin/eosin (Harris modified hematoxylin, Fisher SH 30-500) following manufacturer's instructions, embedded in xylenes, and mounted with permount.

Northern Blots

Northern blots were performed as described.[11] The gels which contained 2.2% agarose BioRad, 1 × MOPS and 6% formaldehyde, were 25 cm long (this is important to resolve the two mRNA populations) and were run until bromophenol blue reached the end of the gel. S1 mapping using a Maxam-Gilbert sequence ladder as marker was as described previously.[10] The probe for S1 mapping was an end-labeled fragment at the DdeI site (position + 265). RNAse H digestion was as described.[12] 20 μg of mature testis RNA was mixed with 1 μg of oligo-dT (12–18) in water (75 μl), heated at 65°C for 2 min and 25 μl of RNase H buffer were added and incubated for 15 min on ice. Two units of RNAse H (Pharmacia 27-0894-0) were then added and the mixture incubated at 37°C for 30 min. This was followed by phenol/chloroform extraction and the RNA was ethanol-precipitated (0.1 vol of 3M Na acetate and 3 ml of ethanol) and the precipitate washed, dried and re-dissolved in water. Various rooster protamine gene probes were prepared as described.[11] The mRNA sizes in the Northern blots were determined by extrapolation using a range of size markers (FIG. 5). The accuracy of the size for each band was estimated to be ± 20 nucleotides for bands **a** and **b**, and ± 15 nucleotides for band **c** (FIG. 5), since this corresponds to the thickness of those bands (contour determined as the intensity representing 95% above that of the peak).

RESULTS

In Situ *Hybridizations*

Hybridization of immature tissue sections with the rooster protamine probe gave only a signal corresponding to background control (FIG. 1). By contrast, under the same hybridization exposure and developing conditions, a markedly increased signal

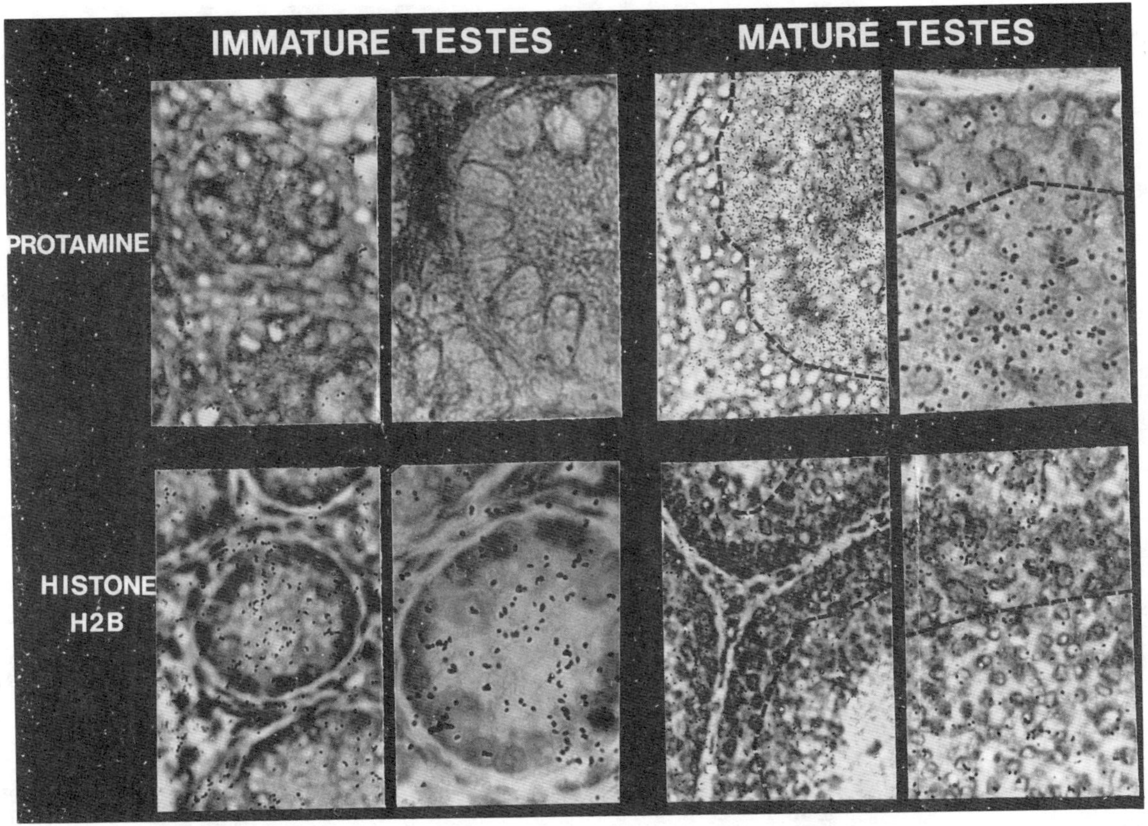

FIGURE 1. *In situ* hybridization of immature (*left panels*) or mature (*right panels*) rooster testis sections with the rooster protamine probe (*top panels*) or histone H2B probe (*bottom panels*). The results are shown in pairs (low magnification at the left and high magnification on the right). For ease of interpretation of the images a black dotted line has been drawn separating the spermatocyte zone from the spermatid region. Background control was 0.16 grains/mm^2 (not shown). The results from these pictures are summarized in FIGURE 2.

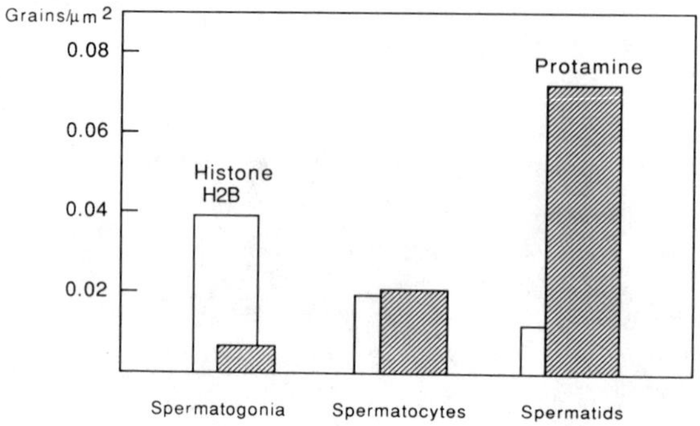

FIGURE 2. Histogram distribution of silver grains over the spermatogonia, spermatocytes or spermatids regions.

is detected in the mature testis sections (FIG. 1, two upper right panels). These results are quantified and summarized in FIGURE 2. It is evident that the silver grains are clustered over the spermatid area indicating strong transcription of the protamine genes at this stage. To eliminate the possibility that the probe might be unable to gain access equally to immature and mature tissue or to spermatocyte and spermatid areas, a control was done with a histone H2B probe. As expected, the rapidly dividing immature tissue (spermatogonia and spermatocytes) showed strong hybridization under the same hybridization, exposure and developing conditions as compared to the protamine probe (FIG. 1). It should also be noted in the mature tissue sections that there is more hybridization with the histone H2B probe over the spermatocytes than the spermatids in keeping with the reduced histone (and DNA) synthesis in spermatids (FIG. 1 and 2).

Effect of Using Different Regions of the Rooster Protamine Gene as Probes on the Northern Blot Pattern in Different Tissues

Northern blot analysis of RNA from different tissues (immature testes, brain and liver) showed no detectable hybridization with the rooster protamine probe (FIG. 3), even when the filters are over-exposed for 2 weeks (not shown). On the other hand mature testis at different stages clearly shows the presence of two protamine mRNAs as indicated by the two bands labeled **a** and **b** in FIGURE 3B but in different proportions in each sample. For example, testis 2 shows a predominance of the upper band, testis 4 approximately equal levels of each band, and testes 1 and 3 a predominance of the lower band. Such differences are likely to arise from the differences in developmental stage of each testis.[11]

FIGURE 3A shows the different regions of the rooster protamine gene that were used in the Northern blots of FIGURES 3B and 5. Identical ratios of bands **a** and **b** were obtained even when different portions of the gene (probes 1, 2 or 3) were used indicating that the two mRNA populations **a** and **b** each contain a full complement of the entire sequence thus ruling out differential splicing and that they must represent transcripts of the same gene. Also different stringency conditions do not have any effect on the relative proportions of population **a** to population **b** (Figure 3B). Thus, the size difference must be due to reasons other than the presence or absence of a region of transcribed sequence. Also the possibility that the two mRNA populations correspond to transcripts of two unrelated genes but with a sufficiently similar nu-

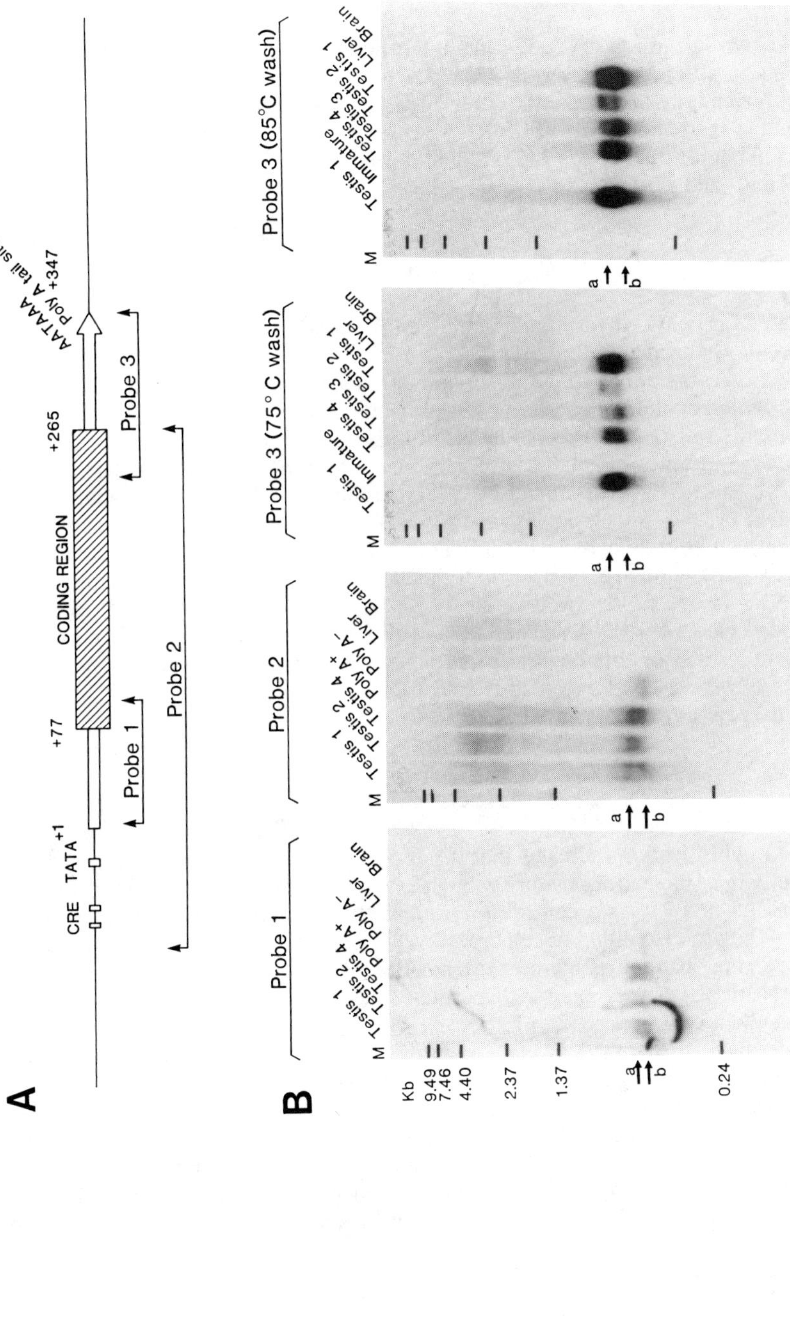

FIGURE 3. Northern blot analysis of RNA from different testis samples and using different regions of the protamine gene as probes. **A:** A scheme is presented indicating the type of probes used in **B**. **B:** Northern blot analysis with the probe 1 (*left*), 2 (*middle*) or 3 (*right*). Labels a and b designate the two mRNA populations respectively.

cleotide composition to cross-hybridize with the chicken protamine probe can also be ruled out.

Mapping of the 3′ Terminus by S1 Analysis

As shown in FIGURE 4A, only one 3′ terminus is detected in the S1 mapping experiments in all the mature testis RNA populations, irrespective of the proportions of mRNA band **a** or **b**. Thus, the same S1 pattern is seen when using testis 2 RNA (enriched in the band **a**) or testis 3 RNA (enriched in band **b**). The site at which the poly-A tail begins (nucleotide 347) coincides precisely with that determined by cDNA sequencing[11] and is shown in FIGURE 4B.

Digestion with RNase H

RNase H is able to digest double-stranded RNA-DNA regions and when oligo-dT is allowed to hybridize with the poly-A region of a mRNA and the complex treated with RNase H, the poly-A-oligo dT double-stranded region is removed. When testis 4 RNA, which contains band **a** of 470 ± 20 nts and band **b** with 430 ± 20 nts, is treated in this way (FIG. 5A), both bands disappear and are replaced by a single band **c** with 345 ± 15 nts. This latter size very accurately matches the distance between the mRNA start (+1) determined by 5′ S1 mapping[10] and the poly A addition site determined by 3′ S1 mapping (FIG. 4) (347 nucleotides). The lengths of poly-A in each band can now be calculated; in band **a**, the poly A is (470 ± 20) − (345 ± 15) = 125 ± 20 while in band **b** it is (430 ± 20) − (345 ± 15) = 85 ± 20 nucleotides. Thus mRNAs **a** and **b** differ by 40 ± 20 poly-A residues. We have previously estimated the sizes of the two mRNA species to be 465 for band **a** and 420 for band **b**[11] and the present results correspond closely with these determinations even though different marker sets were used in each case: Hind III DNA markers in,[11] and the BRL RNA ladder markers in the present work (FIG. 5).

DISCUSSION

In situ hybridization indicates that the rooster protamine gene is expressed predominantly in testis sections mature enough to show regions of post-meiotic spermatid cells (FIGS. 1 and 2). As a control to eliminate the possibility of differential accessibility of the probe to different cell types, we have used a chicken histone H2B probe which reveals a distinctly different pattern of hybridization with the strongest signal over replicating spermatogonia and spermatocytes and not over spermatids (FIG. 1). These results are summarized in FIGURE 2. The conclusion is that the expression of the rooster protamine genes takes place at the genetically haploid stage of spermatogenesis, this result being is good agreement with the preliminary data obtained using Northern blot analysis.[11] Post-meiotic expression of several genes in a variety of mammalian testes has been described including protamines[12] phosphoglycerate kinase-2 isoform,[13,14] and α-tubulin.[15,16] In the case of the rainbow trout protamine mRNA, evidence based on solution hybridization of RNA extracted from separated testis cells[17] indicated the presence of low levels of protamine mRNA in pre-meiotic spermatocytes

A

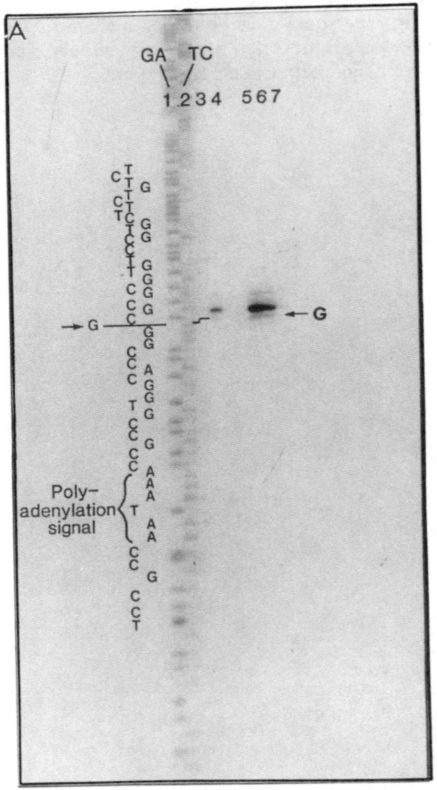

B

```
                                            CRE              CRE                                    -23
CCCGTCCCGA ACGGCCCGGG CGCGTTCGGC TCAGTGACCC GGCCGGCCGT CACAGAGGGC CGCGCGCGGG CGCCTATAAA
                                 ┌→ mRNA start                                             +58
AGCGGCGCGG GGCGCGGAGC GGAGCGGCAC TTCCCGGTCC CGCACGGCTC GGCACCGGCC GCGGGCGCCG TCCCACCGCC
                 +76
GTCCCACCGC AGCCCGGC

ATG GCC CGC TAC CGG CGC AGC AGG ACC CGC AGC CGC AGC CCC CGC AGC CGC CGC CGC CGC CGC+139
 M   A   R   Y   R   R   S   R   T   R   S   R   S   P   R   S   R   R   R   R   R
CGC TCC GGC CGC CGC CGC AGC CCC CGC CGC CGC CGC CGC TAC GGG AGC GCC CGG CGG TCC CGC+2Ø2
 R   S   G   R   R   R   S   P   R   R   R   R   R   Y   G   S   A   R   R   S   R
CGC TCC GTG GGG GGA CGG CGC CGC CGC TAC GGG AGC CGC CGC CGC CGC CGC CGC CGC TAC TGA+265
 R   S   V   G   G   R   R   R   R   Y   G   S   R   R   R   R   R   R   R   Y  Ter
                                                                                   +344
GCCGCCGCCG CCGCCGCTAC TGAGCCGCGC CCGCCCCGCG CCCCGCGCTG CCGCTCCGCC AATAAACCGC CGTGGCACCG
┌→ poly A                                                                          +424
GGCGCGCGTG TCCGTGCTTC TGTCTGCGCC CCGGGGCCGT CCGTGTCCGG CGCTCCCACG GCCCGGGCCG GCACCGTGCG
```

FIGURE 4. A: 3′ S1 mapping of the rooster protamine gene. *Lanes 1* and *2* Maxam and Gilbert reactions for G plus A and T plus C, respectively. *Lane 4*: 10 μg of testis 2 RNA. *Lane 5:* 25 μg of testis 2 RNA. *Lane 6*: 25 μg of testis 3 RNA. *Lane 7:* 5 μg of testis 3 RNA. B: The rooster protamine gene sequence indicating the mRNA start, some of the gene features and the poly A tail site determined by 3′ S1 mapping.

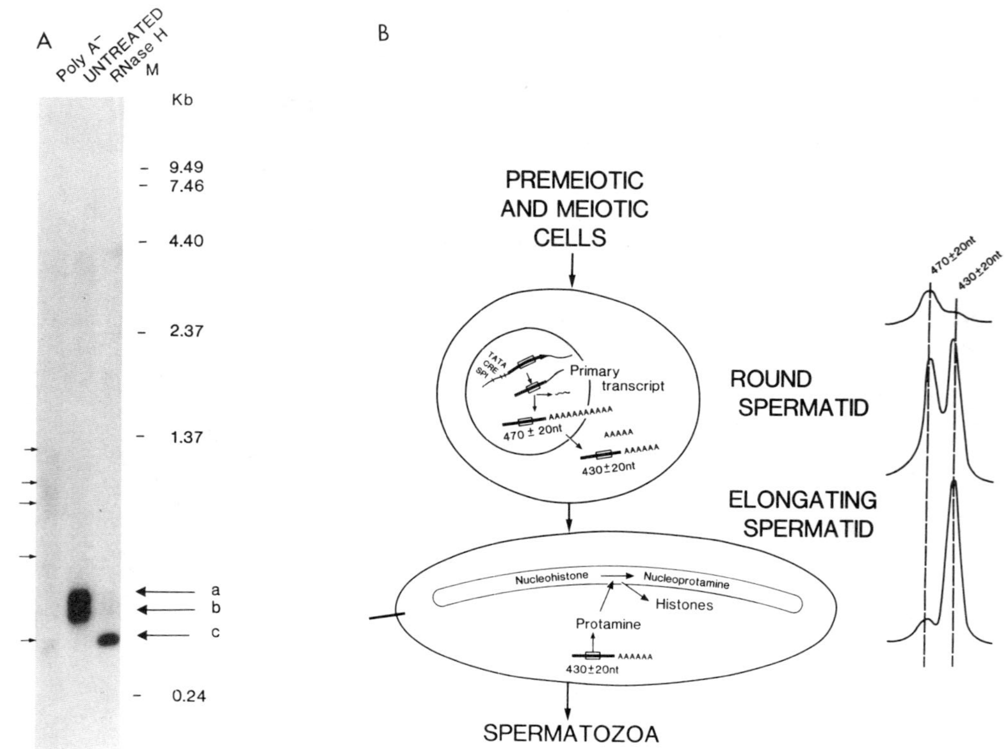

FIGURE 5. **A:** RNase H digestion of mRNA–oligo dT hybrids. mRNA populations a and b present in the untreated sample (lane labeled untreated) yield a single band c (lane labeled "RNase H"). Northern blot analysis of poly A RNA shows several components of weak intensity which are indicated by small arrows (left lane). The probe used was #3 from FIGURE 2a. **B:** Scheme indicating the known steps for protamine mRNA synthesis and processing. The insert at the right corresponds to the relative changes in the protamine mRNA populations of cells separated at unit gravity (11) showing first the appearance of the 470 ± 20 nt population which is then likely to be processed to the 430 ± 20 nt population present in elongated spermatids.

but much larger amounts in post-meiotic spermatids. Recently, *in situ* hybridization[18] of trout testis sections has shown, in fact, that significant protamine mRNA levels can only be found in spermatid cells. The previous observation can probably be explained by contamination of the spermatocyte cell fraction by a small number of spermatids containing high levels of protamine mRNA.

The significance of post-meiotic gene expression has been thought to be important in the phenomenon of transmission rate distortion seen at the t-locus in mice.[19–21] However, using transgenic technology it has been shown that for a mouse protamine 1-human growth hormone (HGh) construct, there is clear evidence of the exchange of the products (mRNAs or HGh) of gene expression through the cytoplasmic bridges connecting spermatids.[22] Therefore, genetically haploid spermatids can behave as if they are phenotypically diploid.

The second issue raised in the present paper is the identification of the difference between the two forms of rooster protamine mRNA (being 470 ± 20 and 430 ± 20 nucleotides in length) with the longer mRNA appearing in round spermatids and the shorter being predominant in elongated spermatids (FIG. 5). The results obtained using a series of DNA probes derived from different regions of the rooster protamine gene, at different hybridization stringencies indicates that each of the two mRNA populations must contain a full complement of identical (or highly similar) sequences which eliminates the possibility of there being two independent mRNAs cross-hybridizing with each other or differing in the length of the transcriptional unit (*e.g.*, because of a deletion or insertion of a sequence during processing). By a combination of S1 analysis to determine the 3′ terminus (FIG. 3) and RNase H removal of the poly-A tails (FIG. 5), it was clear that the longer species **a** had a poly A tail of 125 ± 20 residues whereas the shorter species **b** had a poly A tail of 85 ± 20 nucleotides. The product of RNase H digestion, band **c** in FIGURE 5, had a length of 345 ± 15 nucleotides, which is in excellent agreement with the distance between the 5′ terminus or CAP site (determined by cDNA sequencing[11] and 3′ S1 mapping; FIG. 3).

Despite much experimentation and speculation, the function of the poly A tail on mRNAs is still unclear at present.[29–36] One hypothesis with some experimental support is that the poly-A tail stabilizes mRNA molecules. This would be consistent with the fact that the poly-A-fraction contains a very weak protamine mRNA band of approximately 345 nts migrating in the same position (FIG. 5, small lower left arrow) as the RNase H product (band **c** in FIG. 5). The very small steady-state amount of this poly-A species would be consistent with its rapid degradation following removal of the poly-A tail. There is also a series of faint bands (arrowed at left in FIG. 5) in the poly-A fraction migrating approximately at 560, 800, 900, and 1100 nucleotide lengths which may represent nuclear primary transcripts extending to variable distances 3′ of the gene which are subsequently cleaved and polyadenylated to the two mature poly-A mRNA species. It has been shown in other cases that RNA polymerase II often transcribes well beyond the poly-A site and that these longer transcripts are then cleaved and poly-adenylated.[30,33] They cannot be splicing intermediates since rooster protamine genes do not contain any introns.[10]

In FIGURE 5, a cartoon is presented showing the known steps of protamine mRNA processing in spermatogenesis. It is likely that the larger protamine mRNA of 470 ± 20 nucleotides gives rise to the shorter mRNA of 430 ± 20 nucleotides by the removal of 40–45 A residues although the mechanism of conversion (whether by exonuclease "nibbling" or by endonuclease cleavage of the poly A tract) remains to be determined. In the case of rainbow trout protamine mRNA,[17,23] it has been shown that this messenger existed in two separate pools in trout testis cells. In early spermatids the majority of the mRNA was sequestered in a discrete mRNP particle in the cell supernatant[23] while in later spermatids, protamine mRNP was associated with small polyribosomes and a mRNP particle containing protamine mRNA could be dissociated by EDTA treatment. The longer length of poly-A tails in the cell supernatant mRNP particle was consistent with the idea that the length of the poly-A tail decreased as translation of the mRNA proceeded.

The results presented in this paper prove the universality of the poly-A tail shortening in protamine genes as spermiogenesis proceeds. The opportunity to determine the main function of this event (stabilization of mRNA or transcriptional efficiency?) is now open to study in a model with a natural cessation of endogenous transcription.

SUMMARY

In situ hybridization in immature and mature testis sections shows that the rooster protamine mRNA is transcribed in the post-meiotic stages of spermatogenesis. Two distinct populations of rooster protamine mRNA are expressed as determined by Northern blot analysis. Since there are two copies of the chicken protamine gene per haploid genome, the question was raised of whether the two mRNA populations correspond to the two different genes or was a result of differential mRNA processing. The fact that the two genes differ only in one nucleotide (one extra A in the polyadenylation signal in the second locus) and that random sequencing of several cDNA clones has revealed only one poly-A tail addition site favors the hypothesis that the differences are due to mRNA processing. This is supported by 3′ S1 mapping which shows a single poly-A tail addition site, which in turn suggests that the heterogeneity is due to differences in the length of the poly-A tail. The latter is confirmed by RNAse H digestion of mRNA-Oligo-dT hybrids which shows that the two mRNA populations (470 ± 20 nucleotide (nt) and 430 ± 20 nt respectively) are conerted to a single population of 345 ± 15 nt in good accordance with the poly-A tail site determined by S1 mapping (347 nt). Thus one species has a poly-A tail of 145 nt appearing in round spermatids and the second, a shorter tail of 105 nt present at the later stages of elongated spermatids.

ACKNOWLEDGMENTS

The authors are grateful to Renu Sharma for technical assistance in the S1 mapping experiment, Andrea Seufert for transmitting the method for fixing the tissue, embedding and section cutting in the *in situ* experiments, Manfred Herfort for transmitting the method for dipping the slides in film emulsion for autoradiography and Pepi Albás for typing the manuscript.

REFERENCES

1. Dixon, G. H. 1972. Acta Endocrinol. (Suppl.) **168:** 128–154.
2. Mezquita, C. & C. S. Teng. 1977a. Biochem. J. **164:** 99–111.
3. Mezquita, C. & C. S. Teng. 1977b. Biochem. J. **170:** 203–210.
4. Oliva, R., S. Vidal & C. Mezquita. 1982. Biochem. J. **208:** 269–273.

5. OLIVA, R. & C. MEZQUITA. 1982. Nucleic Acids Res. **10:** 8049–8059.
6. OLIVA, R. & C. MEZQUITA. 1986. Biochemistry **25:** 6508–6511.
7. CHRISTENSEN, M. E. & G. H. DIXON. 1982. Dev. Biol. **93:** 404–415.
8. OLIVA, R., D. BAZETT-JONES, C. MEZQUITA, & G. H. DIXON. 1987. J. Biol. Chem. **262:** 17016–17025.
9. MARUSHIGE, K. & G. H. DIXON. 1971. J. Biol. Chem. **246:** 5799–5805.
10. OLIVA, R. & G. H. DIXON. 1989. J. Biol. Chem. **264:** 12472–12481.
11. OLIVA, R., J. MEZQUITA, C. MEZQUITA & G. H. DIXON. 1988. Dev. Biol. **125:** 332–340.
12. KLEENE, K. C., R. J. DISTEL & N. B. HECHT. 1984. Dev. Biol. **105:** 71–79.
13. ERICKSON, R. P., J. M. KRAUSER, J. RITTENHOUSE & A. SALKELD. 1980. Proc. Natl. Acad. Sci. USA. **77:** 6086–6090.
14. GOLD, B., H. FUJIMOTO, J. M. KRAMER, R. P. ERICKSON & N. B. HECHT. 1983. Dev. Biol. **98:** 392–399.
15. DISTEL, R. J., K. C. KLEENE & N. B. HECHT. 1984. Science **224:** 68–70.
16. KENNEDY, B. P., L. W. CRIM & P. L. DAVIES. 1985. Exp. Cell Res. **158:** 445–460.
17. IATROU, K. & G. H. DIXON. 1977. Cell **10:** 433–411.
18. SENIUK, N. A., W. G. TATTON, P. D. CANNON, A. T. GARBER & G. H. DIXON. 1991. Ann. N.Y. Acad. Sci. **637:** 277–288. This volume.
19. BENNETT, D. 1975. Cell **6:** 441–454.
20. PALMITER, R. D., T. M. WILKIE, H. Y. CHEN & R. L. BRINSTER. 1985. Cell **36:** 869–877.
21. KLEENE, K. C., R. J. DISTEL & N. B. HECHT. 1985. Biochemistry **24:** 719–722.
22. BROWN, R. E., R. R. BEHRINGER, J. J. PESCHON, R. L. BRINSTER & R. D. PALMITER. 1989. Nature **337:** 373–376.
23. GEDAMU, L. K. IATROU & G. H. DIXON. 1977. Cell **10:** 443–451.
24. IATROU, K. & G. H. DIXON. 1978. Fed. Proc. **37:** 2626–2533.
25. HECHT, N. B., P. A. BOWER, K. C. KLEENE & R. J. DISTEL. 1985. Differentiation **29:** 189–193.
26. PESCHON, J. J., R. R. BEHRINGER, R. L. BRINSTER & R. D. PALMITER. 1987. Proc. Natl. Acad. Sci. USA **84:** 5316–5319.
27. IATROU, K., A. W. SPIRA & G. H. DIXON. 1978. Devel. Biol. **64:** 82–98.
28. IATROU, K., L. GEDAMU & G. H. DIXON. 1979. Can J. Biochem. **57:** 945–956.
29. BRAWERMAN, G. 1981. CRC Crit. Rev. Biochem. **10:** 1–38.
30. BIRNSTIEL, M. L., M. BUSSLINGER & K. STRUB. 1985. Cell **41:** 349–359.
31. SHAPIRO, D. J., J. E. BLUME & D. A. NIELSEN. 1987. BioEssays **6:** 221–224.
32. FRIEDMAN, D. I., & J. IMPERIALE. 1987. Ann. Rev. Genet. **21:** 453–488.
33. HUMPHREY, T. & N. J. PROUDFOOT. 1988. Trends Genet. **4:** 243–245.
34. ROSS, J. 1989. Sci. Am. **260:** 48–55.
35. WICKENS, M. 1990. Trends Biochem. Sci. **15:** 320–324.
36. PROUDFOOT, N. 1991. Cell **64:** 671–674.

Expression of Homeobox Genes during Spermatogenesis[a]

DEBRA J. WOLGEMUTH[b,c] CAROLYN M. VIVIANO,[c]
AND FRANÇOISE WATRIN[c,d]

[b]*Department of Genetics and Development*
[c]*The Center for Reproductive Sciences*
Columbia University College of Physicians and Surgeons
630 West 168th Street
New York, New York 10032

[d]*Laboratory of Reproductive Physiology*
University of Paris
4 place Jussieux
75252 Paris Cedex 5, France

HOMEOBOX GENES AND THE REGULATION OF DEVELOPMENT AND DIFFERENTIATION

The homeobox is a highly conserved 183 bp domain found in several classes of development-regulating genes in *Drosophila*.[1-3] Its high level of sequence conservation in the genomes of organisms as evolutionarily diverse as flies, sea urchins, and mammals has provided a direct means for isolating potential development-regulating genes from the complex genomes of higher organisms.[4-7]

Several lines of evidence suggest that homeobox genes may control differentiation by functioning as transcription factors, regulating the expression of other genes, including other homeobox-containing genes. The homeobox domain is rich in basic amino acids and exhibits homology with known yeast and prokaryotic gene regulatory proteins.[8-10] The protein products of several *Drosophila*[11,12] and mouse[13,14] homeobox-containing genes have been localized to the nucleus using antibodies. Proteins containing homeodomains exhibit sequence specific DNA-binding as assayed by protection from DNase I digestion and by electrophoretic mobility shift assays.[15,16] Nuclear magnetic resonance and crystallographic studies on the homeodomain of the *Drosophila Antennapedia* (*Antp*)[17-19] and engrailed[20] genes provide direct evidence for the presence of a helix-turn-helix motif, and hence a potential DNA-binding function. Homeobox domains have been identified in several mammalian tissue-specific transcription factors;[21] for example, in the lymphoid-specific transcription factor OTF-2.[22] In addition, substitution of the homeobox domain from the *prl* gene for the DNA binding and dimerization domains of the *E2A* gene results in the production of a hybrid E2A/prl protein.[23,24] It has been suggested that this mutated form of the *E2A* gene could alter

[a] This work was supported by a grant from the National Institutes of Health (NIH), HD 18122, and a grant from the American Cancer Society.

[b] Author to whom correspondence should be sent; Tel.: (212)305-7900, FAX: (212)305-6084.

its target gene specificity and contribute to the observed acute lymphoblastic leukemia phenotype.

Drosophila homeobox-containing genes have been shown to regulate the expression of one another as well as other classes of development-regulating genes at the genetic and molecular level.[6,25] For example, the levels of expression of *Antp* and *Ultrabithorax* (*Ubx*) in the primordia of parasegments 2, 4, and 6 are dependent upon the proper expression of *fushi tarazu (ftz)*.[26] An intriguing cross-regulatory interaction is exhibited by *ftz* and *even-skipped* (*eve*), in which the absence of *ftz* expression in some neurons results in the elimination of *eve* expression.[27] Direct evidence for cross-regulation is also inferred from the several recent studies in *Drosophila* using *in vitro* binding assays and *in vivo* co-transfection assays.[6,17,25] Nothing is known about a potential cross-regulatory function of mammalian homeobox-containing genes. Since one would predict that cross-regulation via transcription factors would have to occur in a cell-autonomous manner, it will be important to ascertain the cellular site of expression of specific homeobox-containing genes. Spermatogenesis offers an excellent system in which to address this question in the mammal because, as is discussed below, it is possible to define the precise cell types expressing homeobox-containing genes.

CHARACTERIZATION OF MAMMALIAN HOMEOBOX-CONTAINING GENES

More than thirty murine homeobox genes have been identified and the expression of several of these genes has been characterized in embryos and adult tissues. Like their *Drosophila* counterparts, the mammalian homeobox genes exhibit temporal, spatial, and cellular specificity in their expression both during embryogenesis and in adult tissues.[28,29] Mammalian homeobox genes with homology to the *Antp* prototype sequence have been designated *Hox* genes in mouse and *HOX* in humans.[30-32] The homeodomain consists of a conserved arrangement of three helices. Helix three and helix two are thought to be responsible for DNA binding and stabilization, respectively, while helix one may be involved in protein/protein interactions. A comparison of several of the *Antp*-like *Hox* proteins has revealed that their general structure is conserved, with additional regions of homology existing outside of the homeodomain[33,34] (FIG. 1). Substantial conservation is seen in the amino-terminal region of these proteins, in addition to a conserved hexapeptide sequence 5′ to the homeodomain.

Four clusters of these genes have been cloned and mapped to specific chromosomes (FIG. 2). *Hox 1* is located on mouse chromosome 6 and human chromosome 7.[35] The other *Hox* clusters are *Hox 2* on mouse chromosome 11 (human chromosome 17), *Hox 3* on mouse chromosome 15 (human chromosome 12), and *Hox 4* on mouse chromosome 2 (human chromosome 2).[30,36] Although several homeobox genes map close to known developmental mutations, no allelism has yet been proven.[28] The sequence of the homeoboxes within a given cluster differ significantly from each other and from the *Antp* consensus, suggesting that a cluster may have been formed from successive duplications of an ancestral homeobox-containing gene. Subsequent duplication and divergence might then have created the four clusters that exist today.[37,38]

Inter- and intra-cluster comparison of the murine genes has enabled the distinction of subfamilies based on protein identity. The highest degree of conservation is seen between genes occupying the same position within different clusters (for example, *Hox-1.4*, *Hox-2.6*, and *Hox-4.2*). These genes can be referred to as paralogues. Each

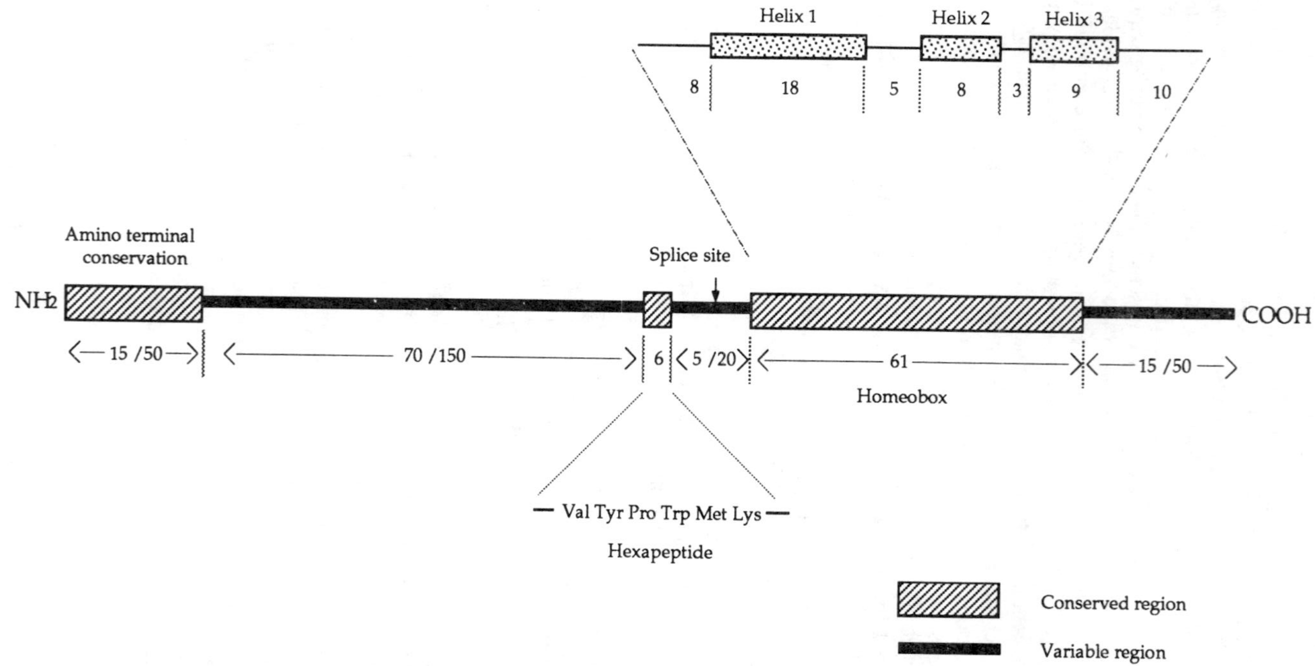

FIGURE 1. Conserved features of vertebrate Hox proteins. Conserved regions are indicated by hatched boxes; numbers indicate approximate sizes (numbers of amino acid residues) of the various domains. The three helices believed to make up the homeobox are shown by stippled boxes. Typically, a splice junction lies 5′ to the homeobox (*arrow*).

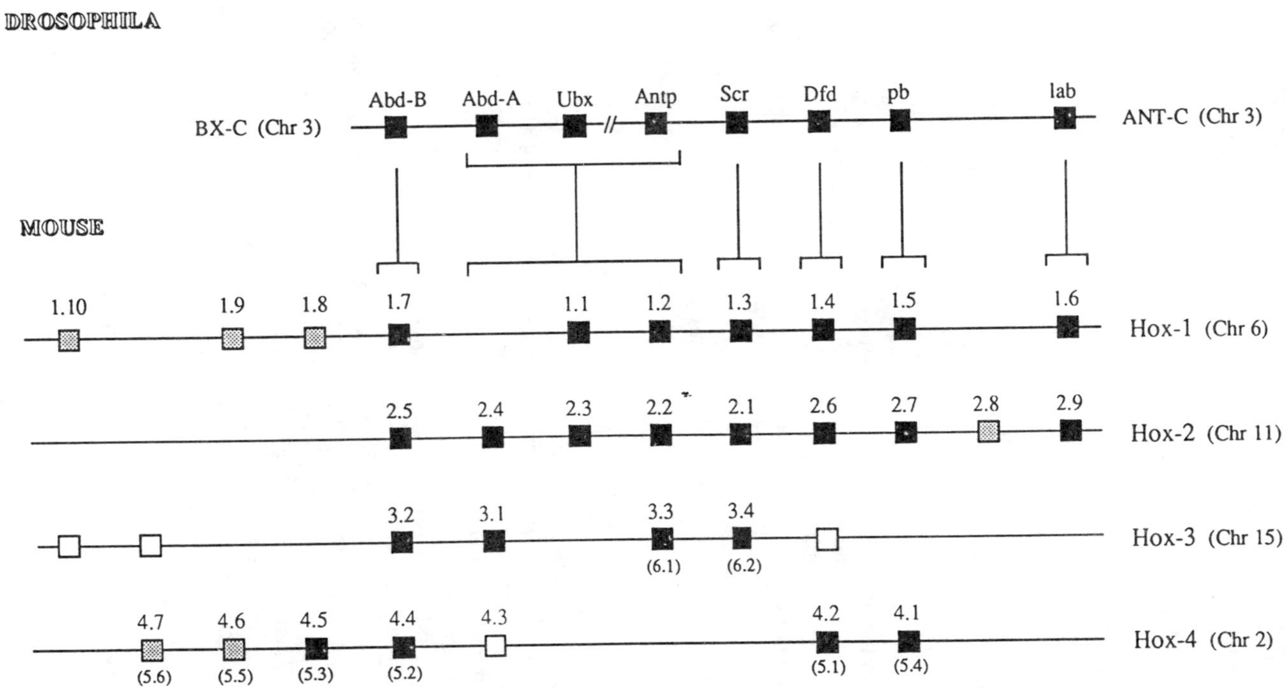

FIGURE 2. Diagram of the nomenclature and organization of vertebrate homeobox genes (Terminology according to refs. 30–32). The number in parentheses after each cluster indicates chromosomal location. The distances between the *Hox* genes have been standardized to facilitate the vertical alignment of paralogous genes. Open boxes represent genes that are predicted from the analysis of human or chicken clusters. Numbers in parentheses below a box indicate its previous designation.[30–32]

set of paralogous murine genes has a *Drosophila* counterpart, as the *Antennapedia* and *bithorax* clusters can be aligned with their vertebrate counterparts according to the same criteria (FIG. 2; for a review, see Kessel and Gruss[29]). These observations are consistent with the theory that the *Drosophila* and murine clusters have evolved from a common ancester.

CORRELATION OF THE STRUCTURAL ORGANIZATION AND THE EXPRESSION OF *Hox* GENES DURING EMBRYOGENESIS AND IN THE ADULT

In the developing embryo mouse *Hox* genes are expressed in ectodermal and mesodermal derivatives along the rostro-caudal axis of the embryo, in a series of partially overlapping domains. As in *Drosophila*, a correlation can be established between the anterior limit of expression of genes along the rostro-caudal axis of the embryo and their relative position within a cluster: genes located at the most 3′ end of a complex being expressed the more anteriorly in the embryo.[33,34,39] This conservation of position within the cluster throughout evolution suggests that maintenance of position may be important for gene regulation. In particular, it has been proposed that the coordinated expression of genes within a cluster (designated as orthologues) along the antero-posterior axis of the embryo could result from the presence of multiple *cis*-acting regulatory elements distributed along the clusters.[33,34] The recent observations that tissue and/or cellular specificity in the mouse embryo might be shared by adjacent members of a cluster would further support the existence of linked *cis*-acting regulatory elements.[39,40]

The relationship between expression boundaries and gene order has recently been shown to have an *in vitro* correlate. Using teratocarcinoma cells, Simeone *et al.*[41] showed that the time-course and level of retinoic acid-inducible expression of genes within the human *HOX2* cluster is related to their 5′ to 3′ order. The most 3′ *HOX2* gene responds to low concentrations of retinoic acid, while increasingly higher concentrations of retinoic acid are needed to induce the expression of more 5′ genes. At a given concentration of retinoic acid, induction of 5′ genes requires a period of days, whereas transcripts from 3′ genes appear in hours.

Comparative analysis on the pattern of expression in the mouse embryo of several sets of paralogous genes has also recently been undertaken. Although stage and tissue-specific differences exist in the pattern of expression, paralogous genes of subfamilies located at the 3′ end of the clusters, such as *Hox-1.4*, *Hox-2.6*, and *Hox-4.2*[40,42] and *Hox-1.3*, *Hox-2.1*, and *Hox-3.4*,[43] display similarities in their antero-posterior boundaries of expression in the embryonic central nervous system and in the prevertebral column. This suggests the conservation of common regulatory elements during the duplication and divergence of the clusters. In contrast, paralogous genes of subfamilies located toward the 5′ end of the clusters, such as *Hox-1.7, Hox-2.5*, *Hox-3.2*, and *Hox-4.4,*[44] and *Hox-1.1* and *Hox-2.3*[45] do not show such similarities in their anterior boundaries of expression in the central nervous system and the prevertebral column.

Several of the mouse homeobox-containing genes have been shown to also be expressed in adult tissues and in specialized cell lineages, including the hematopoietic lineage[46,47] and the germ cell lineage.[48,49] In particular, *Hox-1.4* is expressed abundantly and in a very precise pattern of expression in the male adult germ line[48,50] (see below). Interestingly, the two *Hox-1.4* paralogues, *Hox-2.6* and *Hox-4.2*, have also been reported to be expressed in the adult mouse testis[51,52] as have other members of the *Hox-1* cluster: *Hox-1.1* and *Hox-1.2*;[53,54] *Hox-1.3*;[13] *Hox-1.5* (F. Ruddle, personal communication); and *Hox-1.6*.[55] It will therefore be of interest to consider if regulatory elements that function in the adult lineages are also conserved between paralogues (*e.g.*, *Hox-1.4* and *Hox-2.6*), as evidenced by their similar cellular specificity of expression. Further, the question as to whether there is a temporal or cellular correlation of expression of the orthologous genes needs to be addressed.

SPECIFICITY OF EXPRESSION OF *Hox-1.4* IN THE MALE GERM LINE

The mouse gene now termed *Hox-1.4* was first identified as a cDNA clone pHBT-1, isolated from a library prepared from adult mouse testis RNA.[48] To examine the tissue specificity of expression of *Hox-1.4*, RNA was isolated from a variety of adult tissues, including ovary. Transcripts of 1.4 kb in size were abundant in total RNA of testis but not in any of the other adult tissues examined. Among the murine homeobox genes examined to date, *Hox-1.4* is unique in exhibiting such a tissue-specificity of expression in the adult.

We have used several experimental approaches to show that *Hox-1.4* expression in the testis is restricted to the germ line, specifically to cells that have entered meiotic prophase.[48,50,57] RNA was isolated from testes of a mutant strain of mice carrying the *atrichosis* (*at*) allele, which renders the homozygous animals (*at/at*) sterile because of the absence of germ cells[48] (FIG. 3). *Hox-1.4* transcripts were not detected in RNA from these testes, suggesting that this gene is expressed only in the germinal compartment of the testis. We also took advantage of the developmental progression of spermatogenesis in the embryonic and neonatal mouse, illustrated in FIGURE 4, to determine whether *Hox-1.4* was expressed in pre- or post-meiotic germ cells.[48] As diagrammed in FIGURE 4 and documented in FIGURE 5, neonatal testes from day 7 mice contain spermatogonia, but do not contain meiotic germ cells. Day 17 neonatal testes contain germ cells in all stages of meiotic prophase. Adult testes contain the complete germ cell lineage from spermatogonia to mature spermatozoa. Neonatal and adult testes both contain the complete somatic cell lineage, including Leydig cells, Sertoli cells and peritubular cells. *Hox-1.4* transcripts were not detected in RNA from embryonic or neonatal testes, but were found in samples from adult animals. This strongly suggested that *Hox-1.4* is expressed in the germ line, specifically in cells which have entered into meiotic prophase. *In situ* hybridization analysis confirmed the prediction that *Hox-1.4* was most abundantly expressed in germ cells which had entered the meiotic prophase stage of spermatogenic differentiation (FIG. 5).

To more accurately compare the levels of *Hox-1.4* transcripts in specific cell types, we examined *Hox-1.4* expression by Northern blot hybridization analysis of RNA isolated from enriched populations of spermatogenic cells.[48] *Hox-1.4* transcripts were shown to be present in germ cells from the time they enter meiotic prophase through to the stage where the cytoplasm is shed as the residual body. Using high resolution gel analysis, we detected two different testicular transcripts within the broadly migrating band at ~ 1.4 kb. These transcripts are 1.35 and 1.45 kb in length. The molecular basis of the difference in size of the testicular *Hox-1.4* transcripts has been investigated using an assay based on RNase H sensitivity of double stranded RNA and has revealed that *Hox-1.4* testicular transcripts differ in length of poly(A) tails (C. M.

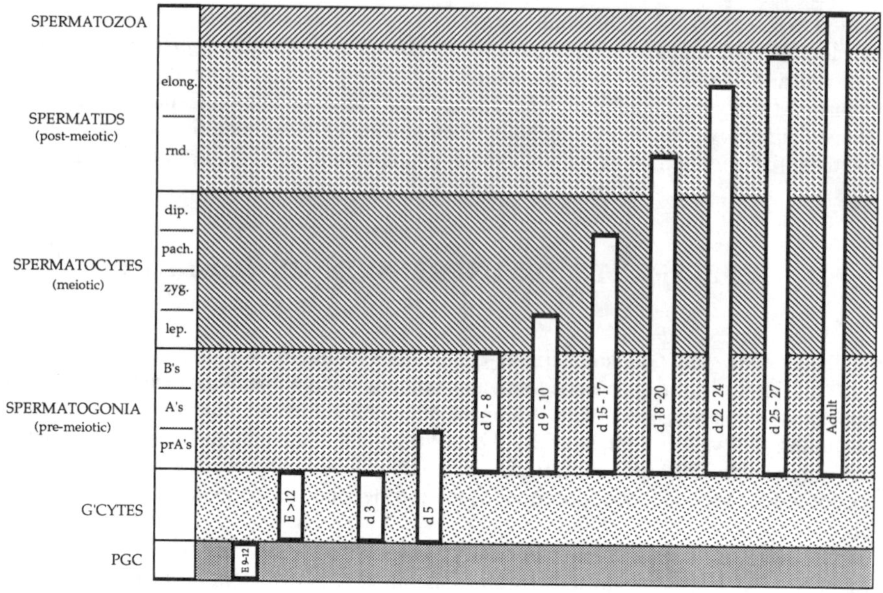

FIGURE 3. Male germ cell populations during the first wave of spermatogenesis in the mouse. The horizontal shaded areas represent the different germ cell populations. The vertical bars indicate which cell types are present at a given stage of pre- or post-natal development. E = embryonic day and d = days post-natal. In the mouse, the progression from spermatogonia to sperm occurs over a period of 35 days.

Viviano and D. J. Wolgemuth, in preparation). The significance of this increase in the length of the poly(A) tail is not known; however, changes in poly(A) tail length have been implicated in stability and translational activation. It is not clear whether a change in poly(A) tail length signals or is concomitant with translational activation. Although speculative, it is possible that the post-meiotic increase in poly(A) tail length of the testicular *Hox-1.4* mRNA reflects translational activation of this message. While localization of the *Hox-1.4* protein may help to clarify this issue, definitive proof would depend upon the identification and testing of sequence elements capable of mediating translational control through cytoplasmic polyadenylation.

Like all of the other mouse homeobox genes characterized to date, *Hox-1.4* is expressed during mid-gestational development of the mouse embryo.[48,49,58-60] The embryonic expression of *Hox-1.4* shows a specific and characteristic pattern. Northern blot and *in situ* hybridization analyses have shown that in the mid-gestation mouse embryo (days 11 to 12.5), *Hox-1.4* mRNAs are most abundant in the developing central nervous system, particularly in the caudal myelencephalon and the rostral spinal cord.[58-60] Other reported sites of embryonic expression include dorsal root ganglia[60] and developing lung and gut.[59,60]

The embryonic versus adult testicular expression of *Hox-1.4* also differs in the size of the transcripts produced: mRNAs of ~ 1.4 kb are observed in the germ line, whereas

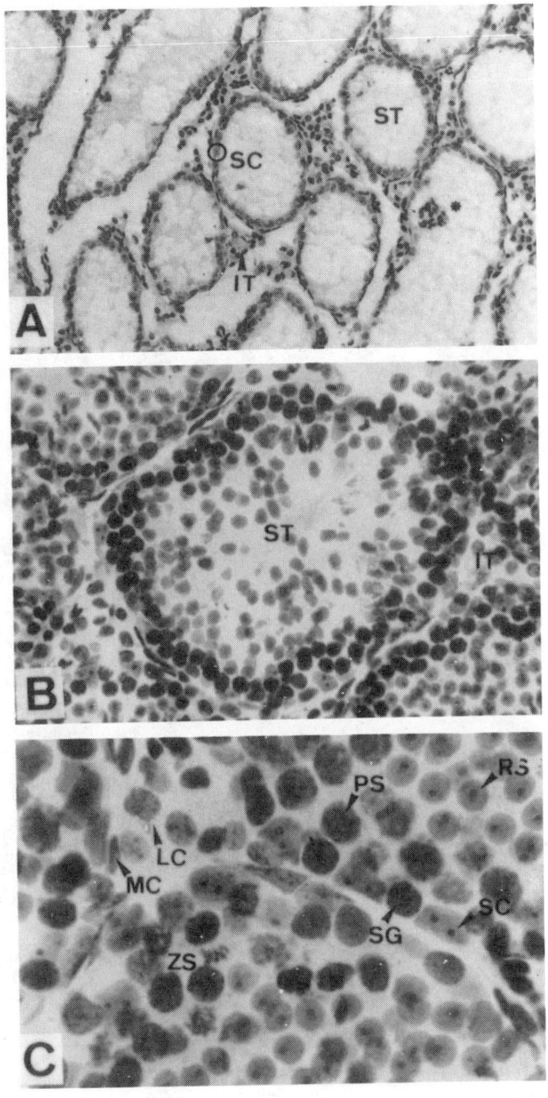

FIGURE 4. Histological analysis of testis sections from normal and mutant adult mice. Testes were fixed with paraformaldehyde, sectioned, and stained with hematoxylin and eosin according to our standard procedures (ref. 50). **A:** section of testis from mice homozygous for the *atriochis* mutation (*at/at*) (×80). **B** and **C** show testicular sections from normal mice, photographed at ×175 (**B**) and ×350 (**C**) magnification. IT = interstial tissue; LC = Leydig cell; MC = peritubular myoid cell; PS = meiotic prophase spermatocyte in the pachytene stage; RS = round spermatid; SC = Sertoli cell; SG = spermatogonium; ST = seminiferous tubule.

the embryonic transcripts are ~1.7 kb in length.[48,50] Direct sequence analysis of genomic and cDNA clones and RNase protection analysis suggest that the embryonic and testicular mRNAs differ at their amino terminal ends (C. M. Viviano and D. J. Wolgemuth, in preparation). The available sequence data also support the hypothesis of the existence of a more 5′ promoter, which may be testis-specific and result in the transcription of an additional small exon. These data also indicate that the *Hox-1.4* protein produced in the testis will *a priori* differ from its embryonic counterpart.

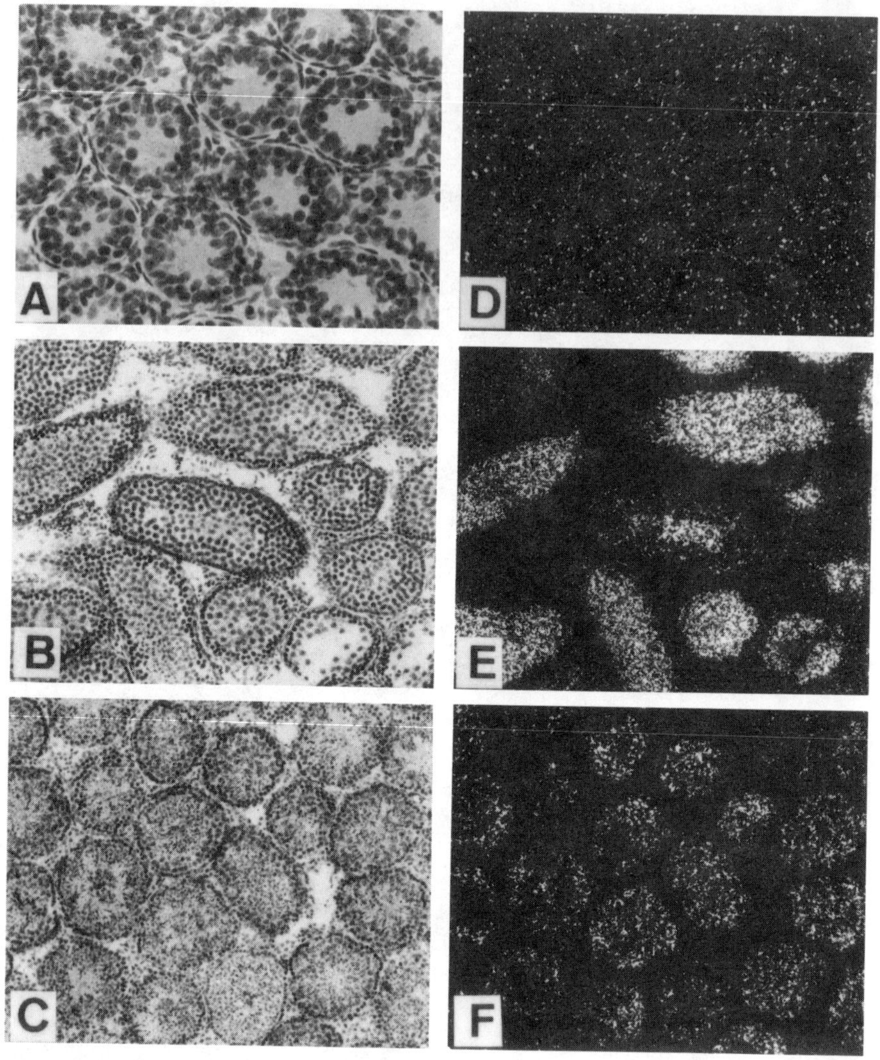

FIGURE 5. Analysis by *in situ* hybridization of the onset of expression of the *Hox-1.4* gene during the first wave of spermatogenesis in the mouse testis. Sections of testes were hybridized with antisense *Hox-1.4* probe p2181 B2 4a (ref. 50) labeled with ^{35}S-UTP. Bright field photographs are shown in **A**, **B**, and **C** and photographs taken with dark field illumination in **D**, **E**, and **F**. Sections were obtained from testes of 7 days (**A** and **D**), 17 days (**B** and **E**), and adult (**C** and **F**) animals.

SUMMARY AND FUTURE STUDIES

The discovery of the evolutionarily conserved homeobox sequence provided a means for isolating potential development regulating genes in vertebrates, and indeed, homeobox-containing genes have now been isolated from a variety of species from *Drosophila* to human. Over thirty homeobox-containing genes have been isolated from mouse alone, and like their *Drosophila* counterparts, they are thought to play an important role in pattern formation during embryonic development. In addition, they appear to be important in the differentiation of several adult tissues including the nervous system, the hematopoietic system, and the germ cell lineage. Conserved features of Hox proteins, their nuclear localization, and their ability to regulate the expression of other genes has suggested that these proteins function as transcription factors.

The generation of transgenic mice in which germ cell specific expression of *Hox-1.4* has been altered while somatic expression remains intact would provide a means of assessing the action of *Hox-1.4* during germ cell development. Once testis-specific promoter elements have been defined for *Hox-1.4*, they could be targeted for mutation by homologous recombination. Alternatively, *Hox-1.4* antisense constructs could be designed such that they would be driven by an appropriate spermatogenic-specific promoter (for example *PGK-2*) and they would produce stable RNAs. Stabilization of the antisense RNAs might be accomplished using sequences from the 3′ untranslated region of the *protamine-1* gene. The antisense experiments are more immediately feasible as the testis specific promoter elements for *Hox-1.4* have not yet been defined. It is important however, that efforts be made to interfere with the expression of this gene as these types of experiments are likely to provide valuable information regarding function during spermatogenesis.

REFERENCES

1. McGinnis, W., M. L. Levine, E. Hafen, A. Kuroiwa & W. J. Gehring. 1984. A conserved DNA sequence in homeotic genes of the *Drosophila Antennapedia* and *Bithorax* complexes. Nature **308:** 428–433.
2. Scott, M. P. & A. J. Weiner. 1984. Structural relationships among genes that control development: Sequence homology between the *Antennapedia*, *Ultrabithorax*, and *fushi tarazu* loci of *Drosophila*. Proc. Natl. Acad. Sci. USA **81:** 4115–4119.
3. Gehring, W. J. 1987. Homeoboxes in the study of development. Science **236:** 1245–1252.
4. McGinnis, W., R. L. Garber, J. Wirz, A. Kuroiwa & W. J. Gehring. 1984. A homologous protein-coding sequence in *Drosophila* homeotic genes and its conservation in other Metazoans. Cell **37:** 403–408.
5. Carrasco, A. E., W. McGinnis, W. J. Gehring & E. M. De Robertis. 1984. Cloning of an *X. laevis* gene expressed during early embryogenesis coding for a peptide region homologous to *Drosophila* homeotic genes. Cell **37:** 409–414.
6. Scott, M. P., J. W. Tamkun & G. W. Hartzell, III. 1989. The structure and function of the homeodomain. BBA Reviews on Cancer **9:** 25–48.
7. Dressler, G. R. & P. Gruss. 1988. Do multigene families regulate vertebrate development? Trends in Genetics **4:** 214–219.
8. Shepherd, J. C. W., W. McGinnis, A. E. Carrasco, E. M. De Robertis & W. J. Gehring. 1984. Fly and frog homeo domains show homologies with yeast mating type regulatory proteins. Nature **310:** 70–71.
9. Pabo, C. O. & R. T. Sauer. 1984. Protein-DNA recognition. Ann. Rev. Biochem. **53:** 293–321.
10. Laughon, A. & M. P. Scott. 1984. Sequence of a *Drosophila* segmentation gene: Protein structure homology with DNA binding proteins. Nature **310:** 25–31.

11. Beachy, P. A., S. L. Helfand & D. S. Hogness. 1985. Segmental distribution of *Bithorax* complex proteins during *Drosophila* development. Nature **313:** 545–551.

12. DiNardo, S., J. M. Kuner, J. Theis & P. H. O'Farrell. 1985. Development of embryonic pattern in *D. melanogaster* as revealed by accumulation of the nuclear *Engrailed* protein. Cell **43:** 59–69.

13. Odenwald, W. F., C. F. Taylor, F. J. Palmer-Hill, V. Friedrich, Jr., M. Tani & R. A. Lazzarini. 1987. Expression of a homeo domain protein in noncontact-inhibited cultured cells and postmitotic neurons. Genes & Dev. **1:** 482–496.

14. Kessel, M., F. Schulze, M. Fibi & P. Gruss. 1987. Primary structure and nuclear localization of a murine homeodomain protein. Proc. Nat. Acad. Sci. USA **84:** 5304–5310.

15. Desplan, C., J. Theis & P. H. O'Farrell. 1985. The *Drosophila* developmental gene, *Engrailed*, encodes a sequence specific DNA binding activity. Nature **318:** 630–635.

16. Odenwald, W. F., J. Garbern, H. Arnheiter, E. Tournier-Lasserve & R. A. Lazzarini. 1989. The *Hox-1.3* homeobox protein is a sequence specific DNA-binding phosphoprotein. Genes & Dev. **3:** 158–172.

17. Muller, M., M. Affolter, W. Leupin, G. Otting, K. Wuthrich & W. Gehring. 1988. Isolation and sequence-specific DNA binding of the *Antennapedia* homeodomain. EMBO J. **7:** 4299–4304.

18. Otting, G., Y. Qian, M. Muller, M. Affolter, W. Gehring & K. Wuthrich. 1988. Secondary structure determination for the *Antennapedia* homeodomain by nuclear magnetic resonance and evidence for a helix-turn-helix motif. EMBO J. **7:** 4305–4309.

19. Billeter, M., Y. Qian, G. Otting, M. Muller, W. J. Gehring & K. Wuthrich. 1990. Determination of the three-dimensional structure of the *Antennapedia* homeodomain from *Drosophila* in solution by ^{1}H nuclear magnetic resonance spectroscopy. J Mol. Biol. **214:** 183–197.

20. Kissinger, C. R., B. Liu, E. Martin-Blanco, T. B. Kornberg & C. O. Pabo. 1990. Crystal structure of an engrailed homeodomain-DNA complex at 2.8 Å resolution: A framework for understanding homeodomain-DNA interactions. Cell **63:** 579–590.

21. Levine, M. & T. Hoey. 1988. Homeobox proteins as sequence-specific transcription factors. Cell **55:** 537–540.

22. Scheidereit, C., J. A. Cromlish, T. Gerster, K. Kawakami, C-G. Balmaceda, R. A. Currie & R. G. Roeder. 1988. A human lymphoid-specific transcription factor that activates immunoglobulin genes is a homeobox protein. Nature **336:** 551–557.

23. Nourse, J., J. D. Mellentin, N. Galili, J. Wilkinson, E. Stanbridge, S. D. Smith & M. L. Cleary. 1990. Chromosomal translocation t(1;19) results in synthesis of a homeobox fusion mRNA that codes for a potential chimeric transcription factor. Cell **60:** 535–545.

24. Kamps, M. P., C. Murre, X. Sun & D. Baltimore. 1990. A new homeobox gene contributes the DNA binding domain of the t(1;19) translocation protein in pre-B ALL. Cell **60:** 547–555.

25. Han, K., M. S. Levine & J. L. Manley. 1989. Synergistic activation and repression of transcription by *Drosophila* homeobox proteins. Cell **56:** 573–583.

26. Ingham, P. W. & A. Martinez-Arias. 1986. The correct activation of *Antennapedia* and *bithorax* complex genes requires the *fushi tarazu gene.* Nature **324:** 592–597.

27. Doe, C. Q., Y. Hironi, W. J. Gehring & C. S. Goodman. 1988. Expression and function of the segmentation gene *fushi tarazu* during *Drosophila* neurogenesis. Science **239:** 170–175.

28. Holland, P. W. H. & B. L. M. Hogan. 1988. Expression of homeobox genes during mouse development: A review. Genes & Dev. **2:** 773–782.

29. Kessel, M. & P. Gruss. 1990. Murine developmental control genes. Science **249:** 374–379.

30. Martin, G. R., E. Boncinelli, D. Duboule, P. Gruss, I. Jackson, R. Krumlauf, P. Lonai, W. McGinnis, F. Ruddle & D. Wolgemuth. 1987. Nomenclature for homeobox-containing genes. Nature 325: 21–22.

31. McAlpine, P. J. & T. B. Shows. 1990. Nomenclature for human homeobox genes. Genomics **7:** 460–461.

32. Duboule, D., E. Boncinelli, E. DeRobertis, M. Featherstone, P. Lonai, G. Oliver & F. H. Ruddle. 1990. An update of mouse and human HOX gene nomenclature. Genomics **7:** 358–359.

33. Duboule, D. & P. Dolle. 1989. The structural and functional organization of the murine *Hox* gene family resembles that of *Drosophila* homeotic genes. EMBO J. **8:** 1497–1505.

34. GRAHAM, A., N. PAPALOPULU & R. KRUMLAUF. 1989. The murine and *Drosophila* homeobox gene complexes have common features of organization and expression. Cell **57:** 367–378.
35. BUCAN, M., T. YANG-FENG, A. M. COLBERG-POLEY, D. J. WOLGEMUTH, J. L. GUENET, U. FRANCKE & H. LEHRACH. 1986. Genetic and cytogenetic localization of the homeo box containing genes on mouse chromosome 6 and human chromosome 7. EMBO J. **5:** 2899–2905.
36. BONCINELLI, E., R. SOMMA, D. ACAMPORA, M. PANNESE, M. D'ESPOSITO, A. FAIELLA & A. SIMEONE. 1988. Organisation of human homeobox genes. Hum. Reprod. **3:** 880–886.
37. FIBI, M., B. ZINK, M. KESSEL, A. M. COLBERG-POLEY, S. LABEIT, H. LEHRACH & P. GRUSS. 1988. Coding sequence and expression of the homeo box gene *Hox-1.3.* Development **102:** 349–360.
38. KAPPEN, C., K. SCHUGHART & F. H. RUDDLE. 1989. Two steps in the evolution of *Antennapedia*-class vertebrate homeobox genes. Proc. Nat. Acad. Sci. **86:** 5459.
39. GAUNT, S. J., P. T. SHARPE & D. DUBOULE. 1988. Spatially restricted domains of homeo-gene transcripts in mouse embryos: Relation to a segmented body plan. *Development* **104**(Suppl.): 169–179.
40. WATRIN, F. & D. J. WOLGEMUTH. 1991. Conserved and unique regulatory elements among *Hox* genes suggested by expression patterns of orthologues and paralogues of the mouse *Hox-1.4* gene. Submitted for publication.
41. SIMEONE, A., D. ACAMPORA, L. ARCIONI, P. W. ANDREWS, E. BONCINELLI & F. MAVILIO. 1990. Sequential activation of Hox 2 homeobox genes by retinoic acid in human embryonal carcinoma cells. Nature **346:** 763–766.
42. GAUNT, S. J., R. KRUMLAUF & D. DUBOULE. 1989. Mouse homeogenes within a subfamily, *Hox-1.4*, *-2.6*, and *-5.1*, display similar anteroposterior domains of expression in the embryo, but show stage- and tissue-dependent differences in their regulation. *Development* **107:** 131–137.
43. GAUNT, S. J., P. L. COLETTA, D. PRAVTCHEVA & P. T. SHARPE. 1990. Mouse *Hox-3.4*: Homeobox sequence and embryonic expression patterns compared with other members of the *Hox* gene network. Development **109:** 329–340.
44. ERSELIUS, J. R., M. D. GOULDING & P. GRUSS. 1990. Structure and expression pattern of the murine *Hox-3.2* gene. Development **110:** 629–642.
45. R. VOGELS, W. DE GRAAFF & J. DESCHAMPS. 1990. Expression of the murine homeobox-containing gene *Hox-2.3* suggests multiple time-dependent and tissue-specific roles during development. Development **110:** 1159–1168.
46. LONAI, P., E. ARMAN, H. CZOSNECK, F. H. RUDDLE & C. BLATT. 1987. New murine homeoboxes: Structure, chromosomal assignment, and differential expression in adult erythropoieses. DNA **6:** 409–418.
47. KONGSUWAN, K., E. WEBB, P. HOUSIAUX & J. M. 1988. Expression of the multiple homeobox genes within diverse mammalian haematopoietic lineages. EMBO J. **7:** 2131–2138.
48. WOLGEMUTH, D. J., E. ENGELMYER, R. N. DUGGAL, E. GIZANG-GINSBERG, G. L. MUTTER, C. PONZETTO, C. M. VIVIANO & Z. F. ZAKERI. 1986. Isolation of a mouse cDNA coding for a developmentally regulated testis-specific transcript containing homeobox homology. EMBO J. **5:** 1229–1235.
49. RUBIN, M. R., L. E. TOTH, M. D. PATEL, P. D'EUSTACHIO & M. C. NGUYEN-HUU. 1986. A mouse homeobox gene is expressed in spermatocytes and embryos. Science **233:** 663–667.
50. WOLGEMUTH, D. J., C. VIVIANO, E. GIZANG-GINSBERG, M. FROHMAN, A. JOYNER & G. R. MARTIN. 1987. Differential expression of the homeo box-containing gene *Hox 1.4* during male germ cell differentiation and embryonic development. Proc. Nat. Acad. Sci USA **84:** 5813–5817.
51. GRAHAM A., N. PAPALOPULU, J. LORIMER, J. H. MCVEY, E. G. D. TUDDENHAM & R. KRUMLAUF. 1988. Characterization of a murine homeo box gene, *Hox-2.6*, related to the *Drosophila Deformed* gene. Genes & Dev. **2:** 1424–1438.
52. FEATHERSTONE, M. S., A. BARON, S. GAUNT, M.-G. MATTEI & D. DUBOULE. 1988. *Hox-5.1* defines a homeobox-containing locus on mouse chromosome 2. Proc. Nat. Acad. Sci. USA **85:** 4760–4764.
53. COLBERG-POLEY, A. M., S. D. VOSS, K. CHOWDHURY & P. GRUSS. 1985. Structural analysis of murine genes containing homeobox sequences and their expression in embryonal carcinoma cells. Nature **314:** 713–718.
54. COLBERG-POLEY, A. M., S. D. VOSS, K. CHOWDHURY, C. STEWART, E. F. WAGNER & P. GRUSS.

1985. Clustered homeoboxes are differentially expressed during murine development. Cell **43:** 39–45.

55. BARON, A., M. S. FEATHERSTONE, R. E. HILL, A. HALL, B. GALLIOT & D. DUBOULE. 1987. Hox-1.6: A mouse homeo-box containing gene member of the *Hox-1* complex. EMBO J. **6:** 2977–2986.
56. BARON, A., M. S. FEATHERSTONE, R. E. HILL, A. HALL, B. GALLIOT & D. DUBOULE. 1987. *Hox-1.6*: A mouse homeo-box-containing gene member of the *Hox-1* complex. EMBO J. **6:** 2977–2986.
57. WOLGEMUTH, D. J., M. MOSTOLLER, C. M. VIVIANO, Z. F. ZAKERI, Y. IWAOKI & G. L. MUTTER. 1988. Temporal and Cellular Specificity of the Murine Homeobox-Containing Gene *Hox-1.4*. *In* Cell to Cell Signals in Mammalian Development. S. W. de Laat, J. G. Bluemink & C. L. Mummery, Eds.: 85–96. Springer-Verlag. Berlin.
58. DUBOULE, D., A. BARON, P. MAHL & B. GALLIOT. 1985. The homeo-box is present in overlapping cosmid clones which define the mouse *Hox-1* locus. EMBO J. **5:** 1973–1980.
59. WOLGEMUTH, D. J., R. R. BEHRINGER, M. P. MOSTOLLER, R. L. BRINSTER & R. D. PALMITER. 1989. Transgenic mice overexpressing the mouse homeobox-containing gene *Hox-1.4* exhibit abnormal gut development. Nature **337:** 464–467.
60. TOTH, L. E., K. L. SLAWN, J. E. PINTAR & M. C. NGUYEN-HUU. 1987. Region-specific expression of mouse homeobox genes in the embryonic mesoderm and central nervous system. Proc. Nat. Acad. Sci. USA **84:** 6790–6794.

Expression of Receptors during the Cycle of the Seminiferous Epithelium[a]

CAROL C. LINDER, LESLIE L. HECKERT, KENNETH P. ROBERTS, KWAN HEE KIM, AND MICHAEL D. GRISWOLD

Department of Biochemistry and Biophysics
Washington State University
Pullman, Washington 99164

INTRODUCTION

The process of spermatogenesis involves a large number of morphologically and biochemically distinct cell types. In any section of the seminiferous tubules from the rat testis, 4 to 5 cell types are found in well-defined patterns of association.[11] These cell types undergo coordinate development toward the formation of spermatozoa. An examination of the patterns of cellular association demonstrate that at any given point in the tubules these associations define a recurring developmental scheme called the cycle of the seminiferous epithelium.[1] Even though this scheme is a continuous developmental process in the rat, the cycle can be separated on the basis of the morphology of the germinal cells, into 14 discrete stages representing 14 different groups of germ cell intermediates. The cellular associations repeat themselves every 12.8 days and the progressive differentiation of a stem cell into a spermatozoan requires the cycle to be traversed approximately 3.7 times over a period of 48 days.[1,2] Sertoli cells not only provide physical and biochemical support to the associated germ cells but also undergo functional changes in response to the cyclical requirements of each of the stages. Cyclic morphological changes in the Sertoli cells associated with different stages have been well documented and information on cyclic biochemical processes is rapidly emerging.[3,4]

USE OF SYNCHRONIZED TESTES

Mammals have evolved asynchronous spermatogenesis because of their need for a continuous supply of sperm. At any given region in the seminiferous tubules of the rat only one stage or pattern of cellular associations is found but in the entire testis all 14 stages are represented many times. This arrangement complicates the determination of cyclic biochemical events in Sertoli cells and has led to the use of specialized experimental techniques. Portions of seminiferous tubules in each stage of

[a] Research for this paper was supported by National Institutes of Health (NIH) grants HD 10808 and HD 25846.

the cycle can be manually dissected from the rat testis and used for biochemical studies.[5] Alternatively, biochemical observations can be made on cross sections of individual tubules using the techniques of immunohistochemistry and *in situ* hybridization.[6] While each of these techniques has been useful, they are limited by the amount of available material and the abundance of the antigen or mRNA. Another approach has been the use of rats with stage-synchronized testes to examine the cyclic activities of Sertoli cells.[6,7] When rats are subjected to a regimen of vitamin A depletion and replacement, spermatogenesis has been demonstrated to be normal except that it is synchronized. Instead of all 14 stages, only 3 to 4 closely related stages are present and sperm are produced approximately every 12.8 days. Since the timing of the cycle remains intact, testes synchronized to defined stages can be obtained simply by sacrificing the rats at various times after retinol replenishment. The advantage of this approach is the availability of large amounts of testicular tissue in defined stages which allows for the characterization of low abundance proteins or mRNAs. We have utilized this technique to examine the cyclic appearance of mRNAs for receptors for hormones, vitamin A and transferrin.

GENERAL PROCEDURES

We have used an established protocol of vitamin A depletion and replacement to obtain rat testes synchronized to specific regions of the cycle of the seminiferous epithelium.[8] The mRNA was then isolated from the testes and subjected to Northern blot analysis. The blots were probed with cDNA probes specific for the transcripts of interest. Autoradiograms of the blots were digitized and quantified by a BioImage data analysis system.

CONTROL FOR AMOUNT OF mRNA

The level of SGP-1 (saposin) mRNA was used to control for the amount of mRNA loaded in each lane. Previous studies using *in situ* hybridization have shown that the SGP-1 mRNA levels change very little across the stages of the cycle.[6] Therefore, all data was normalized to the amount of SGP-1 mRNA in each lane of the Northern blot.

Expression of Results

The integrated densitometric values from the autoradiograms were normalized to the levels of SGP-1 and the highest value for a specific probe was set at 100%. The relative levels of the other samples were then derived. For each sample of synchronized testis the median point and synchronization window were determined.[9] Both of these values can be obtained as a function of the fraction of one cycle and they roughly correspond to the mean ± one standard deviation of the distribution of stages. The median point and synchronization window were plotted against the relative levels of a specific mRNA on a graph template which took into account the relative duration of each stage of the cycle.

TRANSFERRIN RECEPTOR

The transferrin synthesized by Sertoli cells is purportedly utilized in a mechanism which results in the transportation of ferric ions through the Sertoli cells and to the germ cells.[3,10,11] Quantitative *in situ* hybridization and Northern blot hybridization were used in conjunction with stage-synchronized rat testes to show that the amount of transferrin mRNA in Sertoli cells was approximately two fold higher in stages XII–XIV.[6] Transferrin receptor mRNA examined in a similar manner revealed a very different pattern of expression.[12] The levels of transferrin receptor mRNA varied 5- to 7-fold across the cycle with maximal levels in stages VII to XI. Since transferrin receptor mRNA levels are subject to regulation by intracellular iron levels, we propose that Sertoli cells have the lowest intracellular iron levels during stages V to VII of the cycle.[13] These low iron levels may lead to the induction of transferrin receptor mRNA whose protein product can then be used to accumulate iron in Sertoli cells to be delivered to germ cells. The relationship between the levels of these two mRNAs and the proposed iron delivery cycle are illustrated in FIGURE 1.

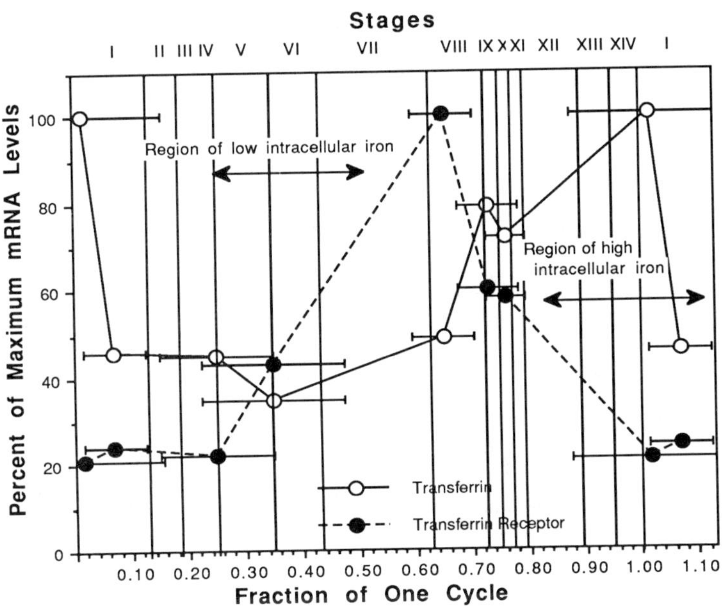

FIGURE 1. Relative levels of transferrin and transferrin receptor mRNA. Stage-synchronized testes were obtained from rats using the VAD depletion-replacement procedure. The distribution of stages (200 tubules) in each testis was determined by light microscopy. The total RNA was isolated from each sample and the mRNA isolated by chromatography over oligo-dT columns. The mRNA (10 μg) from each testis was run on a denaturing agarose gel and blotted to a nylon filter. The blot was probed with ^{32}P-UTP labeled cRNA from plasmids containing the transferrin or transferrin receptor cDNA. The band densities were determined by densitometric scanning of the autoradiographs. The amount of RNA loaded was determined by hybridization to nick-translated cDNA for the SGP-1 sequence.

RETINOIC ACID RECEPTOR

Several forms of receptors specific for retinoic acid have been described.[14] These receptors fall into the general class of DNA-binding proteins which also includes steroid and thyroid hormone receptors. A deficiency of vitamin A results in the cessation of spermatogenesis and the loss of advanced germ cells.[15] The synchronization of spermatogenesis described above is achieved by deprivation of vitamin A followed by the restoration of vitamin A function through the administration of retinol.[7,8] Even though the maintenance and restoration of spermatogenesis requires retinol, it is likely that the biological activity of vitamin A results from retinoic acid which can be formed by the enzymatic oxidation of retinol. We have examined the levels of mRNA for the retinoic acid receptors α and β in the testis, determined the types of transcripts associated with specific cell types and examined the levels of the α transcripts during the cycle of the seminiferous epithelium.[16] Sertoli cells contain a transcript coding for the RARβ (retinoic acid receptor β-2.9 Kb) and transcripts coding for the RARα at 2.7 and 3.4 Kb. The RARβ and the RARα 2.7 Kb transcripts were not found in germinal cells while the RARα 3.4 Kb transcript was also found in spermatocytes. When the RARα transcripts were examined in a series of rats with synchronized testes, the highest levels of both the 2.7 Kb (Sertoli cell) and the 3.4 Kb (Sertoli cell and germinal cell) transcripts were present in stages VIII–XI of the cycle (FIG. 2). It has previously been established that vitamin A deficiency leads to a block in germ cell development

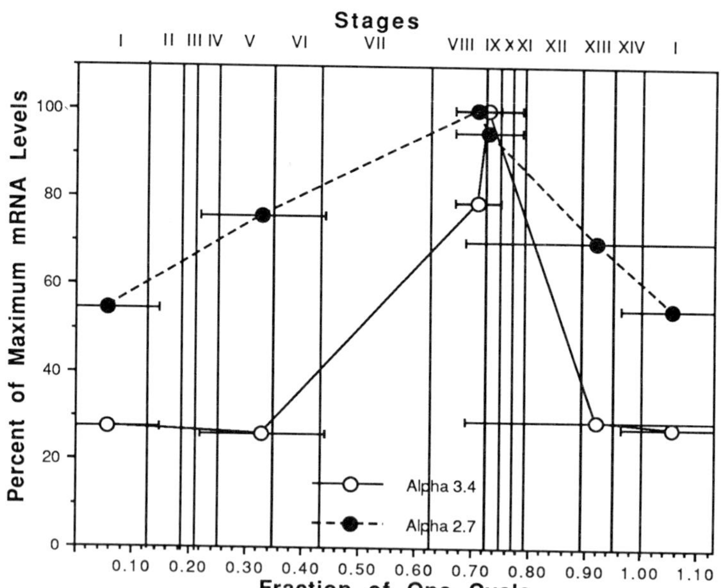

FIGURE 2. Relative levels of retinoic acid receptor α. Procedures were as described in FIGURE 1 except that 4 μg of mRNA were run in each lane and the labeled probe was obtained by random priming of a plasmid containing the cDNA corresponding to retinoic acid receptor α. Note that the 2.7 Kb transcript is localized only in Sertoli cells and the 3.4 Kb transcript is found in both Sertoli cells and germ cells.[16]

near the end of stage VIII and an accumulation of type A1 spermatogonia.[8] Therefore the highest level of transcripts in the synchronized testis appear to correlate well with the stages of the apparent biological block. This result is further corroborated by our data which showed that retinoic acid receptor α mRNA is rapidly induced (2.5-fold) within 30 min of retinol injection into the vitamin A deficient rats whose germ cell development was blocked at stage VIII.[16]

FSH RECEPTOR

Both FSH and testosterone are required for quantitatively normal spermatogenesis in the adult rat. We have used a cDNA probe specific for the FSH receptor (FSHR) in Northern blot analysis to examined the levels of FSH receptor mRNA in rat Sertoli cells.[17] Receptor transcripts of 2.6 (primary transcript) and 4.5 Kb were detected in mRNA isolated from cultured Sertoli cells and whole testes from both prepubertal and adult animals. When the FSH receptor mRNA was analyzed in rats with synchronized testes, it was shown that the levels of the 2.6 Kb transcript varied nearly 5-fold across the cycle with minimal levels in stages VI to IX and maximal levels in stages XIII to II (FIG. 3). These cyclic changes in FSHR mRNA are in agreement with studies

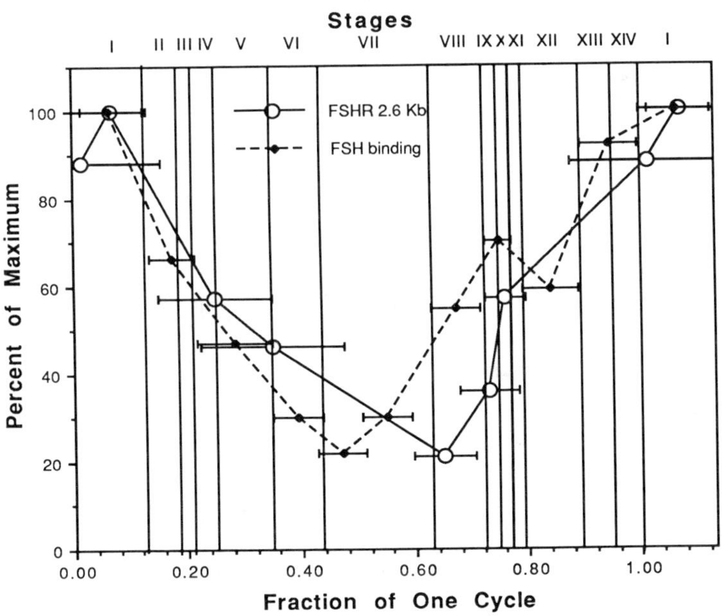

FIGURE 3. Relative levels of FSH receptor mRNA. Procedures were as described in FIGURE 1 except that 10 μg of mRNA were loaded per lane and the probe was generated by random primed replication of a plasmid containing the cDNA for the FSH receptor. Also plotted is the data for the binding of radiolabeled FSH to discrete stages of the cycle. The data were derived from a paper by Kangasniemi *et al.*[19] The horizontal bars in the part of the figure correspond to the stages which were manually dissected from the testis by the authors. These data are included to show the strong correlation between our results on the FSH receptor and the results on binding of FSH reported by Kangasniemi *et al.*

which reported the changes in FSH-induced cAMP levels and FSH binding to receptors as a function of the stages of the cycle.[18,19] The correlation between our studies on mRNA levels and the studies which measured FSH binding and biological activity indicates that FSHR mRNA levels may be a good measure of active receptor levels. In the stages where the FSHR mRNA is highest, FSH, through its actions on the Sertoli cells could influence the mitosis of spermatogonia (stages XII, XIV and I) and the meiotic division of spermatocytes.

ANDROGEN RECEPTOR AND ANDROGEN-BINDING PROTEIN

Androgen is necessary for the completion of meiosis and formation of early spermatids. Attempts to determine the precise sites where the actions of androgens are important in spermatogenesis have led to conflicting and confusing results. Using a cDNA probe specific for the unique 5′ region of the androgen receptor (AR) mRNA we examined the relative levels of AR mRNA in different stages of the cycle of the seminiferous epithelium. We found that the AR mRNA varied approximately twofold across the cycle with the maximal levels in stages XIII to I and the lowest levels in

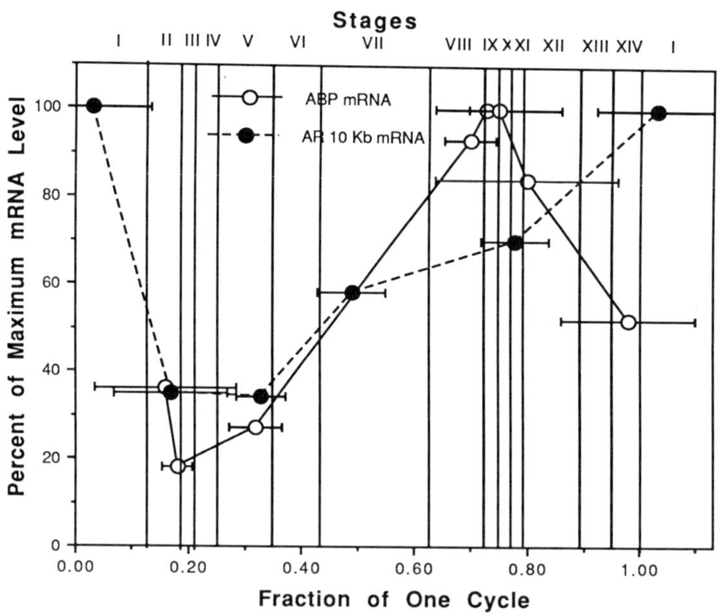

FIGURE 4. Relative levels of androgen receptor mRNA and androgen-binding protein mRNA. Procedures were as described in FIGURE 1 except that one probe was a random primed product from a plasmid containing a 264 BP region in the 5′ end of the cDNA for the androgen receptor. The original cDNA was obtained from C. Chang and S. Liao. The other probe was obtained in a similar manner from a plasmid containing the full-length cDNA originally provided by David Joseph. The gels were originally loaded with 20 μg of mRNA. Although several transcripts are detected for the androgen receptor, only the 10 Kb band was quantified and shown in FIGURE 4. Some of the mRNA for the AR may be derived from peritubular myoid cells or other androgen-responsive cells in the testis.

stages II to VI (FIG. 4). High levels of androgen receptor mRNA were found in the same stages that had the highest levels of FSH receptor mRNA. These stages include the part of the cycle in which the meiotic divisions occur. This analysis was done on mRNA from the whole testis and could be complicated by the cyclic presence of androgen receptors in peritubular myoid cells or elsewhere in the tissue.[20]

Androgen-binding protein is synthesized by Sertoli cells and is supposedly important in the transfer of androgens to the caput epididymis.[21,22] Using a cDNA specific for the rat androgen-binding protein we demonstrated that the mRNA for ABP was highest at stages VIII to XI of the cycle. These mRNA levels corresponded well to the stage-specific secretion of ABP protein that was previously reported to occur during those same stages.[5]

SUMMARY AND CONCLUSIONS

The data presented in this manuscript are all based on some inferences drawn from past experimental observations. The first is that the synchronized testis model is representative of the normal testis. Support for this premise comes from the studies on SGP-2, SGP-1 and transferrin where results using *in situ* hybridization and Northern blots are similar for normal and for synchronized testes.[3,6] The second inference is that normalizing all of the data to the relative levels of SGP-1 mRNA adjusts for the possible differential loading of mRNA samples. The logic of this practice is based on the observation obtained using *in situ* hybridization that SGP-1 mRNA levels did not change across the cycle.[6] The third assumption was that total mRNA levels do not change greatly across the cycle. Wholesale changes in testicular mRNA such as the doubling of all of the mRNA transcripts per testis would not be accounted for by these studies. We feel that this is an unlikely complication because of the strong correlation between much of the data and the known biology. In addition, there is a strong correlation between our data on the FSHR mRNA and the binding data for FSH obtained by another laboratory and different techniques.

The available data in the literature reveals that most of the Sertoli cell products which change in relative concentrations during the cycle of the seminiferous epithelium appear to have a maximum in either stages VII or IX or in stages XIII to III. Thus, the Sertoli cells in the cycle could be described has having two different functional modes. In mode A maximal levels of mRNA for a specific Sertoli cell product are roughly found in stages VII–IX and in mode B the maximal levels are found in stages XIII to III (FIG. 5). The distribution of the receptor mRNA and ABP mRNA can also be described in terms of these two modes of Sertoli cell function. Transferrin receptors, retinoic acid receptors, and androgen-binding protein appear to fall into mode A while FSH and androgen receptors fall into mode B (TABLE 1). Products which have antithetical functions such as FSH and inhibin or cystatin and cathepsin L are found in different modes. We propose that most of the actions of the Sertoli cell during the cycle can be specified by the dual modes described above rather than by an infinite number of operational modes. Mode B which has the highest level of mRNA for androgen receptor and FSH receptor would appear to be the most dependent on hormone action and most likely encompasses functions related to spermatogonial proliferation and meiotic division of spermatocytes. In mode A, the Sertoli cells are concerned with synthesis of proteases and secretion of components of the fluid of the seminiferous tubules. We also propose that the agent or agents which regulate the transition of the

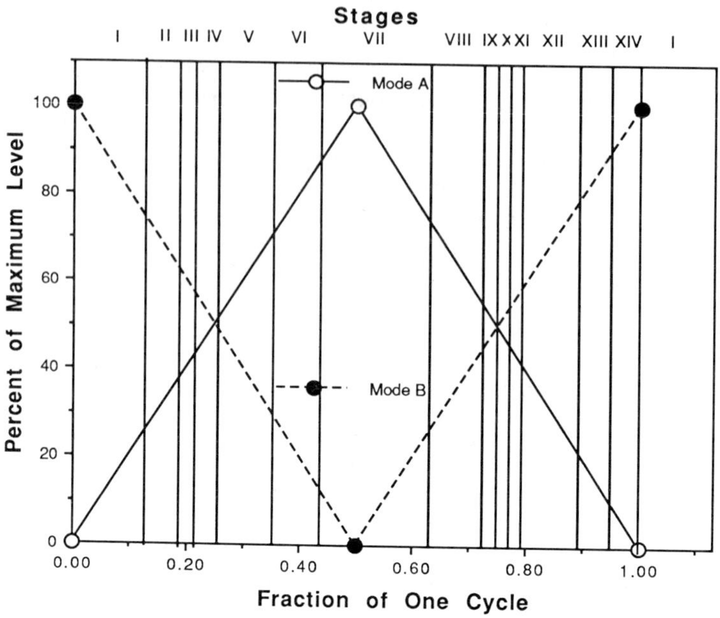

FIGURE 5. Representation of the general areas of functional modes A and B of Sertoli cells during the cycle of the seminiferous epithelium.

TABLE 1. Distribution of Gene Products of Sertoli Cells between the Two Modes of Sertoli Cell Function

Mode A	Mode B
Transferrin receptor	Transferrin
Inhibin[23]	FSH receptor
Cathepsin L[24]	Cystatin (inhibitor of Cathepsin L)[25]
Androgen-binding protein	Androgen receptor
Plasminogen activator[26]	
SGP-2 (Clusterin)[6]	
Retinoic acid receptor α	

Sertoli cells between modes A and B come from the germ cells or from an interaction between the germ cells and the Sertoli cells. We realize that this is a simplistic and rather conspicuous model which does not fit all of the data perfectly but elements of it can be tested experimentally.

REFERENCES

1. LEBLOND, C. P. & Y. CLERMONT. 1952. Definition of the stages of the cycle of the seminiferous epithelium in the rat. Ann. N. Y. Acad. Sci. **55:** 548–573.
2. CLERMONT, Y. 1972. Kinetics of spermatogenesis in mammals. Physiol. Rev. **52:** 198–204.

3. GRISWOLD, M. D., C. MORALES & S. SYLVESTER. 1988. Molecular biology of the Sertoli cell. Ox. Rev. Reprod. Biol. **10:** 124–161.
4. KERR, J. B. & D. M. DEKRETSER. 1975. Cyclic variations in Sertoli cell lipid content throughout the spermatogenic cycle in the rat. J. Reprod. Fertil. **43:** 1–8.
5. PARVINEN, M. 1982. Regulation of the seminiferous epithelium. End. Rev. **3:** 404–417.
6. MORALES, C. R., A. A. ALCIVAR, N. B. HECHT & M. D. GRISWOLD. 1989. Specific mRNAs in Sertoli and germinal cells of testes from stage synchronized rats. Mol. Endocrinol. **3**(4): 725–733.
7. MORALES, C. & M. D. GRISWOLD. 1987. Retinol-induced stage synchronization in seminiferous tubules of the rat. Endocrinology **121:** 432–434.
8. GRISWOLD, M. D., P. D. BISHOP, K.-H. KIM, R. PING, J. E. SIITERI & C. MORALES. 1989. Function of vitamin A in normal and synchronized seminiferous tubules. Ann. N. Y. Acad. Sci. **564:** 154–172.
9. VAN BEEK, M. E. A. B. & M. L. MEISTRICH. 1990. A method for quantifying synchrony in testes of rats treated with vitamin A deprivation and readministration. Biol. Reprod. **42:** 424–431.
10. GRISWOLD, M. D. 1988. Protein secretions of the Sertoli cell. Int. Rev. Cytol. **110:** 133–156.
11. MORALES, C., S. SYLVESTER & M. D. GRISWOLD. 1987. Transport of iron and transferrin synthesis by the seminiferous epithelium of the rat. Biol. Reprod. **37:** 995–1005.
12. ROBERTS, K. & M. D. GRISWOLD. 1990. Characterization of rat transferrin receptor cDNA: The regulation of transferrin receptor mRNA in testes and in Sertoli cells in culture. Mol. Endocrinol. **4:** 531–542.
13. RAO, K., J. B. HARFORD, T. ROUAULT, A. MCCLELLAND, F. H. RUDDLE & R. D. KLAUSNER. 1986. Transcriptional regulation by iron of the gene for the transferrin receptor. Mol. Cell Biol. **6:** 236–240.
14. ZELENT, A., A. KRUST, M. PETKOVICH, P. KLAUSNER & P. CHAMBON. 1989. Cloning of murine α and β retinoic acid receptors and a novel receptor gamma predominantly expressed in the skin. Nature **339:** 714–717.
15. THOMSON, J. N., J. M. HOWELL & G. A. J. PITT. 1964. Vitamin A and reproduction in rats. Proc. R. Soc. Lond. (Biol) **159:** 510–535.
16. KIM, K. H. & M. D. GRISWOLD. 1990. The regulation of retinoic acid receptor mRNA levels during spermatogenesis. Mol. Endocrinol. **4**(11): 1679–1688.
17. HECKERT, L. L. & M. D. GRISWOLD. 1991. Expression of follicle-stimulating hormone receptor mRNA in rat testes and Sertoli cells. Mol. Endocrinol. **5**(5): 670–677.
18. KANGASNIEMI, M., A. KAIPIA, P. MALI, J. TOPPARI, I. HUHTANIEMI & M. PARVINEN. 1990. Modulation of basal and FSH-dependent cyclic AMP production in rat seminiferous tubules stages by an improved transillumination technique. Anat. Rec. **227:** 62–76.
19. KANGASNIEMI, M., A. KAIPIA, J. TOPPARI, A. PERHEENTUPA, I. HUNTANIEMI & M. PARVINEN. 1990. Cellular regulation of follicle-stimulating hormone (FSH) binding in rat seminiferous tubules. J. Androl. **11**(4): 336–343.
20. ANTHONEY, C. T., W. J. KOVACS & M. K. SKINNER. 1989. Analysis of the androgen receptor in isolated testicular cell types with a microassay that utilizes an affinity ligand. Endocrinology **125:** 2628–2635.
21. HAGENAS, L. & E. M. RITZEN. 1975. Sertoli cell origin of testicular androgen-binding protein (ABP). Mol. Cell. Endocrinol. **2:** 339–350.
22. FRENCH, F. S. & E. M. RITZEN. 1973. A high-affinity androgen binding protein (ABP) in rat testis: Evidence for secretion into efferent duct fluid and absorption by epididymis. Endocrinology **93:** 88–95.
23. BHASIN, S., L. A. KRUMMEN, R. S. SWERDLOFF, B. S. MORELOS, W. H. KIM, G. S. DIZEREGA, N. LING, F. ESCH, S. SHIMASAKI & J. TOPPARI. 1989. Stage dependent expression of inhibin α and β-B subunits during the cycle of the rat seminiferous epithelium. Endocrinology **124:** 987–991.
24. WRIGHT, W. W. & M. L. LUZARRAGA. 1986. Isolation of cyclic protein-2 from rat seminiferous tubule fluid and Sertoli cell culture medium. Biol. Reprod. **35:** 761–772.
25. TSURUTA, J. & M. D. GRISWOLD. 1991. In preparation.
26. LACROIX, M., M. PARVINEN & I. B. FRITZ. 1981. Localization of testicular plasminogen activator in discrete portions (stages VII and VIII) of the seminiferous tubule. Biol. Reprod. **25:** 143–146.

Sertoli-Germ Cell Interactions as Determinants of Bidirectional Secretion of Androgen-binding Protein[a]

GLEN L. GUNSALUS AND C. WAYNE BARDIN

The Population Council
1230 York Avenue
New York, New York 10021

At the sixth National Institute of Child Health and Human Development (NICHHD) Workshop on the Testis, held in Houston, Texas (1979), Gunsalus *et al.*[1] reported a series of *in vivo* studies in rats suggesting that androgen-binding protein (ABP) is secreted both from the apex and the base of Sertoli cells into the seminiferous tubular lumen and the interstitial space, respectively. These observations suggested that ABP and possibly other Sertoli cell proteins are secreted bidirectionally by Sertoli cells. Subsequent studies from our own and other laboratories, have supported the view that Sertoli cells, like hepatocytes, can partition their secretory products between two compartments; the vascular compartment and seminiferous tubular lumen in the case of Sertoli cells as compared to blood and bile in the case of hepatocytes.

In an effort to delineate parameters that regulate bidirectional rABP secretion, we have continued to examine the *in vivo* kinetics of ABP release using several models in which germ cell depletion was produced by different mechanisms. TABLE 1 summarizes the studies from our laboratory on this topic. Androgen-binding protein blood level and epididymal content were taken as indices of basal and apical Sertoli cell secretion, respectively.[1] Hormone levels and testicular ABP content were also measured. Of the six hormonal manipulation studies, five resulted in reduction in germ cell number. This included treatment with: LHRH agonist,[2] medroxyprogesterone acetate (MPA),[3] MPA plus testosterone propionate,[3] ethylene dimethanesulfonate (Leydig cell destruction)[4] and neonatal LHRH antiserum (Sertoli cell reduction).[5] Germ cell depletion was also studied in animals with genetic defects,[6,7] and after prenatal γ-irradiation[7] and cold ischemia.[8] Finally, a number of drugs that disrupt seminiferous tubules by a variety of mechanisms were examined. These included: the alkylating agent, busulfan[9]; the DNA inter-calator, doxorubicin[10]; 2, 4-toluenediamine, which blocks fluid outflow from the testis[11]; and lonidamine, which induces shedding of germ cells.[12] In each study, multiple groups of animals were studied for times ranging from 50 to 200 days.

Reduced germ cell number was observed for all treatments and conditions shown in TABLE 1, except the larger dose of testosterone propionate which maintained normal testicular morphology and ABP secretion, even though serum LH and FSH were sup-

[a] This study was supported in part by National Institutes of Health (NIH) grant HD 13541 and by the Mellon Foundation.

TABLE 1. Changes in Testicular (Testis) and Epididymal (Epid) Content and Serum Concentration of Androgen-binding Protein (ABP) in Rats with Conditions or Treatments that Reduce Testicular Sperm Content with or without Changes in Serum Concentrations of LH, FSH, and Testosterone (T)

Condition/Treatment	Hormone Levels			ABP			Reference
	LH	FSH	T	Testis	Epid	Serum	
Hormonal Manipulation							
Neonatal LHRH antiserum	±[a]	±	±	↓	↓	↓	5
Medroxyprogesterone acetate (MPA)	↓	↓	↓	↓	↓	↑	3
Testosterone Propionate (TP)	↓	↓	↑	±	±	±	3
MPA + TP	↓	↓	↑	↓	↓	↑	3
LHRH agonist	↓	↓	↓	↑	↓	↑	2
Ethylene dimethane-sulfonate (EDS)	↑	↑	↓	↓	↓	↑	4
Genetic Defects							
grc/grc	↑	↑	±	↓	↓	±	6
$H^{re/+}$	↑	↑	±	↓	↓	↓	7
Physical Agents							
Prenatal γ irradiation	↑	↑	±	↓	↓	↓	7
Cold ischemia	±	±	±	ND	ND	↑	8
Drug Treatment							
Busulfan	↑	↑	±	↓	↓	↓↑	9
2,4-Toluenediamine	ND	ND	↓	↑	↓	↑	11
Doxorubicin	↑	↑	±	↓	↓	↑↓	10
Lonidamine	±	↑	±	↓	↓	↑	12

[a] ± = Little or no change relative to control animals; ↑ = increase in concentration or content relative to control animals; ↓ = decrease in concentration or content relative to control animals; ↑↓ = biphasic, depending on dose or time after treatment; ND = not determined.

pressed. Regardless of the mechanism used to reduce germ cell number, there was a decrease in apical ABP secretion by Sertoli cells as judged by a marked reduction in the epididymal ABP content. The decline in apical secretion occurred in animals with high or normal LH and FSH and with either normal or low testosterone levels. These observations suggest that the decreased apical ABP secretion was most closely correlated with the loss of germ cells. In all of the studies summarized in TABLE 1, except for neonatal administration of LHRH antiserum, the number of germ cells per Sertoli cell was reduced as was apical ABP secretion by Sertoli cells. Neonatal administration of LHRH antiserum blocked the mitotic effect of FSH on Sertoli cells during the neonatal period. Thus, several rounds of Sertoli cell division were missed by the time the number of Sertoli cells in the testis was fixed and the blood-testis barrier was closed. When these rats matured, their testes were small owing to the reduced number of Sertoli cells. ABP production and germ cell number per Sertoli cell were normal as in the case of Sertoli cell-depleted rats produced by neonatal treatment with cytosine arabinoside.[13]

In contrast to apical release of ABP, basal secretion from Sertoli cells was complex and variable, being increased in seven studies, decreased in three, unchanged in two, and biphasic in two (TABLE 1). Perhaps the two most informative studies were those in which the blood levels of ABP were biphasic (busulfan and doxorubicin, TABLE

1). A single injection of busulfan selectively destroys differentiated spermatogonia so that over time, as the remaining germ cells mature, the cells that would have developed from the destroyed spermatagonia do not appear. The seminiferous epithelium was depleted first of less mature germ cells and this was asssociated with the decline in basal ABP release as evidenced by a decline in blood levels without a change in testicular or epididymal ABP content. Later, all mature germ cells are absent and the newly differentiated spermatogonia begin to repopulate the seminiferous epithelium. As the more mature germ cells were depleted, apical ABP secretion began to fall (as expected from the studies reviewed above), basal secretion increased above normal and was maximal when germ cell depletion was greatest. These studies provide evidence that the basal secretion of ABP is also altered by the particular population of germ cells that are present in the seminiferous tubular epithelium. In experiments using doxorubicin, all four of the doses studied reduced germ cell number and apical ABP secretion. By contrast, a low dose of drug increased ABP basal release, while higher doses depressed it; thus, a given testicular toxin can produce a variety of effects on Sertoli cells.

An examination of the remaining studies listed in TABLE 1 does not provide insight into other regulatory mechanisms of basal ABP secretion except for the observation that reduction of Sertoli cell number by neonatal LHRH antiserum administration or hemi-orchidectomy[1] results in reduced basal secretion. This suggests that in the adult testis the secretion of ABP into blood by Sertoli cells with a full complement of germ cells is relatively constant and that there is no compensatory increase in basal ABP release for the reduction in Sertoli cell number. Furthermore, since there is variable secretion of ABP along the length of the tubule,[14,15] it is not coordinated, as is, for example, LH secretion by the pituitary, so that serum ABP levels are relatively constant.

The reduced basal secretion in $H_re/+$ and prenatal γ-irradiation suggests that marked long-term suppression of the seminiferous epithelium reduces basal as well as apical secretion, although the decrease in the basal secretion was not as great as that at the apex. In this regard the long-term suppression of the testis in grc/grc animals was not associated with modified basal secretion. It is also of note that hormone treatment, regardless of the type, tended to increase basal secretion. The reason for the increased basal secretion of ABP from testes of animals treated with a variety of hormones is of interest but not understood.

Finally, it should be noted that the considerations of apical and basal secretion of ABP as derived from tissue and serum levels are first order approximations since they do not consider independent and divergent variations of ABP synthesis, turnover, and secretion that almost certainly occur with different treatments. In addition, the postulate that serum levels reflect basal secretion is dependent upon the assumption that basal release from Sertoli cells is the only source of blood ABP. We have previously shown that a small amount of ABP can be released into blood from epididymides with inadequate testosterone maintenance.[16] Thus, the increased blood levels of ABP after MPA treatment could represent androgen withdrawal (TABLE 1). However, testosterone propionate treatment of the MPA-treated rats did not prevent the rise in serum ABP, suggesting that the change in basal secretion was an effect of MPA *per se* and that the epididymis did not contribute to serum ABP levels under these conditions.

In conclusion, although FSH and testosterone are important regulators of apical

ABP secretion, germ cells are the major driving force; any treatment that reduces the number of spermatids in the seminiferous epithelium will reduce ABP secretion into the tubular lumen. In the adult testis, the factors that regulate basal secretion are less well understood as evidenced by the fact that serum ABP can increase or decrease independent of LH, FSH, or testosterone levels in serum or of testicular ABP content. The fact that serum ABP levels can be biphasic following some treatments underscores this point. Together, the fourteen studies summarized in TABLE 1 emphasize that Sertoli cell proteins such as ABP can be used to detect subtle differences in the seminiferous tubular epithelium that cannot be detected morphologically and offer promise that testicular proteins can be used to monitor seminiferous tubular function. They further emphasize some of the limitations of *in vitro* studies of Sertoli cell function.

REFERENCES

1. GUNSALUS, G. L., N. A. MUSTO & C. W. BARDIN. 1980. Bidirectional release of a Sertoli cell product, androgen binding protein, into the blood and seminiferous tubule. *In* Testicular Development, Structure, and Function. A. Steinberger & E. Steinberger, Eds.: 291–297. Raven Press. New York.
2. WARD, J. A., B. J. A. FURR, B. VALCACCIA, B. CURRY, C. W. BARDIN, G. L. GUNSALUS & I. D. MORRIS. 1989. Prolonged suppression of rat testis function by a depot formulation of Zoladex, a GnRH agonist. J. Androl. **10:** 478–486.
3. LOBL, T. J., N. A. MUSTO, G. L. GUNSALUS & C. W. BARDIN. 1983. Medroxyprogesterone acetate has opposite effects on the Androgen Binding Protein concentrations in serum and epididymis. Biol. Reprod. **29:** 697–712.
4. MORRIS, I. D., C. W. BARDIN, N. A. MUSTO, R. B. THAU & G. L. GUNSALUS. 1988. Androgen binding protein in serum, testis, and epididymis following treatment with the Leydig cell cytotoxic agent, ethylene dimethanesulfonate. Int. J. Androl. **11:** 153–163.
5. VOGEL, D. L., G. L. GUNSALUS, B. B. BERCU, N. A. MUSTO & C. W. BARDIN. 1983. Sertoli cell maturation is impaired by neonatal passive immunization with antiserum to luteinizing hormone-releasing hormone. Endocrinology 112: 1115–1121.
6. GUNSALUS, G. L., N. A. MUSTO, C. W. BARDIN, H. W. KUNZ & T. J. GILL III. 1985. Rats homozygous for the *grc* complex have defective transport of androgen binding protein to the epididymis, but normal secretion into the blood. Biol. Reprod. **33:** 1057–1063.
7. MUSTO, N. A., C. Y. CHENG, G. L. GUNSALUS, N. ESCOBAR & C. W. BARDIN. 1986. The use of androgen-binding protein and other Sertoli cell products to monitor seminiferous tubular physiology and pathophysiology. *In* Male Reproductive Dysfunction. R. Santen & R. Swerdloff, Eds.: 77–99. Marcel Dekker. New York/Basel.
8. YOUNG, G. P. H., M. GOLDSTEIN, D. M. PHILLIPS, K. SUNDARAM, G. L. GUNSALUS & C. W. BARDIN. 1988. Sertoli-cell-only syndrome produced by hypothermic testicular ischemia. Endocrinology **122:** 1074–1082.
9. MORRIS, I. D., C. W. BARDIN, N. A. MUSTO, R. B. THAU & G. L. GUNSALUS. 1987. Evidence suggesting that germ cells influence the bidirectional secretion of androgen binding protein by the seminiferous epithelium demonstrated by selective impairment of spermatogenesis with busulfan. Int. J. Androl. **10:** 691–700.
10. WARD, J. A., C. W. BARDIN, M. KNIGHT, J. ROBINSON, G. GUNSALUS & I. D. MORRIS. 1988. Delayed effects of doxorubicin on spermatogenesis and endocrine function in rats. Reprod. Toxicol. **2:** 117–126.
11. VARMA, S. K., E. BLOCH, B. GONDOS, V. ROSSI, G. L. GUNSALUS & B. THYSEN. Reproductive toxicity of 2, 4-toluene -diamine in the rat. 3. Effects on androgen binding protein levels, selected seminiferous tubule characteristics and spermatogenesis. J. Toxicol. Environ. Health **25:** 435–451.
12. LOBL, T. J., C. W. BARDIN, G. L. GUNSALUS & N. A. MUSTO. 1981. Effects of lonidamine (AF

1890) and its analogues on follicle-stimulating hormone, luteinizing hormone, testosterone and rat androgen binding protein concentrations in the rat and rhesus monkey. Chemotherapy **27**(Suppl. 2): 61–76.
13. Orth, J. M., G. L. Gunsalus & A. A. Lamperti. 1988. Evidence from Sertoli cell-depleted rats indicates that spermatid number in adults depends on numbers of Sertoli cells produced during perinatal development. Endocrinology. **122:** 787–794.
14. Ritzen, E. E., L. Boitani, M. Parvinen, F. S. French & M. Feldman. 1982. Stage-dependent secretion of ABP by rat seminiferous tubules. Mol. Cell. Endocrinol. **25:** 25–33.
15. Mather, J. P., G. L. Gunsalus, N. A. Musto, C. Y. Cheng, M. Parvinen, W. Wright, V. Perez-Infante, A. Margioris, A. Liotta, R. Becker, D. T. Krieger & C. W. Bardin. 1983. The hormonal and cellular control of Sertoli cell secretion. J. Steroid Biochem. **19:** 41–51.
16. Becker, R. R., G. L. Gunsalus, N. A. Musto & C. W. Bardin. 1984. The epididymis contributes minimally to serum androgen binding protein in the rat: A whole body kinetic study. Endocrinology **114:** 2354–2360.

Mannose 6-Phosphate Receptors: Potential Mediators of Germ Cell–Sertoli Cell Interactions[a]

DEBORAH A. O'BRIEN

Laboratories for Reproductive Biology
Departments of Pediatrics and Cell Biology & Anatomy
University of North Carolina at Chapel Hill
Chapel Hill, North Carolina 27599–7500

CHRISTOPHER A. GABEL

Pfizer Central Research
Department of Immunology and Infectious Diseases
Groton, Connecticut 06340

JEFFREY E. WELCH AND E. M. EDDY

Gamete Biology Section
Laboratory of Reproductive and Developmental Toxicology
National Institute of Environmental Health Sciences
National Institutes of Health
Research Triangle Park, North Carolina 27709

CELL-CELL INTERACTIONS IN THE SEMINIFEROUS EPITHELIUM

Although it is clear that Sertoli cells play a major role in the regulation of germ cell differentiation, precise interactions between spermatogenic and Sertoli cells have not been adequately defined. Sertoli cells form the blood-testis barrier,[1] creating the specialized environment in the adluminal compartment of the seminiferous tubule[2] where later meiotic and haploid germ cells differentiate. There is growing evidence for complex paracrine regulation of spermatogenesis involving reciprocal interactions between Sertoli and germ cells, and between Sertoli cells and the interstitial compartment.[3] Although *in vitro* systems supporting complete mammalian spermatogenesis have not been developed, short-term culture experiments have begun to characterize cell-cell interactions within the seminiferous epithelium (TABLE 1). Spermatogenic cells in culture survive for longer periods in the presence of Sertoli cells and retain limited capacity for differentiation.[4,5] In addition, several Sertoli cell parameters are altered when these cells are co-cultured with spermatogenic cells (TABLE 1). Cyclic variations in several Sertoli secretory products have been demonstrated by culturing

[a] Partial support for these studies was provided by National Institutes of Health (NIH) Grant HD26485 from the National Institute of Child Health and Human Development.

TABLE 1. Germ Cell–Sertoli Cell Interactions

Effects on Germ Cells	Effects on Sertoli Cells
• Limited differentiation in co-cultures[4–6] • ↑ DNA and RNA synthesis[7,8] • ↑ Protein synthesis[9,10] • ↑ Viability and ATP levels[4,5,11,12]	• ↑ Adenylate cyclase activity[13] • ↑ Protein phosphorylation[14] • Alterations in glycoprotein composition[15] • Alterations in membrane proteins[16] • ↑ Transferrin secretion[17–19] • ↑ ABP secretion[17,20–22] • ↓ Estradiol secretion[21,22] • Cyclic variations in secretory products[23–25]

tubule segments at different stages of the cycle of the seminiferous epithelium,[23–25] suggesting stage-specific interactions between germ cells and Sertoli cells.

Potential mediators of germ cell-Sertoli cell interactions include direct cell contact and secretory products. Multiple junctional specializations have been identified between germ cells and Sertoli cells, including desmosome-like junctions, gap junctions, and ectoplasmic specializations adjacent to condensing spermatids.[26] At least one of these junctional specializations, the desmosome-like junctions which increase during meiosis *in vivo*, forms *in vitro* between Sertoli cells and pachytene spermatocytes.[27] Isolated spermatogenic cells, particularly pachytene spermatocytes, also adhere specifically to cultured Sertoli cells prior to the appearance of junctions.[27–30] A glycoprotein on the surface of rat pachytene spermatocytes with an apparent molecular weight of 80,000 appears to mediate this adhesion.[30]

Sertoli cells secrete a wide array of products that may influence germ cell differentiation. Sertoli cell production of metabolic substrates such as lactate and pyruvate, which are used preferentially by spermatogenic cells *in vitro*, may be an important component in the nutritional maintenance of germ cells.[31] In addition, Sertoli cells secrete a variety of proteins and glycoproteins, including hormones, growth factors, basement membrane components, enzymes, transport proteins, and proteins with unknown functions[32] (TABLE 2). Polypeptide factor(s) in conditioned medium from mouse Sertoli cells maintain ATP levels of pachytene spermatocytes and round spermatids for at least two days in culture.[11,12] Thus far, specific effects of individual Sertoli secretory proteins on spermatogenic cells have not been determined. The best characterized model of secretory interactions in the seminiferous epithelium is the delivery of iron via Sertoli cell transferrin to the adluminal compartment where it binds to transferrin receptors on spermatogenic cells.[32] Other receptor-mediated processes may operate within the seminiferous epithelium to integrate secretory signals from Sertoli cells and possibly from germ cells.[18,19,22] Our recent studies have focused on mannose 6-phosphate receptors as potential mediators of germ cell-Sertoli cell interactions.

Two secretory products of rat Sertoli cells, transforming growth factor-β (TGF-β) precursor[33,34] and procathepsin L,[24,45] have been identified as glycoproteins bearing the mannose 6-phosphate (M6P) recognition marker.[59,60] TGF-β inhibits Leydig cell steroidogenesis[61] and modulates peritubular cell shape, contractility,[62] and protein secretion.[34] Although effects on spermatogenic cells have not been reported, it is interesting to note that TGF-β stimulates meiotic maturation of rat oocytes.[63] Procathepsin L is a lysosomal cysteine protease, but is also the major excreted protein (MEP) of transformed mouse fibroblasts.[60,64] Synthesis and secretion of MEP is stimulated

TABLE 2. Proteins Secreted by Sertoli Cells[a]

Hormones or Growth Factors	Enzymes
TGF-β precursor[33,34]	Procathepsin L (cyclic protein 2)[24,46]
Anti-Müllerian hormone (MIS)[35R,36]	Plasminogen activator[47,48]
Inhibin[37R]	
TGF-α[38]	**Transport proteins**
EGF-like growth factor[39]	Androgen-binding protein[49R,50]
Basic FGF-like growth factor[40]	Transferrin[32R,51]
Seminiferous growth factor[41]	Ceruloplasmin[52]
IGF-I[42]	
Interleukin-1-like factor[43]	**Other**
Leydig cell stimulatory factor[44]	Sulfated glycoprotein 1 (prosaposin)[53,54]
Basement Membrane Components	Sulfated glycoprotein 2 (clusterin)[53,55,56]
Type IV collagen[45]	Testibumin[57]
Laminin[45]	Testins[58]

[a] Table modified from Griswold, 1988.[32] Review articles are indicated by an R after the reference number.

by viral transformation, tumor promoters, and growth factors.[65,66] In the testis procathepsin L (cyclic protein 2) is maximally secreted by rat Sertoli cells at stages VI and VII of the cycle of the seminiferous epithelium,[24] and is postulated to play a role in the release and movement of spermatids toward the tubule lumen.[46] Other glycoproteins secreted by Sertoli cells bear the M6P recognition signal (see below), and could include additional members of the TGF-β family such as inhibin and anti-Müllerian hormone.[67]

MANNOSE 6-PHOSPHATE RECEPTORS

Mannose 6-phosphate receptors (MPRs) mediate the specific targeting of acid hydrolases to lysosomes and also function at the cell surface.[68] Lysosomal enzymes which bear the M6P recognition marker bind to MPRs in the Golgi apparatus and are transported to a prelysosomal compartment. Following receptor-ligand dissociation in this acidic compartment, the enzymes are packaged into lysosomes and the unoccupied receptors recycle to the Golgi apparatus.[68] Two distinct MPRs, both capable of directing acid hydrolases to lysosomes, have been purified from mammalian tissues.[69,70] Characteristics of these two receptors are compared in TABLE 3.

TABLE 3. Characteristics of Mannose 6-Phosphate Receptors

	CI-MPR	CD-MPR
Targets lysosomal enzymes	Yes	Yes
Mediates endocytosis	Yes	No
Distinct binding site for IGF-II	Yes	No
Signal transduction—IGF-II, M6P growth factors (TGF-β precursor, proliferin)	Yes	?
Approximate molecular weight	275,000	46,000
Dominant transcript size	~10 kb	2.4 kb

cDNA and predicted amino acid sequences determined for both bovine and human MPRs indicate that the two receptors are products of distinct genes that may be evolutionarily related.[71-75] The larger receptor, the cation-independent (CI) form, has an approximate molecular weight of 275,000 and is identical to the receptor for insulin-like growth factor II (IGF-II).[76] The smaller cation-dependent (CD) MPR has a subunit molecular weight of ~46,000, exhibits higher binding affinities in the presence of divalent cations,[77] and does not bind IGF-II.[78,79] Sequence analyses suggest that each of the MPRs is composed of four structural domains—a signal sequence, an extracytoplasmic domain that binds ligand, a membrane-spanning domain, and a short cytoplasmic tail which lacks a tyrosine kinase domain.[71,80]

Both MPRs are localized predominantly on intracellular membranes, although 10–20% of each is found on fibroblast plasma membranes under steady-state conditions.[81,82] The cell surface receptors are in equilibrium with intracellular receptors, indicating that the receptors move between different subcellular compartments.[83,84] Although both MPRs are found at the cell surface, only the CI-MPR efficiently mediates endocytosis of extracellular M6P-bearing ligands.[85,86] Furthermore, surface CI-MPRs are available to bind to IGF-II and M6P-containing growth factors such as proliferin[87] and the TGF-β precursor.[59] A recent study suggests that activation of the latent TGF-β precursor requires binding to the CI-MPR.[88] M6P-containing ligands and IGF-II bind to distinct sites on the CI-MPR and may exert reciprocal effects on ligand binding, receptor-mediated endocytosis, and redistribution of CI-MPRs to the cell surface.[68]

Recent studies have provided evidence that the CI-MPR is linked to signal transduction mechanisms which respond both to IGF-II and M6P-containing growth factors. In Balb/c 3T3 cells IGF-II stimulates calcium influx via a transmembrane signaling system that includes the CI-MPR, a G_i guanine nucleotide-binding protein and a calcium-permeable cation channel.[89,90] In addition, IGF-II stimulates the production of inositol 1,4,5-trisphosphate (IP_3) and diacylglycerol by apparent activation of phospholipase C in kidney membranes, an effect that is potentiated by M6P.[91] Although M6P alone and β-galactosidase (a M6P-containing lysosomal enzyme) do not elicit effects in either system, M6P-containing growth factors (TGF-β precursor and proliferin) stimulate IP_3 production.[92,93]

MPRs IN ISOLATED SPERMATOGENIC AND SERTOLI CELLS

To determine the distribution of the CI- and CD-MPRs in cells within the mouse seminiferous epithelium, radiolabeled receptors have been isolated from germ cells and Sertoli cells by phosphomannan-Sepharose affinity chromatography.[94] Thus far, MPRs have been characterized in pachytene spermatocytes, round spermatids, and Sertoli cells.

Pachytene spermatocytes and round spermatids were isolated from adult seminiferous cell suspensions by unit gravity sedimentation with purities and viabilities exceeding 90%.[95,96] These cells were cultured at 32°C for periods up to 24 h in Eagle's minimal essential medium (MEM) supplemented with antibiotics, 6 mM sodium L-lactate, 1 mM sodium L-pyruvate, 15 mM HEPES, and 10% fetal bovine serum. Germ cells cultured under these conditions retained viabilities >90% as measured by trypan blue exclusion, exhibited incorporation of radiolabeled amino acids and sugars that was linear and proportional to isotope concentration, and synthesized multiple stage-specific proteins.[97]

Sertoli cells were isolated from the testes of 17-day old mice by sequential enzymatic dissociation.[95,96] The cells were cultured in serum-free MEM supplemented with antibiotics, lactate, pyruvate and HEPES as described above, plus insulin, transferrin, epidermal growth factor, retinol, testosterone, and growth hormone.[94,98] After two days in culture, germ cells were removed by hypotonic lysis.[99] Contamination by peritubular myoid cells was <10% as monitored by alkaline phosphatase histochemistry.[100] The Sertoli cells displayed typical morphological features[94] and secreted transferrin and sulfated glycoproteins 1 and 2 (SGP-1 and SGP-2, see below).

Germ cells and Sertoli cells were cultured overnight (16–18 h) in the presence of [^{35}S]methionine. To isolate metabolically labeled MPRs, membrane proteins were extracted from the radiolabeled cells and were applied to a phosphomannan-Sepharose column.[94] Proteins eluted from the column were separated on SDS-polyacrylamide gels and were visualized by autoradiography (FIG. 1). The major [^{35}S]methionine-labeled protein eluted specifically with M6P from pachytene spermatocyte and round spermatid samples co-migrated with the CD-MPR purified from bovine liver. Both pachytene spermatocytes and round spermatids also synthesized lower quantities of a protein that co-migrated with the bovine liver CI-MPR. To our knowledge, this is the first study to purify receptors from spermatogenic cells by affinity chromatography and to demonstrate that these receptors are synthesized by germ cells.

Unlike spermatogenic cells, primary Sertoli cell cultures synthesized the CI-MPR almost exclusively (FIG. 1). As determined by pronase solubilization of the radioactive bands, the ratio of [^{35}S]methionine incorporated into the two receptors (CI:CD) was 1:7 for pachytene spermatocytes, 1:3 for round spermatids, and 17:1 for Sertoli cells. It is likely that these marked differences in expression of the CI- and CD-MPRs reflect differential roles of the two MPRs in the seminiferous epithelium. In addition to their potential role in germ cell–Sertoli cell interactions, these receptors (particularly the CD-MPR which is abundant in early spermatids) may mediate targeting of hydrolytic enzymes to the acrosome.

Recently, we have examined CI- and CD-MPR mRNAs in isolated spermatogenic and Sertoli cells by northern blot analysis using [^{32}P] labeled cDNA probes specific for each receptor (kindly provided by Peter Lobel, Center for Advanced Biotechnology and Medicine, Piscataway, NJ, USA).[101] To detect the CI-MPR, which is less abundant in germ cells, poly(A)$^+$ mRNA was isolated from testes, germ cells and Sertoli cells. A single CI-MPR mRNA, comparable in size to the 9.5 kb CI-MPR mRNA in calf liver,[74] was detected by autoradiography on northern blots of poly(A)$^+$ RNA from pachytene spermatocytes, round spermatids and Sertoli cells probed with a mouse CI-MPR cDNA fragment. Higher levels of CI-MPR mRNA were apparent in Sertoli cells compared to germ cells, as anticipated from studies examining the synthesis of MPRs.

When northern blots of poly(A)$^+$ or total RNA were probed at high stringency with a restriction fragment of the bovine CD-MPR cDNA, multiple transcripts were detected in germ cells. In addition to the 2.4 kb mRNA found in somatic tissues, a 1.2 kb transcript was detected in pachytene spermatocytes and a 1.4 kb transcript in round spermatids. Multiple polyadenylation signals are present in the cDNA sequence for the bovine CD-MPR,[71,72] suggesting that germ cells may use alternate polyadenylation signals to produce transcripts of different sizes. The larger 2.4 kb CD-MPR

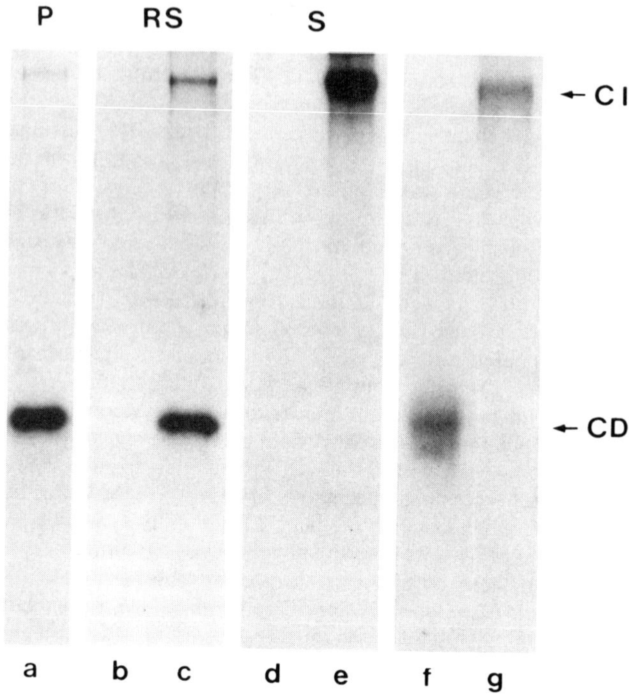

FIGURE 1. Mouse spermatogenic and Sertoli cells synthesize different proportions of the two mannose 6-phosphate receptors (MPRs). [^{35}S]Methionine-labeled MPRs were isolated from membrane preparations by phosphomannan-Sepharose affinity chromatography and were analyzed by SDS gel electrophoresis and autoradiography. MPRs were eluted from the affinity column with mannose 6-phosphate (*lanes a, c, e*), but not with glucose 6-phosphate (*lanes b, d*). Both pachytene spermatocytes (P) and round spermatids (RS) synthesized predominantly the cation-dependent (CD) MPR and lower levels of the cation-independent (CI) MPR (*lanes a, c*). In contrast, Sertoli cells (S) synthesized the CI-MPR, but very little CD-MPR (*lane e*). Purified bovine liver CD-MPR and CI-MPR stained with Coomassie blue are shown in *lanes f* and *g* for comparison. (From O'Brien *et al.*[94] Reprinted with permission from *Endocrinology.*)

transcript also was prominent in RNA isolated from cultured Sertoli cells. Since little CD-MPR protein has been detected in Sertoli cells cultured under identical conditions, expression of this receptor may be regulated by posttranscriptional mechanisms.

M6P RECEPTOR-MEDIATED ENDOCYTOSIS IN SERTOLI AND GERM CELLS

In order to monitor M6P receptor-mediated endocytosis, pachytene spermatocytes, round spermatids and Sertoli cells were cultured overnight with a mixture of [^{125}I]M6P-bearing lysosomal enzyme precursors (M6P-ligands) or with purified M6P-bearing [^{125}I]β-glucuronidase.[94] Both germ cells and somatic cells accumulated these radiolabeled ligands by a process that was time-dependent, proportional to cell number,

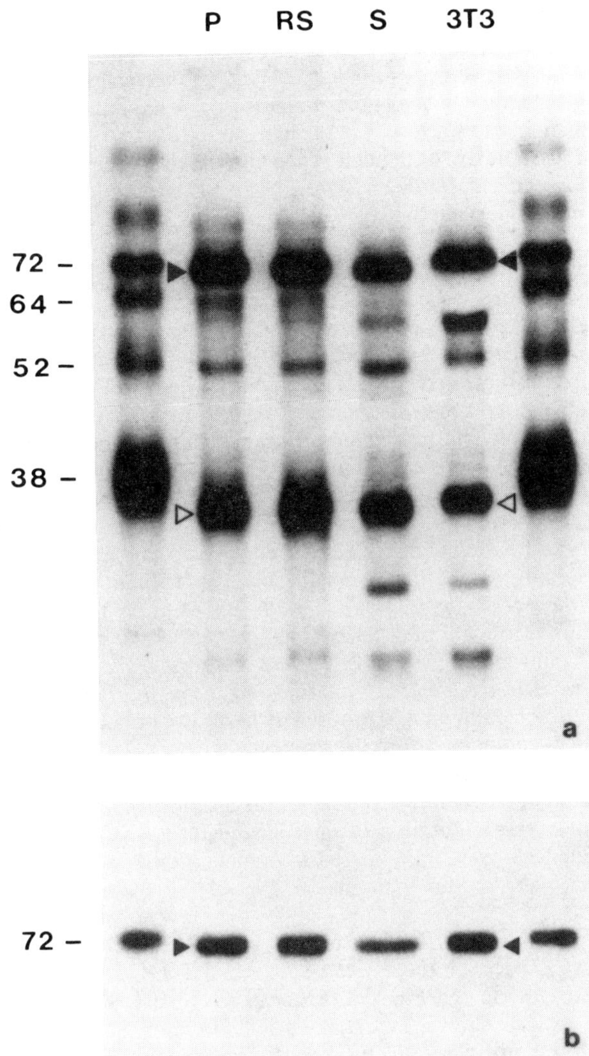

FIGURE 2. Cell-associated M6P-ligands are processed to mature enzymes with lower molecular weights. Cells were incubated overnight with a mixture of [^{125}I]M6P-ligands isolated from the secretions of J774 macrophages (**a**) or with purified [^{125}I]β-glucuronidase (**b**). Cell-associated proteins were extracted with Triton X-100 and were characterized by SDS polyacrylamide gel electrophoresis and autoradiography. The autoradiograms show the input ligand preparations (first and last lanes, apparent molecular weights (M_r) $\times$ 10^{-3} indicated on the left), and cell-associated proteins extracted from pachytene spermatocytes (P), round spermatids (RS), Sertoli cells (S) and 3T3 fibroblasts (3T3). The 68,000 M_r mature form of β-glucuronidase (▶) and a 35,000 M_r species processed from the 38,000 M_r input protein (▷) are identified. Proteolytic maturation of the input proteins is apparent in all samples. (From O'Brien *et al.*[94] Reprinted with permission from *Endocrinology*.)

and inhibited by M6P. Monosaccharide competition studies indicated that M6P was the most effective inhibitor of ligand uptake, reducing [^{125}I]β-glucuronidase accumulation by >97% for pachytene spermatocytes, round spermatids and 3T3 fibroblasts, and 94% for Sertoli cells. Glucose 6-phosphate also caused partial inhibition of ligand uptake, while mannose, galactose 6-phosphate and glucose 6-sulfate had little or no effect on this process in any of the cell types tested. These results suggest that phosphorylated oligosaccharides attached to the M6P-ligands mediate binding to the cell surface, presumably via the CI-MPR which is responsible for endocytosis in other cell types.[85]

Both spermatogenic cells and Sertoli cells accumulated <10% of the amount of [^{125}I]M6P-ligands internalized by 3T3 fibroblasts. The low levels of ligand internalized by germ cells were consistent with the relatively small amounts of CI-MPR synthesized by these cells. However, Sertoli cells synthesized substantial levels of the CI-MPR. Comparisons between the accumulation of [^{125}I]M6P-ligands by intact cells and ligand binding to total cell membranes suggest that Sertoli cells produce large amounts of the CI-MPR, but may express little of this receptor on the cell surface.[94]

Radiolabeled M6P-ligands accumulated by germ cells and Sertoli cells were analyzed by SDS-polyacrylamide gel electrophoresis and autoradiography to verify that the observed accumulation of M6P-ligands correlated with an internalization process and not simply with binding to the cell surface.[94] Proteolytic maturation of lysosomal enzyme precursors to mature enzymes with lower molecular weights is a characteristic feature of the endocytic pathway.[102] Radioactive proteins detected in the cell-associated fractions from cultured pachytene spermatocytes, round spermatids, Sertoli cells and 3T3 fibroblasts were smaller than the input proteins (FIG. 2), providing evidence that the M6P-ligands were internalized through an endocytic process and modified to lower molecular weight forms. Furthermore, proteins recovered from cultured germ cells were distinct from the processed proteins isolated from Sertoli and 3T3 cells. These differences indicate that endocytosis detected in germ cell populations was not due to Sertoli cell contamination. In addition, the electrophoretic profiles suggest that proteolytic maturation of internalized lysosomal enzymes may be less efficient in isolated germ cells compared to somatic cells.

SERTOLI CELL SECRETION OF M6P-CONTAINING GLYCOPROTEINS THAT ARE ENDOCYTOSED BY SPERMATOGENIC CELLS

To determine if mouse Sertoli cells secrete glycoproteins bearing the M6P recognition marker (M6P-glycoproteins), conditioned medium was fractionated by CI-MPR affinity chromatography.[94,103] Sertoli cells were cultured overnight with [^{35}S]methionine in serum-free reduced-methionine medium. The conditioned medium was collected and centrifuged to remove any cellular material, concentrated by ultrafiltration using membranes with a molecular weight cutoff of 30,000, and equilibrated with phosphate-buffered saline. Proteins were then fractionated on an affinity column containing the bovine liver CI-MPR coupled to Affi-Gel 10 or Affi-Prep 10 as described previously.[104] Three peaks were obtained from the column: the flowthrough peak (A) containing >80% of the recovered cpm, a low affinity peak (B) eluted without changing the column buffer, and the M6P-glycoprotein peak (C) eluted with M6P.

Proteins in these peaks were separated on one- and two-dimensional (2D) gels and were visualized by fluorography.[103] In the M6P-glycoprotein fraction (peak C), at least ten glycoproteins with molecular weights (M_r) between 30,000 and 135,000 were resolved. Two of these proteins (30,000 and 35,000 M_r) apparently had lower affinities for the CI receptor and were partially eluted in peak B before the application of M6P to the column. On 2D gels, the M6P-glycoproteins had isoelectric points <6.5 and exhibited characteristic charge and molecular weight heterogeneity.

To determine if any of these M6P-glycoproteins correspond to known Sertoli secretory products, we have begun to identify proteins on immunoblots from 2D gels according to procedures used in our previous studies.[105] We have verified that SGP-1 and SGP-2 are major secretory products of cultured mouse Sertoli cells using antibodies kindly provided by S. Sylvester and M. Griswold (Washington State University, Pullman, WA, USA). The location of transferrin and the SGP-2 subunits on 2D gels suggests that these proteins are not members of the M6P-containing subset of secretory proteins. However, a protein similar to SGP-1 in molecular weight and isoelectric point is present in the M6P-containing fraction (peak C), and is absent in the protein fraction that does not bind to the CI-MPR affinity column (peak A). Initial efforts to immunoprecipitate SGP-1 from the M6P-glycoprotein fraction have been inconclusive. Immunoprecipitation experiments have detected procathepsin L in both the low affinity (peak B) and M6P-glycoprotein (peak C) fractions isolated from Sertoli cell-conditioned medium. Elution of procathepsin L in multiple peaks is consistent with its lower affinity for the CI-MPR than other lysosomal enzyme precursors.[104] Other potential constituents of the Sertoli M6P-glycoprotein fraction include the TGF-β precursor[34] and testins,[58] previously shown to be secreted by rat Sertoli cells.

Since the CI-MPR is identical to the IGF-II receptor, IGF-II is also a potential ligand for this receptor in the seminiferous epithelium. IGF-II in the concentration range detected in rat serum has multiple effects on cultured rat Sertoli cells.[106,107] mRNA for IGF-II was not detected in the adult rat testis,[108] although others have reported IGF-II in human seminal fluid[109] and fetal testes,[110] and in the testes of immature rats following hypophysectomy.[111] IGF-II expression in mouse testes may be higher during development as in other mammalian tissues[112] or may be confined to specific cell types.

Recent studies have determined that isolated germ cells endocytose Sertoli M6P-glycoproteins and process them to lower molecular weight forms.[113] Pachytene spermatocytes or round spermatids were incubated with [^{125}I]Sertoli M6P-glycoproteins for 17 h (± competing monosaccharides) and cell-associated radioactivity was determined. Germ cell accumulation of Sertoli M6P-ligands was inhibited by M6P, but not by mannose, mannose 1-phosphate or galactose 6-phosphate. Like lysosomal enzyme precursors (see above), the Sertoli M6P-glycoproteins were modified to lower molecular weight forms following endocytosis by spermatogenic cells. The observed decreases in molecular weight did not result from extracellular proteolysis since radiolabeled Sertoli glycoproteins recovered from the culture supernatants were identical to the input glycoproteins. Further studies are needed to determine if the endocytosed Sertoli M6P-glycoproteins are targeted to specific organelles and/or affect germ cell function.

SUMMARY

These studies have demonstrated that mouse pachytene spermatocytes, round spermatids, and Sertoli cells synthesize mannose 6-phosphate receptors and that the proportions of the CI- and CD-MPRs vary markedly between cell types.[94] Isolated spermatogenic cells synthesize predominantly the CD-MPR and lower levels of the CI-MPR. In contrast, cultured Sertoli cells selectively synthesize the CI-MPR, even though transcripts for the CD-MPR have been detected in these cells. These striking differences in the expression of MPRs suggest that these receptors may serve multiple roles during germ cell differentiation. We have hypothesized that MPRs in the seminiferous epithelium mediate interactions between germ cells and Sertoli cells, and participate in the targeting of hydrolytic enzymes to the acrosome.[94]

In support of the first hypothesis, we have shown that functional MPRs are localized on the surface of spermatogenic cells and Sertoli cells where they mediate the endocytosis of M6P-containing ligands.[94] As in other somatic cells,[85,86] the CI-MPR is likely to be responsible for M6P receptor-mediated endocytosis in the seminiferous epithelium. Recent studies have shown that Sertoli cells in culture synthesize and secrete at least ten M6P-containing glycoproteins.[104] Furthermore, pachytene spermatocytes and round spermatids endocytose these Sertoli M6P-glycoproteins and process them to lower molecular weight forms that persist during 17 h culture periods.[112] The identification of relevant ligands for mannose 6-phosphate receptors in the seminiferous epithelium may help define new regulatory mechanisms in cell differentiation. Current efforts to determine if Sertoli M6P-glycoproteins modulate germ cell function should confirm the significance of surface MPRs and clarify their roles in signal transduction and/or the endocytosis of Sertoli cell products.

ACKNOWLEDGMENTS

The authors thank Dr. Peter Lobel for providing cDNA probes for the mannose 6-phosphate receptors and Drs. Steven Sylvester and Michael Griswold for providing antibodies to sulfated glycoproteins 1 and 2. We also are grateful for the excellent technical assistance of Douglas Rockett and Arles Taylor.

REFERENCES

1. Dym, M. & D. W. Fawcett. 1970. Biol. Reprod. **3:** 308–326.
2. Waites, G. M. H. & R. T. Gladwell. 1982. Physiol. Rev. **62:** 624–671.
3. Saez, J. M., N. H. Perrard-Sapori, P. G. Chatelain, E. Tabone & M. A. Rivarola. 1987. J. Steroid Biochem. **27:** 317–329.
4. Tres, L. L. & A. L. Kierszenbaum. 1983. Proc. Natl. Acad. Sci. USA **80:** 3377–3381.
5. Hadley, M. A., S. W. Byers, C. A. Suarez-Quian, H. K. Kleinman & M. Dym. 1985. J. Cell Biol. **101:** 1511–1522.
6. Parvinen, M., W. W. Wright, D. M. Phillips, J. P. Mather, N. A. Musto & C. W. Bardin. 1983. Endocrinology **112:** 1150–1152.
7. Rivarola, M. A., P. Sanchez & J. M. Saez. 1985. Endocrinology **117:** 1796–1802.
8. Fradin, S., P. Barbey & M. A. Drosdowsky. 1989. Mol. Reprod. Dev. **1:** 122–128.
9. Jutte, N. H. P. M., R. Jansen, J. A. Grootegoed, F. F. G. Rommerts & H. J. van der Molen. 1983. J. Reprod. Fertil. **68:** 219–226.
10. Boitani, C., F. Palombi & M. Stefanini. 1983. Cell Biol. Int. Rep. **7:** 383–393.
11. O'Brien, D. A., A. Frøysa & D. L. Rockett. 1986. J. Cell Biol. **103:** 485a.
12. O'Brien, D. A. & D. L. Rockett. 1987. J. Cell Biol. **105:** 84a.
13. Welsh, M. J., M. E. Ireland & G. J. Treisman. 1985. Biol. Reprod. **33:** 1050–1056.
14. Ireland, M. E. & M. J. Welsh. 1987. Endocrinology **120:** 1317–1326.
15. Galdieri, M., B. M. Zani, L. Monaco, E. Ziparo & M. Stefanini. Exp. Cell Res. **145:** 191–198.
16. Galdieri, M. & L. Monaco. 1986. Cell Differentiation **18:** 51–55.

17. JANECKI, A., A. JAKUBOWIAK & A. STEINBERGER. 1988. J. Androl. **9:** 126–132.
18. DJAKIEW, D. & M. DYM. 1988. Biol. Reprod. **39:** 1193–1205.
19. LE MAGUERESSE, B., C. PINEAU, F. GUILLOU & B. JEGOU. 1988. J. Endocrinol. **118:** R13–R16.
20. GALDIERI, M., L. MONACO & M. STEFANINI. 1984. J. Androl. **5:** 409–415.
21. LE MAGUERESSE, B. & B. JEGOU. 1988. Endocrinology **122:** 1672–1680.
22. LE MAGUERESSE, B. & B. JEGOU. 1988. Mol. Cell. Endocrinol. **58:** 65–72.
23. PARVINEN, M. 1982. Endocrine Rev. **3:** 404–417.
24. WRIGHT, W. W., M. PARVINEN, N. A. MUSTO, G. L. GUNSALUS, D. M. PHILLIPS, J. P. MATHER & C. W. BARDIN. 1983. Biol. Reprod. **29:** 257–270.
25. SHABANOWITZ, R. B., R. M. DEPHILIP, J. A. CROWELL, L. L. TRES & A. L. KIERSZENBAUM. 1986. Biol. Reprod. **35:** 745–760.
26. RUSSELL, L. D. & R. N. PETERSON. 1985. Int. Rev. Cytol. **94:** 177–211.
27. ZIPARO, E., R. GEREMIA, M. A. RUSSO & M. STEFANINI. 1980. Am. J. Anat. **159:** 385–388.
28. DEPHILIP, R. M. & D. G. DANAHEY. 1987. Biol. Reprod. **37:** 1271–1282.
29. ENDERS, G. C. & C. F. MILLETTE. 1988. J. Cell Sci. **90:** 105–114.
30. D'AGOSTINO, A. & M. STEFANINI. 1990. Mol. Reprod. Dev. **25:** 172–176.
31. GROOTEGOED, J. A., R. JANSEN & H. J. VAN DER MOLEN. 1984. Biochim. Biophys. Acta **767:** 248–256.
32. GRISWOLD, M. D. 1988. Int. Rev. Cytol. **110:** 133–156.
33. BENAHAMED, M., C. COCHET, M. KERAMIDAS, M. A. CHAURIN & A. M. MORERA. 1988. Biochem. Biophys. Res. Commun. **154:** 1222–1231.
34. SKINNER, M. K. & H. L. MOSES. 1989 Mol. Endocrinol. **3:** 625–634.
35. JOSSO, N., J.-Y. PICARD & D. TRAN. 1980. *In* Testicular Development, Structure, and Function. A. Steinberger & E. Steinberger, Eds.: 21–31. Raven Press. New York.
36. CATE, R. L., J. MATTALIANO, C. HESSION, R. TIZARD, N. M. FARBER, A. CHEUNG, E. G. NINFA, A. Z. FREY, D. J. GASH, E. P. CHOW, R. A. FISHER, J. M. BERTONIS, G. TORRES, B. P. WALLNER, K. L. RAMACHANDRAN, R. C. RAGIN, T. F. MANGANARO, D. T. MACLAUGHLIN & P. K. DONAHOE. Cell **45:** 685–698.
37. DE JONG, F. H. & D. M. ROBERTSON. 1985. Mol. Cell. Endocrinol. **42:** 95–103.
38. SKINNER, M. K., K. TAKACS & R. J. COFFEY. 1989. Endocrinology **124:** 845–854.
39. HOLMES, S. D., SPOTTS G. & R. G. SMITH. 1986. J. Biol. Chem. **261:** 4076–4080.
40. SMITH, E. P., S. H. HALL, L. MONACO, F. S. FRENCH, E. M. WILSON & M. CONTI. 1989. Mol. Endocrinol. **3:** 954–961.
41. FEIG, L. A., M. KLAGSBRUN & A. R. BELLVÉ. 1983. J. Cell Biol. **97:** 1435–1443.
42. SMITH, E. P., M. J. SVOBODA, J. J. VAN WYK, A. L. KIERSZENBAUM & L. L. TRES. 1987. Endocrinology **120:** 186–193.
43. SYED, V., O. SODER, S. ARVER, M. LINDH, S. KHAN & E. M. RITZEN. 1988. Int. J. Androl. **11:** 437–447.
44. VERHOEVEN, G. & J. CAILLEAU. 1986. J. Steroid Biochem. **25:** 393–402.
45. SKINNER, M. K., P. S. TUNG & I. B. FRITZ. 1985. J. Cell Biol. **100:** 1941–1947.
46. ERICKSON-LAWRENCE, M., S. ZABLUDOFF & W. W. WRIGHT. 1990. J. Cell Biol. **111:** 107a.
47. LACROIX, M., F. E. SMITH & I. B. FRITZ. 1977. Mol Cell. Endocrinol. **9:** 227–236.
48. VIHKO, K. K., P. KRISTENSEN, K. DANO & M. PARVINEN. 1988. Dev. Biol. **126:** 150–155.
49. TINDALL, D. J., D. R. ROWLEY, L. MURTHY, L. I. LIPSHULTZ & C. H. CHANG. 1985. Int. Rev. Cytol. **94:** 127–149.
50. JOSEPH, D. R., S. H. HALL, M. CONTI & F. S. FRENCH. 1988. Mol. Endocrinol. **2:** 3–13.
51. SKINNER, M. K. & M. D. GRISWOLD. 1980. J. Biol. Chem. **255:** 9523–9525.
52. SKINNER, M. K. & M. D. GRISWOLD. 1983. Biol. Reprod. **28:** 1225–1229.
53. SYLVESTER, S. R., M. K. SKINNER & M. D. GRISWOLD. 1984. Biol. Reprod. **31:** 1087–1101.
54. COLLARD, M. W., S. R. SYLVESTER, J. K. TSURUTA & M. D. GRISWOLD. 1988. Biochemistry **27:** 4557–4564.
55. COLLARD, M. W. & M. D. GRISWOLD. 1987. Biochemistry **26:** 3297–3303.
56. CHENG, C. Y., C.-L. CHEN, Z.-M. FENG, A. MARSHALL & C. W. BARDIN. 1988. Biochem. Biophys. Res. Commun. **155:** 398–404.
57. CHENG, C. Y. & C. W. BARDIN. 1986. Biochemistry **25:** 5276–5288.
58. CHENG, C. Y., J. GRIMA, M. S. STAHLER, R. A. LOCKSHIN & C. W. BARDIN. 1989. J. Biol. Chem. **264:** 21386–21393.

59. Purchio, A. F., J. C. Cooper, A. M. Brunner, M. N. Lioubin, L. E. Gentry, K. S. Kovacina, R. S. Roth & H. Marquardt. 1988. J. Biol. Chem. **263:** 14211–14215.
60. Sahagian, G. G. & M. M. Gottesman. 1982. J. Biol. Chem. **257:** 11145–11150.
61. Lin, T., J. Blaisdell & J. F. Haskell. 1987. Biochem. Biophys. Res. Commun. **146:** 387–394.
62. Ailenberg, M., P. S. Tung & I. B. Fritz. 1990. Biol. Reprod. **42:** 499–509.
63. Feng, P., K. J. Catt & M. Knecht. 1988. Endocrinology **122: 181**–186.
64. Mason, R. W., S. Gal & M. M. Gottesman. 1987. Biochem. J. **248:** 449–454.
65. Gottesman, M. M. & M. E. Sobel. 1980. Cell **19:** 449–455.
66. Prence, E. M., J. Dong & G. G. Sahagian. 1990. J. Cell. Biol. **110:** 319–326.
67. Sporn, M. B., A. B. Roberts, L. M. Wakefield & R. K. Assoian. 1986. Science **233:** 532–534.
68. Kornfeld, S. & I. Mellman. 1989. Annu. Rev. Cell Biol. **5:** 483–525.
69. Hoflack, B. & S. Kornfeld. 1985. J. Biol. Chem. **260:** 12008–12014.
70. Stein, M., H. E. Meyer, A. Hasilik & K. von Figura. 1987. Biol. Chem. Hoppe-Seyler **368:** 927–936.
71. Dahms, N. M., P. Lobel, J. Breitmeyer, J. M. Chirgwin & S. Kornfeld. 1987. Cell **50:** 181–192.
72. Pohlmann, R., G. Nagel, B. Schmidt, M. Stein, G. Lorkowski, C. Krentler, J. Cully, H. E. Meyer, K.-H. Grzeschik, G. Mersmann, A. Hasilik & K. von Figura. 1987. Proc. Natl. Acad. Sci. USA **84:** 5575–5579.
73. Lobel, P., N. M. Dahms, J. Breitmeyer, J. M. Chirgwin & S. Kornfeld. 1987. Proc. Natl. Acad. Sci. USA **84:** 2233–2237.
74. Lobel, P., N. M. Dahms & S. Kornfeld. 1988. J. Biol Chem. **263:** 2563–2570.
75. Oshima, A., C. M. Nolan, J. W. Kyle, J. H. Grubb & W. S. Sly. 1988. J. Biol. Chem. **263:** 2553–2562.
76. Roth, R. A. 1988. Science **239:** 1269–1271.
77. Hoflack, B. & S. Kornfeld. 1985. Proc. Natl. Acad. Sci. USA **82:** 4428–4432.
78. Tong, P. Y., S. E. Tollefsen & S. Kornfeld. 1988. J. Biol. Chem. **263:** 2585–2588.
79. Kiess, W., G. D. Blickenstaff, M. Sklar, C. Thomas, S. P. Nissley & G. G. Sahagian. 1988. J. Biol. Chem. **263:** 9339–9344.
80. Morgan, D. O., J. C. Edman, D. N. Standring, V. A. Fried, M. C. Smith, R. A. Roth & W. J. Rutter. 1987. Nature **329:** 301–307.
81. Fischer, H. D., A. Gonzalez-Noriega & W. S. Sly. 1980. J. Biol. Chem. **255:** 5069–5074.
82. Stein, M., T. Braulke, C. Krentler, A. Hasilik & K. von Figura. 1987. Biol. Chem. Hoppe-Seyler **368:** 937–947.
83. Braulke, T. C., A. Gartung, A. Hasilik & K. von Figura. 1987. J. Cell Biol. **104:** 1735–1742.
84. Duncan, J. R. & S. Kornfeld. 1988. J. Cell Biol. **104:** 1735–1742.
85. Stein, M., J. E. Zijderhand-Bleekemolen, H. Geuze, A. Hasilik & K. von Figura. 1987. EMBO J. **6:** 2677–2681.
86. Wantanabe, H., J. H. Grubb & W. S. Sly. 1990. Proc. Natl. Acad. Sci. USA **87:** 8036–8040.
87. Lee, S.-J. & D. Nathans. 1988. J. Biol. Chem. **263:** 3521–3527.
88. Dennis, P. A. & D. B. Rifkin. 1991. Proc. Natl. Acad. Sci. USA **88:** 580–584.
89. Nishimoto, I., Y, Hata, E. Ogata & I. Kojima. 1987. J. Biol. Chem. **262:** 12120–12126.
90. Nishimoto, I., Y. Murayama, T. Katada, M. Ui & E. Ogata. 1989. J. Biol. Chem. **264:** 14029–14038.
91. Rogers, S. A. & M. R. Hammerman. 1989. J. Biol. Chem. **264:** 4273–4276.
92. Rogers, S. A., A. F. Purchio & M. R. Hammerman. 1990. J. Biol. Chem. **265:** 9722–9727.
93. Okamoto, T., I. Nishimoto, Y. Murayama, Y. Ohkuni & E. Ogata. 1990. Biochem. Biophys. Res. Commun. **168:** 1201–1210.
94. O'Brien, D. A., C. A. Gabel, D. L. Rockett & E. M. Eddy. 1989. Endocrinology **125:** 2973–2984.
95. Bellvé, A. R., C. F. Millette, Y. M. Bhatnagar & D. A. O'Brien. 1977. J. Histochem. Cytochem. **25:** 480–494.
96. O'Brien, D. A. 1987. Biol. Reprod. **37:** 147–157.
97. Gerton, G. L. & C. F. Millette. 1986. Biol. Reprod. **35:** 1025–1035.
98. Tres, L. L., E. P. Smith, J. J. van Wyk & A. L. Kierszenbaum. 1986. Exp. Cell Res. **162:** 33–50.
99. Galdieri, M., E. Ziparo, F. Palombi, M. A. Russo & M. Stefanini. 1981. J. Androl. **5:** 249–254.
100. Palombi, F. & C. Di Carlo. 1988. Biol. Reprod. **39:** 1101–1109.

101. O'Brien, D. A., J. E. Welch, A. A. Taylor, Jr. & E. M. Eddy. 1990. J. Cell Biol. **111:** 109a.
102. Kornfeld, S. 1987. FASEB J. **1:** 462–468.
103. O'Brien, D. A., C. A. Gabel, D. L. Rockett & E. M. Eddy. 1989. J. Cell Biol. **109:** 68a.
104. Lazzarino, D. & C. A. Gabel. 1990. J. Biol. Chem. **265:** 11864–11871.
105. O'Brien, D. A., G. L. Gerton & E. M. Eddy. 1988. Biol. Reprod. **38:** 955–967.
106. Skinner, M. K. & M. D. Griswold. 1983. Cell Biol. Int. Rep. **7:** 441–446.
107. Borland, K., M. Mita, C. L. Oppenheimer, L. A. Blinderman, J. Massague. P. F. Hall & M. P. Czech. 1984. Endocrinology **114:** 240–246.
108. Murphy, L. J., G. I. Bell & H. G. Friesen. 1987. Endocrinology **120:** 1279–1282.
109. Ramasharma, K., C. M. Cabrera & C. H. Li. 1986. Biochem. Biophys. Res. Commun. **140:** 536-542.
110. Voutilainen, R. & W. L. Miller. 1988. DNA **7:** 9–15.
111. Closset, J., A. Gothot, B. Sente, M. L. Scippo, A. Igout, M. Vanderbroeck, D. Dombrowicz & G. Hennen. 1989. Mol. Endocrinol. **3:** 1125–1131.
112. Daughaday, W. H. & P. Rotwein. 1989. Endocrine Rev. **10:** 68–91.
113. O'Brien, D. A., C. A. Gabel & E. M. Eddy. 1991. Biol. Reprod. **44**(Suppl. 1): 93.

Spermatids Are Regulators of Sertoli Cell Function[a]

BERNARD JÉGOU

Groupe d'Etude de la Reproduction chez le Mâle
INSERM/CJF 91-04
Université de Rennes I
Campus de Beaulieu
35042 Rennes Cédex, France

INTRODUCTION

There is considerable evidence that Sertoli cells play an essential role in the control of germ cell division, differentiation, and metabolism.[1-3] Understanding Sertoli cell regulation is therefore crucial to a fuller understanding of spermatogenesis.

It is now well established that, in addition to FSH, paracrine factors such as testosterone and P-Mod-S (which originate in the Leydig and peritubular cells, respectively) exert a positive influence on Sertoli cell function.[1-3] Moreover, our own studies and those of other laboratories have recently demonstrated that germ cells also contribute greatly to the control of Sertoli cell activity.[3,4] In this chapter, we describe data acquired from morphological observations and from experiments conducted both *in vitro* and *in vivo*, and establish a specific feature of paracrine control of Sertoli cells by germ cells, namely the influence of spermatids on Sertoli cell function.

THE MORPHOLOGICAL POINT OF VIEW

The spermatogenetic process can be divided into three phases: the spermatogonial proliferation phase, the meiotic phase (spermatocytes), and spermiogenesis, which corresponds to the metamorphosis of spermatids into spermatozoa. This metamorphosis is a unique phenomenon which comprises extensive changes in the shape of the spermatid, within the cytoplasm, and in the nucleus of this cell type.[1] These morphological events, combined with the fact that the ratio of spermatids per Sertoli cell is higher than the ratio of any other germ cell category per Sertoli cell,[5] explain why, of all the germ cell types, it is the spermatid which exerts the greatest work stress on the Sertoli cell.

Spermatids communicate physically and chemically with Sertoli cells through the existence of a unique variety of structural devices which are summarized in TABLE 1. These anatomical structures can be separated on a functional basis into two groups: 1) the desmosome-like junctions, the ectoplasmic specializations, and the tubulobulbar

[a] Part of these studies were funded by l'INSERM (Paris, grants 844010, 874010, 900406), la Fondation pour la Recherche Médicale (Paris), la Fondation de France (Paris) and le Ministère de la Recherche et de la Technologie (D.R.R.T. N° 89 H 0112).

complexes that play an important role in the cytoarchitecture of the seminiferous tubules; and 2) the gap-junctions, the Sertoli cell processes, the tubulobulbar complexes, and the residual bodies which are involved in the transfer of materials from one cell type to another.

THE FUNCTIONAL POINT OF VIEW

The fact that elongating and elongated spermatids cannot be isolated in mammals without causing great damage, and that early spermatids do not survive well in culture,[18,19] has long hampered studies into the relationship between spermatids and Sertoli cells. This reflects the intimate interdependence of these two cell categories.

In an attempt to obviate these major experimental obstacles, our group has developed the following complementary approaches: 1) selective removal of sub-classes of germ cells and study of the consequences on Sertoli cell function; 2) culture and coculture of Sertoli cells and of germ cells; and 3) use of a non-mammalian model: the dogfish (*S. Canicula*).

The present review will be essentially restricted to the results obtained with the first two approaches.

Influence of Spermatids on Sertoli Cell Function in the Immature Rat

In Vivo *Experiment*

Since the pioneer studies of Piana and Savarese,[20] demonstrating that experimental cryptorchidism induces the degeneration of germ cells, this model has probably been

TABLE 1. Structural Relationships of Spermatids and Sertoli Cells

Structure	Steps of Spermiogenesis	Presumed Function	Selected References[a]
Desmosome-like junctions	1–7 (rat)	• Attachment devices	6, 7
Gap-junctions	1–7 (rat)	• Passage of small MW molecules	8
Sertoli cell processes	8–16 (mouse)	• Transfer of materials	9
Ectoplasmic specializations	1–18 (rat)	• Prevention of premature sloughing of spermatids • Role in sperm release and possibly in acrosome shaping	6, 7, 10, 11
Tubulobulbar complexes	18–19 (rat)	• Elimination of excess cytoplasm of late spermatids • Anchor late spermatids • May trigger sperm release mechanism • Indirectly engineer the formation of residual bodies	12, 13
Residual bodies	Spermiation cytoplasm	• Elimination of late spermatid • Role in the coordination of spermatogenesis	14–17

[a] For a more complete list of references see the recent review of de Kretser and Kerr.[1]

the most extensively used to explore testicular function. In a study that we performed several years ago, cryptorchidism was surgically induced in 14-day-old rats and allowed to persist until they were 35 days old. These animals, and sham-operated rats of the same age, were then killed to assess testicular function.[21]

In the 35-day old controls, the most advanced stage of spermatogenesis was the early spermatid stage (FIG. 1A). In the testis of the cryptorchid animals, on the other hand, there was a marked decrease in the number of early spermatids and a moderate reduction in the number of primary spermatocytes (FIG. 1B). Most of the remaining early spermatids had pyknotic nuclei and formed multinucleate collections in the lumen of the seminiferous tubules. Sertoli cell function appeared severely altered: the ABP production rate was decreased whereas serum FSH levels, which are often used to indirectly monitor inhibin production, were increased (FIG. 2). These results therefore suggest that early spermatids, and maybe pachytene spermatocytes, affect Sertoli cell function in the prepubertal rat.

In Vitro *Experiment*

That ABP and inhibin production by Sertoli cells from immature rats is markedly influenced by pachytene spermatocytes and by early spermatids (steps 1–8 of spermiogenesis) is evidenced by the results obtained when we added isolated pachytene spermatocytes or early spermatids to Sertoli cells recovered from 20-day-old rats: both ABP and inhibin production were very significantly stimulated (FIG. 3). Moreover, at least part of the effects of germ cells observed in coculture originates from

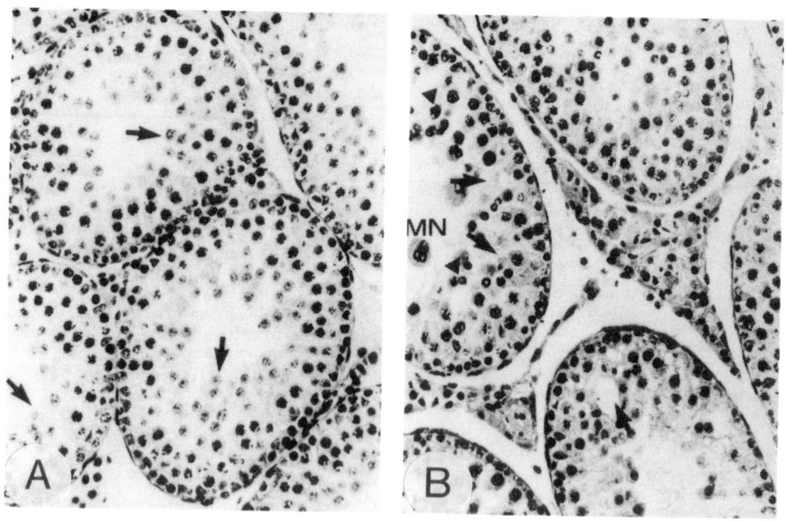

FIGURE 1. A: Photomicrograph of testis from 35 day old normal rat. Note most advanced cell type the early spermatid (*arrows*). **B:** Photomicrograph of testis from 35 days old cryptorchid rat. Note depopulation of epithelium (*arrows*). Pyknotic spermatocytes and spermatids (*arrowheads*) and multinucleate cells (MN). Also note prominent intertubular tissue. (From Jégou *et al.*[21] with permission from *Biology of Reproduction*.)

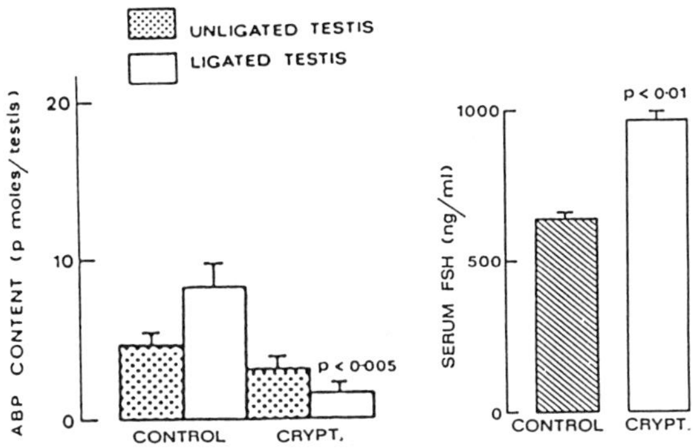

FIGURE 2. The effect of cryptorchidism in immature rats on ABP content and accumulation following unilateral efferent duct ligation 16 h previously and on serum FSH levels. Values represent mean ± SEM for 5–7 rats/group. (From Jégou *et al.*[21] with permission from *Biology of Reproduction*.)

secreted factor(s), since spermatocyte and spermatid conditioned media also significantly enhanced the levels of these Sertoli cell parameters.[19,24] It is notable that, whereas pachytene spermatocytes were generally found to be more potent regulators of ABP production than early spermatids,[19,22,23] the reverse situation was observed for inhibin.[24] The purification of the germ cell protein(s) involved in the regulation of Sertoli cell function is in progress in several laboratories.

In conclusion, given the results of these *in vivo* and *in vitro* experiments, the existence of a close temporal relationship *in vivo* between the development of the secretion of many Sertoli cell products, and the appearance and increase of primary spermatocytes and early spermatids,[4] we hypothesize that these two germ cell categories play a major role in the initiation of Sertoli cell function in the mammalian testis, either in conjunction or sequentially as they appear in the tubules.

Influence of Spermatids on Sertoli Cell Function in the Adult Rat

In Vivo *Experiments*

We have shown that when cryptorchidism is induced in rats less than 20 days old (i.e., well before the body-testis temperature gradient observed in the adult is reached[25]), the germ cell complement progressively decreases (see above). In contrast, the translocation of the testis into the abdominal cavity after puberty results in very rapid germ cell degeneration and loss,[26,29] and precise study of the relationship between germ cells and Sertoli cells becomes impossible. Interestingly, Steinberger and co-workers have demonstrated that after brief exposure of the adult rat scrotum to heat, a specific sequence of germ cell damage occurs.[30-32] We therefore adopted one of the treatments described by these authors: the application of a temperature of 43 °C for 15 min to the scrotum of anesthetized adult rats.

We confirmed that moderate heat essentially causes pachytene spermatocytes and early spermatids to deteriorate, which in turn provokes a progressive reduction in the number of late spermatids, through a maturation-depletion process (FIG. 4). It appeared that contrary to what had been observed previously in the immature testis (see above), the loss of most pachytene spermatocytes and of early spermatids had no major effect on Sertoli cell activity. However, a decline of ABP production rate

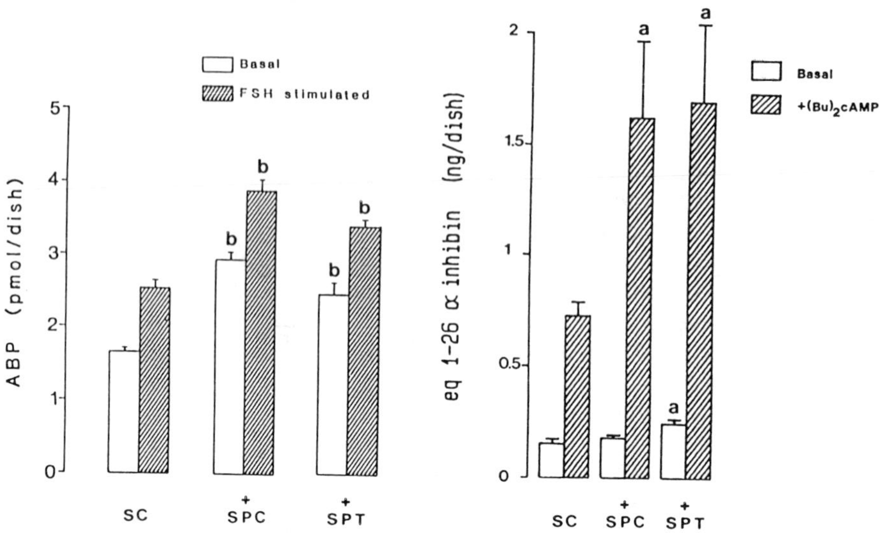

FIGURE 3. Effect of enriched fractions containing pachytene spermatocytes (SPC) or early spermatids (SPT) on ABP and inhibin secretion by rat Sertoli cells. Values for ABP are mean ± SEM. a, $p < 0.005$; b, $p < 0.001$; when compared with respective Sertoli cell control (SC) (basal or + FSH for ABP or + $(BU)_2$ cAMP for inhibin). (ABP: From Le Magueresse *et al.*[22] with permission from *Journal of Reproduction and Fertility*; inhibin: From Pineau *et al.*[24] with permission from *Molecular Cellular Endocrinology*.)

occurred 14 days post-heating and reached a nadir at 26 days, when late spermatids were the only category of germ cells whose number was greatly reduced. This change in Sertoli cell secretory activity was totally reversible, with full restoration of spermatogenesis (FIG. 4). Since the same relationship was found between the number of late spermatids and other parameters of Sertoli cell function (*e.g.*, tubular fluid, the number of FSH receptors, and inhibin levels—indirectly estimated by serum FSH levels), we concluded that in the adult rat "late spermatids may interact with the Sertoli cell."[33]

To investigate this hypothesis further, we developed several radiation protocols; differences concerned: the mode of exposure (chronic or acute), the type of energy (gamma or neutrons plus gamma) and the irradiation dose.[34-36] When gamma rays were administered continuously and at a low dose-rate of 7 cGy/day, A spermatogonia were specifically damaged[34-36] (FIG. 5A). The loss of these cells created a "gap" in the spermatogenic process which resulted in a very progressive and sequential dose-related reduction in the subsequent stages of spermatogenesis. In contrast, the number of Sertoli cells was unchanged[34-36] (FIG. 5A). All spermatogonia were not destroyed, however; at the end of irradiation, we observed sequential repopulation of the seminiferous tubules by the different germ cell types. Spermatogenesis was fully restored at about 12 weeks post-irradiation[36] (FIG. 5A). In these experimental conditions, depopulation and repopulation patterns of the different germ cell categories did not overlap. The effect of altered germ cell complement on Sertoli cell morphology and function could therefore be analyzed with precision. This highlights the particular value of this protocol.

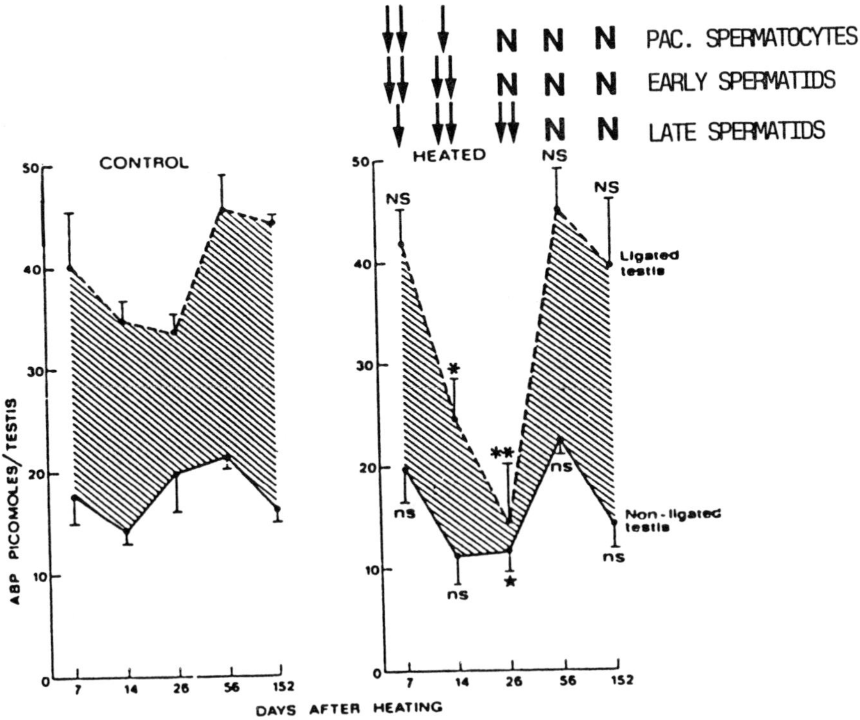

FIGURE 4. The effect of heating on ABP content in cytosols from the non-ligated and ligated testis following 16 h of efferent duct ligation. The shaded area represents the ABP accumulation over the 16 h period. Values represent the mean ± SEM for 5 rats per group. ↓ = decrease in numbers of germ cells. N = normal appearance. (From Jégou *et al.*[33] with permission from *International Journal of Andrology*).

We have demonstrated that Sertoli cells can sustain the disappearance of most spermatogonia, preleptotene spermatocytes, pachytene spermatocytes and round spermatids, with no significant change in secretory activity[35,36] (FIG. 5,B&C), nor in ultrastructural appearance.[35] Conversely, as shown above after heating the testes, Sertoli cell activity declined, in close parallel to the decrease in the number of late spermatids, as evidenced by reduced ABP production and increased plasma FSH levels (FIG. 5,B&C). At the same time, vacuoles appeared in the Sertoli cells, while the number of cytoplasmic organelles decreased. These morphological changes were followed by thickening and folding of the peritubular tissue.[35] Interestingly, no significant changes in ABP and FSH levels were observed until day 42 post-irradiation, whereas germ cells had repopulated the tubules to the early spermatid stage. In contrast, the progressive reappearance of late spermatids between days 42 and 86 post-irradiation was closely associated with the recovery of Sertoli cell activity (FIG. 5,B&C). When all the parameters from individual groups (killed on a given day) were correlated using standard linear regression analysis, a highly positive significant correlation between the number

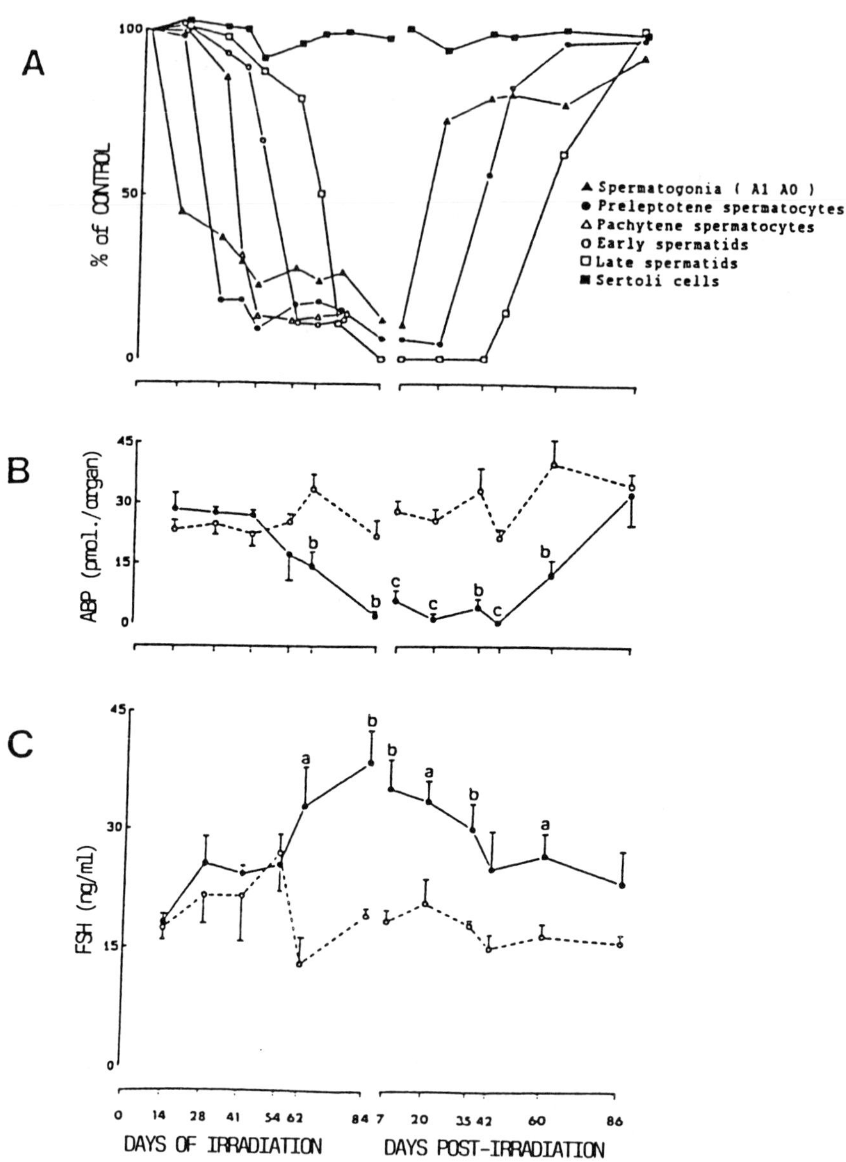

FIGURE 5. A: Temporal changes in the number of Sertoli and germ cells per testis during chronic gamma-irradiation. B and C: The effect of chronic gamma irradiation on epididymal ABP content and plasma FSH concentrations. Values (○, control; ●, irradiated) represent the mean ± SEM for 5 rats/group. a, $p < 0.005$; b, $p < 0.01$; c, $p < 0.001$, compared to the time-matched control. (From Pineau *et al.*[36] with permission from *Endocrinology*.)

of late spermatids and ABP levels as well as a negative significant correlation between the numbers of this germ cell type and FSH levels were found.[36]

We have demonstrated that the decline in ABP levels was not related to the total radiation dose administered,[35] and that there is a close relationship between Sertoli cell function and late spermatids when spermatogenesis was disrupted using factors as different as heat,[33] procarbazine,[37] methoxy-acetic acid (MAA),[38–40] and X rays.[41] Consequently, the changes observed at the Sertoli cell level did not result directly from exposure to gamma rays. Late spermatids therefore seem to be a major factor in the control of Sertoli cell function.

It is highly probable that other germ cell types may also modulate Sertoli cell activity in the adult testis in light of the evidence presented by Parvinen *et al.*[41–43] and as suggested by other studies.[36] However, the fact that Sertoli cells may be able to compensate, within certain limits, for the loss of pachytene spermatocytes,[44] whereas they never adapt to the loss of late spermatids, provides conclusive proof that late spermatids play a predominant role in the paracrine control of Sertoli cell function by germ cells in the adult rat. This is also likely to exist in man: in a study involving both the quantitative analysis of different germ cell types in testicular biopsy specimens obtained from men undergoing varicocelectomy and the measurement of circulating FSH levels, the authors concluded that "except for late spermatids, no correlations between FSH and germ cell counts could be demonstrated."[45]

Moreover, we have found an important relationship between Sertoli cell function and the last steps of spermiogenesis in the dogfish (*S. canicula*),[46] which belongs to the cartilaginous fishes that appeared at least 350 millions years ago. This proves that the interaction between late spermatids and the Sertoli cell has survived throughout evolution and therefore constitutes a major aspect of the paracrine regulation of spermatogenesis.

As stated earlier,[4] whereas pachytene spermatocytes and early spermatids appear to be essential regulators of Sertoli cell function in the immature rat, our studies in the adult rat found no correlation between these germ cell type counts and Sertoli cell activity. This might indicate that at each step of the development of testicular function, the regulation of Sertoli cell activity is essentially taken over by the most advanced generation(s) of germ cell present within the seminiferous epithelium.

MECHANISMS OF SPERMATID ACTION ON SERTOLI CELLS

Early Spermatids

The effects of early spermatids on Sertoli cell function are most probably mediated through different pathways: the secretion of one or several factors (see above), surface molecules that mediate cell to cell adhesion and plasma membrane specializations (TABLE 1).

In an *in vitro* system in which enriched preparations of germ cells were added to cultures of Sertoli cells, it was found that in the rat, a lower proportion of early spermatids than pachytene spermatocytes and than residual bodies/cytoplasts from elongated spermatids (RB/CES), adhere to Sertoli cells.[22,23,48] Our studies have also established that in Sertoli cell–germ cell membrane recognition, the governing mechanisms: 1) vary with the age of the Sertoli cell donors, early spermatids adhering twice as much to Sertoli cells from 45-day-old rats as to Sertoli cells from younger animals (10 or 20 days of age); and 2) are influenced by FSH. Cameron and Muffly[49] have recently shown that both FSH and testosterone are necessary to achieve maximal spermatid binding to Matrigel-supported Sertoli cells in culture. According to these authors, the involvement of FSH may consist of inducing a junction-related structural competence of the Sertoli cell, whereas testosterone only stimulates spermatid binding to Sertoli cells rendered competent by FSH.

In the mouse, using a different *in vitro* assay system, Enders and Millette[50] have demonstrated that the number of early spermatids and pachytene spermatocytes binding sites on the Sertoli cell monolayers were similar, but that binding kinetics were different.

To date, the nature of the cell surface components involved in spermatid-Sertoli cell adhesion is unknown. However, Byers *et al.*[51] and Cyr *et al.*[52] have recently demonstrated that at least one member of the cadherin family (neural cadherin[52]), composed of structurally and functionally related molecules which participate in calcium-dependent homotypic intercellular adhesion,[53] is found in the testis and the seminiferous tubules of the rat. In particular, a testicular cadherin is probably present where Sertoli cell ectoplasmic specializations are localized.[51]

Since cell-cell adhesion molecules (CAMs) are morphoregulators thought to be responsible for the epigenic regulation of tissue and function, experiments in this field should rapidly lead to the identification of new important paracrine regulatory factors of the spermatogenic process.

Late Spermatids

As is the case for early spermatids, very little is known on the mechanisms underlying the control of Sertoli cell function by late spermatids. Gene expression occurs in late spermatids.[54] To date, there is, however, no evidence that late spermatids gene products are secreted. In contrast, genes of these cells and RNAs transcribed from earlier stages present in their cytoplasm, can code for stuctural proteins,[54] like actin and tubulin (including testicular isotypes). Owing to the role that these proteins can play in cell shaping and cytoarchitecture, they may contribute to the interaction between germ cells and the Sertoli cell.

Moreover, as indicated at the beginning of this chapter (TABLE 1), several important types of plasma membrane specializations between late spermatids and Sertoli cells exist and recent studies from our laboratory have demonstrated the high ability of late spermatids and RB/CES to adhere to Sertoli cells at different ages.[22,55] The fact that early spermatid binding was much lower than that of pachytene spermatocytes and of RB/CES, indicates that changes occur in the binding characteristics and/or in the nature of the adhesion molecules at the cell surface, during meiosis and spermiogenesis. We also found that *in vitro*: 1) the binding kinetics of RB/CES to rat Sertoli cells in culture is not influenced by the age of the Sertoli cell donors (20 or 45 days of age); 2) FSH accelerates RB/CES binding; 3) FSH markedly reduces RB/CES phagocytosis; and 4) peritubular cells only marginally influence RB/CES binding.[55]

Two main hypotheses, which are not mutually exclusive, can be formulated to explain how late spermatids regulate the Sertoli cell. The first hypothesis may also apply to other germ cell stages; it is based on the model presented by Bissel and Barcellos-Hoff[56] and presumes that the influence of late spermatids on Sertoli cells is communicated through modifications in the Sertoli cell cytoskeleton, which may modulate gene expression via the nuclear matrix. This hypothesis has not been investigated yet. However, it is very likely that the marked changes which occur in the Sertoli cell shape during the seminiferous epithelium cycle[1] and following germ cell depletion (Sertoli cells collapse, particularly after the loss of late spermatids), have important consequence on Sertoli cell functional integrity. A structure-function relationship has recently been suggested in Sertoli cells when cultured on different extracellular matrix substrates.[57]

The second hypothesis only applies to the later spermatid stage; it supposes that residual bodies shed during spermiation and subsequently phagocytosed by the Sertoli cell,[14,58,59] play a key role in coordinating spermatogenesis in mammals. This hypothesis was first proposed by Roosen-Runge;[17] it is based on the coincidence between the formation and phagocytosis of the residual bodies and the occurrence of major events such as: 1) mitosis of the type A spermatogonia; 2) spermatocyte entry into the meiotic prophase; 3) the rapid transformation of the young spermatids; and 4) drastic morphological changes of Sertoli cells.[60] The hypothetical role of the residual bodies in spermatogenesis was further developed by Lacy,[61] in reports on the appearance of lipids in the Sertoli cell cytoplasm, in parallel to residual body digestion. This hypothesis was however subsequently abandoned on the grounds that the cyclical adult pattern of the seminiferous epithelium emerges well before the first generation of spermatozoa is released into the lumen of the tubules.[60] However, in our opinion, a key role for residual bodies in the synchronization of spermatogenesis process is not limited to the existence of earlier regulatory mechanism(s) that may be sequentially assumed by younger generations of germ cell as they appear in the tubules, during testicular maturation (see above).

We have identified two possible complementary pathways by which residual bodies may influence Sertoli cell function and earlier generations of germ cells: 1) through the translation of mRNA released after the lysis of residual bodies in the Sertoli cell cytoplasm, since they contain RNA;[62–66] and 2) through the induction of the synthesis and the release of Sertoli cell factor(s) by residual body surface components and by the phagocytic process itself. This is only speculation. However, we have developed an *in vitro* model to explore RB/CES–Sertoli cell interactions.[22,55] We have also recently demonstrated[67] that Sertoli cells, like other phagocytic cells,[68] produce interleukin-1 α which is known to stimulate spermatogonial and meiotic DNA synthesis.[69–71] We therefore have the means as well as the clues to reactivate the hypothesis concerning the role played by residual bodies in the coordination of spermatogenesis.

SUMMARY

Spermatids are major regulators of Sertoli cell function. Specific anatomical structures exist between spermatids and Sertoli cells. Their nature evolves during spermiogenesis and they are essential mediators in the interaction between these two cell types. Spermatids play a crucial role in Sertoli cell gene expression and secretory function at different ages. Early spermatid effect is partly mediated through the secretion of soluble factor(s). The influence of late spermatids on Sertoli cell secretion in the adult testis is conserved throughout evolution and may be mediated via their implication in the conformational changes on Sertoli cells that occur during spermatogenesis and through phagocytosis of the residual bodies.

ACKNOWLEDGMENTS

The author thanks Mrs. L. Fornari, Dr. F. Bauché, Mrs. A. M. Touzalin and Mr. L. Communier for their help during the preparation of this manuscript.

REFERENCES

1. DE KRETSER, D. M. & J. F. KERR. 1988. The cytology of the testis. *In* The Physiology of Reproduction. E. Knobil, J. D. Neill, *et al.*, Eds. Vol. **1:** 837–932. Raven Press. New York.
2. BARDIN, W., C. Y. CHENG, N. A. MUSTO & G. L. GUNSALUS. 1988. The Sertoli cell. *In* The Physiology of Reproduction. E. Knobil, J. D. Neill, *et al.*, Eds. Vol. **1:** 933–974. Raven Press. New York.
3. SKINNER, M. K. 1991. Cell-cell interactions in the testis. Endocr. Rev. **12:** 45–78.
4. JÉGOU, B., B. LE MAGUERESSE, P. SOURDAINE, C. PINEAU, J. F. VELEZ DE LA CALLE, D. H. GARNIER, F. GUILLOU & C. BOISSEAU. 1988. Germ cell-Sertoli cell interactions in vertebrates. *In* Molecular and Cellular Endocrinology of the Testis. B. A. Cooke & R. M. Sharpe, Eds. Serono Symposia Publications. Vol. **30:** 255–270. Raven Press. New York.
5. WING, T. Y. & A. K. CHRISTENSEN. 1982. Morphometric studies on rat seminiferous tubules. Am. J. Anat. **165:** 13–25.
6. BRÖKELMANN, J. 1963. Fine structure of germ cells and Sertoli cells during the cycle of the seminiferous epithelium in the rat. Z. Zellforsch. Mikroskop. Anat. **59:** 820–850.
7. RUSSELL, L. D. 1977. Movement of spermatocytes from the basal to adluminal compartment of the rat testis. Am. J. Anat. **148:** 313–328.
8. MCGINLEY, D. M., Z. POSALAKI, M. PORVAZNIK & L. D. RUSSELL. 1979. Gap-junctions between Sertoli and germ cells of rat seminiferous tubules. Tissue & Cell **4:** 741–754.
9. SAKAI, Y., T. NAKAMOTO & S. YAMASHINA. 1988. Dynamic changes in Sertoli cell processes invading spermatid cytoplasm during mouse spermatogenesis. Anat. Rec. **220:** 51–57.
10. RUSSELL, L. D. 1979. Further observations on tubulo-bulbar complexes formed by late spermatids and Sertoli cells in the rat testis. Anat. Rec. **194:** 213–232.
11. ROSS, M. H. 1976. The Sertoli cell junctional specialization during spermiogenesis and at spermiation. Anat. Rec. **186:** 79–104.
12. RUSSELL, L. D. & Y. CLERMONT. 1976. Anchoring device between Sertoli cells and late spermatids in rat seminiferous tubules. Anat. Rec. **185:** 259–278.
13. GRAVIS, C. J. 1980. Ultrastructural observations on spermatozoa retained within the seminiferous epithelium after treatment with dibutyryl cyclic AMP. Tissue & Cell **12:** 309–322.
14. REGAUD, C. 1901. Etudes de la structure des tubes séminifères et sur la spermatogénèse chez les mammifères. Arch. Anat. Microscop. Morphol. Exptl. **4:** 101–156 (a) & 231–380 (b).
15. CHEMES, H. 1986. The phagocytic function of Sertoli cells: A morphological, biochemical, and endocrinological study of lysosomes and acid phosphatase localization in the rat testis. Endocrinology **119:** 1673–1681.
16. CLERMONT, Y., C. MORALES & L. HERMO. 1987. Endocytic activities of Sertoli cells in the rat. Ann. N.Y. Acad. Sci. **513:** 1–15.
17. ROOSEN-RUNGE, E. C. 1952. Kinetics of spermatogenesis in mammals. Ann. N.Y. Acad. Sci. **55:** 574–584.
18. JUTTE, N. H. P. M., J. A. GROOTEGOED, F. F. G. ROMMERTS & H. J. VAN DER MOLEN. 1981. Exogenous lactate is essential for metabolic activities in isolated rat spermatocytes and spermatids. J. Reprod. Fertil. **62:** 399–405.
19. LE MAGUERESSE, B. & B. JÉGOU. 1988. Paracrine control of immature Sertoli cells by adult germ cells, in the rat (an *in vitro* study). Cell-cell interactions within the testis. Mol. Cell. Endocrinol. **58:** 65–72.
20. PIANA, G. & G. SAVARESE. 1891. Su alcuni studii anatomopatologici. Clin. Vet. Milano. **14:** 50–51.
21. JÉGOU, B., R. A. PEAKE, D. C. IRBY & D. M. DE KRETSER. 1984. Effects of the induction of experimental cryptorchidism and subsequent orchidopexy on testicular function in immature rats. Biol. Reprod. **30:** 179–187.

22. LE MAGUERESSE, B., F. LE GAC, M. LOIR & B. JÉGOU. 1986. Stimulation of rat Sertoli cell secretory activity *in vitro* by germ cells and residual bodies. J. Reprod. Fertil. **77:** 489–498.
23. LE MAGUERESSE, B. & B. JÉGOU. 1988. *In vitro* effects of germ cells on the secretory activity of Sertoli cells recovered from rats of different ages. Endocrinology **122:** 1672–1680.
24. PINEAU, C., R. M. SHARPE, P. T. K. SAUNDERS, N. GÉRARD & B. JÉGOU. 1990. Regulation of Sertoli cell inhibin production and of inhibin α-subunit mRNA levels by specific germ cell types. Mol. Cell. Endocrinol. **72:** 13–22.
25. KORMANO, M. 1967. Development of the rectum-testis temperature difference in the post-natal rat. J. Reprod. Fertil. **14:** 427–437.
26. PARVINEN, M. 1973. Observations on freshly isolated and accurately identified spermatogenic cells of the rat. Early effects of heat and short-time experimental cryptorchidism. Virchows Arch. Abt. B. Zellpathol. **13:** 38–47.
27. WALSH, P. C. & R. S. SWERDLOFF. 1973. Experimental cryptorchidism: Effect on serum LH and FSH in the rat. Urol. Res. **1:** 22–26.
28. JÉGOU, B., G. P. RISBRIDGER & D. M. DE KRETSER. 1983. Effects of experimental cryptorchidism on testicular function in adult rats. J. Androl. **4:** 88–94.
29. JÉGOU, B., A. O. LAWS & D. M. DE KRETSER. The effect of cryptorchidism and subsequent orchidopexy on testicular function in adult rats. J. Reprod. Fertil. **69:** 137–145.
30. STEINBERGER, E. & W. J. DIXON. 1959. Some observations on the effect of heat on the testicular germinal epithelium. Fertil. Steril. **10:** 578–595.
31. CHOWDHURY, A. K. & E. STEINBERGER. 1964. A quantitative study of the effect of heat on germinal epithelium of rat testes. Am. J. Anat. **115:** 509–524.
32. CHOWDHURY, A. K. & E. STEINBERGER. 1970. Early changes in the germinal epithelium of rat testes following exposure to heat. J. Reprod. Fertil. **22:** 205–212.
33. JÉGOU, B., A. O. LAWS & D. M. DE KRETSER. 1984. Changes in testicular function induced by short-term exposure of the rat testis to heat: Further evidence for interaction of germ cells, Sertoli cells and Leydig cells. Int. J. Androl. **7:** 244–257.
34. PINON-LATAILLADE, G., M. C. VIGUIER-MARTINEZ & J. MAAS. 1985. Endocrinological changes induced by continuous low dose gamma-irradiation of the rat testis. Acta Endocrinol. (Copenhagen) **109:** 558–562.
35. PINON-LATAILLADE, G., J. F. VELEZ DE LA CALLE, M. C. VIGUIER-MARTINEZ, D. H. GARNIER, R. FOLLIOT, J. MAAS & B. JÉGOU. 1988. Influence of germ cells upon Sertoli cells during continuous low-dose rate gamma-irradiation of adult rats. Mol. Cell. Endocrinol. **58:** 51–63.
36. PINEAU, C., J. F. VELEZ DE LA CALLE, G. PINON-LATAILLADE & B. JÉGOU. 1989. Assessment of testicular function after acute and chronic irradiation: Further evidence for an influence of late spermatids on Sertoli cell function in the adult rat. Endocrinology **124:** 2720–2728.
37. VELEZ DE LA CALLE, J. F., J. CL. SOUFIR, F. CHODORGE, C. BOISSEAU, H. KERCRET & B. JÉGOU. 1988. Reproductive effects of the anti-cancer drug procarbazine in male rats at different ages. J. Reprod. Fertil. **83:** 51–61.
38. BARTLETT, J. M., J. B. KERR & R. M. SHARPE. 1988. The selective removal of pachytene spermatocytes using methoxy acetic acid as an approach to the study *in vivo* of paracrine interactions in the testis. J. Androl. **9:** 31–40.
39. SHARPE, R. M. 1989. Possible role of elongated spermatids in control of stage-dependent changes in the diameter of the lumen of the rat seminiferous tubules. J. Androl. **10:** 304–310.
40. ALLENBY, G., P. M. D. FOSTER & R. M. SHARPE. 1991. Evidence that secretion of immunoactive inhibin by seminiferous tubules from the adult testis is regulated by specific germ cell types: Correlation between in vivo and in vitro studies. Endocrinology **128:** 467–476.
41. KANGASNIEMI, M., A. KAIPIA, J. TOPPARI, A. PERHEENTUPA, I. HUHTANIEMI & M. PARVINEN. 1990. Cellular regulation of follicle-stimulating hormone (FSH) binding in rat seminiferous tubules. J. Androl. **11:** 336–343.
42. PARVINEN, M. 1982. Regulation of the seminiferous epithelium. Endocr. Rev. **3:** 404–417.
43. VIKHO, K. K., J. J. O. SUOMINEN & M. PARVINEN. 1984. Cellular regulation of plasminogen activator secretion during spermatogenesis. Biol. Reprod. **31:** 383–389.
44. PINON-LATAILLADE, G., M. C. VIGUIER-MARTINEZ, A. M. TOUZALIN, J. MAAS & B. JÉGOU. 1991. Effect of a single exposure of adult rat testes to gamma rays on germ cells and on Sertoli and Leydig cell functions. Reprod. Nut. Dev. In press.

45. Rodriguez-Rigaud, L. J., Z. Zukerman, D. B. Weiss, K. D. Smith & E. Steinberger. 1980. Hormone control of spermatogenesis in man: Comparison with the rat. *In* Testicular Development, Structure and Function. A. Steinberger & E. Steinberger, Eds.: 139–146, Raven Press. New York.
46. Sourdaine, P., D. H. Garnier & B. Jégou. 1990. The adult dogfish (*Scyliorhinus canicula L*) testis: A model to study stage-dependent changes in steroid levels during spermatogenesis. J. Endocrinol. **127:** 451–460.
47. Le Magueresse, B., C. Pineau, F. Guillou & B. Jégou. 1988. Influence of germ cells upon transferrin secretion by rat Sertoli cells *in vitro.* J. Endocrinol. **118:** R13-R16.
48. Ziparo, E., R. Geremia, M. A. Russo & M. Stefanini. 1980. Surface interactions *in vitro* between Sertoli cells and germ cells at different stages of spermatogenesis. Am. J. Anat. **159:** 385–388.
49. Cameron, D. F. & K. E. Muffly. 1991. Hormonal stimulation of spermatid binding to Sertoli cells *in vitro. In* Proceedings of the 11th North American Testis Workshop, The Male Germ Cell: Spermatogonium to Fertilization, Montréal. Abstract **35:** 60.
50. Enders, G. C. & C. F. Millette. 1988. Pachytene spermatocyte and round spermatid binding to Sertoli cells *in vitro.* J. Cell. Sci. **90:** 105–114.
51. Byers, S. W., B. Jégou & O. W. Blaschuk. 1991. Localization of cadherins in the testis by conventional and confocal microscopy. Proceedings of the 11th North American Testis Workshop, The Male Germ Cell: Spermatogonium to Fertilization, Montréal. Abstract **39:** 64.
52. Cyr, D. G., B. Robaire & O. W. Blaschuk. 1991. Development pattern of steady-state mRNA for placental and neural cadherin in the rat testis. Proceedings of the 16th Annual Meeting of The American Society of Andrology. J. Androl. January/February (Suppl.) **A2:** 25.
53. Takeichi, M. 1990. Cadherins: A molecular family important in selective cell-cell adhesion. Ann. Rev. Biochem. **59:** 237–252.
54. Hecht, N. B. 1988. Haploid gene expression and the regulation of post-meiotic structural genes. *In* Development and Function of the Reproductive Organs. M. Parvinen, I. Huhtaniemi & L. J. Pelliniemi, Eds. Vol. **14:** 325–334. Serono Symposia Review, Ares Serono Symposia. Rome, Italy.
55. Pineau, C., B. Le Magueresse, J. L. Courtens & B. Jégou. 1991. Study *in vitro* of the phagocytic function of Sertoli cells in the rat. Cell Tissue Res. **264:** 589–598.
56. Bissel, M. J. & M. H. Barcellos-Hoff. 1987. The influence of extracellular matrix on gene expression: Is structure the message? J. Cell. Sci. (Suppl. 8): 327–343.
57. Dym, M., S. Lamsam-Casalotti, M. C. Jia, H. K. Kleinman & V. Papadopoulos. 1991. Basement membrane increases G-protein levels and follicle-stimulating hormone responsiveness of Sertoli cell adenyl cyclase activity. Endocrinology **128:** 1167–1176.
58. Von Ebner, H. 1888. Zur Spermatogenese bein den Säugetieren. Arch. Mikrosk. Anat. Entwicklungsmech. **31:** 236–247.
59. Fawcett, D. W. 1975. Ultrastructure and function of the Sertoli cell. *In* Handbook of Physiology, Section 7, Endocrinology. Male Reproductive System. D. W. Hamilton & R. O. Greep, Eds. Vol. **5:** 21–55. Williams and Wilkins. Baltimore.
60. Roosen-Runge, E. C. 1962. The process of spermatogenesis in mammals. Biol. Rev. **37:** 343–377.
61. Lacy, D. 1960. Light and electron microscopy and its use in the study of factors influencing spermatogenesis in the rat. J. R. Microsc. Soc. **79:** 209–225.
62. Daoust, R. & Y. Clermont. 1955. Distribution of nucleic acids in germ cells during the cycle of the seminiferous epithelium in the rat. Am. J. Anat. **96:** 255–279.
63. Lacy, D. 1962. Certain aspects of testis structure and function. Br. Med. Bull. **18:** 205–208.
64. Firlitt, C. F. & J. R. Davis. 1965. Morphogenesis of the residual body of the mouse testis. Quart. J. Micr. Sci. **106:** 93–98.
65. Monesi, V. 1964. Ribonucleic acid synthesis during mitosis and meïosis in the mouse testis. J. Cell. Biol. **22:** 521–532.
66. Monesi, V. 1965. Synthetic activities during spermatogenesis in the mouse. Exp. Cell. Res. **39:** 197–224.
67. Gérard, N., V. Syed, W. Bardin, N. Genetet & B. Jégou. 1991. Sertoli cells are the site of IL-1 α synthesis in rat testis. Submitted.
68. Dinarello, C. A. 1988. Biology of interleukin 1. FASEB J. **2:** 108–115.

69. PÖLLANEN, P., O. SÖDER & M. PARVINEN. 1989. Interleukin-1 α stimulation of spermatogonial proliferation *in vivo.* Reprod. Fertil. Dev. **1:** 85–87.
70. SÖDER, O., V. SYED, G. V. CALLARD, J. TOPPARI, P. PÖLLANEN, M. PARVINEN, B. FRÖYSA & E. M. RITZÉN. 1991. Production and secretion of an interleukin-1-like factor. Int. J. Androl. **14:** 223–231.
71. PARVINEN, M., O. SÖDER & E. M. RITZÉN. 1991. Interleukin-1 α regulates DNA synthesis during spermatogenesis. Proceedings of the 11th North American Testis Workshop, The Male Germ Cell: Spermatogonium to Fertilization, Montréal. Abstract **9:**34.

Cell-Cell Interactions and the Regulation of Testis Function

MICHAEL K. SKINNER,[a] JOHN N. NORTON,
BRIAN P. MULLANEY, MARINELLA ROSSELLI,
PATRICIA D. WHALEY, AND
CATHERINE T. ANTHONY

Department of Pharmacology
Vanderbilt University School of Medicine
Nashville, Tennessee 37232–6600
and
Reproductive Endocrinology Center
University of California, School of Medicine
San Francisco, California 94143-0556

INTRODUCTION

The testis is an endocrine-responsive tissue that requires a number of important cell-cell interactions for the maintenance and control of cellular growth and differentiation. The Sertoli cells form the seminiferous tubules and provide the cytoarchitectural support and microenvironment required for the developing spermatogenic cells. Peritubular myoid cells surround the tubule and are separated from the basal surface of the Sertoli cells by a complex extracellular matrix. In the interstitium of the testis are numerous cell types including the Leydig cells that are responsible for the production of androgens. Previous investigation of testicular cell-cell interactions have primarily utilized Leydig, peritubular, Sertoli, and germinal cells. Other cell types such as the lymphatic endothelium, testicular macrophages, lymphocytes, and stromal cells will likely be involved in local cell-cell interactions, but these require further elucidation. Interactions between Leydig, peritubular, Sertoli, and germinal cells will be the focus of the current review.

The types of interactions that occur between cells are numerous and have previously been categorized into environmental, nutritional and regulatory interactions.[1] Structural interactions mediated by extracellular matrix components or cell adhesion molecules are examples of an environmental interaction. The delivery of an essential metabolite or nutritional substance between cells is an example of a nutritional interaction. The production and subsequent action of a paracrine or autocrine agent to elicit a signal transduction event to influence cellular functions on a molecular level is an example of a regulatory interaction. Although environmental and nutritional interactions are critical for normal cellular physiology, regulatory interactions are needed to alter and maintain cellular function and differentiation. The current review will

[a] Address correspondence to Dr. Skinner at the University of California; Tel.: (415)476-4295.

focus on regulatory interactions and the specific factors involved. The interactions reviewed will also be discussed in reference to the endocrine regulation of testis function.

SPECIFIC INTERACTIONS

Sertoli Cell–Germinal Cell Interactions

In 1865, Enrico Sertoli described specialized branched cells within the tubules which were later determined to be essential for both germinal cell development and spermatogenesis.[2] Sertoli cells are columnar epithelial cells which extend from the basal to apical surface of the seminiferous tubule.[3] Germinal cells at all stages of development require the physical support provided by the Sertoli cells and these environmental interactions between Sertoli cells and germinal cells are essential for testis function. Tight junctions are formed between Sertoli cells to prevent the passage of macromolecules from the interstitial space into the lumen of the tubule. Sertoli cells, therefore, provide energy metabolites, such as lactate and pyruvate, to support germinal cell metabolism[4] and binding proteins such as transferrin and ceruloplasmin to transport iron and copper to germinal cells.[5,6] Although these environmental and nutritional interactions are essential for the maintenance of spermatogenesis, regulatory interactions are required to control cell function on a molecular level.

Investigation of the potential presence of regulatory interactions directed at germinal cells initially utilized co-culture experiments. The presence of Sertoli cells has been shown to increase germinal cell RNA and DNA synthesis, induce the appearance of germinal cell surface antigens and maintain spermatogenic cell glutathione synthesis.[7–9] Consideration of potential regulatory agents that act on germinal cells have focused on several growth factors produced by the Sertoli cell. Insulin-like growth factor-I (IGF-I) is a somewhat ubiquitous factor that is produced by Sertoli cells.[10] IGF-I receptors have been localized on spermatogenic cells, indicating that IGF-I may act on these cells.[11] The epidermal growth factor-like substance transforming growth factor-alpha (TGF-α) is also produced by Sertoli cells. Germinal cells do not appear to express the EGF receptor; therefore, the paracrine function of TGF-α is unclear.[12] The growth inhibitor transforming growth factor-beta (TGF-β) is also produced by Sertoli cells; however, the actions of TGF-β on germinal cells remain to be elucidated.[13] Another apparent Sertoli cell product is interleukin-1 (IL-1), a cytokine which may stimulate germinal cell growth.[14] Although a number of potential paracrine factors are produced by Sertoli cells (TABLE 1), the direct actions of these factors on germinal cells remain to be established.

Investigation of regulatory interactions directed at Sertoli cells have also utilized co-culture of germinal and Sertoli cells. Spermatogenic cells, particularly pachytene spermatocytes and early stage round spermatids, can influence Sertoli cell function. Germinal cell conditioned medium has been shown to stimulate phosphorylation of specific proteins and gamma-glutamyl transpeptidase activity in Sertoli cells.[15,16] Conditioned medium also can increase ABP production, increase transferrin gene expression and production, decrease estradiol synthesis, and decrease RNA synthesis.[7,17–19] Preliminary characterization of the active components in germinal cell conditioned medium has determined that the activity is heat and trypsin sensitive.[17] Partial purification of the activity has demonstrated that a fraction containing three polypeptides between 10 and 30 kDa has the ability to influence Sertoli cells.[19] Further pur-

TABLE 1. Potential Regulatory Agents Involved in Testicular Cell–Cell Interactions[a]

Potential Paracrine Factor	Proposed Site Production	Proposed Site Action	Proposed Actions/Function	Site Synthesis	Secretions	Characterization	Actions	Physiology
Sertoli Cell–Germinal Cell Interactions								
IGF-1	Sertoli	Germinal	? Growth/Metabolism	X	X	X		
TGF-β	Sertoli	Germinal	? Growth/Differentiation	X	X	X		
IL-1	Sertoli	Germinal	? Growth	X	X			
IGF-2	Sertoli	Germinal	? Metabolism/Growth			X		
SGF/SCSGF	Sertoli	GC/SC	? Growth	X	X			
NGF	Germinal	Sertoli	? Growth	X				
Peritubular Cell–Sertoli Cell Interactions								
PModS	Peritubular	Sertoli	Differentiation	X	X		X	
TGF-α	PC/SC	PC/?SC	Growth	X	X	X	X	
TGF-β	PC/SC	PC/SC	Growth/Differentiation	X	X	X	X	
Sertoli Cell–Leydig Cell								
Androgen	Leydig	Sertoli	Differentiation	X	X	X	X	X
POMC Peptides β-END, MSH, ACTH	Leydig	Sertoli	Alter FSH Action	X	X	X	X	
Stimulatory Factor (?)	Sertoli	Leydig	Steroidogenesis	X	X		X	
Inhibitory Factor (?)	Sertoli	Leydig	Steroidogenesis	X	X		X	
LHRH-like Factor	Sertoli	Leydig	Steroidogenesis	X	X		X	
IL-1	Sertoli	Leydig	Steroidogenesis	X	X		X	
Estrogen	SC/LC	Leydig	Steroidogenesis	X	X	X		
TGF-α	SC/?LC	LC/SC	Growth/Steroidogenesis	X	X	X	X	
TGF-β	SC/?LC	LC/SC	Growth/Steroidogenesis	X	X	X	X	
Inhibin	SC/LC	LC/?SC	Steroidogenesis	X	X	X		
Leydig Cell–Peritubular Cell								
Androgen	Leydig	Peritubular	Differentiation	X	X	X	X	X

[a] Potential paracrine factors in the testis with their proposed site of production and action designated, as well as proposed action/function. (?) denotes a postulated cell type or function with negligible data currently available. The inset box designates with an (X) experimental investigation of the site of synthesis, cellular secretion, biochemical characterization, action(s) and physiological relevance for the various paracrine factors with an open box indicating the lack of available information or experimental analysis.

ification and characterization of the active components is needed to identify or define the unique properties of the paracrine factor(s) and to determine if these factors are actively secreted by the germinal cells or are released as a consequence of poor cell viability and cell lysis. A growth factor that may potentially be involved in germinal cell–Sertoli cell interactions is nerve growth factor (NGF). NGF immunoreactivity and β-NGF gene expression have been observed in spermatocytes and early spermatids.[20] NGF receptor gene expression has been identified in Sertoli cells under androgen regulation.[21] Although this indicates that NGF may be a paracrine factor for these cells, further investigation is necessary to identify its exact function.

The potential paracrine control of Sertoli and spermatogenic cell function (TABLE 1) can be influenced by the endocrine system. Follicle-stimulating hormone acts through receptors on the Sertoli cell to effect cellular differentiation and function. Therefore, FSH may indirectly effect germinal cell development by altering the interactions between the Sertoli and germinal cell populations.[22]

Peritubular Cell–Sertoli Cell Interactions

The mesenchymal (*i.e.*, stromal)-derived peritubular-myoid cells contribute to the exterior wall of the seminiferous tubule and are separated from the epithelial-like Sertoli cells by an extracellular matrix. While peritubular cells are important in maintaining the structural integrity of the seminiferous tubule, they also appear to produce paracrine factors that may be important in regulatory interactions in the tubule. Initial observations with co-cultures of peritubular and Sertoli cells indicated that the presence of peritubular cells can alter Sertoli cell morphology and enhance Sertoli cell function, including the production of transferrin and ABP.[23,24]

Potential regulatory agents that may mediate interactions between Sertoli and peritubular cells include growth factors. Both Sertoli and peritubular cells produce TGF-α and TGF-β.[12,13,24] Functional EGF receptors are expressed on peritubular cells and possibly Sertoli cells.[12,26] TGF-α/EGF can stimulate peritubular cell but not midpubertal Sertoli cell growth.[12] While EGF has been shown to influence Sertoli cell function,[27] little effect is seen in highly purified preparations of Sertoli cells.[12] Further molecular analysis of EGF receptor localization and TGF-α action are necessary to elucidate the local interactions mediated by the TGF-α. TGF-β does not appear to have dramatic effects on Sertoli cell growth or function; however, TGF-β can inhibit TGF-α–induced peritubular cell proliferation. Peritubular cell differentiation may also be induced by TGF-β, as indicated by increased production of specific proteins such as matrix components and antiproteases.[13,28] TGF-β also promotes peritubular cell chemotaxis and colony formation.[13] Therefore, morphogenesis of the seminiferous tubule may be dependent on this factor. Both Sertoli and peritubular cells produce insulin-like growth factor I (IGF-I). IGF-I can stimulate growth of peritubular and immature Sertoli cells and may also stimulate Sertoli cell function, however, high levels of IGF-I are present in the interstitial fluid available to both cell types.

Potential paracrine factors that primarily influence cellular differentiation are also important in mediating peritubular-Sertoli cell interactions. Peritubular cells have been shown to produce a nonmitogenic factor which modulates Sertoli cell function, termed PModS.[29,30] The apparent production of PModS is under androgen control, thus allowing for an indirect mechanism for gonadotropin/androgen action in the testis.[29,30] PModS has been purified into two biologically related forms, PModS(A) and PModS(B), and purified PModS enhances a number of Sertoli cell functions, including transferrin production.[31] PModS can stimulate many Sertoli cell functions to a greater extent than any known regulatory agent, including FSH.[31,32] Interestingly, peritubular cell-Sertoli cell interactions provide an example of a mesenchymal (*i.e.*, stromal)-epithelial cell interaction. PModS may provide an example of a mesenchymal inducer substance that can influence the differentiation of the adjacent epithelial cell. It is postulated that PModS may have an important role in the induction and maintenance of Sertoli cell differentiation. Further molecular characterization of PModS and analysis of *in vivo* actions of PModS is required.

Leydig Cell–Sertoli Cell Interactions

Regulatory interactions between Leydig cells and Sertoli cells were among the first cell-cell interactions investigated in the testis. The identification of androgen production by Leydig cells and the ability of androgens to maintain the process of spermatogenesis prompted considerable research on the actions of androgens on Sertoli cells. Sertoli cells express the androgen receptor gene; however, the effects of androgens on Sertoli cell function *in vitro* are absent or less than those obtained with FSH. Since peritubular cells enhance the actions of androgens on Sertoli cells, highly purified preparations of Sertoli cells should be used to investigate the actions of androgens.[30] The role direct actions of androgen have on Sertoli cells remains to be elucidated.

In addition to androgens, a number of peptides and proteins have been localized to Leydig cells. Several peptides derived from proopiomelanocortin (POMC) appear to be produced by Leydig cells, including beta-endorphin (βEND), alpha-melanocyte stimulating hormone (α-MSH), and adrenocorticotropin (ACTH)[33] and it has been speculated that these are involved in the regulation of Sertoli cell function.[34] Endorphin receptors have been localized on Sertoli cells, and βEND can inhibit the actions of FSH.[34,35] Further work is required to determine the physiological significance of Leydig cell derived peptides and their role in mediating regulatory interactions between Leydig cells and Sertoli cells.

The ability of Sertoli cells or seminiferous tubules to influence Leydig cell function also has been the object of intense investigation. Damage to the seminiferous tubule by cytotoxic agents, vitamin A deficiency, fetal irradiation or cryptorchidism alters Leydig cell morphology. These morphologic studies imply that a regulatory interaction may exist between Sertoli cells and Leydig cells. Observations have been extended with co-culture of the two cell types or co-culture of Leydig cells with specific stages of the seminiferous epithelium. When studies were performed using Sertoli cell–conditioned media both increases[6,37] and decreases[38,39] in Leydig cell steroidogenesis were demonstrated. An interesting study which utilized spent media from seminiferous tubules isolated from both normal and cryptorchid testis revealed that under normal conditions predominately inhibitory activity was present while cryptorchidism induced the appearance of stimulatory activity.[38] The active components apparently secreted by Sertoli cells that influence Leydig cell steroidogenesis remain to be purified and characterized.

Several Sertoli cell secretory products have also been identified that can potentially mediate regulatory interactions between Sertoli cells and Leydig cells (TABLE 1). Estrogen, has an inhibitory influence on Leydig cell steroidogenesis and is produced by Sertoli cells.[40] Leydig cells, however, also produce high levels of estrogen which could act in an autocrine manner on the cell. Inhibin, a peptide hormone produced by Sertoli cells and its related protein, activin, both can influence Leydig cell steroidogenesis.[41,42] Leydig cells, however, have also been shown to produce both inhibin and activin.[43] Several growth factors produced by Sertoli cells that can influence Leydig cells include; IGF-I[44] TGF-α,[45,46] and TGF-β.[47] The potential production of these growth factors by Leydig cells,[48] however, questions the importance of paracrine interactions with these growth factors. Additional regulatory agents apparently produced by Sertoli cells that can influence Leydig cell function include an interleukin-1 type molecule[49] and an LHRH-like substance.[50] The Sertoli cell appears to produce a number of regulatory agents that can influence Leydig cells (TABLE 1) and an investigation of their physiological importance is now required.

The majority of Sertoli cell products that may influence Leydig cell function have been identified through the ability to effect Leydig cell steroidogenesis. Although the production of androgen by Leydig cells and subsequent actions of androgen on the seminiferous tubule is essential for the maintenance of testis function, the physiological requirement to modulate steroidogenesis in the adult must be critically evaluated. The concentration of androgen present in the adult testis is significantly higher than the concentration needed to maintain germinal cell development.[51,52] Although an active regulation of Leydig cell androgen production may be needed during embryonic and pubertal development, local transient alteration in androgen production in the adult may not have major effects on Sertoli cell or germinal cell development. In particular, stimulation of androgen production would not appear to be important for testis function in the adult testis. Factors produced by Leydig cells, other than androgens, however, may need to be actively regulated.

Leydig Cell–Peritubular Cell Interactions

Growth factors are potential paracrine factors that may mediate interactions between Leydig cells and peritubular cells. Leydig cells respond to several growth factors shown to be produced by peritubular cells including IGF-I, TGF-α and TGF-β. Although IGF-I, TGF-α and TGF-β have been shown to be produced by peritubular cells, the production of these growth factors in the interstitium has not been thoroughly assessed; therefore, the significance of growth factor–mediated paracrine interactions is unclear.

The primary regulatory agent produced by Leydig cells that has been shown to influence peritubular cells is androgen. Androgen receptors are present in high numbers in peritubular cells and peritubular cell differentiation appears to be dependent on the presence of androgen.[53] Androgens increase the apparent production of the paracrine factor PModS by peritubular cells which subsequently can influence Sertoli cell function.[29] These potential indirect actions of androgens on the Sertoli cells through peritubular cells are speculated to be important for the control and maintenance of spermatogenesis.[1] The indirect role of androgen action may be that luteinizing hormone influences Leydig cells to produce androgen which stimulates PModS secretion from peritubular cells that then acts to influence Sertoli cell functions vital for the maintenance and control of spermatogenesis. The dramatic effects of PModS on Sertoli cell function and differentiation observed *in vitro* and the lack of major androgen effects on purified Sertoli cell cultures support this postulated interaction. Further investigation of the hormonal regulation of PModS production and the *in vivo* actions of PModS, however, is required. The potential ability of LH to influence this series of cell-cell interactions provides an example of how the endocrine regulation of testis function may be indirectly mediated through local cell-cell interactions.

SUMMARY

Regulatory interactions have been shown to occur between all the testicular cell types considered. The paracrine factors mediating these interactions generally influ-

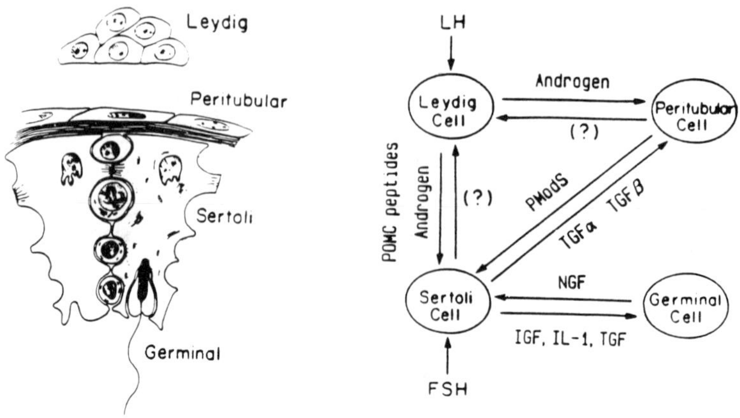

FIGURE 1. Postulated cell-cell interactions in the testis with the appropriate paracrine factors speculated to be involved. Note the potential indirect effects of gonadotropins on various cell types via local cell-cell interactions.

ence either cellular growth or differentiation. The regulation of cellular growth is essential in the developing testis and is required for the maintenance of spermatogenesis in the adult testis. The rapid rate of germinal cell proliferation and the continuous but slowed growth of the peritubular cells and Leydig cells requires the presence of specific growth factors in the adult. Therefore, cell-cell interactions have evolved that involve growth factors such as IGF, TGF-α, TGF-β and NGF (FIG. 1). Other growth factors such as FGF or less characterized components like the seminiferous growth factor (SGF) also may be involved in the paracrine regulation of testis cell growth.[54] An alternate cellular parameter to cell growth to consider is the regulation of cellular function and differentiation. A number of endocrine agents and locally produced paracrine factors have been shown to control and maintain testis cell function and differentiation (FIG. 1). Cell-cell interactions mediated by factors such as androgens, POMC peptides, and PModS are all primarily directed at the regulation of cellular differentiation. Therefore, the agents which mediate cell-cell interactions in the testis can generally be categorized into factors that regulate cell growth or those which influence cellular differentiation. The specific cell-cell interactions identified (FIG. 1) will likely be the first of a large number of cellular interactions yet to be investigated. Although a number of potentially important cell-cell interactions have been identified, future research will require the elucidation of the *in vivo* physiological significance of these interactions.

The existence of different cell types and potential cell-cell interactions in a tissue implies that the actions of an endocrine agent on a tissue will not simply involve a single hormone and single cell. The endocrine regulation of testis function will have effects on cell-cell interactions and be affected by local cell-cell interactions. The ability of LH to influence Leydig cell androgen production promotes a cascade of interactions mediated through several cell types to maintain the process of spermatogenesis. FSH actions on Sertoli cells also promote cell-cell interactions that influence germinal cell development, peritubular myoid cell differentiation and Leydig cell function. Therefore, elucidation of the endocrine regulation of testis function requires an understanding of the local cell-cell interactions in the testis.

REFERENCES

1. SKINNER, M. K. 1987. Cell-cell interactions in the testis. Ann. N.Y. Acad. Sci. **513:** 158–171.
2. SERTOLI, E. 1865. On the existence of special branched cells in the seminiferous tubules of the human testis. Morgagni **7:** 31–39.
3. FAWCETT, D. W. 1975. The ultrastructure and functions of the Sertoli cell. *In* Handbook Physiol, Vol. 5, Section 7. R. Greep & E. Hamilton, Ed. Washington, D.C. 21–55 Am. Physiol. Soc.: 21–55.
4. JUTTE, N. H. P. M., R. JANSEN, J. A. GROOTEGOED, F. F. G. ROMMERTS & H. J. VAN DER MOLEN. 1983. FSH stimulation of the production of pyruvate and lactate by rat Sertoli cells may be involved in hormonal regulation of spermatogenesis. J. Reprod. Fertil. **68:** 219–226.
5. SKINNER, M. K. & M. D. GRISWOLD. 1980. Sertoli cells synthesize and secrete a transferrin-like protein. J. Biol. Chem. **255:** 9523–9525.
6. SKINNER, M. K. & M. D. GRISWOLD. 1983. Sertoli cells synthesize and secrete a ceruloplasmin-like protein. Biol. Reprod. **28:** 1225–1229.
7. RIVAROLA, M. A., P. SANCHEZ & J. M. SAEZ. 1985. Stimulation of ribonucleic acid and deoxyribonucleic acid synthesis in spermatogenic cells by their co-culture with Sertoli cells. Endocrinology **117:** 1796–1802.
8. VAN DER DONK, J. A., A. L. DE RUITER-BOOTSMA, A. M. ULTEE-VAN GESSEL & P. J. WAUBEN-PENRIS. 1986. Cell-cell interaction between rat Sertoli cells and mouse germ cells *in vitro.* Exp. Cell Res. **164:** 191–198.
9. LI, L. Y., A. P. SEDDON, A. MEISTER & M. S. RISLEY. 1989. Spermatogenic cell-somatic cell interactions are required for maintenance of spermatogenic cell glutathione. Biol. Reprod. **40:** 317-331.
10. SMITH, E. P., M. E. SVOBODA, J. J. VAN WYK, A. L. KIERSZENBAUM & L. L. TRES. 1987. Partial characterization of a somatomedin-like peptide from the medium of cultured rat Sertoli cells. Endocrinology **120:** 186–193.
11. VANNELLI, B. G., T. BARNI, C. ORLANDO, A. NATALI, M. SERIO & G. G. BALBONI. 1988. Insulin-like growth factor-I (IGF-I) and IGF-I receptor in human testis: An immunohistochemical study. Fertil. Steril. **49:** 666–669.
12. SKINNER, M. K., K. TAKACS & R. J. COFFEY. 1989. Cellular localization of transforming growth factor-alpha gene expression and action in the seminiferous tubule: Peritubular cell-Sertoli cell interactions. Endocrinology **124:** 845–854.
13. SKINNER, M. K. & H. L. MOSES. 1989. Transforming growth factor-beta gene expression and action in the seminiferous tubule: peritubular cell-Sertoli cell interactions. Mol. Endocrinol. **3:** 625–634.
14. POLLANEN, P., O. SODER & M. PARVINEN. 1989. Interleukin-1 alpha stimulation of spermatogonial proliferation *in vivo* Reprod. Fertil. Dev. **1**(1): 85–87.
15. IRELAND, M. E. & M. J. WELSH. 1987. Germ cell stimulation of Sertoli cell protein phosphorylation. Endocrinology **120:** 1317–1326.
16. SCHTEINGART, H. F., M. A. RIVAROLA & S. B. CIGORRAGA. 1989. Hormonal and paracrine regulation of gamma-glutamyl transpeptidase in rat Sertoli cells. Mol. Cell. Endocrinol. **67:** 73–80.
17. LE MAGUERESSE, B., C. PINEAU, F. GUILLOU & B. JEGOU. 1988. Influence of germ cells upon transferrin secretion by rat Sertoli cells *in vitro.* J. Endocrinol. **118:** R13-R16.
18. DJAKIEW, D. & M. DYM. 1988. Pachytene spermatocyte proteins influence Sertoli Cell function. Biol. Reprod. **39:** 1193–1205.
19. STALLARD, B. J. & M. D. GRISWOLD. 1990. Germ cell regulation of Sertoli cell transferrin mRNA levels. Mol. Endocrinol. **4:** 393–401.
20. AYER-LELIEVRE, C., L. OLSON, T. EBENDAL, F. HALLBÖÖK & H. PERSSON. 1988. Nerve growth factor mRNA and protein in the testis and epididymis of mouse and rat. Proc. Natl. Acad. Sci. USA **85:** 2628–2632.
21. PERSSON, H., C. AYER-LELIEVRE, O. SODER, M. J. VILLAR, M. METSIS, L. OLSON, M. RITZEN

& T. Hokfelt. 1990. Expression of beta-nerve growth factor receptor mRNA in Sertoli cells downregulated by testosterone. Science **247:** 704–707.
22. Fritz, I. B. 1978. Sites of action of androgens and follicle stimulating hormone on cells of the seminiferous tubule. *In* Biochemical Actions of Hormones. G. Litwack, Ed. Acad. Press. New York. Vol. V: 249–281.
23. Tung, P. S. & I. B. Fritz. 1980. Interactions of Sertoli cells with myoid cells *in vitro*. Biol. Reprod. **23:** 207–217.
24. Hutson, J. C. & D. M. Stocco. 1981. Peritubular cell influence on the efficiency of androgen-binding protein secretion by Sertoli cells in culture. Endocrinology **108:** 1362–1368.
25. Benahmed, M., G. Esposito, T. C. Sordoille, E. dePeretti, M. A. Chauvin, C. Ghiglieri, A. Revol & A. M. Morera. 1989. Transforming growth factor β and its related peptides in the testis: An intragonadal polypeptide control system. Persp. Androl. **53:** 191–201.
26. Suarez-Quian, C. A., M. Dai, M. Onoda, R. M. Kriss & M. Dym. 1989. Epidermal growth factor receptor localization in the rat and monkey testes. Biol. Reprod. **41:** 921–932.
27. Morris, P. L., W. W. Vale, S. Cappel & C. W. Bardin. 1988. Inhibin production by primary Sertoli cell-enriched cultures: Regulation by follicle-stimulating hormone, androgens, and epidermal growth factor. Endocrinology **122:** 717–725.
28. Nargolwalla, C., D. McCabe & I. B. Fritz. 1990. Modulation of levels of messenger RNA for tissue-type plasminogen activator in rat Sertoli cells, and levels of messenger RNA for plasminogen activator inhibitor in testis peritubular cells. Mol. Cell. Endocrinol. **70:** 73–80.
29. Skinner, M. K. & I. B. Fritz. 1985. Testicular cells secrete a protein under androgen control that modulates Sertoli cell function. Proc. Natl. Acad. Sci. USA **82:** 114–118.
30. Skinner, M. K. & I. B. Fritz. 1985. Androgen stimulation of Sertoli cell function is enhanced by peritubular cells. Mol. Cell. Endocrinol. **40:** 115–122.
31. Skinner, M. K., P. M. Fetterolf & C. T. Anthony. 1988. Purification of a paracrine factor, PModS, produced by testicular peritubular cells that modulates Sertoli cell function. J. Biol. Chem. **263:** 2884–2890.
32. Norton, J. N. & M. K. Skinner. 1989. Regulation of Sertoli cell function and differentiation through the actions of a testicular paracrine factor PModS. Endocrinology. **124:** 2711–2719.
33. Margioris, A. N., A. Liotta, H. Vaudry, C. W. Bardin & D. T. Krieger. 1983. Characterization of immunoreactive proopiomelanocortin-related peptides in rat testis. Endocrinology **113:** 663–671.
34. Fabbri, A., G. Knox, E. Buczko & M. L. Dufau. 1988. Beta-endorphin production by the fetal Leydig cell: Regulation and implications for paracrine control of Sertoli cell function. Endocrinology **122:** 749–755.
35. Orth, J. M. 1986. FSH-induced Sertoli cell proliferation in the developing rat is modified by β-endorphin produced in the testis. Endocrinology **119:** 1876–1878.
36. Benahmed, M., C. Grenot, E. Tabone, P. Sanchez & A. M. Morera. 1985. FSH regulates cultured Leydig cell function via Sertoli cell proteins: An in vitro study. Biochem. Biophys. Res. Commun. **132:** 729–734.
37. Janecki, A., A. Jakubowiak & A. Lukaszyk. 1985. Stimulatory effect of Sertoli cell secretory products on testosterone secretion by purified Leydig cells in primary culture. Mol. Cell. Endocrinol. 1985: **42:** 235–243.
38. Syed, V., S. A. Khan & E. M. Ritzen. 1985. Stage-specific inhibition of interstitial cell testosterone secretion by rat seminiferous tubules in vitro. Mol. Cell. Endocrinol. **40:** 257–264.
39. Benahmed, M., A. M. Morera & M. A. Chauvin. 1986. Evidence for a Sertoli cell, FSH-suppressible inhibiting factor(s) of testicular steroidogenic activity. Biochem. Biophys. Res. Commun. **139:** 169–178.
40. Dorrington, J. H., I. B. Fritz & D. T. Armstrong. 1978. Control of testicular estrogen synthesis. Biol. Reprod. **18:** 55–64.
41. Hsueh, A. J., K. D. Dahl, J. Vaughan, E. Tucker, J. Rivier, C. W. Bardin & W. Vale. 1987. Heterodimers and homodimers of inhibin subunits have different paracrine action in the modulation of luteinizing hormone-stimulated androgen biosynthesis. Proc. Natl. Acad. Sci. USA **84:** 5082–5086.
42. Lin, T., J. K. Calkins, P. L. Morris, W. Vale & C. W. Bardin. 1989. Regulation of Leydig cell function in primary culture by inhibin and activin. Endocrinology **125:** 2134–2140.
43. Risbridger, G. P., J. Clements, D. M. Robertson, A. E. Drummond, J. Muir, H. G. Berger

& D. M. de Kretser. 1989. Immuno- and bioactive inhibin and inhibin alpha-subunit expression in rat Leydig cell cultures. Mol. Cell. Endocrinol. **66:** 119–122.

44. Handelsman, D. J., J. A. Spaliviero, C. D. Scott & R. C. Baxter. 1985. Identification of insulin-like growth factor-I and its receptors ind the rat testis. Acta Endocrinol. (Copenhagen) **109:** 543–549.

45. Ascoli, M. 1981. Regulation of gonadotropin receptors and gonadotropin responses in a clonal strain of Leydig tumor cells by epidermal growth factor. J. Biol. Chem. **256:** 179–183.

46. Welsh, T. H., Jr. & A. J. W. Hsueh. 1982. Mechanism of the inhibitory action of epidermal growth factor on testicular androgen biosynthesis in vitro. Endocrinology **110:** 1498–1506.

47. Avallet, O., M. Vigier, M. H. Perrard-Sapori & J. M. Saez. Transforming growth factor β inhibits Leydig cell functions. Biochem. Biophys. Res. Commun. **146:** 575–581.

48. Teerds, K. J., F. F. Rommerts & J. H. Dorrington. 1990. Immunohistochemical detection of transforming growth factor-alpha in Leydig cells during the development of rat testis. Mol. Cell. Endocrinol. **69:** R1–R6.

49. Calkins, J. H., H. Guo, M. M. Sigel & T. Lin. 1990. Differential effects of recombinant interleukin-1α and β on Leydig cell function. Biochem. Biophys. Res. Commun. **167:** 548–553.

50. Sharpe, R. M., Fraser, H. M., I. Cooper & F. F. Rommerts. 1981. Sertoli-Leydig cell communication via an LHRH-like factor. Nature **290:** 785–787.

51. Sun, Y-T., D. C. Irby, D. M. Robertson & D. de Kretser. 1989. The effects of exogenously administered testosterone on spermatogenesis in intact and hypophysectomized rats. Endocrinology **25:** 1000–1010.

52. Santulli, R., R. L. Sprando, C. A. Awoniyi, L. L. Ewing & B. R. Zirkin. 1990. To what extent can spermatogenesis be maintained in the hypophysectomized adult rat testis with exogenously administered testosterone? Endocrinology **126:** 95–102.

53. Hovatta, O. 1972. Effect of androgens and antiandrogens on the development of the myoid cells of the rat seminiferous tubules (organ culture). Z. Zellforsch. **131:** 299–308.

54. Bellve, A. R. & W. Zheng. 1989. Growth factors as autocrine and paracrine modulators of male gonadal functions. J. Reprod. Fertil. **85:** 771–793.

Spermatozoa Are Exposed to a Complex Microenvironment as They Traverse the Epididymis[a]

T. T. TURNER

Departments of Urology and Anatomy and Cell Biology
University of Virginia School of Medicine
Charlottesville, Virginia 22908

INTRODUCTION

Spermatozoa arriving in the caput epididymidis from the testis have little to no capacity for progressive motility or fertility; however, by the time the sperm reach the cauda epididymidis they have matured and acquired the capacity for both motility and fertility.[1,2] It is generally accepted that the specialized microenvironment provided within the epididymal lumen is important for these developments. There is current debate about the ability of the obstructed epididymis to allow sperm maturation with minimal epididymal transient,[2] but this debate is tangential to consideration of the normal microenvironment to which sperm are exposed within the unobstructed epididymis. It is this latter topic to which this report is addressed.

CHARACTERISTICS OF EPIDIDYMAL INTRALUMINAL FLUIDS

The epididymal microenvironment is in reality a series of microenvironments. The inorganic and organic constituents of the epididymal lumen fluid change as the epididymal lumen content (sperm + fluid) progresses along the epididymal tubule, and since the exposure of the sperm to this ever-changing milieu is important to sperm maturation, scientists have been interested in characterizing the fluids in the various regions of the mammalian epididymis and in understanding the epididymal epithelial functions which construct the intraluminal microenvironment.

Prior to the advent of *in vivo* micropuncture techniques, the work of several investigators had progressed using post-mortem epididymidal tissues and surface collection of fluids expressed from tubules after needle-stick or incision. Important early studies by Crabo,[3] for example, demonstrated that sperm concentrations in fluids collected in this manner generally increased from proximal to distal epididymis while Na^+ and Cl^- concentrations generally decreased. At least one organic secretory product of the epididymal epithelium, glycerylphosphorylcholine (GPC), also increased in concentration from proximal to distal epididymis.[3]

The problems associated with the use of excised tissues and with the lack of ability

[a] This work supported by NIH grants HD 09490 and HD 18252.

to collect uncontaminated fluids from specific compartments of the epididymis were first overcome by Levine and Marsh.[4] These investigators used *in vivo* micropuncture of rat epididymal tubules to examine electrolyte transport, osmolality, and spermatocrit in intraluminal fluids collected from the caput, corpus, and cauda epididymidis of the rat. That study demonstrated that in the *in vivo* epididymis intraluminal Na^+ concentrations and Cl^- concentrations decreased and K^+ and pH increased as the fluid moved from caput to cauda epididymidis. The reabsorption of Na^+ and Cl^- was shown to be against an electrochemical gradient and it became clear that the epididymal epithelium was an active agent in the production of a ". . . series of progressive concentration changes which begin in the head and reach their full extent somewhere near the tail or vas deferens itself."[4] *In vivo* micropuncture techniques were soon being used in other laboratories[5-7] and it became clear that both the inorganic and organic constituents of fluids collected from the epididymal lumen were variably subject to secretion and reabsorption by the epididymal epithelium. The rat has been the most common species studied.

Intraluminal sperm concentrations increase from proximal to distal epididymis (FIG. 1A), though the pattern of increase may differ from species to species.[3] Sperm concentrations increase because of fluid reabsorption, a phenomenon especially active in the initial segment (FIG. 1B). Approximately 90% of the fluid leaving the rete testis is reabsorbed by the time the intraluminal content reaches the rat caput epididymidis.[8] Sixty-two percent of the fluid remaining in the caput is reabsorbed by the time the luminal content reaches the distal cauda epididymidis; thus sperm concentrations increase through the length of the epididymal duct. Fluid reabsorption is primarily driven by Na^+ and Cl^- reabsorption, *i.e.*, active antiluminal transport by the epididymal epithelium,[4,9] and this reabsorption has implications beyond causing the increase in intraluminal sperm concentrations.

FIGURES 2 and 3 illustrate intraluminal concentrations of selected inorganic and organic constituents, respectively, in the rat epididymis. A rise in the concentration of a selected constituent between two sites along the duct (*e.g.*, FIG. 2 K; FIG. 3B, ABP) does not imply that the constituent is secreted into the lumen between these two points. Rather, the effect of fluid reabsorption on the concentration of intraluminal substance must be considered to determine whether secretion or reabsorption has occurred.

The formulae below allow for such consideration and allow one to calculate the amount of substance secreted or absorbed between proximal and distal epididymal zones.

$$\widehat{\mathrm{Conc_D}} = \mathrm{Conc_P} \times \frac{\mathrm{SC_D}}{\mathrm{SC_P}} \tag{1}$$

Where $\widehat{\mathrm{Conc_D}}$ = predicted mean value for the concentration of a substance in a distal zone given a known concentration in a proximal zone; $\mathrm{SC_D}$ = sperm concentration in any distal zone; $\mathrm{SC_P}$ = mean sperm concentration in any proximal zone; and $\mathrm{Conc_P}$ = concentration of substance in proximal zone.

$$\Delta_{\mathrm{Conc}} = \mathrm{Conc_D} - \widehat{\mathrm{Conc_D}} \tag{2}$$

Where $\mathrm{Conc_D}$ = mean concentration of any substance in a distal zone; $\widehat{\mathrm{Conc_D}}$ = predicted mean concentration of the substance in the distal zone; and Δ_{Conc} = the difference between the predicted value and the value actually found upon analysis, thereby indicating a net secretion (+) or reabsorption (−) of the substance per amount of distal zone fluid volumes.[8]

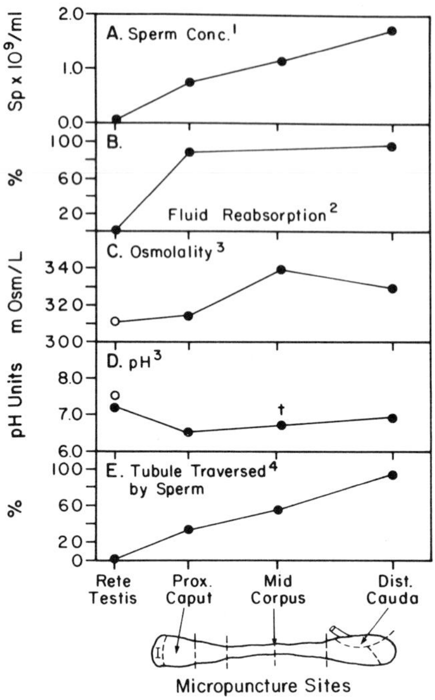

FIGURE 1. Features of tubule fluid in the proximal through distal rat epididymis. Values for caput, corpus, and cauda epididymidal fluid are indicated, but where possible, values used are from the proximal caput, mid-corpus, and distal cauda epididymidis. Rete testis values are included to reflect changes that occur in the efferent ducts and initial segment (I). Open circles (○) indicate serum values. **A:** Sperm concentration in the lumen of the excurrent ducts. **B:** Fluid reabsorption as a percentage of the fluid leaving the rete testis. **C:** Osmolality of serum and intraluminal fluids. Note the hypertonicity of epididymal fluids. **D:** pH of intraluminal fluids. Note that the fluids become acidic after leaving the testis. **E:** The percentage of pre-vas excurrent tubule traversed by intraluminal spermatozoa at each point reported. Superscripts 1–4 indicate source of information. ([1] Turner & Cesarini. 1983. J. Androl. **4:** 197; [2] Turner. 1984. J. Reprod. Fertil. **72:** 509; [3] Levine & Marsh. 1971. J. Physiol. **213:** 557; [4] Turner *et al.* 1990. J. Androl. **11:** 422.) † Data point from B. T. Hinton (personal communication). The schematic outline of the rat epididymis illustrates typical micropuncture points to obtain fluids for study from the proximal caput, mid-corpus, and distal cauda epididymidis of the rat. Dotted lines on schematic of rat epididymis indicate approximate demarcation of typical micropuncture zones 1–8.

By using these simple calculations, one can determine, for example, that while sodium concentration decreases and potassium increases in intraluminal content from proximal-to-distal epididymis, they both undergo net reabsorption by the initial segment and epididymal epithelium.[8] Similarly, while GPC, inositol, and carnitine all increase in concentration along the epididymal duct (FIG. 3A), GPC and inositol experience net reabsorption between caput and cauda epididymidis, while carnitine is secreted between those same regions.[8,10,11]

Intraluminal total protein concentrations remain relatively constant between caput and cauda epididymidis (FIG. 3C), being approximately one-third of the protein concentration found in serum. Calculations using the above formulae indicate a net protein reabsorption along the epididymal duct,[8] but it is also clear from electrophoretic studies of intraluminal protein that individual proteins are both secreted into and reabsorbed from the epididymal lumen fluid.[12,13] The changing intraluminal protein microenvironment is thought to be important to the development of maturing spermatozoa because: 1) these proteins variably associate and disassociate from sperm cell membranes during epididymal transit,[14-16] 2) interference with normal epididymal protein secretion decreases sperm fertility,[17,18] and 3) sperm-egg binding is increased by exposure of pre-epididymal sperm to proteins extracted from the epididymal tubules.[19] It also is possible that some intraluminal proteins are important not because of their direct effect on spermatozoa, but because of their effects on the epididymal epithelium.

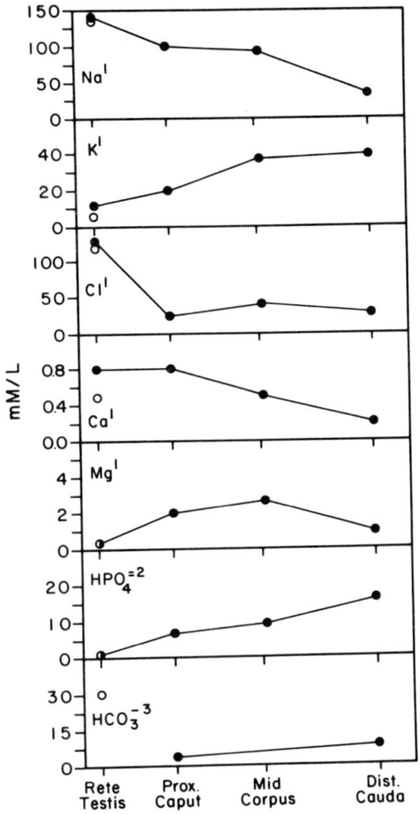

FIGURE 2. Selected inorganic constituents of the rete testis and epididymal luminal fluids of the rat. See FIGURE 1 for notes on site selection. Open circles (○) indicate serum values. Superscripts 1–3 indicate source of information. ([1] Jenkins *et al.* 1980. Biol. Reprod. **23:** 981; [2] Hinton & Setchell. 1980. J. Reprod. Fertil. **58:** 401; [3] Levine & Marsh. 1971. J. Physiol. **213:** 557.)

Specific proteins have been detected in the epididymal lumen of several species and are secreted by the epididymal epithelium; among them are Clusterin (SGP-2), immobilin, acrosomal stabilizing factor, α-lactalbumin-like protein, and several enzymes important in carbohydrate, steroid, and protein biochemistry. While space does not allow full review of these works, they are mentioned to emphasize the complexity of the protein microenvironment in the epididymal lumen.

There is evidence from several laboratories recently reviewed elsewhere,[2,20] that human epididymides secrete region-specific proteins, that these proteins bind to spermatozoa, and sperm from the more distal regions of the unobstructed human epididymis have an increased capacity for sperm-egg binding and fertility.

Intraluminal proteins in the cauda epididymidis also appear to be important in sperm storage, at least in some species. A proteinaceous sperm motility inhibiting factor was found in the rat cauda epididymidis,[21] isolated and termed immobilin,[22] and found to immobilize sperm by its high viscoelastic property.[22,23] Nevertheless, some species do not use a highly viscoelastic cauda lumen fluid to suppress cauda sperm motility.[24] Human sperm are essentially immotile in the cauda epididymidis, yet the fluid there is not highly viscous.[24] It is possible that human sperm, like bull sperm, are

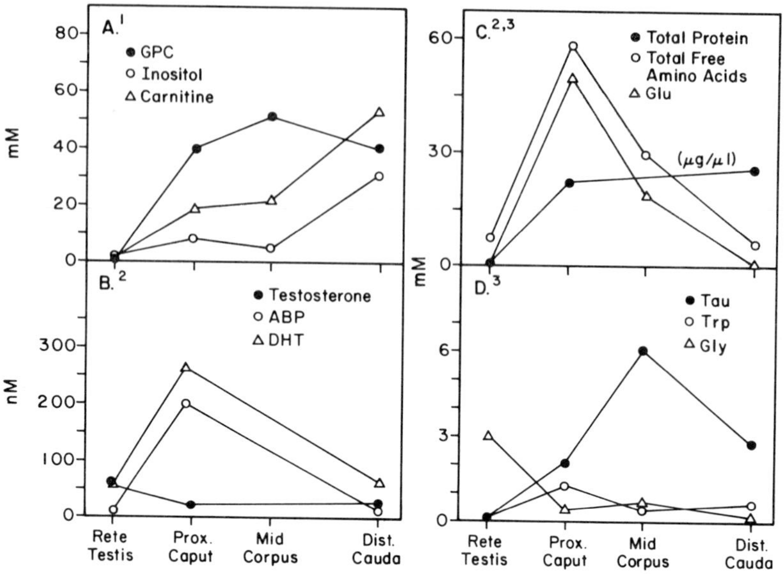

FIGURE 3. Selected organic constituents of rete testis fluid and luminal fluids of the rat epididymis. See FIGURE 1 for notes on micropuncture site selection. **A:** Three small organic molecules appearing in the epididymal lumen. **B:** Two androgens and androgen-binding proteins (ABP). **C:** Total protein, total free amino acids, and glutamate (GLU), the major intraluminal free amino acid. **D:** Three other intraluminal amino acids which appear in high concentrations in lumen fluid relative to 14 other amino acids. Note that different amino acids show different patterns of appearance. Superscripts 1–3 indicate source of information. ([1] Hinton. 1980. Invest. Urol. **18:** 1; [2] Turner *et al.* 1984. Endocrinology **115:** 1925; [3] Hinton. 1990. J. Androl. **11:** 498.)

quiescent in the cauda epididymidis owing to the proposed interaction of a quiescence factor in the cauda lumen fluid and the maintenance of an acidic intracellular pH in the spermatozoan.[25]

Free amino acids make up 20% of the intraluminal osmolytes and are concentrated most highly in the caput lumen.[26] Glutamate appears in the highest concentration (FIG. 3C), but others appear in mM concentrations as well (FIG. 3D).[26] The roles of these specific amino acids in their specific patterns of appearance are unknown.

FLUID MOVEMENT THROUGH THE EPIDIDYMIS

The fluid movement rate through an actively secreting or absorbing tubule can have a profound effect on the constitution of the intraluminal fluid. In the epididymis, conditions which significantly alter fluid flow rate could also have a significant effect on the epididymal microenvironment to which maturing sperm are exposed. Fluid movement rates for oil droplets spanning the epididymal lumen diameter were recently determined in the rat.[27] Fluid flow rates declined from proximal to distal epididymis (TABLE 1), consistent with the progressive reabsorption of lumen fluid along the duct. The proportionate length of each epididymal zone was determined by micro-

TABLE 1. Oil Droplet Movement in the Lumen of the Rat Epididymis

Region	Zone	Net Movement (mm/h)	Max:Min[b] (mm/h)
Proximal caput	2	18.5 ± 3.7*,[a]	31:5
Proximal corpus	4	16.4 ± 1.4*	20:11
Proximal cauda	6	9.0 ± 1.4**	12:5
Distal cauda	8	2.5 ± 0.5***	6:0

[a] Means ± SE's sharing the same superscript are not significantly different ($p < .05$).
[b] Maximum and minimum net distances traveled by intraluminal oil drops from point of injection in different epididymides.

dissection and measurement (FIG. 4), and the duration of sperm transit through the caput, corpus, and cauda epididymides were determined (2.1 days, 0.8 days, and 9.8 days, respectively).[27] The total time of epididymal transit (~12 days) is consistent with previous estimates using other techniques.[1] These data indicate that sperm arrive in the proximal cauda epididymidis relatively quickly, thus, that the pre-cauda maturational events also occur relatively quickly. This fact, plus the pendular movement of lumen fluid which allows for some degree of sperm mixing, especially in areas where net progressive movement is reduced, might contribute to the apparent fertility of some sperm collected from the obstructed proximal human epididymis.

It was also demonstrated that epididymal obstruction by vasectomy significantly reduced intraluminal fluid flow as far back as the caput epididymidis.[27] Obstruction persistent after vasovasostomy maintained the reduction in intraluminal fluid flow.[27] Since the intraluminal microenvironment is the product of the secretory and absorptive rates of the surrounding epithelium and the luminal fluid flow rate, alteration in flow necessarily affects the sperm cell's microenvironment. This might contribute to the mixed prognosis for fertility in human males after vasovasostomy.

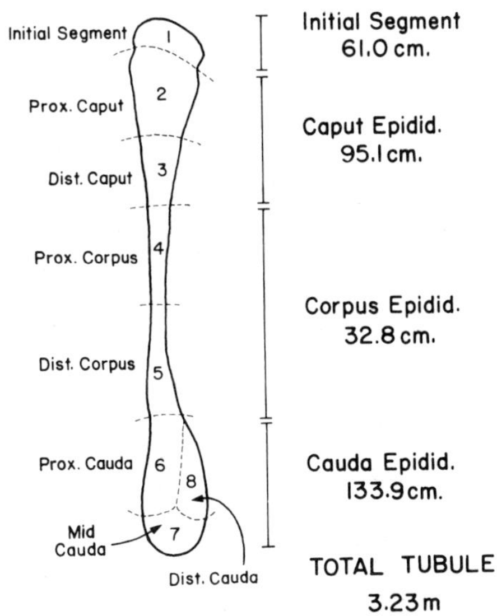

FIGURE 4. Micropuncture zones (1–8) of the rat epididymis; estimated length of the initial segment, caput, corpus, and cauda epididymidis, and estimated total epididymal length. (Illustration adapted from ref. 27.)

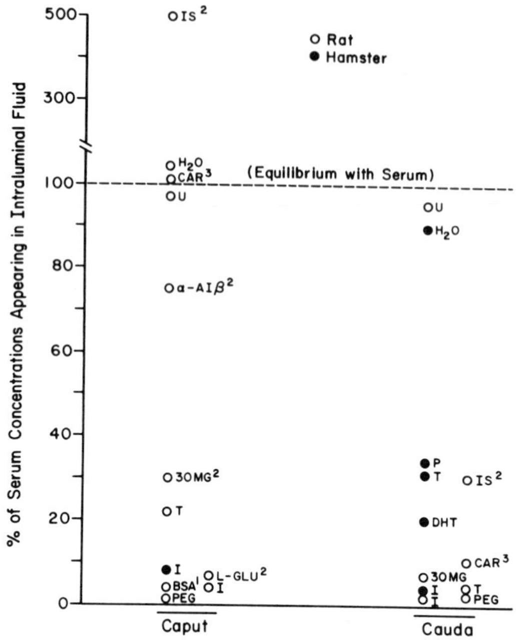

FIGURE 5. Availability of biological molecules in serum to the luminal microenvironment of the epididymis. Compounds isotopically labeled with ^{14}C, ^{3}H, or ^{125}I were infused systemically. Serum and epididymal fluids were subsequently collected by *in vivo* micropuncture, and radioactivity of intraluminal fluids was compared to radioactivity of serum collected at the same times. Values reflect only net movement of molecules from blood-to-lumen, and are the plateau concentrations found in intraluminal fluids within 2–3 h experimental periods, except as noted. [1] Plateau not noted, max value 2 h post-infusion. [2] Plateau not noted, max value 3 h post-infusion. [3] Plateau not noted, value 12 h post-infusion. I: inulin; IS: inositol; CAR: carnitine; U: urea; α AIB: α-aminoisobutyric acid; T: testosterone; L-GLU: L-glucose; 3OMG: 3-O-methyl-D-glucose; PEG: polyethyleneglycol; BSA: bovine serum albumin; DHT: 5 α-dihydrotestosterone; P: progesterone. (Data sources: BSA, PEG, U: Hinton and Howards (1981) J. Reprod. Fertil. **63:** 95; 3OMG, α-AIB, L-GLU, IS: Hinton and Howards (1982) Biol. Reprod. **27:** 1181; PEG: Turner *et al.* (1989) Biol. Reprod. **41:** 143; CAR: Hinton and Setchell (1980) *Carnitine Biosynthesis, Metabolism, and Functions.* Academic Press, New York, p. 237; I: Turner *et al.* (1987) Biol. Reprod. **36:** 926; Turner *et al.* (1981) Invest. Urol. **19:** 81; 3OMG: Turner *et al.* (1980) J. Reprod. Fertil. **60:** 285; U: Turner and Howards (1978) Invest. Urol. **16:** 237; H_2O: Turner *et al.* (1979) J. Reprod. Fertil. **55:** 237; T, P, DHT: Turner *et al.* (1981) Biol. Reprod. **25:** 342; Turner (1988) Biol. Reprod. **39:** 399.)

THE BLOOD EPIDIDYMAL BARRIER

Cell-cell tight junctions near the apical border of the epididymal epithelial cells provide a zonula occludens which prevents or restricts pro-luminal movement of some blood-borne substances.[1] These cell-cell tight junctions restrict the movement of molecules approaching the epididymal lumen by the paracellular route; however, substances which diffuse or are transported into the cell cytoplasm also often experience restricted entry into the lumen. *In vivo* micropuncture experiments have illustrated the tenacity of the blood-epididymal barrier,[28] and results from different laboratories and species have demonstrated the varying availability of serum substances to the epididymal lumen (FIG. 5).

The net blood-to-lumen movement of compounds is sometimes different between caput and cauda epididymidis (FIG. 5). Water, carnitine, and urea all reach unity with serum in the caput epididymidal lumen; *i.e.*, intraluminal concentrations become equivalent to serum concentrations, but carnitine entry into the cauda lumen is much more limited, only approaching 10% of serum values. Large molecules like albumin

(67,000 kD) polyethyleneglycol (PEG; 6,000 kD) or inulin (5,000 kD) are largely excluded in both the caput and cauda epididymidis since they cross neither the cell-cell tight junctions nor the cell membranes. Interestingly, albumin (FIG. 5, BSA) and IgG[29,30] both show very restricted movement from blood-to-epididymal lumen, but electrophoretic analysis shows significant albumin present in the lumen of all epididymal zones,[12,13] and IgG is detected by western blot in all zones (T. Turner and C. Spann, unpublished data).

Inositol is transported from blood into the caput lumen against a concentration gradient, but experiences only restricted net movement (reaching approximately 30% of serum concentrations) into the cauda lumen. 3-O-methyl-D-glucose (3OMG), a nonmetabolizable glucose analog, reaches equilibrium with blood in neither the caput nor cauda epididymidis, but availability of this glucose is much more restricted in the cauda lumen where sperm are stored than in the caput lumen (FIG. 5). Carnitine, inositol, and 3OMG are three examples of how the blood-epididymal barrier (or lack thereof) to serum components can be different in different regions of the epididymis, and illustrate another way the epididymal epithelium maintains its specialized microenvironment *in vivo*. Also, carnitine, inositol, GPC, and proteins are examples of substances synthesized and secreted or transported into epididymal fluid by the epididymal epithelium and whose concentrations cannot be accounted for by only the cell-cell tight junctions of the morphological blood-epididymal barrier.

The net effects of the secretory and absorptive functions of the epididymal epithelium as well as the intraluminal flow characteristics and blood-epididymal barrier are generalized in FIGURE 6, absent androgens which are discussed below. The above review focuses on aspects of the epididymal microenvironment which have been studied primarily through the use of *in vivo* micropuncture and associated techniques. These techniques allow the acquisition of information about the intraluminal fluids not attainable by other means, but it is important to note that investigators using other methods of fluid and tissue collection and a variety of analytical techniques have contributed significant information about epididymal physiology and the luminal microenvironment. Their important contributions are impossible to address in this focused review, but have been comprehensively reviewed most recently by Robaire and Hermo.[1]

THE ANDROGEN MICROENVIRONMENT OF MATURING SPERMATOZOA

The epididymis is an androgen target tissue, and its metabolism and epithelial secretion depend on the presence of androgens; consequently, epididymal sperm maturation does not occur in the absence of androgens.[1,31] Androgen concentrations in epididymal tissue extracts are high relative to serum, especially in the caput epididymides of several species[32,33] including the human,[34] and caput epididymidal lumen fluid androgen concentrations are higher still.[35] It has been a primary goal of our laboratory in recent years to understand the mechanism by which the intraluminal androgen microenvironment is maintained, and secondly, to understand why such intraluminal androgen concentrations are necessary to normal epithelial function. Using a combination of *in vivo* micropuncture techniques and a rapid centrifugation method to collect intraluminal reproductive tract fluids, Turner *et al.*[35] have shown that intraluminal androgens leave the testes primarily in the form of testosterone (approximately 60 nM) but appear in the lumen of the caput epididymidis in much higher

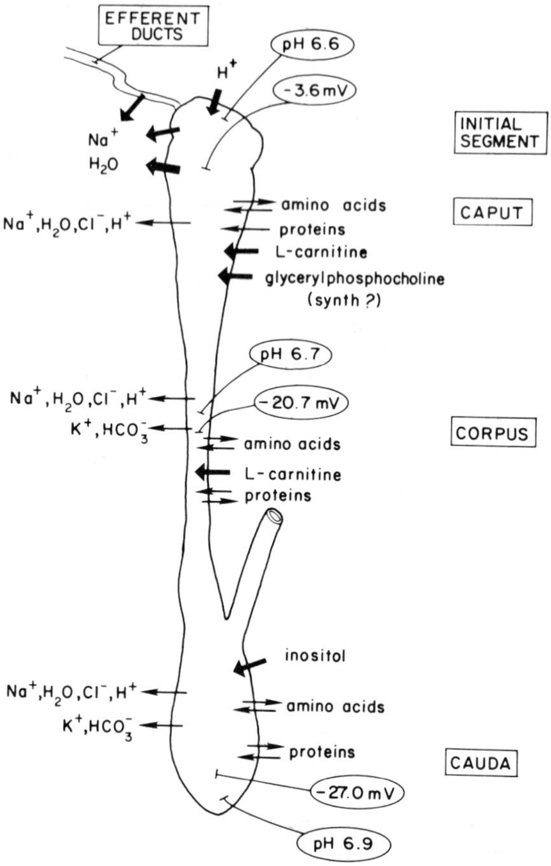

FIGURE 6. Net movement of water, ions, organic solutes, and macro- into and out of the rat epididymal lumen. Thickness of arrow reflects degree of movement. In the case of proteins, glycerylphosphorylcholine, and possibly inositol, synthesis by the epididymal epithelium is required. (Illustration modified from ref. 11.)

concentrations of 5 α-dihydrotestosterone (DHT, approximately 200 nM; see FIG. 7). 5 α-Reductase, known to be highly active in the caput epididymidis,[1] converts the luminal testosterone to DHT, but since the 5 α-reductase enzyme is only known to be localized within the epithelial cells, indeed mostly within the cell nuclei, the mechanism of this luminal conversion is unknown.

Androgen-binding protein (ABP), a Sertoli cell product under the regulation of testosterone and FSH,[36,37] also increases in intraluminal concentrations between the rete testis and caput epididymidis.[8,35] Relevant to the previous discussion of secretion and absorption, the increase in ABP concentrations between the rete testis and caput epididymidis (from 60–266 nM) is not as much as would have been expected owing to fluid reabsorption alone (562 nM), therefore, the Δ_{Conc} for ABP in the rat caput epididymidis is −296 nM/L caput fluid.[35] This implies a large amount of ABP catabolism or reabsorption in the efferent ducts or proximal caput tubule. In fact, immunocytochemical studies in other laboratories have shown reabsorption to occur.[38]

Intraluminal ABP concentrations are at near unity with total androgens (for the

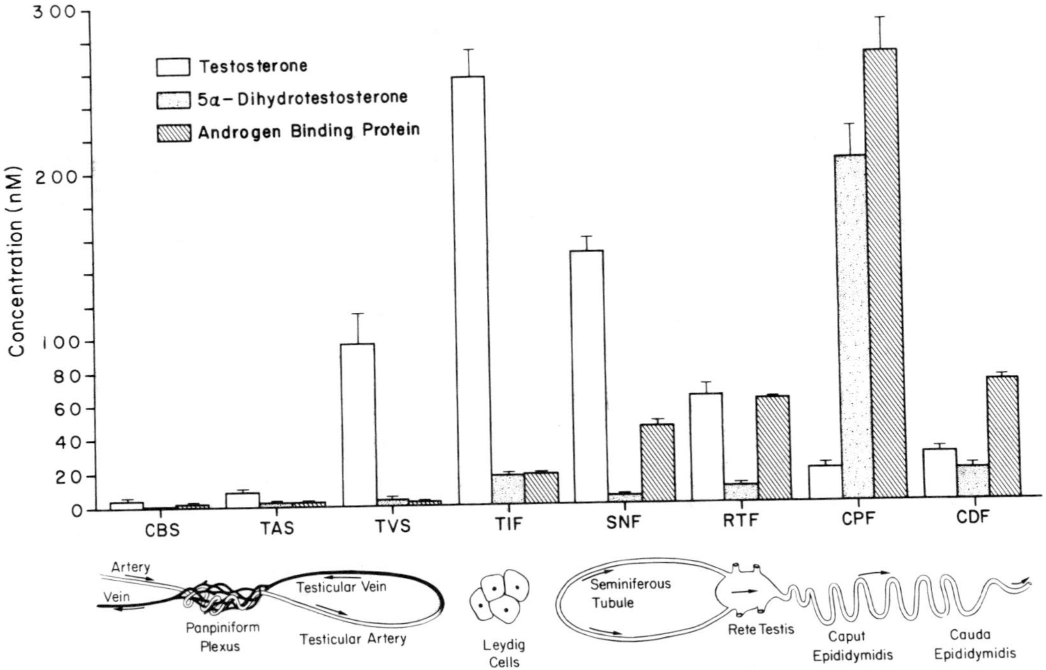

FIGURE 7. Concentrations of testosterone, DHT, and ABP in sera and reproductive tract fluids of the adult male rat. ABP concentrations were calculated on the basis of 1 μleq immunoassayable ABP = 8 fmol ABP (Gunsalus *et al.* (1978) Int. J. Androl. Suppl. **2:** 482–493). Arrows in schematic indicate direction of intraluminal flow. CBS: cardiac blood serum; TAS: testicular arterial serum; TVS: testicular venous serum; TIF: testicular interstitial fluid; SNF: seminiferous tubule fluid; RTF: rete testis fluid; CPF: caput epididymidal fluid; CDF: cauda epididymidal fluid. (Figure from ref. 34, used with permission.)

present purposes, testosterone + DHT; see FIG. 7) in the caput and cauda epididymidal lumina.[35] Also, between the rete testis and caput epididymidis large amounts of androgens leave the excurrent ducts until androgen concentrations no longer exceed intraluminal ABP concentrations. These facts suggest that ABP is important in maintaining the high androgen concentrations detected in caput lumen fluid; *i.e.*, once the intraluminal androgen (as testosterone or DHT) leave the rete testis via the efferent ducts the steroids begin diffusing out of the excurrent duct lumen, but the androgens stop diffusing out of the lumen when they reach a concentration equivalent to the ABP concentration. The remaining androgen (now DHT) is bound to the intraluminal binding molecule. Thus, while the epididymal lumen contains high DHT concentrations, the bulk of the steroid is bound to ABP and is not free steroid. Recently, Veeramachaneni *et al.*[39] have also found intraluminal ABP concentrations in the ram caput epididymidis to be very high relative to ABP concentrations in ram rete testis fluid or cauda epididymidal fluid. Intraluminal androgen concentrations in other species have not been reported.

While the report of Turner *et al.*[35] characterized the concentrations of androgens in serum and the peritubular and intraluminal fluids of the male rat reproductive tubules, many aspects of the tissue and cellular endocrinology of the tubules remained unclear. Especially, there was little resolution about local mechanisms that regulate androgen availability to the apical or basal membranes of the reproductive tract epithelial cells. For example, the richest source of androgen for Sertoli cells is across their basal membrane whereas the richest source of androgen for caput epithelial cells is across their apical membrane (FIG. 7). On the other hand, much of the intraluminal androgen in the seminiferous tubule lumen is apparently free while that in the epididymal lumen is largely bound (FIG. 7).

In order to study this compartmentalization of androgens in the testis and epididymis of the rat, we have used *in vivo* tubule perifusion, tubule perfusion, and micropuncture techniques to control the molecular environment presented to either the basal or apical aspects of the seminiferous and epididymal epithelia.[40] In the perifusion experiments, ^{3}H-testosterone has been perifused around the tubules since testosterone is the primary peritubular androgen *in vivo*. It is recognized that over time the ^{3}H-testosterone is variably metabolized to other androgens *in vivo*, primarily to ^{3}H-DHT in the epididymis[40]; thus, the interstitial and intraluminal radiolabeled steroids we report are referred to simply as ^{3}H-androgens.

^{3}H-androgens at physiological concentrations (266 nM) in the testicular interstitium enter the seminiferous tubule in a restricted manner (FIG. 8).[40,41] These findings are consistent with data from earlier experiments where ^{3}H-testosterone, ^{3}H-progesterone, and ^{3}H-DHT had been infused into the systemic circulation of the hamster and exhibited little net appearance in seminiferous tubule fluid (see FIG. 5). Net movement of ^{3}H-androgens into the seminiferous tubule lumen is not subject to competitive inhibition with unlabeled androgen (FIG. 8).[41] In contrast, net ^{3}H-androgen movement into the caput and cauda epididymidal tubules occurs against an apparent concentration gradient and is subject to competitive inhibition with unlabeled testosterone (FIG. 8). Interestingly, this antigrade androgen movement into the caput lumen is not evident when ^{3}H-androgens are presented via the vasculature,[40] implying that androgen binding in the vascular or interstitial space is a factor in androgen compartmentalization within the epididymis.

The antigrade movement of ^{3}H-androgen from interstitial-to-intraluminal space in the epididymis was confirmed by dry-mount autoradiography after *in vitro* incu-

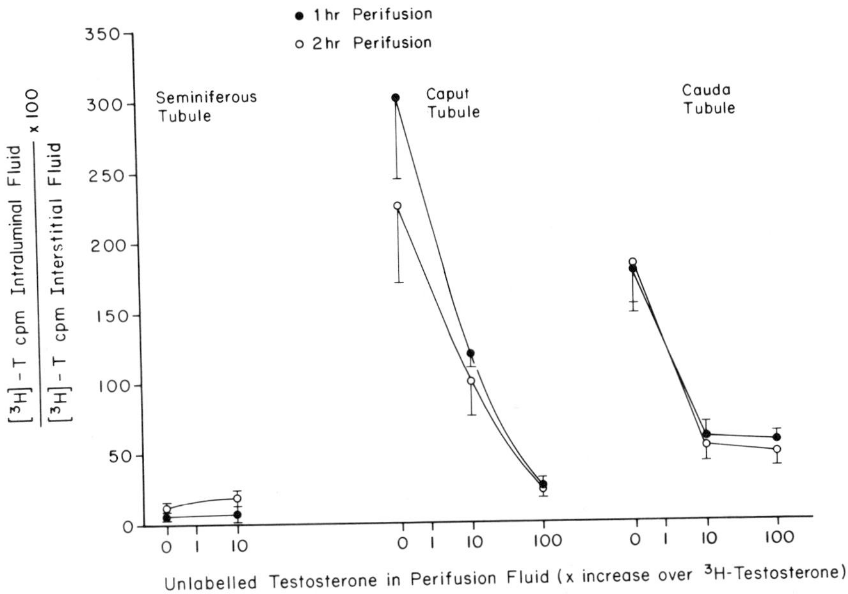

FIGURE 8. Net proluminal movement of isotope perifused into testicular and epididymal interstitial space as ^3H-testosterone. As illustrated perifusion fluid in some experiments contained unlabeled testosterone at 10 or 100× the concentration of labeled testosterone. The ordinate value of 100 indicates unity of intraluminal and peritubular concentrations. One-hour and 2-h perifusion data were similar indicating that intraluminal values had reached equilibrium. (Figure adapted from ref. 41.)

bation of caput epididymidal tubules with ^3H-DHT. Intraluminal grain counts in the caput autoradiograms were 250% of interstitial grain counts, data consistent with the *in vivo* perifusion experiments where intraluminal isotope concentrations were 200–300% of intraluminal isotope concentrations. The dry-mount autoradiography experiments also showed that grain localizations occurred in cell-free portions of lumen fluid as well as in those areas containing spermatozoa and that the *in situ* caput sperm do not bind the ^3H-androgen. Steady-state gel electrophoresis of 1 μl aliquots of cell-free intraluminal fluid demonstrated that there is only one ^3H-androgen binding component in seminiferous, caput, and cauda epididymidal lumen fluids and that this ABP activity is higher in the caput epididymidal lumen than in other areas.[41] This binding activity data is consistent with data on immunoreactive ABP determined by radioimmunoassay.[35]

The data collected to this point were consistent with the hypothesis that high intraluminal androgen concentrations in the epididymis are maintained by androgens arriving via the efferent ducts plus movement of free androgens from the peritubular fluids. Intraluminal ABP was hypothesized to be important to the antigrade ^3H-androgen movement detected. It was hypothesized that the ^3H-androgen movement was due to simple diffusion across the epididymal epithelium followed by binding of the ^3H-androgen to intraluminal ABP, with the ^3H-androgen competing with the native unlabeled steroid for binding sites.

ABP is secreted from Sertoli cells under the influence of FSH and testosterone; therefore, subsequent experiments examined the effect of gonadotropin deprivation on proluminal ^{3}H-androgen movement in the caput epididymidis. Hypophysectomy of adult male rats eliminated antigrade ^{3}H-androgen movement across the caput epididymidal epithelium, and gonadotropin replacement to hypophysectomized rats returned caput proluminal ^{3}H-androgen movement to normal.[42] At both 1 and 2 hours after initiation of ^{3}H-androgen perifusion around caput tubules, control intraluminal ^{3}H-androgen concentrations were 275–315% of interstitial androgen concentrations, but in hypophysectomized animals, the intraluminal values were reduced to 44–91% of interstitial ^{3}H-androgen concentrations. Both FSH and LH (24 μg/day for 10 days) returned net proluminal ^{3}H-androgen movement to normal (intraluminal ^{3}H-androgen concentrations = 250–400% of peritubular ^{3}H-androgen concentrations).[42] These data were consistent with the stated hypothesis that intraluminal ABP was important to the antigrade movement of ^{3}H-androgens across the epididymal epithelium, but did not prove the hypothesis directly. To determine if intraluminal ABP specifically effects ^{3}H-androgen uptake by caput epididymidal tubules, a different approach was necessary.

A microperfusion technique was developed which allows placement of fluids and molecules of choice within the epididymal lumen and subsequent analysis of the tubule lengths for ^{3}H-androgen uptake.[43] Lengths of caput epididymidal tubule were dissected free and tied with 8-0 silk suture at either end of 2 cm segments. These tubules contained native lumen content. Other lengths of tubule were dissected free from adjacent tubule coils and perfused at a rate of 2 μl/min with either fresh rat rete testis fluid which contained ABP or an artificial medium containing no ABP. The latter fluid (MKB) did contain BSA in concentrations equivalent to the total protein concentration in rete testis fluid. After completing the perfusion, the tubules were closed with 8-0 silk as above. The tubule lengths were incubated *in vitro* for 2.5 h in 35° MEM containing 2 ng/ml ^{3}H-testosterone and trace amounts of ^{14}C-PEG to act as a contamination marker. Tubules containing rete testis fluid (with ABP) took up 137% of the ^{3}H-androgen taken up by tubules not containing ABP, and the ^{3}H-androgen uptake was subject to competitive inhibition.[43] Additionally, 95% pure rat ABP was generously provided by Dr. Benjamin Danzo, Vanderbilt University, and in a subsequent series of experiments, 2 cm lengths of caput tubule were perfused with fresh caput fluid, MKB alone, or MKB containing 5.0 or 50.0 ng ABP/μl. Perfusing caput tubules with MKB significantly reduced caput tubule uptake of ^{3}H-androgen from the medium, but increasing intraluminal ABP concentrations caused step-wise increases in caput tubule uptake of ^{3}H-androgens (FIG. 9A). If it is assumed that perfusion with MKB removed 100% of the lumen-associated binding activity of caput tubules, then intraluminal concentrations of purified ABP at 5.0 and 50.0 ng/μl returned caput tubule ^{3}H-androgen uptake to 31% and 71% of control values (FIG. 9B). The difficulty in obtaining net ^{3}H-androgen uptake values more nearly approximating those of tubules perfused with native lumen content might be due to errors in achieving appropriate ABP concentrations at this small scale, or to some change induced in the epididymal epithelium due to absence of other factors in artificial perfusion medium. These experiments demonstrate that purified ABP does stimulate ^{3}H-androgen uptake by caput tubules from the surrounding fluid environment.

When seminiferous and caput epididymidal tubules were perifused *in vivo* with increasing concentrations of ^{3}H-androgen, the movement of ^{3}H-androgen into the

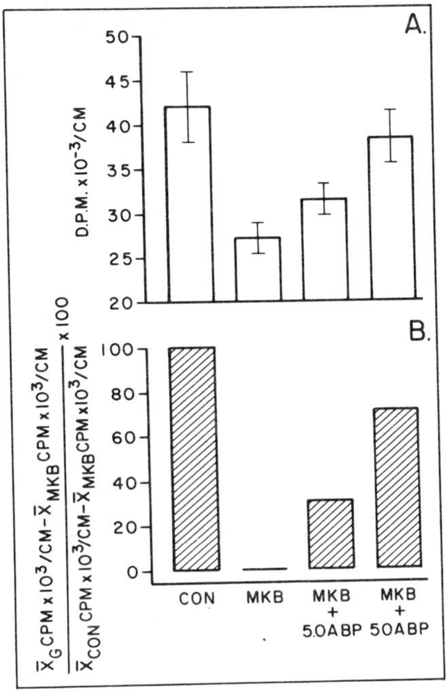

FIGURE 9. The effect of tubule perfusion and replacement of intraluminal ABP on caput tubule uptake of ^{3}H-androgens *in vitro.* A: ^{3}H-androgen uptake in tubules perfused with fresh caput lumen fluid (CON), MKB containing no ABP, or MKB containing ABP at 5.0 or 50 ng/μl. B: Percentage return of ^{3}H-androgen uptake capacity in tubules perfused with fluids as above. The calculation on the ordinate is based on the assumption that tubules perfused with MKB lost 100% of their lumen-associated androgen binding capacity. Increasing intraluminal ABP concentrations increased ^{3}H-androgen uptake by perfused tubules. (Illustration adapted from ref. 43.)

seminiferous tubules was linear with the increasing peritubular ^{3}H-androgen concentrations, confirming pro-luminal movement by diffusion (FIG. 10A), but similar experiments with the *in vivo* caput epididymal tubule (FIG. 10B) again illustrated the striking difference between androgen movement into the two types of tubule.[44] The best-fit model for ^{3}H-androgen movement into rat caput epididymidal tubules was the hyperbolic regression described by the equation $Y = AX/B+X$ where A (342.6 nM) expresses the capacity for the binding event in the mechanism of movement from one compartment to another and B (63.1 nM) is equivalent to the concentration of interstitial ^{3}H-androgen at which intraluminal values are half maximal. Intraluminal caput ABP concentrations detected by radioimmunoassay have previously been reported to be approximately 270 nM (FIG. 7) and this is sufficiently close to the calculated binding capacity in the present experiments (340 nM) to suggest consistency with the hypothesis that intraluminal ABP sets intraluminal androgen concentration in the rat epididymis.

The hypothesis that ^{3}H-androgens cross the epididymal epithelium by simple diffusion is not supported by the data in FIGURE 10B, however. If diffusion alone was the mechanism of movement across the epithelium, intraluminal ^{3}H-androgen concentrations should have continued to rise linearly as interstitial ^{3}H-androgen concentrations increased after the saturation of available intraluminal binding sites. This did not occur. The net movement of ^{3}H-androgens into the caput epididymidal lumen plateaued at high concentrations (~340 nM) of interstitial ^{3}H-androgens. These data appear to be consistent with an active transport system exhibiting a transport maximum rather than the hypothesized diffusion followed by intraluminal binding to ABP.

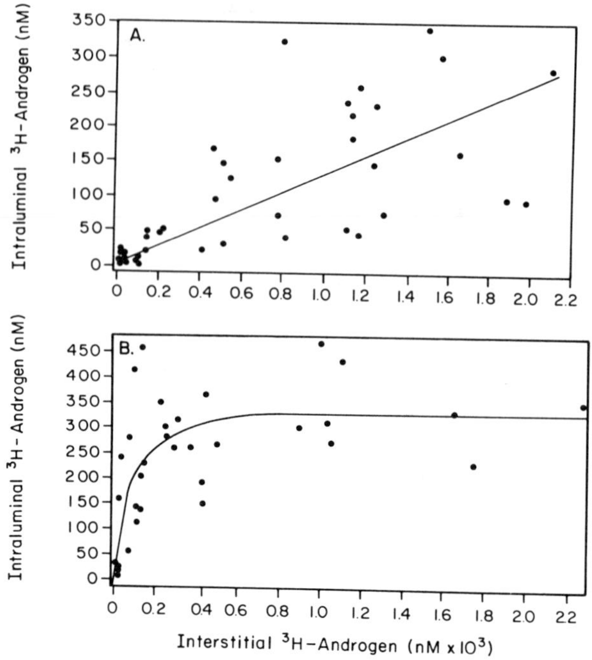

FIGURE 10. A: Intraluminal ^{3}H-androgen concentrations in rat seminiferous tubules at 10 nM–2,000 nM interstitial ^{3}H-androgen concentrations 1 h after initiation of perifusion. Intraluminal ^{3}H-androgens averaged 17.6% of interstitial values at all concentrations. Residuals around the linear regression line were randomly distributed. **B:** Intraluminal ^{3}H-androgen concentrations in rat caput lumen fluid at 10 nM–2,000 nM interstitial ^{3}H-androgen concentrations. Intra-luminal ^{3}H-androgen concentrations increased hyperbolically with increasing interstitial concentrations. Intraluminal ^{3}H-androgen concentrations plateaued at approximately 340 nM even though maximal interstitial values exceeded 2,000 nM. Residuals around the hyperbolic regression line ($y = AX/B+X$) were randomly distributed.

These results not only conflicted with our hypothesis about androgen compartmentalization in the epididymis, but conflict as well with the basic dogma that steroids simply diffuse across cell membranes and epithelia. These results caused us to undertake a series of experiments wherein caput tubules were exposed *in vivo* to metabolic inhibitors.

Perifusion of caput tubules with 0.1 mM 2,4-dinitrophenol (DNP) and potassium cyanide (KCN) decreased both caput tissue ATP concentrations and proluminal ^{3}H-androgen movement (FIGS. 11A,B).[44]

The finding that proluminal ^{3}H-androgen movement is inhibited by uncouplers of oxidative phosphorylation was unexpected, based on previous experience.[41] We subsequently determined that intraluminal ABP concentrations in these treated caput tubules had not been affected by the metabolic inhibitors (data not shown). Thus, caput epididymal tubules with normal intraluminal ABP concentrations, but with a metabolically inhibited epithelium, did not allow the movement of ^{3}H-androgens against an apparent concentration gradient.

Our results present two lines of evidence: one which indicates that intraluminal

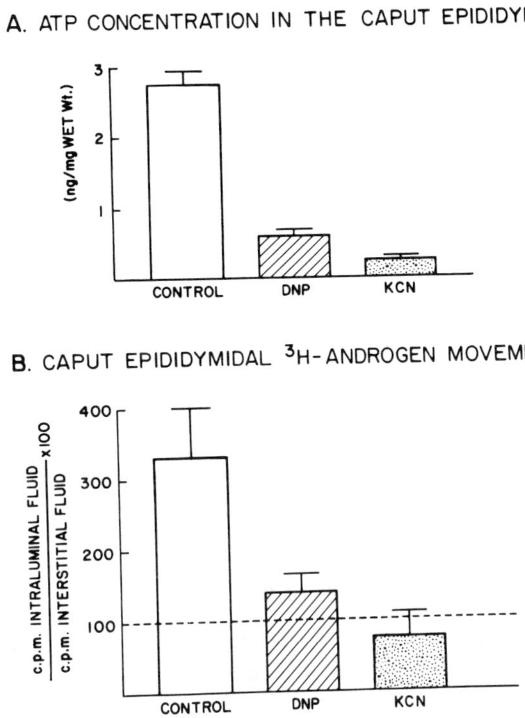

FIGURE 11. Effects of 2,4-dinitrophenol (DNP) and potassium cyanide (KCN) on (A) caput tissue ATP content and (B) net proluminal ^{3}H-androgen movement. Dashed line indicates value expected from diffusion of ^{3}H-androgen alone. (Illustration adapted from ref. 44.)

ABP concentrations set intraluminal ^{3}H-androgen concentrations and another indicating that ^{3}H-androgens move into the caput lumen by an energy-requiring, active transport process. If ^{3}H-androgens move into the caput epididymidal lumen by an active transport process, then the tubule lumen without ABP present should accumulate ^{3}H-androgens against a concentration gradient as did the lumen containing native lumen fluid. To determine if this was the case, caput epididymidal tubules were perfused with artificial caput fluid (ACF) while being perifused with the perifusion fluid containing ^{3}H-androgen. Data from these experiments were compared to data from *in vivo* perifusion experiments done in the usual manner where the native lumen content is unaltered prior to micropuncture (see FIG. 12, control and ACF). One hour perifusion of caput tubules with ^{3}H-androgen resulted in intraluminal ^{3}H-androgen concentrations which were 323% of interstitial values in control perifusions, and this value was reduced to 100% of interstitial ^{3}H-androgen concentrations when native lumen content was replaced with ACF containing no ABP (FIG. 12).[44] Thus, caput tubules perfused with artificial caput fluid while being perifused with ^{3}H-androgens did not exhibit antigrade, proluminal ^{3}H-androgen movement. It is important to realize that the perifusion fluid in these experiments was exactly the same as in the control experiments, and that the signal difference in the experiments was that in

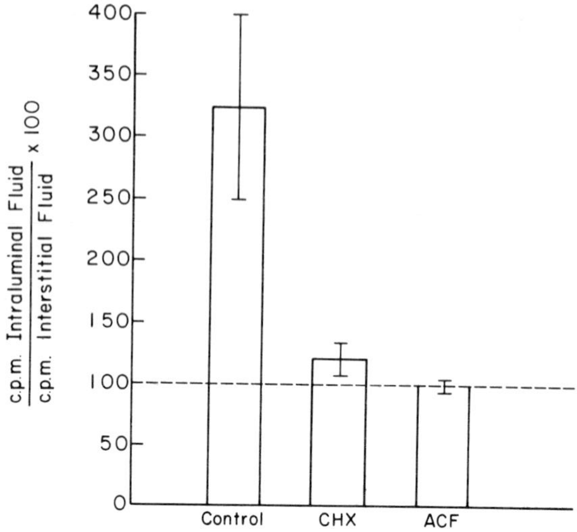

FIGURE 12. Proluminal ^{3}H-androgen movement into caput epididymidal lumen fluid after tubules were perifused *in vivo* for 1 h with fluid containing 240 nM ^{3}H-testosterone. Control: Tubule contained native lumen content. ACF: Tubules perfused with artificial caput fluid. CHX: Tubules perifused with fluid containing 240 nM ^{3}H-testosterone + 100 μg/ml cyclohexamide. (Illustration adapted from ref. 44.)

the experiments where the native lumen content was perfused with artificial caput fluid, the tubule lumen contained no ABP. Antigrade ^{3}H-androgen movement does not occur in the caput epididymidis in the absence of intraluminal ABP.

Nevertheless, some energy-dependent process is important in maintaining antigrade androgen movement in the presence of native lumen content (FIG. 11). Caput tubules were subsequently perifused with 100 μg/ml cyclohexamide (CHX) included in the perifusion fluid along with the ^{3}H-testosterone. This was done to determine if the important energy expenditure occurs in a mechanism requiring the synthesis of intracellular proteins. Perifusion of caput tubules with CHX did significantly inhibit both ^{35}S-methionine incorporation into TCA precipitable proteins (data not shown) and proluminal ^{3}H-androgen movement (FIG. 12). These data indicate that continuing synthesis of intracellular proteins is important to the ability of peritubular androgens to pass against a concentration gradient into the intraluminal microenvironment. Protein synthesis is an energy requiring process, and this perhaps accounts for metabolic deprivation inhibiting proluminal ^{3}H-androgen movement.

How intracellular proteins affect the movement of ^{3}H-androgens from the basal to the apical aspect of the epididymal epithelium is unknown. A general inhibition of protein synthesis can produce effects that range from altered cytoskeleton assembly to perturbations of apical and baso-lateral membrane synthesis. Further investigations are required to determine which intracellular protein syntheses are important to the compartmentalization of androgens between the peritubular fluids, the intracellular fluids, and the intraluminal microenvironment.

The experiments detailed above have demonstrated that the rat epididymis maintains a high intraluminal concentration of androgen, primarily DHT, and that intraluminal ABP is important in that maintenance. As we have stated, however, intraluminal androgens are bound, not free, and are not available to intraluminal spermatozoa which apparently do not bind steroids in any case.[41] The important question then is of what importance is the high intraluminal ABP or ABP:DHT complex to the epididymal epithelium?

As already discussed, ABP can be localized in the epithelium of the rat efferent ducts and the epididymal epithelium.[38] Reabsorption from the lumen appears to be by receptor-mediated endocytosis,[45] and ABP still appears to retain its androgen when it is internalized into the epithelial cell.[46] Data from the ram epididymis[46] is consistent with the findings in the rat. Anthony *et al.*[48] have found the presence of intraluminal ABP to be associated with sperm fertility, and earlier workers have found that some intraluminal product of the testis other than androgens is necessary for morphological maintenance of the initial segment[48] and caput epididymidal tubule.[49,50] If ABP is a testicular product destined for a function in the epididymis, it is unclear whether it is the ABP or the DHT it carries with it that is important in the maintenance of the epididymal epithelium. Current studies in our laboratory are attempting to determine the effect of intraluminal ABP on nuclear androgen localization in caput epididymidal cells. These studies are carried out with intraluminal perfusion of ABP alone or the ABP-DHT complex when the epididymal tubule is surrounded *in vivo* with radiolabeled androgens.

In an early study, Tindall *et al.*[51] found that epididymal cytoplasmic androgen receptor exhibited increased androgen binding in the presence of ABP, and Lobl *et al.*[52] later proposed that ABP might function as an intracellular androgen transporter in the epididymis. It is possible that high intraluminal concentrations of the ABP:DHT complex are important for androgen regulation of the epididymal epithelium, and that this circuit is important in order that a testicular product be directly involved with the regulation of the luminal microenvironment to which new sperm are being exposed. Proluminal androgen movement as observed in our *in vivo* experiments with ^{3}H-testosterone may be the result of steroid movement into the epididymal lumen merely to keep the ABP charged with DHT; however, intracellular trafficking of androgens may be more complex than has previously been thought, and unknown factors there may account for the effects of metabolic inhibition on proluminal ^{3}H-androgen movement.

Finally, preliminary studies in our laboratory indicate that differential binding of ^{3}H-androgens to molecules in the testicular and caput epididymidal interstitial space can also affect availability of peritubular androgens to the intraluminal microenvironment (T. Turner and M. Yamamoto, unpublished data). Androgen availability at specifically the basal or apical aspects of reproductive tract epithelial cells could well be important features of the cellular endocrinology of the male reproductive tract and the regulation of the intraluminal microenvironments in which sperm maturation occur.

REFERENCES

1. Robaire, B. & L. Hermo. 1988. Efferent ducts, epididymis, and vas deferens: Structure, functions, and their regulation. *In* The Physiology of Reproduction. E. Knobil & J. Neil, Eds. Vol. **1:** 999–1079. Raven Press. New York.
2. Cooper, T. 1990. In defense of the human epididymis. Fertil. Steril. **54:** 965–975.
3. Crabo, B. 1965. Studies on the composition of epididymal content in bulls and boars. Acta Vet. Scand. **6** (Suppl. 5):1–94.
4. Levine, N. & D. J. Marsh. 1971. Micropuncture studies of the electrochemical aspects of fluid and electrolyte transport in individual seminiferous tubules, the epididymis, and the vas deferens in rats. J. Physiol. **213:** 557–570.
5. Howards, S. S., A. Johnson & S. Jessee. 1975. Micropuncture and microanalytical studies of the rat testis and epididymis. Fertil. Steril. **26:** 13–19.

6. TURNER, T. T., P. K. HARTMAN & S. S. HOWARDS. 1979. *In vivo* sodium and potassium and sperm concentrations in the rat epididymis. Fertil. Steril. **28:** 191–194.
7. HINTON, B. T., H. M. DOTT & B. P. SETCHELL. 1979. Measurement of the motility of rat spermatozoa collected by micropuncture from the testis and from different regions along the epididymis. J. Reprod. Fertil. **55:** 167–172.
8. TURNER, T. T. 1984. Resorption versus secretion in the rat epididymis. J. Reprod. Fertil. **72:** 509–514.
9. WONG, P. Y. D., C. L. AU & H. K. NGAI. 1978. Electrolyte and water transport in rat epididymis: Possible role in sperm maturation. Int. J. Androl. (Suppl. 2):608–628.
10. SETCHELL, B. P. & B. T. HINTON. 1981. The effects on spermatozoa of changes in the composition of luminal fluid as it passes along the epididymis. Prog. Reprod. Biol. **8:** 58–66.
11. HINTON, B. T. & T. T. TURNER. 1988. Is the epididymis a kidney analog? News Physiol. Sci. **3:** 28–31.
12. TURNER, T. T., J. L. PLESUMS & C. L. CABOT. 1979. Luminal fluid proteins of the male rat reproductive tract. Biol. Reprod. **21:** 883–890.
13. OLSON, G. E. & B. T. HINTON. 1985. Regional differences in luminal fluid polypeptides of the rat testis and epididymis revealed by two-dimensional gel electrophoresis. J. Androl. **6:** 20–34.
14. VERNON, R. B., C. H. MULLER, J. C. HERR, F. A. FEUCHTER & E. M. EDDY. 1982. Epididymal secretion of a mouse sperm surface component recognized by a monoclonal antibody. Biol. Reprod. **26:** 523–535.
15. VOGLMAYR, J. K., R. F. SAWYER & J. L. DACHEUX. 1985. Glycoproteins—A variable factor in surface transformation of ram sperm during epididymal transit. Biol. Reprod. **33:** 165–176.
16. CORNWALL, G. A., J. T. VREEBURG, M. K. HOLLAND & M. C. ORGEBIN-CRIST. 1990. Interactions of labelled epididymal secretory proteins with spermatozoa after injection of ^{35}S-methionine in the mouse. Biol. Reprod. **43:** 121–129.
17. ORGEBIN-CRIST, M. C. & N. JAHAD. 1979. The maturation of rabbit epididymal spermatozoa in organ culture: Inhibition by anti-androgens and inhibitors of ribonucleic acid and protein synthesis. Endocrinology **103:** 46–53.
18. FOURNIER-DELPECH, S., M. COUROT & M. P. DUBOIS. 1985. Decreased fertility and motility of spermatozoa from rats immunized with prealbumin epididymal specific glycoprotein. J. Androl. **6:** 246–250.
19. ORGEBIN-CRIST, M. C. & S. FOURNIER-DELPECH. 1982. Sperm-egg interaction: Evidence for maturational changes during epididymal transit. J. Androl. **3:** 429–433.
20. ROSS, P., F. W. K. KAN, P. ANTAKI, N. VIGNEAULT, A. CHAPDELAINE & K. D. ROBERTS. 1990. Protein synthesis and secretion in the human epididymis and immunoreactivity with sperm antibodies. Mol. Reprod. **26:** 12–23.
21. TURNER, T. T. & R. D. GILES. 1982. A sperm motility inhibiting factor in the rat epididymis. Am J. Physiol. **242:** R199-R203.
22. USSELMAN, M. C. & R. A. CONE. 1983. Rat sperm are mechanically immobilized in the cauda epididymidis by "immobilin," a high molecular weight glycoprotein. Biol. Reprod. **29:** 1241–1253.
23. TURNER, T. T. 1987. The influence of proteins in the rat cauda epididymidal lumen fluid on cauda sperm motility. Gam. Res. **18:** 267–278.
24. TURNER, T. T. & G. W. REICH. 1985. Cauda epididymidal sperm motility: A comparison among five species. Biol. Reprod. **32:** 120–129.
25. ACOTT, T. S. & D. W. CARR. 1984. Inhibition of bovine spermatozoa by caudal fluid: II. Interaction of pH and a quiescence factor. Biol. Reprod. **30:** 926–935.
26. HINTON, B. T. 1990. The testicular and epididymal luminal amino acid microenvironment in the rat. J. Androl. **11:** 498–505.
27. TURNER, T. T., J. L. GLEAVY & J. M. HARRIS. 1990. Fluid movement in the lumen of the rat epididymis. Effect of vasectomy and subsequent vasovasostomy. J. Androl. **11:** 422–428.
28. TURNER, T. T. & S. S. HOWARDS. 1985. The tenacity of the blood-testis and blood-epididymal barriers. *In* Male Fertility and Its Regulation. T. Lobl & E. S. E. Hafez, Eds. MTP Press. Boston, MA.
29. WONG, P. Y. D., A. Y. F. TSANG, W. O. FU & H. K. LAU. 1983. Restricted entry of an anti-rat epididymal protein IgG into the rat epididymis. Int. J. Androl. **6:** 275–282.
30. WEININGER, R. B., S. FISHER, J. RIFKIN & J. M. BEDFORD. 1982. Experimental studies on the passage of specific IgG to the lumen of the rabbit epididymis. J. Reprod. Fertil. **66:** 251–258.
31. BROOKS, D. E. 1983. Epididymal functions and their hormonal regulation. Aust. J. Biol. Sci. **36:** 205–221.

32. BOUJARD, D., D. THOMAS & D. H. GARNIER. 1982. Regional distribution of steroids in the dog epididymis. Reprod. Nutr. Develop. **22:** 931–939.
33. PUJOL, A., F. BAYARD, J. P. LOUVET & C. BOULARD. 1976. Testosterone and dihydrotestosterone concentrations in plasma, epididymal tissue, and seminal fluids of rats. Endocrinology **98:** 383–392.
34. DELARMINAT, M. A., M. J. HINRICHSEN, C. SCORTICATI, J. M. GHIRLANDA, J. A. BLAQUIER & R. S. CALANDRA. 1980. Uptake and metabolism of androgen in the human epididymis in vitro. J. Reprod. Fertil. **59:** 397–402.
35. TURNER, T. T., C. E. JONES, S. S. HOWARDS, L. L. EWING, B. ZEGEYE & G. L. GUNSALUS. 1984. On the androgen microenvironment of maturing spermatozoa. Endocrinology **115:** 1925–1932.
36. HANSSON, V., S. C. WEDDINGTON, F. S. FRENCH, W. MCLEAN, A. SMITH & S. N. NEYFEH. 1976. Secretion and role of androgen-binding proteins in the testis and epididymis. J. Reprod. Fertil. Suppl. **24:** 17–33.
37. DANZO, B. J., S. N. PAVLOU & H. L. ANTHONY. 1990. Hormonal regulation of androgen binding protein in the rat. Endocrinology **127:** 2829–2838.
38. PELLINIEMI, J., M. DYM, G. L. GUNSALUS, N. A. MUSTO, W. BARDIN & D. W. FAWCETT. 1981. Immunocytochemical localization of androgen binding protein in the male rat reproductive tract. Endocrinology **108:** 925–931.
39. VERRAMACHANENI, D. N. R., R. AMANN, J. S. PALMER & B. T. HINTON. 1990. Proteins in luminal fluid of the ram excurrent ducts: Changes in composition and evidence for differential endocytosis. J. Androl. **11:** 140–154.
40. TURNER, T. T. 1988. Transepithelial movement of ^{3}H-androgen in seminiferous and epididymal tubules: A study using *in vivo* micropuncture and *in vivo* microperfusion. Biol. Reprod. **39:** 399–408.
41. TURNER, T. T., C. E. JONES & M. S. RODDY. 1989. On the proluminal movement of ^{3}H-androgen across the rat epididymal epithelium. Biol. Reprod. **41:** 143–152.
42. YAMAMOTO, M. & T. T. TURNER. 1989. Proluminal movement of ^{3}H-androgen across the epididymal epithelium in the rat after hypophysectomy and gonadotropin supplementation. Biol. Reprod. **41:** 474–479.
43. TURNER, T. T. & M. S. RODDY. 1990. Intraluminal androgen binding protein alters ^{3}H-androgen uptake by rat epididymal tubules *in vitro.* Biol. Reprod. **43:** 414–419.
44. TURNER, T. T. & M. YAMAMOTO. 1991. Different mechanisms are responsible for ^{3}H-androgen movement across the rat seminiferous and epididymal epithelium *in vivo.* Biol. Reprod. **45:** 358–364.
45. GUEANT, J. L., S. FREMONT, J. KHANFRI, A. GERARD, G. GRIGNON, J. P. NICHOLAS & H. GERARD. 1988. Biochemical evidences for receptor mediated uptake of rat androgen binding protein by epididymis. Steroids **52:** 347–348.
46. GERARD, A., J. KHANFRI, J. L. GUEANT, J. P. FREMONT, J. P. NICHOLAS, G. GRIGNON & H. GERARD. 1988. Electron microscope radiographic evidence of *in vivo* androgen binding protein internalization of the rat epididymis principal cells. Endocrinology **122:** 1297–1307.
47. ANTHONY, C. T., B. J. DANZO & M. C. ORGEBIN-CRIST. 1984. Investigations on the relationship between sperm fertilizing ability and androgen binding protein. Endocrinology **114:** 1413–1418.
48. FAWCETT, D. W. & R. P. HOFFER. 1979. Failure of exogenous androgens to prevent regression of the initial segments of the rat epididymis after efferent duct ligation or orchiectomy. Biol. Reprod. **20:** 162–181.
49. ROBAIRE, Bα(B. R. ZIRKIN. 1981. Hypophysectomy and simultaneous testosterone replacement: Effects on male rat reproductive tract and epididymal Δ^4H-5 α-reductase and 3 α-hydroxysteroid dehydrogenase. Endocrinology **109:** 1225–1233.
50. TURNER, T. T., L. L. EWING, C. E. JONES, S. S. HOWARDS & B. ZEGEYE. 1985. Androgens in the male reproductive tract fluids: Hypophysectomy and steroid replacement. Am. J. Physiol. **248:** E274-E280.
51. TINDALL, D. J., V. HANSSON, M. SAR, W. E. STUMPF, F. S. FRENCH & S. N. NEYFEH. 1974. Further studies on the accumulation and binding of androgen in the rat epididymis. Endocrinology **95:** 1119–1128.
52. LOBL, T. J., J. A. CAMPBELL, D. J. TINDALL, G. R. CUNNINGHAM & A. R. MEANS. 1980. A model for the mechanism of androgen binding, transport, and translocation to the nucleus. *In* Testicular Development, Structure, and Function. A. Steinberger & E. Steinberger, Eds.: 323–330. Raven Press. New York.

Differential Patterns of Regulated Gene Expression in the Adult Rat Epididymis[a]

JAMES DOUGLASS,[b] SUSANNE H. GARRETT, AND JAMES E. GARRETT

The Vollum Institute
Oregon Health Sciences University
3181 SW Sam Jackson Park Road
Portland, Oregon 97201

INTRODUCTION

The epididymis represents an important component of the excurrent duct system within the mammalian male reproductive tract. The main function of the tissue is to receive immature sperm from the testis, modify them by the interaction of secreted peptide products, and store functional sperm for release to the vas deferens. The organ is made up of a single continuous, highly convoluted tubule. The major epithelial cell type lining the tubule has been classified as a principal cell. These cells are highly secretory in nature, and are continuous throughout the organ.

Polarized principal cells lining the caput tubule share many common characteristics; for example, the presence of microvilli, the lack of secretory granules, and a similar localization within the tubule. However, a variety of morphological and biochemical criteria have confirmed the concept of specialization among this class of cells. Morphologically, the size and shape of principal cells changes throughout the caput epididymis.[1,2] Principal cells are large and highly columnar in the tubule of the proximal caput, while cells are much smaller and cuboid in shape within the tubule of the distal caput. Additional morphological variation within the caput epididymis is observed regarding the diameter of the tubule lumen and the number of spermatozoa located within the lumen. Although variation in tissue and cellular morphology is suggestive of specialized cellular function, such correlations are often difficult to demonstrate. Direct evidence of principal cell specialization, however, is reflected in studies documenting alterations in the protein composition of luminal fluid from different regions of the epididymis.[3-8] Such differences are presumably the result of regional specialization regarding the synthesis and secretion of proteins from principal cells. It is at least partially through this mechanism that spermatozoa are exposed to differing biochemical environments as they traverse the length of the tubule.

The studies described here document regional specialization regarding transcriptional activity of several genes within the efferent duct/caput epididymis. Such spe-

[a] These studies were supported by USPHS Grant HD-25970 (to J.D.), and F32-NS08068 (to J.E.G.).
[b] Author to whom correspondence should be addressed.

cialized mRNA synthesis supports the concept that region-specific patterns of transcriptional expression along the epididymal tubule serve as the major molecular basis underlying region-specific patterns of luminal proteins within the tubule. Additionally, multiple testicular factors appear to regulate expression of these mRNAs, suggesting that a complex array of nuclear events and signals received by the principal cells determine the transcriptional status of genes expressed within this epididymal cell type.

REGIONAL SPECIFICITY OF GENE EXPRESSION IN THE EPIDIDYMIS

Four genes which are transcriptionally active within the epididymis were chosen for analysis. One gene (whose cDNA is designated as IB15 throughout the text) encodes the enzyme peptidyl-prolyl *cis-trans* isomerase (PPI), also referred to as cyclophilin. PPI is thought to function in directing the folding of nascent proteins within the cell,[9] thus PPI mRNA is abundantly expressed in nearly all rat tissue and cell types examined, and is well conserved across a broad phylogenetic spectrum.[10] Moreover, IB15 mRNA appears to be constitutively expressed in nearly every cell type examined, making it an excellent control transcript for nonregulated expression.

A second gene encodes an epididymis-specific protein secreted by principal cells, protein B/C. In the caput epididymis, this secreted protein accounts for approximately 10% of the total luminal fluid protein, and is dependent on androgen for its expression.[3,11,12] Protein B/C is not glycosylated and does not appear to directly interact with epididymal spermatozoa. Its amino acid sequence has served to assign it to the $\alpha_{2\mu}$-globulin family of proteins,[13] suggesting that it may function as a retinoic acid binding protein.

The third gene examined encodes another epididymis-specific protein secreted by principal cells, protein D/E. As with protein B/C, protein D/E also accounts for nearly 10% of the total luminal fluid protein, and is dependent on androgen for its expression.[14,15] This glycoprotein has been shown to adhere to the head of epididymal spermatozoa,[16] and may serve a functional role in the fertilization process. The primary sequence of protein D/E bears limited homology to that of carboxypeptidase Y, suggesting that it may function to post-translationally modify luminal or sperm-associated proteins.[14]

The final gene examined encodes the opioid peptide precursor, proenkephalin (for review, see ref. 17). In the central nervous system, proenkephalin is proteolytically processed to generate the enkephalin pentapeptides, Met- and Leu-enkephalin. These peptides are stored in secretory granules, released into the synapse, and function as neurotransmitters and neuromodulators following high affinity binding to the μ and δ subclass of opioid receptors. Proenkephalin is also expressed in non-neuronal tissues such as the pituitary, adrenal, heart, ovary, uterus, testis, vas deferens, and epididymis. Non-neuronal cell types such as glial cells and lymphocytes also express the proenkephalin precursor. In the majority of these tissue and cell types, however, it appears that proenkephalin is not proteolytically processed to the small enkephalins. Rather, large fragments of the protein appear to be secreted. This has led to speculation that in non-neuronal cells, large forms of proenkephalin are secreted and perform as yet undefined functional roles via a non-opioid receptor mediated mechanism.

To determine the site of transcriptional expression of these genes within the epi-

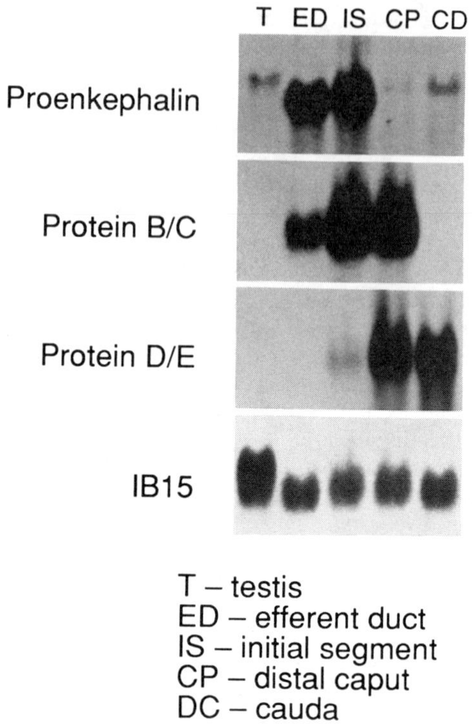

FIGURE 1. Regional distribution of specific mRNAs in the rat epididymis. RNAs (20 μg in each lane) prepared from dissected regions of the adult rat reproductive tract were analyzed by Northern blot. ^{32}P-radiolabeled cRNA probes to rat proenkephalin, protein B/C, protein D/E, and IB15 (cyclophilin) were used to detect the corresponding species of mRNA. (Adapted from J. E. Garrett *et al.*,[18] with permission from *Molecular Endocrinology.*)

didymis, Northern blot analysis was first employed (FIG. 1). Total RNA was extracted from rat testis, efferent duct, epididymal initial segment, distal caput epididymis and cauda epididymis. The RNA was separated by size on a denaturing formaldehyde/agarose gel, and transferred to nylon membrane. The membrane was then incubated with ^{32}P-labeled cRNA probes to rat PPI, protein B/C, protein D/E and proenkephalin mRNA, followed by washing and autoradiography.[18]

As expected, PPI mRNA is present at equivalent levels in all regions of the epididymis. Proenkephalin mRNA is present at relatively high levels in the efferent duct and initial segment regions, and detectable at much lower levels in all other regions. Within the initial segment, we estimate that proenkephalin transcripts make up as much as 5% of the total cellular pool of poly(A) mRNA. Protein B/C transcripts are abundant in total RNA isolated from the efferent duct, initial segment, and caput epididymis, with no observable transcripts localized to the cauda. Protein D/E transcripts are present at high levels in the caput and cauda epididymis, observable in the initial segment region, and absent in the efferent duct. Thus, each species of mRNA examined reveals a unique pattern of transcriptional expression within the adult rat epididymis.

In situ histochemical analysis of tissue sections from adult rat epididymis was also employed to define more accurately the region of the tissue, as well as the epididymal cell type(s), expressing the transcripts. The tissue was prepared, sectioned and incubated with ^{35}S-radiolabeled cRNA probes as described elsewhere.[18] Sections were hybridized and washed under stringent conditions, and emulsion-coated slides were exposed at 4°C for 6–16 days. The sections were then analyzed for silver grain density by both dark field and light field microscopy. A description of the hybridization pattern observed for each probe is given below, with a pictorial representation shown in FIGURE 2.

Radiolabeled proenkephalin cRNA grain density was highly localized to a small region of the initial segment of the epididymis, adjacent to the connection with the efferent duct. No hybridization was observed within the efferent duct, suggesting that efferent duct mRNA analyzed by Northern blot contained mRNA from the initial segment as well. Hybridization was also specific to the principal cell population, suggesting that proenkephalin-derived products may be secreted into the luminal fluid. Within the initial segment, two distinct patterns of hybridization are observed. Beginning at the junction of the efferent duct and initial segment, every principal cell around the circumference of the tubule contains a high density of silver grains. Moving distally, a lower percentage of principal cells within the tubule contain a high density of silver grains. The molecular or cellular basis underlying this differential pattern of expression is unknown. There are no hybridization-positive cells observed in the caput epididymis distal to the end of zone 1.

The silver grain density profile resulting from hybridization of the protein D/E cRNA probe is dramatically different from that described above. No hybridization-positive cells are observed within the efferent duct, initial segment and proximal caput through zone 2. Weak hybridization begins near the end of zone 3 caput, and becomes uniformly strong in tubules representing the proximal region of zone 4. This strong hybridization pattern extends through the length of the caput epididymis. Silver grain densities are localized to the principal cells of the tubule. In these distinct hybridization positive areas, every principal cell within the tubule appears to express the protein D/E transcript, and little heterogeneity is observed regarding the silver grain density per cell. In the caput, protein D/E is located predominantly in the lumen of the epididymal tubule beyond the flexure of the organ well into zone 4,[19] and the *in situ* histochemical results identifying epithelial cells containing protein D/E mRNA correlate well with this observation.

When the protein B/C cRNA probe is used for *in situ* histochemical analysis, strong uniform silver grain density is observed over tubules throughout the entire caput epididymis, from zone 1 through zone 5. Some hybridization also occurs within the junctional segment of the efferent duct. Again, in these hybridization positive areas, every principal cell within the tubule appears to express the protein B/C transcript, and little heterogeneity is observed regarding the silver grain density per cell. The *in situ* histochemical pattern described here is indeed quite similar to the immunohistochemical pattern described previously.[19] One notable exception, however, is the observation that protein B/C mRNA is synthesized in zone 1, while neither immunochemical nor culturing techniques have demonstrated secretion of protein B/C into tubules of this region. One possible explanation for this observation is that protein B/C is secreted from zone 1 epithelial cells at a rate faster than that from more distal epithelial cells. Alternatively, region specific patterns of degradation or absorption could account for this observation.

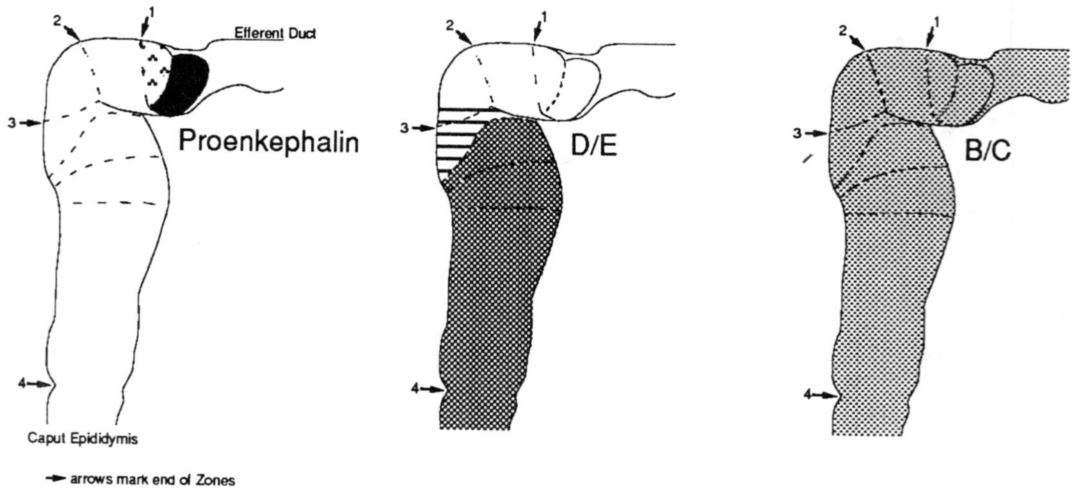

FIGURE 2. Pictorial diagram of specific patterns of gene expression within the adult rat efferent duct/caput epididymis following *in situ* hybridization analysis. Sites of transcription of the proenkephalin, protein B/C, and protein D/E genes are diagrammed. For each cRNA probe employed, solid areas represent regions exhibiting strong patterns of *in situ* hybridization, while patched areas represent regions of decreasing *in situ* hybridization intensities. Differences in shading intensities are not intended to represent differences in silver grain densities between any two species of cRNA probe.

TRANSCRIPTIONAL REGULATION OF GENE EXPRESSION WITHIN THE EPIDIDYMIS

In common with other mammalian male reproductive tissues, the epididymis is dependent upon androgens for its normal development, as well as the maintenance of proper structure and physiological function in the adult.[20] Androgen receptors have been localized mainly to epithelial principal cells,[21] suggesting that this specific epididymal cell type is dependent on androgen for maintenance of function. For example, androgen-dependent transcription of the protein B/C and protein D/E genes within epididymal principal cells has been previously documented.[11-15]

There is also evidence to suggest that the biosynthesis of certain epididymal products is dependent upon testicular factors other than androgen. This dependence on putative gonadal factors is most evident in the initial segment region, and is suggested by several observations. In bilaterally castrated animals given androgen replacement therapy, only partial prevention of regression of principal cell morphology is observed.[22] Also, in efferent duct–ligated animals, where circulating androgen levels remain normal, there is partial regression of initial segment principal cells, suggesting the need for testicular factors in addition to androgen.[22] Similar experimental paradigms have examined the dependence of epididymal protein synthesis on non-androgen testicular factors. In castrate animals, a number of proteins synthesized in the initial segment are absent from luminal fluid. Androgen replacement can maintain the synthesis of some proteins, but a number are still absent, suggesting the necessity of testicular factors other than androgen.[7] In the studies described below, the dependence on various testicular factors for transcriptional expression of the PPI, protein B/C, protein D/E and proenkephalin genes within the epididymis is examined by Northern blot analysis.

Castration/Androgen Replacement

To determine the direct effect of androgen on transcriptional expression, adult rats were bilaterally or unilaterally castrated. Androgen replacement in some bilaterally castrate animals was achieved by subcutaneous implant of silastic tubing containing testosterone (T). The bilaterally castrate adults provide an experimental paradigm in which all testicular factors are absent. Bilaterally castrate animals given continuous T replacement allows the assessment of androgen effects in the absence of additional gonadal factors. Unilaterally castrate animals then allow for the assessment of additional gonadal effects. Serum androgen levels were determined by radioimmunoassay (RIA), and found to be greatly reduced in bilaterally castrate animals, normal in unilaterally castrate and control animals, and two- to threefold higher than control in T-replaced animals. The animals were sacrificed 7 days following the surgical manipulation, the initial segment/caput epididymis removed, and total RNA from the tissue was subject to Northern blot analysis (FIG. 3).

As expected, PPI (*i.e.*, IB15) mRNA levels were unaltered following any surgical manipulation, indicating that castration does not have a generalized effect upon principal cell gene expression. Protein B/C and protein D/E mRNA levels, on the other hand, were significantly reduced compared to control values in the epididymis from bilaterally castrate animals. Androgen replacement, however, prevented completely this decline, suggesting a direct effect of androgen on transcription of these genes.

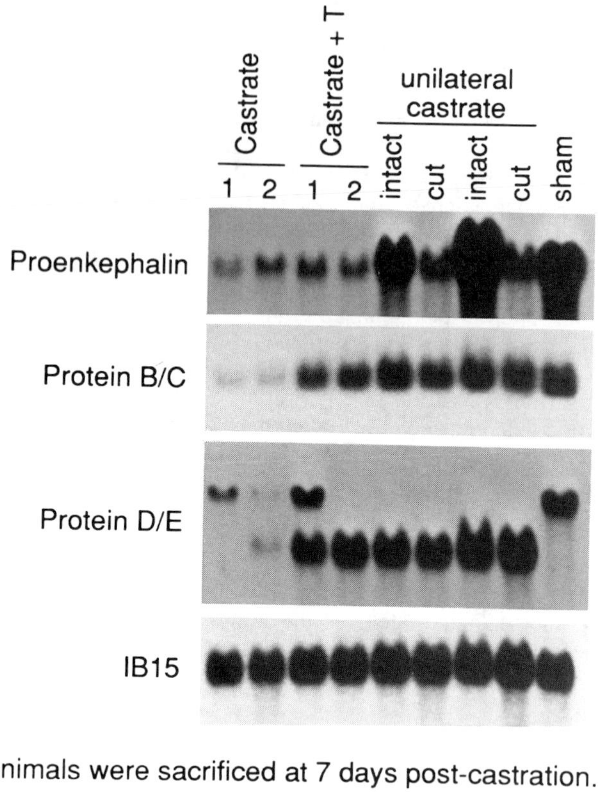

FIGURE 3. Castration differentially regulates the levels of specific epididymal transcripts. Northern blot analysis was performed on total RNA (20 μg) from initial segment/caput epididymis following specific surgical and pharmacological manipulations. Animals (adult Sprague-Dawley rats) were sacrificed 7 days after the noted manipulations. ^{32}P-radiolabeled cRNA probes to rat proenkephalin, protein B/C, protein D/E, and IB15 (cyclophilin) were used to detect the corresponding species of mRNA. (Adapted from J. E. Garrett *et al.*[18] with permission from *Molecular Endocrinology.*)

Additionally, no difference in mRNA levels was observed in either cut or intact epididymis from unilaterally castrate animals, suggesting that non-androgen testicular factors do not contribute to correct transcriptional expression of these genes in the epididymis. Proenkephalin mRNA levels revealed yet another distinct pattern of transcriptional expression. mRNA levels were dramatically reduced in bilaterally castrate animals, with androgen replacement unable to prevent the decline. This observation implies that the proenkephalin gene is not directly regulated by androgen. Rather, a non-androgen testicular factor appears to positively affect transcription of the gene. This is suggested by the observation that mRNA levels in unilaterally castrate animals were significantly reduced in the epididymis from the castrate side, but normal in the epididymis isolated from the intact side.

Thus, three distinct patterns of transcriptional expression emerge from this study. One pattern, represented by IB15 mRNA, is that of constitutive expression, unaffected by any gonadal factor. A second pattern is that of androgen-regulated transcription, exemplified by expression of protein B/C and protein D/E mRNA. A third pattern suggests the involvement of a non-androgen testicular factor(s) on transcriptional expression, and is exemplified by proenkephalin gene expression in the initial segment.

Efferent-Duct Ligation

The unilateral castration experiment suggested that an intact connection between the testis and epididymis allows for the transport of a testicular factor into the epididymal tubule, resulting in the maintenance of proenkephalin gene expression within the initial segment. If this is indeed the case, then unilateral ligation of the efferent duct should reduce proenkephalin mRNA levels within the epididymis of the ligated side, while having no effect on mRNA levels within non-ligated epididymis. FIGURE 4 represents the results of such an experiment.

Adult rats were anesthetized, and a suture was tightly wrapped twice around the efferent ducts. Care was taken to avoid the vasculature entering the testis in close proximity to the efferent ducts. As a control, the efferent ducts on the contralateral side of the same animal were loosely wrapped with a suture, so as not to impede the flow of testicular fluid. At 1, 3, and 6 days following surgery the animals were sacrificed, epididymis from the ligated and intact sides removed, and total RNA subjected to Northern blot analysis. No change in IB15, protein B/C, and protein D/E (not shown) mRNA levels was observed, confirming that expression of these genes is not dependent on the presence of a non-androgen testicular factor. However, proenkephalin mRNA levels were dramatically reduced in a time-dependent fashion within the ligated epididymis. Twenty-four hours following duct ligation, proenkephalin mRNA levels had begun to drop, and at 6 days following ligation the mRNA was barely detectable. No changes were observed within epididymis from the non-ligated controls. These data serve to strengthen the notion that a non-androgen testicular factor controls proenkephalin gene expression in the initial segment.

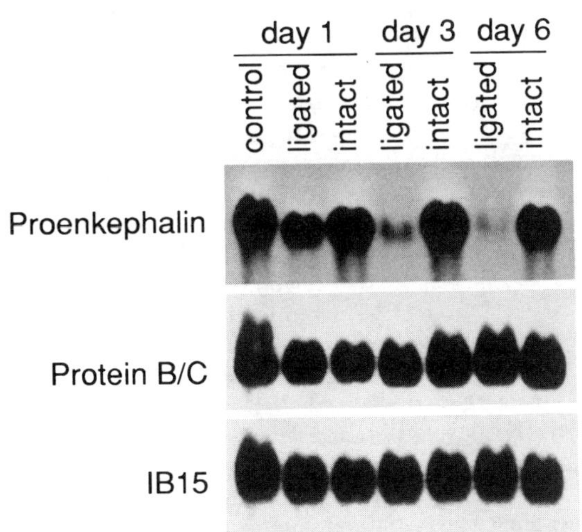

FIGURE 4. Ligation of the efferent duct leads to a rapid decline in proenkephalin mRNA levels in the epididymis. Northern blot analysis was performed on total RNA (20 μg) from initial segment tissue removed from ligated or intact sides at 1, 3, or 6 days following efferent duct ligation. ^{32}P-radiolabeled cRNA probes to rat proenkephalin, protein B/C, and IB15 (cyclophilin) were used to detect the corresponding species of mRNA. (Adapted from J. E. Garrett *et al.*,[18] with permission from *Molecular Endocrinology.*)

Developmental Aspects of Gene Expression

In order to gain insight regarding the nature of the testicular factor controlling epididymal proenkephalin gene expression, the developmental profile of expression was studied. The time course of rat gonadal development has been well characterized. Androgen production by testicular Leydig cells and germ cell proliferation show pronounced increases at 20–25 days of age.[23] Additionally, androgen receptors are first present in epididymal epithelial cells at day 20.[24] Day 44 of postgestational male rat development corresponds to the time at which spermatozoa are first released from the seminiferous tubules and enter the epididymal lumen.[2] The number of spermatozoa within the epididymis increases from day 44, finally reaching adult steady state levels at day 100.[25]

To determine if epididymal proenkephalin gene expression is correlative with any of these time-dependent events, total RNA from efferent duct/caput epididymis was isolated from animals at 15, 20, 22, 24, 26, 28, 30, 34, 40, 44, 50, and 90 days following birth, and subjected to Northern blot analysis (FIG. 5). IB15 mRNA levels appeared to be equivalent at all times studied, again indicating that this is a constitutively expressed gene. Protein B/C and protein D/E mRNA levels became apparent at day 20, were dramatically increased at day 22, and appeared to reach steady-state levels by day 26–30. This time course of appearance correlates well with the establishment of the androgen/androgen receptor system within the reproductive tract. In contrast, epididymal proenkephalin mRNA levels, while detectable, remain relatively low through the first 40 days of development. At 44 days of age a dramatic increase in mRNA levels was observed, and these levels continued to rise from day 44 to 90. This time course of expression closely follows that of the arrival and subsequent increase of testicular spermatozoa within the epididymis, suggesting the involvement of spermatozoa in the regulation of epididymal proenkephalin gene expression.

Effects of Busulfan on Epididymal Gene Expression

To more directly test the aforementioned hypothesis, a pharmacological agent that produces a transient depletion of spermatozoa from the testis and epididymis was employed. Busulfan is an alkylating agent which, at the appropriate dose, results in the destruction of the earliest stages of proliferating spermatogonia.[26] Later germ cell stages are unaffected by busulfan treatment and complete development. Approximately 5 weeks following busulfan treatment the germinal epithelium recovers and the process of spermatogenesis proceeds in a normal fashion. Busulfan treatment thus provides a means of depleting the adult epididymis of spermatozoa from approximately weeks 7 through 12 following the administration of the drug.

Adult rats were injected i.p. with a single dose of busulfan (10 mg/kg) and sacrificed at 6, 11, and 15 weeks following treatment. An oil-injected animal was sacrificed at 6 weeks and served as a control. Total RNA was then isolated from the initial segment of the epididymis and subjected to Northern blot analysis, with the results shown in FIGURE 6. As expected, IB15, protein B/C and protein D/E (not shown) epididymal mRNA levels were unaffected by the treatment. Proenkephalin mRNA levels, on the other hand, were dramatically negatively affected by busulfan treatment. At both 6 and 11 weeks following treatment, mRNA levels were greatly reduced. Microscopic evaluation of luminal contents revealed the presence of spermatozoa at the 6 week

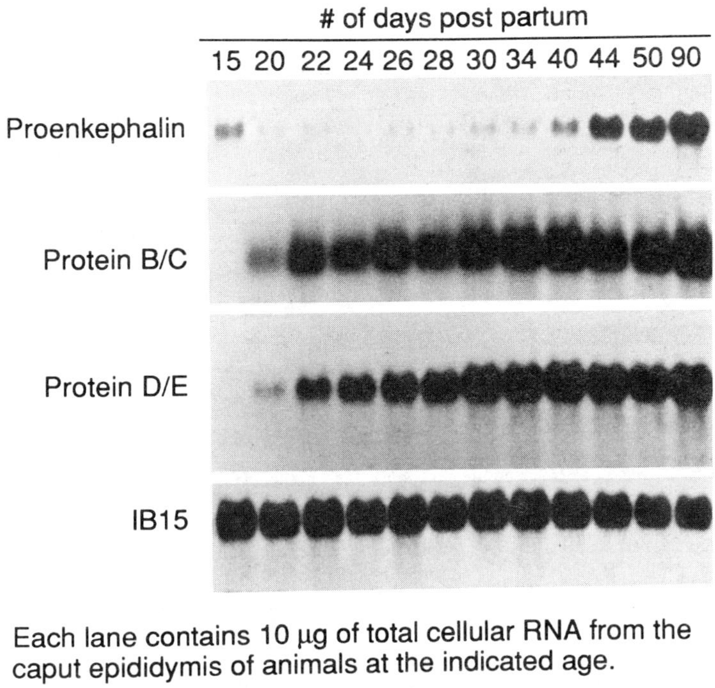

FIGURE 5. Developmental profile of epididymal gene expression. Total RNA was prepared from efferent duct/caput epididymis tissue obtained from Sprague-Dawley rats at the indicated days of age. Northern blot analysis was then performed on 20 µg RNA samples, using ^{32}P-radiolabeled cRNA probes to detect rat proenkephalin, protein B/C, protein D/E, and IB15 (cyclophilin) mRNA. An increase of proenkephalin mRNA levels in the epididymis coincides with the entry of spermatozoa into the epididymal lumen. (Adapted from J. E. Garrett *et al.*,[18] with permission from *Molecular Endocrinology.*)

time point (although no attempt was made to quantitate the number of spermatozoa), while at the 11 week time point virtually no spermatozoa were observed. At 15 weeks, spermatozoa were again present in the epididymis, and proenkephalin mRNA levels, although still reduced compared to control values, were greatly elevated relative to the earlier time point. Although we cannot rule out the possibility of a direct effect of busulfan on testicular somatic cells or epididymal epithelial cells, the close correlation of the decline and reappearance of proenkephalin mRNA in the initial segment with the decline and reappearance of spermatozoa is highly suggestive of a direct regulatory relationship.

FATE OF PROENKEPHALIN SYNTHESIZED IN THE INITIAL SEGMENT

The functional role of protein products of several genes investigated here is either known, or can be suggested based on sequence homology with other characterized

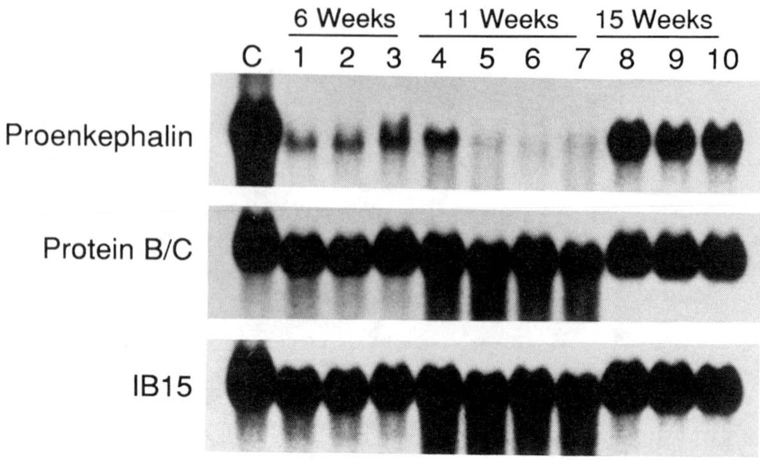

FIGURE 6. Effects of the alkylating agent, busulfan, on the levels of specific epididymal transcripts. Total RNA was prepared from initial segment tissue at the times noted following a single injection of busulfan. An oil-injected control was sacrificed at 6 weeks following injection. Northern blot analysis was then performed on 20 μg RNA samples, using ^{32}P-radiolabeled cRNA probes to detect rat proenkephalin, protein B/C, and IB15 (cyclophilin) mRNA. (Adapted from J. E. Garrett *et al.*,[18] with permission from *Molecular Endocrinology.*)

proteins. PPI functions within the cell to help direct the proper folding of nascent proteins.[9] The amino acid sequence of protein B/C has assigned it to the $\alpha_{2\mu}$-globulin family of proteins,[13] and suggests that it may function as a retinoic acid binding/carrier protein within the luminal fluid. Also, the amino acid sequence of protein D/E reveals limited homology with metalloproteins such as carboxypeptidase Y,[14] suggesting that it may serve to modify sperm-associated and/or luminal proteins.

Determination of the functional role of epididymal proenkephalin-derived product(s), however, presents a challenge. The gene is highly transcriptionally active within principal cells of the initial segment, suggesting that the cells are capable of synthesizing large amounts of the proenkephalin precursor. Kilpatrick and co-workers have also shown that proenkephalin mRNA in the caput epididymis is present on high molecular weight polysomes,[27] suggesting that the mRNA is efficiently translated. The same group also used Sephadex G-75 chromatography to show that the majority of epididymal proenkephalin is proteolytically processed to large molecular weight forms between 10–30 kD in size.[27] Very little, if any, free Met-enkephalin pentapeptide was observed in the caput epididymis.

To better determine the fate of epididymal proenkephalin, Met-enkephalin levels were determined by radioimmunoassay (RIA) of protein extracts from various regions of the epididymis, as well as various components of the epididymis. The extracts were assayed both before and after trypsin/carboxypeptidase B (CPB) treatment in order to estimate relative levels of the various forms of proenkephalin-derived products within the tissue.[28,29] The antibody used in these studies was to the Met-enkephalin pentapeptide. When the Met-enkephalin moiety is contained within larger processed forms of the proenkephalin precursor, however, the antibody is unable to recognize and interact with the epitope. If, though, the large forms are treated with the enzymes trypsin and CPB, the Met-enkephalin moieties contained within the large fragments are liberated, and can then be detected by the Met-enkephalin antibody. Thus, immunoreactive material detected without enzymatic treatment represents *free* Met-enkephalin, while that detected prior to enzymatic treatment represents *cryptic* Met-enkephalin, or that contained within larger proenkephalin-derived products.

TABLE 1 shows the levels of free and cryptic Met-enkephalin immunoreactivity (per gram of wet weight tissue) in various regions of the rat epididymis compared to that found in rat brain. In the latter tissue, relatively high levels of free Met-enkephalin are present, as trypsin/CPB treatment only increases levels approximately twofold. Of the various regions of the epididymis examined, the initial segment had the highest levels of free Met-enkephalin immunoreactivity. This value, however, was at least 20-fold lower than that observed for brain. Treatment of initial segment extracts with trypsin/CPB dramatically increased Met-enkephalin levels; an approximately 30-fold increase was observed. Met-enkephalin levels in other regions of the epididymis also increased following treatment, although not nearly as dramatically. These data suggest that the initial segment indeed contains relatively high levels of large proenkephalin-derived peptides, with very little free Met-enkephalin present. These levels rapidly decline in regions distal to the initial segment, suggesting rapid degradation of any and all forms of proenkephalin in these areas.

A second study was aimed at determining the specific epididymal component containing initial segment-derived proenkephalin products. As above, the epididymis was dissected into various regions; initial segment, caput epididymis, and cauda epididymis. From these regions, specific components were isolated; the tubule and constituent cells, spermatozoa, and luminal fluid. Protein extracts from these components were then assayed by RIA for Met-enkephalin content. As before, the extracts were assayed both before and after trypsin/CPB treatment in order to estimate relative levels of the various forms of proenkephalin-derived products. The results are depicted in FIGURE 7 as the percentage of total epididymal Met-enkephalin immunoreactivity present in each epididymal region and component.

The first bar represents the previously stated observation that the majority of epididymal proenkephalin products are localized to the initial segment, and present as

TABLE 1. Localization of Proenkephalin Products in the Adult Rat Epididymis[a]

	Met-enkephalin ir (p mol/g wet wt. tissue)	
Tissue	Free (−T/CPB)	Cryptic (+T/CPB)
Initial segment	3.8	111.6 ± 36
Caput epididymus	<0.5	4.4 ± 0.8
Corpus epididymus	<0.5	3.9 ± 0.9
Cauda epididymus	<0.5	1.7 ± 0.5
Brain	72.8	166.4 ± 59

[a] Adult Sprague-Dawley rats were sacrificed, followed by immediate removal of tissue. The tissue was dissected, frozen on dry ice, and weighed. Total protein was extracted as previously described.[28] Some of the extract was treated with TPCK-trypsin and carboxypeptidase B (CPB) as described,[28] to liberate any Met-enkephalin moieties which may be contained within large fragments of proenkephalin. Samples were assayed for Met-enkephalin content by radioimmunoassay using previously characterized antisera to synthetic Met-enkephalin. Met-enkephalin measured without trypsin/CPB treatment is referred to as Free, while that observed following trypsin/CPB treatment is referred to as Cryptic.

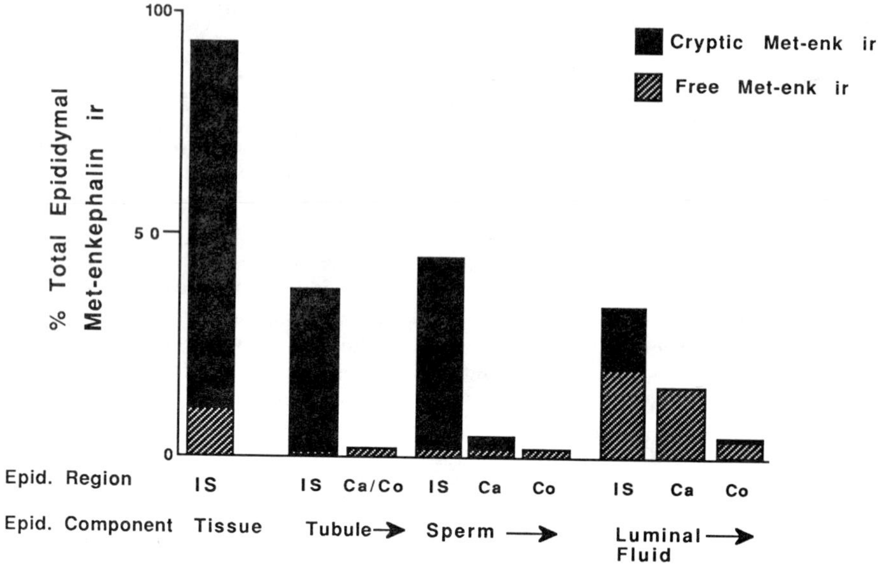

FIGURE 7. Fate of proenkephalin in the rat epididymis. Specific epididymal regions (initial segment, IS; caput epididymis, Ca; corpus epididymis, Co) and components (whole tissue, tubule and component cells, spermatozoa, and luminal fluid) were isolated, and total protein extracted.[28] Some of the extract was treated with TPCK-trypsin and carboxypeptidase B (CPB) as described[28] to liberate any cryptic Met-enkephalin moieties. Samples were assayed for Met-enkephalin content by radioimmunoassay using previously characterized antisera to synthetic Met-enkephalin. The values are presented as percent total epididymal Met-enkephalin immunoreactivity, both free and cryptic, present in each epididymal region and component.

cryptic Met-enkephalin. As predicted from the *in situ* histochemical analysis, when extracts from the epididymal tubule and constituent cell types are assayed, virtually all of the immunoreactive material is found in the initial segment as cryptic Met-enkephalin. However, the immunoreactive material represents only approximately one third of that found within the intact tissue. When protein extracts from purified luminal spermatozoa are analyzed, again virtually all of the immunoreactive material is localized to the initial segment as cryptic Met-enkephalin. Little material is associated with caput or cauda spermatozoa. This observation suggests that large form(s) of proenkephalin are released from initial segment principal cells, and interact with luminal spermatozoa. When protein extracts from luminal fluid are examined, the majority of the immunoreactive material is still found in the initial segment, but this time larger quantities are found in the caput and cauda luminal fluid. Also, the ratio of cryptic to free Met-enkephalin changes when luminal fluid is analyzed, with much higher levels of free Met-enkephalin now observed.

When taken together, these data suggest the following fate of proenkephalin synthesized within principal epithelial cells of the initial segment. A portion of the synthesized protein is secreted in the form of high molecular weight proenkephalin products, some of which then becomes associated with luminal spermatozoa. The cryptic/free Met-enkephalin ratio is similar in these initial segment components, implying that initially the material associated with spermatozoa is of a high molecular weight. However, once spermatozoa reach the caput epididymis, the large proenkephalin products no longer appear to be associated with this cell type. Proenkephalin products within the luminal fluid are apparently rapidly degraded. Low levels of cryptic Met-enkephalin are found in initial segment fluid; most is present as free Met-enkephalin. Trace amounts of free Met-enkephalin are observed in luminal fluid from regions distal to the initial segment, suggesting complete degradation of all proenkephalin-derived products.

These descriptive studies still leave the question of potential function unanswered. Virtually no proenkephalin-derived products are found in any component of the epididymis distal to the initial segment. This suggests that any functional consequence of proenkephalin synthesis is transient in nature, and lies in the initial segment and adjacent caput epididymis. The observation that cryptic Met-enkephalin products interact with initial segment spermatozoa may be suggestive of a potential functional role regarding this specific cell type and localization.

SUMMARY

Specialization among the principal epithelial cells of the epididymal tubule is documented following the analysis of transcriptional activity of four distinct species of mRNA. *In situ* histochemical analysis revealed a unique pattern of expression for each transcript. This observation supports the concept that region-specific patterns of transcriptional expression along the epididymal tubule serve as the major molecular basis underlying region-specific patterns of luminal proteins within the tubule. Additionally, multiple testicular factors appear to regulate expression of these mRNAs. The transcript encoding peptidyl-prolyl *cis-trans* isomerase is constitutively expressed. Those encoding the major secretory proteins, protein B/C and protein D/E, are directly regulated by testicular androgen. That encoding the opioid peptide precursor, proenkephalin, is regulated by a non-androgen testicular factor(s), specifically, spermatozoa or a spermatozoa-related factor. Thus, a complex array of nuclear events and signals received by the principal cells serve to determine the transcriptional status of genes expressed within this epididymal cell type.

REFERENCES

1. Reid, B. L. & K. W. Clelend. 1957. Aust. J. Zool. **5:** 223–246.
2. Hamilton, D. W. 1975. *In* Handbook of Physiology. R. Greep & E. Astwood, Eds. Vol. **5:** 303–317. American Physiology Society. Washington, D.C.
3. Brooks, D. E. & S. J. Higgins. 1980. J. Reprod. Fertil. **59:** 363–375.
4. Olson, G. E. & B. T. Hinton. 1985. J. Androl. **6:** 20–35.
5. Bartlett, R. J., O. A. Lea, E. C. Murphy & F. S. French. 1984. Ann. N. Y. Acad. Sci. **438:** 29–38.
6. Flickinger, C. J. 1981. Biol. Reprod. **25:**871–883.
7. Brooks, D. E. 1983. Mol. Cell Endocrinol. **29:** 255–270.
8. Holland, M. K. & M.-C. Orgebin-Crist. 1988. Biol. Reprod. **38:** 487–496.
9. Takahashi, N., T. Hayano & M. Suzuki. 1989. Nature **337:** 473–475.
10. Danielson, P. E., S. Forss-Peter, M. A. Brow, L. Calavetta, J. Douglass, R. J. Milner & J. G. Sutcliffe. 1988. DNA **7:** 261–267.
11. Brooks, D. E. 1987. Mol. Cell Endocrinol. **53:** 59–66.
12. Brooks, D. E., A. R. Means, E. J. Wright, S. P. Singh & K. K. Tiver. 1983. J. Biol. Chem. **11:** 4956–4961.

13. BROOKS, D. E. 1987. Biochem. Int. **14:** 235–240.
14. BROOKS, D. E., A. R. MEANS, E. J. WRIGHT, S. P. SINGH & K. K. TIVER. 1986. Eur. J. Biochem. **161:** 13–18.
15. CHAREST, N. J., D. R. JOSEPH, E. M. WILSON & F. S. FRENCH. 1988. Mol. Endocrinol. **2:** 999–1004.
16. BROOKS, D. E. & K. TIVER. 1983. J. Reprod. Fertil. **69:** 651–657.
17. AKIL, H., S. J. WATSON, E. YOUNG, M. E. LEWIS, H. KHACHATURIAN & J. M. WALKER. 1984. Ann. Rev. Neurosci. **7:** 223–255.
18. GARRETT, J. E., S. H. GARRETT & J. DOUGLASS. 1990. Mol. Endocrinol. **4:** 108–118.
19. BROOKS, D. E. 1987. Ann. N. Y. Acad. Sci. **513:** 179–194.
20. ORGEBIN-CRIST, M.-C., B. J. DANZO & J. DAVIES. 1975. *In* Handbook of Physiology. R. Greep & E. Astwood, Eds. Vol. **5:** 319–337. American Physiology Society. Washington, D.C.
21. SAR, M., V. E. QUARMBY, D. B. LUBAHN, D. R. JOSEPH, E. M. WILSON & F. S. FRENCH. 1988. *In* Regulation of Testicular Function: Signalling Molecules and Cell-Cell Communication. Abstracts from the 10th Annual Testis Workshop. Baltimore, MD. Abst. 11.
22. FAWCETT, D. W. & A. P. HOFFER. 1979. Biol. Reprod. **20:** 162–181.
23. STEINBERGER, E. & A. STEINBERGER. 1975. *In* Handbook of Physiology. R. Greep & E. Astwood, Eds. Vol. **4:** 325–334. American Physiology Society. Washington, D.C.
24. CALANDRA, R. S., E. J. PODESTA, M. A. RIVAROLA & J. A. BLAQUIER. 1974. Steroids **24:** 507–518.
25. ROBB, Q. W., R. P. AMANN & G. J. KILLIAN. 1978. J. Reprod. Fertil. **54:** 103–107.
26. JACKSON, H., Ed. 1966. Antifertility Compounds in the Male and Female. Charles C Thomas. Springfield, IL.
27. KEW, D., D. F. JIN, F. KIM, T. LADDIS & D. L. KILPATRICK. 1989. Mol. Endocrinol. **3:** 1191–1196.
28. THOMAS, G., L. THOMAS, B. A. THORNE & E. HERBERT. 1988. Biochime **70:** 89–97.
29. LINDBERG, I. & G. THOMAS. 1990. Endocrinology **126:** 480–487.

Developmental Regulation of Epithelial- and Placental-Cadherin mRNAs in the Rat Epididymis[a]

DANIEL G. CYR AND BERNARD ROBAIRE[b]

Department of Pharmacology and Therapeutics
Centre for the Study of Reproduction
McGill University
3655 Drummond Street
Montréal, Québec, H3G 1Y6 Canada

INTRODUCTION

During postnatal development the epididymis undergoes substantial changes. From day 8 to day 21 after birth the principal cells of the convoluted tubule will form junctional complexes which may lead to the formation of the blood-epididymal barrier.[1] Once the Leydig cells in the testis begin to secrete testosterone (days 28–35), the epididymis will undergo a dramatic growth phase, between 28 and 91 days of age, during which this tissue will increase 9-fold in weight.[2] It is not until day 49 that sperm will enter the caput epididymidis and day 56 when sperm will begin to be stored in the cauda epididymidis.[2] While the epididymis contains different cell types (principal, narrow, basal, halo, and clear cells), cell-cell interaction in the epididymis is still poorly understood.[3-5]

The interaction between principal cells in the formation of the blood-epididymal barrier has been shown histologically[1,6-10] and its integrity has been assayed using various exclusion markers.[6,11-13] The biochemical characterization of the factors which mediate the formation and maintenance of this barrier is not known.

Cadherins are a family of transmembrane proteins which mediate calcium-dependent intercellular adhesion.[14-17] Three cadherins were initially identified: epithelial cadherin (E-Cad), neural cadherin (N-Cad), and placental cadherin (P-Cad). It has recently been reported that two other cadherins (truncated cadherin[18] and retinal cadherin[17] have also been isolated; it has further been proposed that there may be other cadherins yet to be isolated.[17] Cadherins mediate homotypic intercellular adhesion and have been implicated in the formation of adherens and tight junctions[18-21] (FIG. 1).

Since junctional complexes between principal cells found in the epididymis are mediated in a calcium-dependent manner, as determined by cell separation studies,[22-25] we propose that these complexes are mediated by cadherins. Since cadherins have been shown to be important during embryonic organogenesis,[14,15,26] a developmental

[a] This study was supported by grants from the Medical Research Council of Canada. D. G. C. is an MRC-Ciba Geigy postdoctoral fellow.

[b] Author to whom correspondence should be addressed.

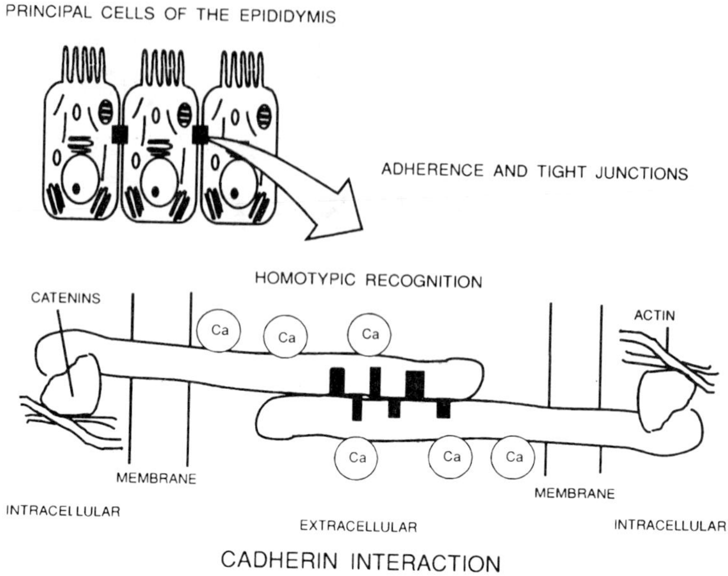

FIGURE 1. A schematic diagram demonstrating a hypothetical homotypic cadherin interaction between two principal cells of the epididymis.

study was done to determine which cadherin mRNAs are present in the epididymis, and whether it (they) is (are) regulated during postnatal epididymal development.

MATERIALS AND METHODS

Animals

Sprague-Dawley rats (300–325 g) were purchased from Charles River Canada, Inc. (St. Constant, QC). Rats were maintained under a 14 h-light: 10 h-dark photoperiod regime and received food and water *ad libitum.* Timed pregnant female rats were brought into the lab one week prior to giving birth. Within 24 hours after birth, the pups were randomized and female pups were removed from the litters. New litters of 10 male rats were placed with each lactating rat. Rats were weaned at 24 days of age. Male rats were randomly removed and killed at weekly or biweekly intervals. Rats were ether-anesthetized and killed by cervical dislocation. Epididymides were dissected free of other tissues and subdivided into four different sections to assess the longitudinal distribution: initial segment (section 1), caput (sections 2–3), corpus (section 4), and cauda (sections 5–6), as previously described.[27] For the developmental study, RNA was isolated from the caput-corpus epididymidis (sections 1–4). This was done in order to obtain sufficient tissue from the young animals. Following the dissection, tissues were immediately frozen in liquid nitrogen and subsequently stored at −80°C. At each time point, between 3 and 30 rats were killed and tissues were pooled for RNA isolation. Each experiment was done in triplicate using three independent tissue pools.

RNA Isolation

Frozen tissues were pulverized under liquid nitrogen using a mortar and pestle. Total cellular RNA was isolated using the guanidinium isothiocyanate method and centrifugation in cesium chloride as described by Sambrook *et al.*[28] The concentration of RNA recovered from these tissues was determined spectrophotometrically.

Northern Blot Transfers

RNA samples (10 μg) were fractionated by electrophoresis on 1.2% Agarose-formaldehyde gels at 30 V for 20 h in 5× running buffer (80 mM boric acid, 16 mM sodium borate, 1 mM EDTA, pH 8.3). Following electrophoresis the gel was soaked in sterile water for 5 min and placed on an LKB vacuum-transfer apparatus. The gel was hydrolyzed in 50 mM NaOH, 10 mM NaCl for 30 min with a vacuum of 50 cm H_2O and then neutralized in 0.1 M Tris-Cl (pH 7.4) for 30 min. The RNA was transferred for 90 min in a 10× sodium citrate buffer (20× sodium citrate: 3 M NaCl, 30 mM sodium citrate; pH 7.0, SSC) onto a nylon membrane (Genescreen-plus, DuPont Canada Inc., Missassauga, ON). Following the RNA transfer the gel was removed and the membrane washed for 5 min in 5× SSC. The membrane was then baked at 80°C under vacuum for 2 h.

cDNA Probes

All three cadherin cDNA probes were kindly provided by M. Takeichi, Kyoto University. The mouse E-Cad probe is composed of two fragments of 0.6 and 2.5 kb covering the whole coding region as described by Nagafuchi *et al.*[29] The N-Cad cDNA clone was identical to the mn-2 clone described by Myatani *et al.*[30] The P-Cad probe is a 0.6 kb Hinc II-Hinc II fragment of clone 28 described by Nose *et al.*[31] Each of the denatured probes (50 ng/reaction) was labeled by random priming (Oligolabeling Kit, Pharmacia, Montréal, QC) using ^{32}P-labeled deoxycytosine triphosphate (^{32}P-dCTP, specific activity: 3000 Ci/mmol, Amersham Canada, Inc., Oakville, ON). The labeled probe was separated from non-incorporated free phosphorus using a Sephadex column (Sephadex G–50, Pharmacia) equilibrated in a Tris-EDTA buffer.[28]

18S RNA Probe

Northern blots were standardized for the amount of RNA loaded in each lane using a synthetic oligonucleotide probe recognizing the 18S RNA sequence.[32] The probe was labeled with gamma-ATP (specific activity 3000 Ci/mmol, Amersham Canada, Inc.) using the end-labeling method described by Sambrook *et al.*[28]

Hybridizations

Hybridizations of nylon membranes with the cadherin cDNA probes were done in hybridization buffer (50% formamide, 1% dextran sulfate, 1% sodium dodecyl sulfate (SDS), and 1 M NaCl) at 42°C. Membranes were prehybridized for 30 min in hybridization buffer and then hybridized with 100 μg/ml of denatured sheared salmon sperm DNA (Sigma Chemicals, St. Louis, MO) and 1–5 × 10^6 cpm of probe for 18–20 h. At the end of the hybridization period, membranes were washed twice for 5 min in 2× SSC at room temperature followed by a 60 min wash at 68°C in 2× SSC, 1% SDS, and a final wash in 0.2× SSC for 30 min at room temperature. Membranes were packed with a Kodak X-OMAT R X-ray film between 2 intensifying screens for radioautography at −80°C.

In order to reprobe the Northern blots, membranes were stripped of the cDNA probe using a solution of 0.02× SSC, 1% SDS for 30 min at 100°C. The membranes were then prepared for hybridization with the 18S oligonucleotide probe. Membranes were prehybridized in 30 ml of hybridization buffer B (6× SSC, 1× Denhardt's (100× is 10 g polyvinylpyrrolidone, 10 g bovine serum albumin, 10 g Ficoll 400, in 500 ml H_2O), 0.05% pyrophosphate, 0.5% SDS and 100 μg of salmon sperm DNA) at 42°C for 30 min. The probe (0.8 ng/ml) was then added to the hybridization buffer and the membrane was hybridized overnight at 42°C. The membrane was subsequently washed twice at room temperature in 6× SSC, 0.05% pyrophosphate and two more times in the same buffer with 1% SDS at 55°C. Membranes were packed for radioautography as previously described.

RNA Quantification

Radioautograms were scanned using an LKB laser densitometer and the integrated area under the curve for each signal was standardized against the signal for the 18S oligonucleotide probe. The linearity of the densitometric scan was determined for the apparatus and all readings presented in these experiments are within the linear range for the absorbance of the signal.

RESULTS

Longitudinal Distribution

In order to determine the presence and longitudinal distribution of cadherin mRNAs in the rat epididymis, RNA was isolated from the initial segment, caput, corpus, and cauda epididymidis from adult rats. The rat epididymis contains an mRNA transcript of 4.5 kb for E-Cad (FIG. 2). The steady-state mRNA concentrations for E-Cad are greatest in the caput and corpus epididymidis; these concentrations are fourfold higher than those in the initial segment and almost fivefold higher than those in the cauda epididymidis.

A P-Cad 4.3 kb transcript was also present in the epididymis, and its longitudinal distribution was different from that of E-Cad. Steady-state mRNA concentrations for P-Cad were distributed evenly throughout the epididymis (FIG. 2). No signal was ob-

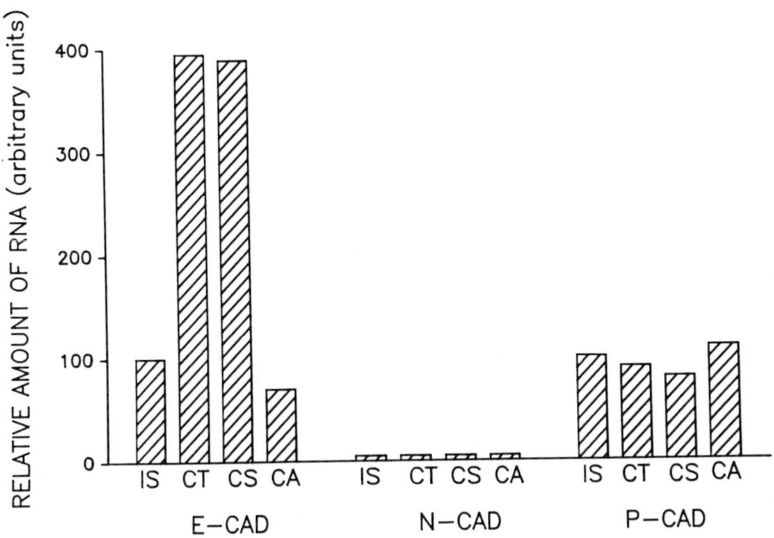

FIGURE 2. Longitudinal distribution of cadherin mRNAs in the adult rat epididymis. Total RNA (10 μg) was isolated from the initial segment, caput, corpus, and cauda epididymidis and subjected to Northern blot analysis. Each blot was standardized for the amount of RNA loaded in each lane using an oligonucleotide probe recognizing the 18S ribosomal RNA sequence and the relative concentrations were obtained by laser densitometry. Data are expressed as a % of the initial segment.

served for N-Cad in the epididymis although the cDNA probe could hybridize to two mRNA species of 4.3 and 3.5 kb in the rat brain (data not shown).

Developmental Changes in E-Cad mRNA

Having determined that the rat epididymis contained an mRNA transcript for E-Cad, a developmental study was undertaken to determine the exact nature of the developmental regulation of steady-state E-Cad mRNA. Epididymides were removed from rats from 7 to 91 days of age and total RNA was isolated from the caput-corpus region of the epididymis. Steady-state E-Cad mRNA concentrations were lowest at 7 days of age and increased to peak concentrations by day 42 (FIG. 3). A dramatic decrease in steady-state mRNA concentrations occurred from 42 to 49 days of age. This coincides with the entry of sperm into the epididymis.[33] E-Cad mRNA concentrations subsequently increased to approximately 65%, on day 56, of the peak obtained on day 42 and remained relatively constant until day 91 (FIG. 3).

Developmental Changes in P-Cad mRNA

Unlike E-Cad mRNA whose greatest concentrations were in the caput and corpus epididymidis, P-Cad mRNA concentrations were equal throughout the epididymis.

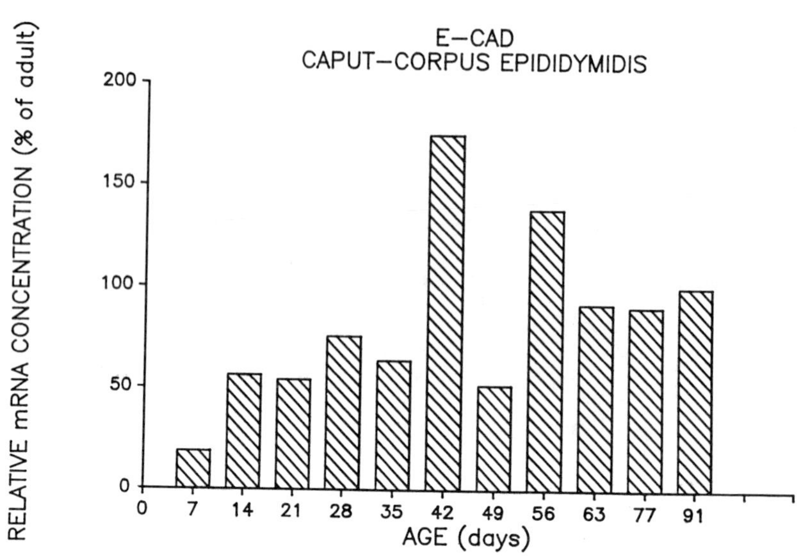

FIGURE 3. E-Cad mRNA concentrations in the caput-corpus epididymidis at different ages during post-natal development in the rat. Total RNA (10 μg) was isolated from the caput-corpus epididymidis and subjected to Northern blot analysis. Each blot was standardized for the amount of RNA loaded in each lane using an oligonucleotide probe recognizing the 18S ribosomal RNA sequence and the relative concentrations were obtained by laser densitometry. Data are expressed as a % of the 91-day-old rats.

The developmental pattern for steady-state P-Cad mRNA concentrations was also different from that of E-Cad. P-Cad mRNA concentrations in the caput-corpus epididymidis was highest in 7- and 14-day-old rats (FIG. 4). P-Cad mRNA concentrations subsequently decreased gradually as development proceeded. A slight increase was observed in the 42-day-old rats, but this appeared to be transient and steady-state concentrations subsequently decreased until day 91 (FIG. 4).

DISCUSSION

The presence of adherens and tight junctions between principal cells in the mammalian epididymis, as well as their role in formation of the blood-epididymal barrier is well documented.[1,9] The biochemical mechanisms responsible for the formation of these important cell contacts in the epididymis remain poorly understood. In the present study, we report that the rat epididymis contains specific mRNA transcripts for two cadherin molecules (E-Cad and P-Cad) which have been shown, for other cells, to be responsible for mediating the formation of adherens and tight junctions.[19-21]

The principal cells of the epididymis are epithelial cells.[3] Since previous studies have reported the presence of E-Cad in other epithelial cells,[19,21,34-36] it is not surprising to find E-Cad mRNA transcripts in the epididymis. Steady-state mRNA concentrations for E-Cad were highest in the caput and corpus epididymidis. While the blood-epididymal barrier appears to be intact throughout the epididymis, it is interesting

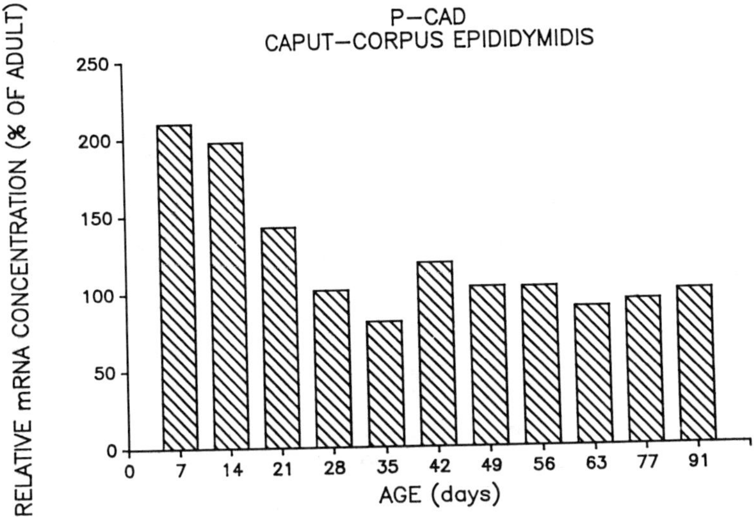

FIGURE 4. P-Cad mRNA concentrations in the caput-corpus epididymidis at different ages during post-natal development in the rat. Total RNA (10 μg) was isolated from the caput-corpus epididymidis and subjected to Northern blot analysis. Each blot was standardized for the amount of RNA loaded in each lane using an oligonucleotide probe recognizing the 18S ribosomal RNA sequence and the relative concentrations were obtained by laser densitometry. Data are expressed as a % of the 91-day-old rats.

that the steady-state mRNA concentrations for E-Cad are not equivalent throughout the different segments of this tissue. Physiologically, the caput secretes many different proteins which are thought to be important in the process of sperm maturation; the corpus, which also secretes proteins, acts mainly as a conduit to the cauda epididymidis where spermatozoa are stored.[3,37] Perhaps these functional differences may be important in understanding the differences in the longitudinal distribution of steady-state E-Cad mRNA concentrations which are most elevated in those segments of the epididymis that have highest secretory activity.

The initial isolation of P-Cad was done from mouse placental tissue.[31] It was therefore surprising that the epididymis should also contain RNA transcripts for P-Cad. Previous reports have shown that the bovine kidney contains a high concentration of P-Cad.[38] Since both the epididymis and kidney are embryologically derived from the mesonephric duct, perhaps the ability of these tissues to produce P-Cad is the result of their common embryonic origin. Unlike E-Cad, P-Cad is distributed in equal concentrations throughout the different segments of the epididymis. This contrast between these two cadherins reflects the complexity of cadherins and the potential role that different cadherins may play in mediating cell contacts within a single organ. No signal was detected for N-Cad in these experiments, suggesting that N-Cad is either not present in the epididymis or present in concentrations below the level of detection.

The developmental pattern of E-Cad mRNA concentrations in the caput-corpus epididymidis suggests that E-Cad is low shortly after birth and increases to a peak at day 42. This increase in steady-state E-Cad mRNA concentrations parallels closely the increase previously reported in specific activity for the enzyme 4-ene steroid 5-α-reductase[2] which is responsible for converting testosterone to its active metabolite dihydrotestosterone (DHT).[39] These changes would suggest that steady-state E-Cad mRNA concentrations are dependent on either serum or intraluminal concentrations of DHT. Following peak E-Cad mRNA concentrations on day 42, a dramatic decrease was observed on day 49. This was followed by a subsequent increase in E-Cad mRNA concentrations on day 56 which then leveled off until day 91. The decrease in E-Cad mRNA concentrations observed on day 49 coincides with the first appearance of sperm in the rat epididymis.[33] While the physiological mechanism responsible for this decrease in E-Cad mRNA concentrations is unknown, perhaps the appearance of sperm in the epididymis may somehow stress the junctions, resulting in an increase in the turnover of E-Cad mRNA to protein, and therefore lower steady-state E-Cad mRNA concentrations. This effect appears to be transient as E-Cad mRNA concentrations were elevated in the subsequent weeks following this trough in E-Cad mRNA concentrations.

The developmental pattern of P-Cad mRNA concentrations was different from that of E-Cad. P-Cad mRNA concentrations were high shortly after birth, on days 7 and 14, and subsequently decreased to lower levels thereafter. The elevated levels of P-Cad mRNA would suggest a role for P-Cad early in epididymal development. It is possible that the role of P-Cad in the epididymis may be linked to cell recognition as opposed to the formation of junctional complexes. This would be supported by the fact that E-Cad mRNA concentrations increase with development as P-Cad mRNA concentrations are decreasing. The decrease in steady-state P-Cad mRNA concentrations following day 14 onward coincides with the change from the period of cellular undifferentiation to differentiation in the rat epididymis.[5] During the period of differentiation, principal cells become the dominant cell of the epididymal epithelium, narrow cells appear in the epithelium, as do basal cells.[5] It is therefore possible that the decrease in steady-state P-Cad mRNA concentrations is related to P-Cad being present in a particular cell type whose relative abundance in the epididymis decreases following the period of cellular differentiation. This would suggest that P-Cad mRNA is present in undifferentiated cells but that, during differentiation, perhaps only one of the two cell types, columnar cells or narrow cells, retains the ability to express P-Cad. A second possibility is that P-Cad mRNA concentrations are related to changes in circulating levels of estradiol. Serum levels of estradiol are low in the adult but high shortly after birth and would be correlated with decreasing P-Cad mRNA concentrations.[40]

The decrease in P-Cad mRNA concentrations from day 21 onward is in marked contrast to the increase in E-Cad mRNA concentrations which occurs from day 21 onward. This would suggest that the epididymis as a whole is "switching-over" from one cadherin to another during postnatal development. These "switch-overs" have been observed during embryonic development[14–16] and are deemed to be important for cell segregation during organogenesis.[14] Since the "switch-over" occurs during the period shortly after the formation of the blood-epididymal barrier (8–14 days), these changes may be important in the formation and maintenance of the barrier.

Results from this study indicate that the rat epididymis contains specific mRNA transcripts for both E-Cad and P-Cad. Based on the physiological function of cadherins in mediating cell adhesion, it is likely that these molecules play a role in the formation and maintenance of the blood-epididymal barrier and perhaps in cell-cell interactions between the different cell types in the epididymis. The developmental patterns for each of the transcripts in the caput-corpus epididymidis indicate that these molecules are regulated during development, and that the nature of this regulation may be occurring via different sex steroids or by changes in relative abundance in different epididymal cell types.

ACKNOWLEDGMENTS

Dr. M. Takeichi is thanked for his generous gift of cDNA probes. Mr. R. S. Viger is thanked for his assistance.

REFERENCES

1. Agarwal, A. & A. P. Hoffer. 1989. Ultrastructural studies on the development of the blood-epididymis barrier in immature rats. J. Androl. **10:** 425–431.
2. Scheer, H. & B. Robaire. 1980. Steroid Δ^4-5α-reductase and 3α-hydroxysteroid dehydrogenase in the rat epididymis during development. Endocrinology **107:** 948–953.
3. Robaire, B. & L. Hermo. 1988. Efferent ducts, epididymis, and vas deferens: Structure, functions, and their regulation. *In* The Physiology of Reproduction. E. Knobil & J. Neill, Eds.: 999–1079. Raven Press Ltd. New York.
4. Sun, E. L. & C. J. Flickinger. 1982. Proliferative activity in the rat epididymis during postnatal development. Anat. Rec. **203:** 273–284.
5. Sun, E. L. & C. J. Flickinger. 1979. Development of cell types and of regional differences in the postnatal rat epididymis. Am. J. Anat. **154:** 27–55.
6. Hinton, B. T. 1985. The blood-epididymis barrier. *In* Male Fertility and Its Regulation. T. J. Lobl & E. S. E. Hafez, Eds.: 371–382. MTP Press Ltd. Boston, MA.
7. Hoffer, A. B. & B. T. Hinton. 1984. Morphological evidence for a blood epididymis barrier and the effects of gossypol on its integrity. Biol. Reprod. **30:** 991–1004.
8. Greenberg, J. & W.-G. Forssman. 1983. Studies of the guinea pig epididymis. II. Intercellular junctions of principal cells. Anat. Embryol. **168:** 195–209.
9. Friend, D. S. & N. B. Gilula. 1972. Variations in tight junctions and gap junctions in mammalian tissues. J. Cell Biol. **53:** 758–776.
10. Suzuki, F & T. Nagano. 1978. Development of tight junctions in the caput epididymal epithelium of the mouse. Dev. Biol. **63:** 321–334.
11. Hinton, B. T. & S. S. Howards. 1981. Permeability characteristics of the epithelium in the rat caput epididymis. J. Reprod. Fertil. **63:** 95–99.
12. Hinton, B. T. 1983. The epithelium of the caput epididymidis: Its permeability and its role in the formation of a specialized microenvironment. Ann. N.Y. Acad. Sci. **383:** 462–463.
13. Turner, T. T. & S. S. Howards. 1989. The tenacity of the blood-testis and blood-epididymal barriers. *In* Male Fertility and Its Regulation. T. J. Lobl & E. S. E. Hafez, Eds.: 383–393. MTP Press Ltd. Boston, MA.
14. Takeichi, M. 1990. Cadherins: A molecular family important in selective cell-cell adhesion. Ann. Rev. Biochem. **59:** 237–252.
15. Takeichi, M. 1987. Cadherins: A molecular family essential for selective cell-cell adhesion and animal morphogenesis. TIG **3:** 213–217.
16. Takeichi, M. 1991. Cadherin cell adhesion receptors as a morphogenetic regulator. Science **251:** 1451–1455.
17. Takeichi, M. 1988. The cadherins: Cell-cell adhesion molecules controlling animal morphogenesis. Development **102:** 639–655.
18. Ranscht, B. & M. Bronner-Fraser. 1991. T-Cadherin expression alternates with migrating neural crest cells in the trunk of the avian embryo. Development **111:** 15–22.
19. Vestweber, D., R. Kemler & P. Ekblom. 1985. Cell-adhesion molecule uvomorulin during kidney development. Dev. Biol. **112:** 213–221.
20. Gumbiner, B. & K. Simons. 1986. A functional assay for proteins involved in establishing an

epithelial occluding barrier: Identification of a uvomorulin-like polypeptide. J. Cell Biol. **102:** 457–468.
21. Bollier, K., D. Vestweber & R. Kemler. 1985. Cell-adhesion molecule uvomorulin is localized in the intermediate junctions of adult intestinal epithelial cells. J. Cell Biol. **100:** 327–332.
22. Robaire, B. & L. J. Buchanan. 1985. The use of epididymal cell and organ culture in toxicology. Concepts Toxicol. **3:** 114–129.
23. Byers, S. W., N. A. Musto & M. Dym. 1985. Culture of ciliated and nonciliated cells from rat ductuli efferentes. J. Androl. **6:** 271–278.
24. Klinefelter, G. R., R. P. Amann & R. H. Hammerstedt. 1982. Culture of principal cells from the caput epididymidis. Biol. Reprod. **26:** 885–901.
25. Klinefelter, G. R. & R. P. Amann. 1980. Isolation of principal cells and basal cells by elutriation of suspensions of rat epididymal tissue. Int. J. Androl. **3:** 287–300.
26. Hatta, K. & M. Takeichi. 1986. Expression of N-cadherin adhesion molecule associated with early morphogenic events in chick development. Nature **320:** 447–449.
27. Hales, B. F., C. Hachey & B. Robaire. 1980. The presence and longitudinal distribution of the glutathione S-transferases in rat epididymis and vas deferens. Biochem. J. **189:** 135–142.
28. Sambrook, J., E. F. Fritsch & T. Maniatis. 1989. Molecular Cloning. Cold Spring Harbor Laboratory Press. Cold Spring Harbor, NY.
29. Nagafuchi, A., Y. Shirayoshi, K. Okazaki, K. Yasoda & M. Takeichi. 1987. Transformation of cell adhesion properties by exogenously introduced E-Cadherin cDNA. Nature **129:** 341–343.
30. Miyatani, S., K. Shimamura, M. Hatta, A. Nagafuchi, A. Nose, M. Matsunaga, K. Hatta & M. Takeichi. 1989. Neural cadherin: Role in selective cell-cell adhesion. Science **245:** 631–634.
31. Nose, A., A. Nagafuchi & M. Takeichi. 1987. Isolation of placental cadherin cDNA: Identification of a novel gene family of cell-cell adhesion molecules. EMBO J. **6:** 3655–3661.
32. Szyf, M., D. S. Milstone, B. P. Schimmer, K. L. Parker & J. G. Seidman. 1990. Cis modification of the steroid 21-hydroxylase gene prevents its expression in the mouse adrenocortical tumor cell line. Mol. Endocrinol. **4:** 1144–1152.
33. Robaire, B., H. Scheer & C. Hachey. 1981. Regulation of epididymal steroid metabolizing enzymes. *In* Bioregulators of Reproduction. G. Jagiello & H.J. Vogel, Eds.: 487–498. Academic Press. New York.
34. Ringwald, M., R. Shuh, D. Vestweber, H. Eistetter, F. Lottspeich, J. Engel, R. Dolz, F. Jahnig, J. Epplen, S. Mayer, C. Muller & R. Kemler. 1987. The structure of cell adhesion molecule uvomorulin. Insights into the mechanism of Ca-dependent cell adhesion. EMBO J. **6:** 3647–3653.
35. Ogou, S. I., C. Yoshida-Noro & M. Takeichi. 1983. Calcium-dependent cell-cell adhesion molecules common to hepatocytes and teratocarcinoma stem cells. J. Cell Biol. **97:** 944–948.
36. Sorkin, B. C., J. J. Hemperly, G. M. Edelman & B. A. Cunningham. 1988. Structure of the gene for the liver cell adhesion molecule, L-CAM. Proc. Natl. Acad. Sci. USA **85:** 7617–7621.
37. Flickinger, C. J. 1981. Regional differences in synthesis, intracellular transport, and secretion of protein in the mouse epididymis. Biol. Reprod. **25:** 871–883.
38. Liaw, C. W., C. Cannon, M. D. Power, P. K. Kiboneka & L. L. Rubin. 1990. Identification and cloning of two species of cadherins in bovine endothelial cells. EMBO J. **9:** 2701–2707.
39. Robaire, B., L. L. Ewing, B. R. Zirkin & D. C. Irby. 1977. Steroid Δ^4-5α-reductase and 3α-hydroxysteroid dehydrogenase in the rat epididymis. Endocrinology **101:** 1379–1390.
40. Orgebin-Crist, M.-C. 1981. The influence of testicular function on related reproductive organs. *In* Comprehensive Endocrinology: The Testis. H. Burger & D. de Kretser, Eds.: 239–253. Raven Press. New York.

Characteristics of Sperm Motility

DAVID F. KATZ

Departments of Obstetrics and Gynecology, School of Medicine and Chemical Engineering
University of California
Davis, California 95616

INTRODUCTION

Flagellar motion is a fundamental expression of the vitality of a sperm cell, and is essential for its reproductive function. This motion results from complex intracellular processes, which are influenced by the sperm's environment. Mammalian spermatozoa utilize their motile capacity during migration from the site of insemination to the site of fertilization, and in penetration of the ovum vestments. Thus, an understanding of sperm motility can contribute to an understanding of sperm cell biology, and the mechanisms of sperm transport and fertilization. From a practical standpoint, sperm motility can be a useful biomarker of the potential fertility of a male, and its alterations. The latter may relate to therapies for infertility, contraceptive action, or exposure to external toxicants. This syllabus is a brief review of salient knowledge about mammalian sperm motility, emphasizing those species with a mucus-laden cervix, *i.e.*, primates and ruminants. The presentation of comparative information here is intended to provide a perspective relevant, as much as possible, to the human. It should be emphasized that the motion of spermatozoa is very much dependent upon not just their biological state, but also the conditions of observation.[1] For example, the physical properties of the suspending fluid and the depth of the observation chamber are known to affect flagellar motion and the subsequent swimming trajectory of a spermatozoon. Likewise, different methods of measurement delineate the motions of the flagellum and/or head with different degrees of accuracy, precision and biological incisiveness. These issues are addressed here, to some extent. For further information on biomedical aspects of sperm motility, the reader is referred to several reviews: on sperm transport;[2-4] on automated semen analysis;[5] and on sperm forces and videomicroscopy.[1,6]

THE GENERATION OF SPERM MOTION

The active mechanism of flagellar motion involves a complex set of coupled chemical, electrochemical and mechanochemical processes which culminate in movement of the flagellar axial filament complex or axoneme. This consists of nine microtubular doublets, circularly arranged to form a cylinder around a central pair of single microtubules (FIG. 1).[7] The "nine plus two" pattern has been highly conserved and is found throughout eukaryotic organisms in other flagellae and cilia. Each doublet has two subfibers: subfiber A is a complete microtubule and is circular. Subfiber B is incomplete, and is C-shaped. Both subfibers, and the central microtubular singlets, consist of dimers of the protein tubulin. Divergent arms of dynein, a protein with adenosine triphosphatase (ATPase) activity, project from each subfiber A. Slender bridges of nexin connect each of the nine microtubular doublets to its adjacent neighbor, linking subfiber A of one doublet to subfiber B of the next. The microtubules in the central pair are connected by more bridges, arranged like the rungs of a ladder, and are surrounded by a helical sheath from which radial links extend to join each peripheral doublet. In the middle piece of the flagellum, the axoneme is surrounded by an outer cylinder of nine dense fibers. Around this cylinder is a discontinuous helix of individual, elongated mitochondria enclosed by a fibrous sheath. The entire structure is encased in the cell membrane. The annulus forms the junction between the middle and the principal pieces of the flagellum. The principal piece lacks the mitochondrial helix, and here, the axoneme is covered only by a relatively thin fibrous sheath and cell membrane. The principal piece is about ten times the length of the middle piece, and it terminates in the tail endpiece. The total length of a human sperm flagellum is about 45 μm.

The electro-mechano-chemical mechanisms responsible for sperm motility are complex and incompletely understood. They involve processes intrinsic and extrinsic to the cell.[8-10] Intrinsic processes relate to the sperm's metabolic activity, the structure of its axoneme, membrane integrity, and transport phenomena. Extrinsic factors include substrate availability, ionic signals, and the physical properties of the sperm's microenvironment. In the presence of appropriate ionic signals, mitochondrial adenosine triphosphate (ATP) is hydrolyzed by the dynein arms to induce sliding movements between microtubular doublets in the axoneme. A sequence of principal and reverse bends ensues, but the precise means whereby such sliding is transformed into bending are not well understood.

Our understanding of the mechanisms of flagellar motion distinguishes between the pattern and vigor of such motion. To some extent, different processes dominate the control of these two basic kinematic features. For example, under controlled conditions, flagellar beat frequency and, thus, bend propagation rate are linked to ATP dephosphorylation.[11,12] Flagellar beat amplitude and wavelength depend, in some instances, upon the effective viscosity of the surrounding environment.[13,14] Although each of these examples has been introduced with a caveat, the basic distinction between pattern and vigor is quite useful in characterizing sperm motion, whatever the biomedical questions being asked.

THE BIOLOGICAL IMPORTANCE OF SPERM MOTILITY

Sperm motility is essential for transport through the female tract and for fertilization. There is variation among mammals in the details of sperm transport and fertilization. However, from a large body of research on these subjects, a number of concepts and themes emerge:[4]

1. Vigorous motility is necessary in certain sites and at certain times to insure successful sperm migration to the site of fertilization and transit through the granulosa cell investments and zona pellucida of the oocyte. Thus, the motility of spermatozoa recovered from the female reproductive tract depends not just upon the site of recovery but upon the time post insemination.

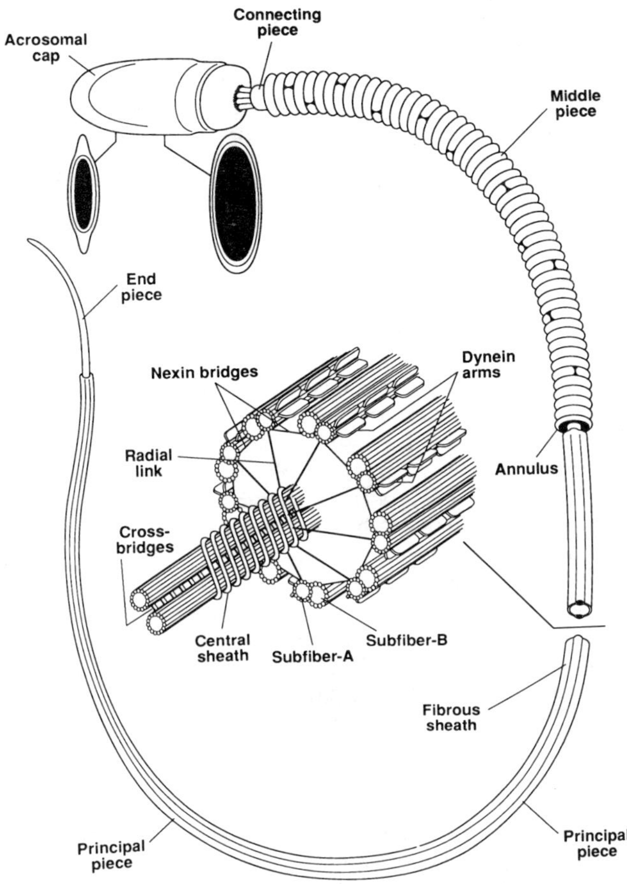

FIGURE 1. Basic structure of a mammalian spermatozoon. (From Boyers *et al.*, 1989,[5] with permission).

2. However necessary, motility alone is not sufficient as an active sperm-transporting mechanism. The physical and chemical activity of the female viscera, and ciliary activity, are also required.

3. The kinematics of flagellar bending are not constant during the natural history of the sperm cells. The epithelial surfaces and secretions of the female tract, as well as the egg investments, appear to modulate sperm motility and may coordinate the transport and union of the gametes. Inhibition of flagellar activity may be associated with the temporary retention of sperm in anatomical reservoirs of the female tract, while resumption of vigorous motion is coincident with the continuation of sperm migration.

The evidence is not conclusive, but it is currently believed that active motility may contribute to sustained, if not initial sperm entry and escape from the mucus-laden cervix. Active motility might contribute to passage through the uterotubal junction, and migration along the oviductal isthmus and ampulla; but these are processes difficult to study experimentally, and the justification for such a role is far from complete. Active motility undoubtedly contributes to passage through the cumulus oophorus and zona pellucida. In the following sections, the nature and role of motility during sperm-cervical mucus interaction, and in the oviduct, will be discussed.

HUMAN SPERM MOTILITY IN SEMEN AND DURING INTERACTION WITH CERVICAL MUCUS

Human semen is remarkable for its diversity of sperm motions and of morphology. Such diversity generally exists even in the specimens of highly fertile men; there can be significant variability in both the vigor and pattern of motion amongst spermatozoa. Thus, some sperm cells may progress rapidly along trajectories that are relatively straight (generally due to flagellar beats that are three dimensional; see below), while others may appear vigorous but exhibit asymmetric beats and highly curved, erratic trajectories. The distinguishing characteristics of "normal" human spermatozoa in semen are not known, and the relationships between human semen quality and fertility are not yet well developed.[5] Increased motile vigor and directionality of movement are associated with semen of increased quality, as interpreted clinically. Spermatozoa identified as morphologically normal have more vigorous motility than those with abnormal morphology.[15] Generally speaking, putatively normal human spermatozoa in semen exhibit flagellar beats of moderate amplitude and curvature, with relatively little bending of the midpiece.[16] The shape of such beats is qualitatively different from those occurring later in sperm transport, *e.g.*, during interaction with cervical mucus or during capacitation.

Cervical mucus is a gel, consisting of a network of glycoprotein macromolecules and a plasma component containing soluble proteins, inorganic salts and other chemical species.[17,18] The physical properties of mucus are viscoelastic, and depend primarily upon the concentration of the protein, the pH and the strengths of other ions in the mucus plasma.[19] Sperm penetrability of mucus is maximal during the periovulatory period, when mucus hydration is maximal, although some penetrability is possible outside this time interval in the reproductive cycle. When sperm enter periovulatory mucus from low viscosity fluid, their motility changes conspicuously (FIG. 2). There is much less bending of the proximal flagellum and, thus, much less lateral displacement of the sperm head. The sperm trajectory is nearly a straight line. These changes in sperm motion reflect the response of the flagellar bending mechanism to the viscoelastic properties of mucus. This response, as in the cumulus oophorus, involves the interaction of the sperm body with the macromolecular network of the mucus gel; and its electro-chemico-mechanical details are just now beginning to be studied.[20] If the mucus has been sheared in a particular direction, as in the loading of a capillary tube, the mucus microstructure is aligned in that direction, with the consequence that sperm trajectories tend to become a set of parallel quasi-straight lines. Strictly speaking, human sperm motion in stretched human mucus is different from that in mucus that has not been subjected to such orientation, as on a plane microscopic slide. In stretched mucus, there is more bending along the proximal flagellum, and the beat is three di-

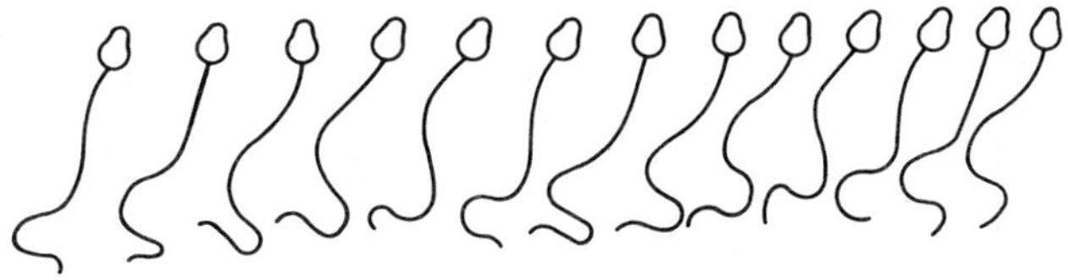

FIGURE 2. Typical flagellar beat patterns of a human spermatozoon swimming in semen (left) and in human cervical mucus (right). (From Katz and Berger, 1980, with permission).

mensional. In the non-aligned mucus, the motion is planar. It has been postulated that at least some of the mucus within the cervix *in vivo* is aligned, thereby providing directionality to sperm migration which might lead the cells to sites of *storage* in the cervical crypts.[21] It has also been postulated that active motility may enable or help sperm to escape from the cervical reservoir, but the details of such a process have not been established. What is clear is that sperm motility changes conspicuously upon escape from mucus *in vitro*. Bending now increases in curvature along the proximal flagellum, and the overall motion can be quite vigorous. This *in vitro* observation is consistent with the vigorous motility seen in sperm collected directly from the uterus.

SPERM MOTILITY IN THE UTERUS AND OVIDUCT

The vigorous motility seen in sperm which have swum out of cervical mucus may relate to the early stages of capacitation, which could be initiated by removal of seminal factors that inhibit this process.[22] It is noteworthy that relatively few observations have been made of the motility of sperm collected from the uterus, but such sperm, too, generally exhibit vigorous motion.[23,24] There are a few observations that small subpopulations of uterine sperm may exhibit *hyperactivated* motion, a motile behavior more generally associated with the final stages of capacitation and sperm function in the oviduct (see below).[25]

There is evidence in a number of species that sperm exhibit subdued flagellar activity after arrival in the lower oviductal isthmus, involving very low amplitude flagellar bending.[26,27] Such motion may be associated with retention of these cells in an isthmic reservoir.[3] Reinvigoration of isthmic sperm has been observed in cells recovered from the rabbit[28] and directly through the lumen of the mouse oviduct.[27,29] Such renewed motile activity is associated with escape of these sperm from the isthmus and transit to the ampulla. During this time the kinematics of motion change, resulting in a visually striking pattern referred to as *hyperactivation*.

Hyperactivated Sperm Motion

Although the term hyperactivation had yet to be coined, this distinct motility pattern was first described for hamster spermatozoa which had been capacitated *in vitro*.[30–32] A few years later, asymmetric beat patterns were described for mouse sperm collected from the oviduct.[33] There followed the identification of motility hyperactivation in the spermatozoa of most mammals studied, whether they were undergoing capacitation *in vitro* after collection from the male, or *in vivo* following recovery from the inseminated female.[1] The motivation for studying hyperactivation has been twofold: 1) it is a useful biological marker as related to capacitation; and 2) it may mechanically promote a number of sperm functions, including transport through the oviduct, and penetration of the cumulus and zona pellucida.

As the term implies, hyperactivated sperm move very rapidly in a simple medium, often in complex, jerky paths. Early descriptions were subjective and included such terms as *bobbing*, *whiplash*, *serpentine* and *dancing*. Direct micrographic recording techniques (see below) enabled later investigators to define measures which more objectively characterize the changes in motility which accompany capacitation and which culminate in hyperactivation. For motion as complex and diversified as hyperactivation, such measures are larger in number and often more difficult to obtain than for the more symmetrical motions characteristic of sperm in semen and cervical mucus (see below). In general, hyperactivation involves not only an increase in the curvature of flagellar bends; the beat shape becomes more asymmetrical because the flagellar bends in one direction have greater curvature than those in the other direction (FIG. 3). Sperm normally have somewhat asymmetric beat shapes, but they continue to move progressively by rolling about the axis of propulsion. During hyperactivation, the flagellar beats become more planar, and this, together with increasing asymmetry of the flagellar beat, causes free swimming sperm to move in nonlinear trajectories. The asymmetry may become so extreme that the sperm are completely nonprogressive and move in circles, or even figure-of-eight shaped trajectories. Typically, these increases in bend curvature and beat asymmetry are accompanied by a significant increase in the curvilinear velocity of the head and a decrease in the linearity of the sperm track, while the beat frequency may actually decrease. Such changes in sperm motion are the hallmarks of hyperactivation.

However, the transition to hyperactivated motion, and the motion itself can depend upon the conditions of sperm collection and/or culture as well as the microscopic preparation within which the cells are observed. For example, rabbit sperm collected from the oviductal isthmus are initially quite subdued. Their reinvigoration involves two intermittent episodes of motion: rapid forward swimming, with rolling of the sperm head due to a clearly three-dimensional beat; and figure of eight trajectories due to planar, highly asymmetric beats of high midpiece curvature.[23,28] These two episodes of motion are quite distinct visually. The impression from experiment is that the latter becomes more prevalent in sperm that are more fully capacitated (either owing to incubation time or site of collection in the female). Such distinct patterns of motion have also been described in hamster sperm. Precapacitated hamster sperm tend to swim with planar moderately asymmetric beats. A transitional mode of motion during capacitation *in vitro* involves more three dimensional flagellar beats, causing pronounced rolling of the sperm head in a helical path, and such motion has been termed *helical*.[34] The majority of fully capacitated hamster sperm in simple medium are marked by the full figure-of-eight trajectories due to planar beats. The intermittency between beat types is less obvious in the freely swimming sperm of this species than for the rabbit. However, direct observations of hamster sperm during cumulus and zona penetration indicate that such intermittency does exist.[35,36] The movements of such sperm are constrained by the increased viscoelasticity of the ovum vestments. Nonetheless, hamster sperm videorecorded during penetration of the zona pellucida, intermittently switch between large amplitude beats of lower frequency, and smaller amplitude beats of higher frequency.[36] The former appear much like the beats of a cilium.

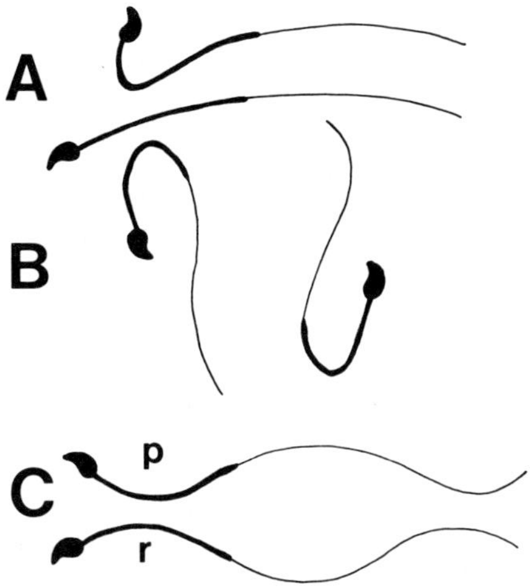

FIGURE 3. Types of flagellar bends and waves seen in hyperactivated hamster sperm. A. The two sperm show extreme positions of the asymmetric waveform produced by an extreme principal bend in the proximal midpiece. B. Extreme reverse bends initiated in the distal midpiece are propagated along the flagellum followed by principal bends of very low curvature. The resulting asymmetrical waveform, displayed by some hyperactivated sperm in low viscosity medium, may produce star-shaped or figure-of-eight-shaped trajectories. C. Sinusoidal-like waves are symmetrical because principal bends (p) are propagated along the flagellum followed by reverse bends (r) of equal curvature. These beats are usually three-dimensional. (From Drobnis and Katz, 1991, with permission).

Human sperm exhibit hyperactivated motion during capacitation and this has the same qualitative features as such motion in other species.[37–39] Human sperm hyperactivation is now the subject of great interest as a biomarker of fertilizing capacity, *e.g.*, in the context of diagnosis and prognosis in *in vitro* fertilization programs. The great majority of data for the human depict motions of the sperm head, as measured by CASA (computer-assisted sperm analysis, see below). There is relative little information on flagellar motions of hyperactivated human sperm.[37,40] The CASA data are almost exclusively obtained under sampling conditions which do not fully delineate the kinematics of the sperm head,[41–44] *e.g.*, the video framing rates are too low and/or the analysis intervals are too short. Nonetheless, these studies of the hyperactivated movements of the human sperm head have begun to define objective, quantitative criteria for its identification that have not generally existed for other species.[45] A transitional phase of motion, during the onset of full hyperactivation, has been defined for human sperm, and is associated with increased curvilinear swimming velocity, increased lateral displacements of the sperm head about its swimming path, but a relatively straight average shape of this path (see below for definitions of these kinematic features of swimming). Whether or not this transitional phase consists of planar flagellar beats, distinguishing it from the three dimensional *helical* motions of hamster sperm that precede full hyperactivation,[34] is not yet understood. The final phase of human sperm hyperactivation resembles the highly asymmetric movement seen in other species, involving considerable curvature of the average path. Sperm exhibiting such full hyperactivation may actually display several distinct subtypes of motion, with differing degrees of curvature[37] and a new set of metaphors has arisen to describe its attributes, including such descriptors as *star spin* and *thrashing*. Such details may depend upon the conditions of incubation and observation of human sperm,[42] and are in need of further study.

CHARACTERIZATION OF SPERM MOTILITY

The overall motion of a swimming sperm can be thought of as consisting of two components: the flagellar bending mechanism produces *undulatory* (propulsive) motions; and the entire sperm body (flagellum plus head) moves with a resultant *rigid-body* velocity (that may contain angular as well as linear components). The swimming velocity of the sperm is just such that the hydrodynamic *drag* on the sperm body equals the flagellar *thrust* (allowing, also, for a balance of the applied *moment* or torque on the sperm body). Sperm *kinematics* refers to the time-dependent geometries of these motions. The history of sperm motion analysis contains studies focusing upon either flagellar beat kinematics, the kinematics of the sperm head or, occasionally, both. The choice of movement characteristics is generally dictated by the measurement technology available (see below), and the biomedical questions being asked.

Strictly speaking, full characterization of flagellar kinematics is a challenging task. Different points on the flagellum move with different velocities at different times within a beat cycle. Thus, a rigorous mathematical representation requires a formalism that delineates the movement of each such flagellar point at each time, and this can be complex and cumbersome. When there is consistency, and especially periodicity, in flagellar motions, this formalism is greatly simplified. For example, if the flagellar beat were a simple traveling sine wave, then algebraic formulas and simple quadratures (here, mathematical integrals of trigonometric functions) would suffice to prescribe its motion. These expressions would contain parameters, such as amplitude, wavelength and the number of waves, which collectively delineate beat shape, and also beat frequency, a measure of rate or vigor (FIG. 4). The wave propagation speed along the flagellum, another measure of vigor, could then be computed as a quadrature involving beat frequency and beat shape parameters. The spermatozoa of some marine invertebrates, such as sea urchins and star fish, exhibit beats that are sine-like.[46] However, this is seldom, if ever, the case for mammalian spermatozoa. Precapacitated, mature mammalian sperm, in low viscosity fluid, tend to exhibit flagellar motions that are periodic, but which usually contain motions in three dimensions.[47–49] (It is the torque produced by the motions outside the plane of microscopic focus that causes the sperm head to roll about its axis of propulsion.) The three dimensionality increases distally along the flagellum, and movements of the midpiece are very nearly planar. The distal tip of the flagellum moves in an arc whose cross section perpendicular to

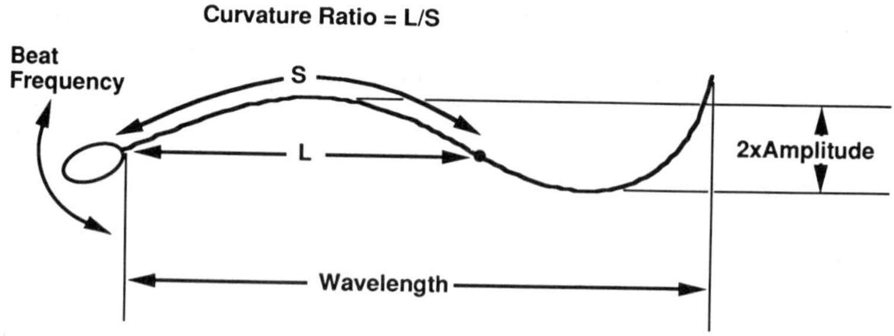

FIGURE 4. Definition of parameters of flagellar motion. These are generally determined at an instant in which the beat displays its most sinusoidal-like form and the head-midpiece junction is on the axis of propulsion.

the plane of microscopic focus is an ellipse. Under some conditions of observation, *e.g.*, when the sperm are near flat surfaces, these motions are nearly two dimensional. It should be remembered that such sperm seldom exhibit flagellar beats that are truly symmetrical about the net axis of propulsion, even if that axis, or *average path* (see below), is relative straight. Nonetheless, various investigators have characterized such motions in terms of sine-like waves that vary in amplitude and wavelength as the bends propagate distally along the flagellum.[47,50] For purposes of kinematic classification, such approaches have been useful. However, their absolute accuracy when hydromechanical quantities (e.g., power output, flagellar thrust) are being computed is less well understood (see below). Moreover, the magnitude and significance of the motions in the third dimension are not well appreciated, and are very difficult to measure. To some extent, the rolling frequency of the sperm head is a measure of the three dimensionality of the beat; *i.e.*, the higher the ratio (rolling frequency/flagellar beat frequency), the more three dimensional the beat. This phenomenon is apparent, for example, in observing human sperm as they begin to capacitate.

When the flagellar motion becomes more asymmetric (as with the onset of hyperactivation), then the sine wave approach becomes less accurate and discriminatory. One facet of hyperactivation is the increased bending of the flagellar midpiece. An *ad hoc* method for quantitating such bending is to approximate a net radius of maximum curvature for it.[28] A more recent alternative is based upon identification of the arc length along the midpiece from the head-midpiece junction to the first distal geometric inflection point (FIG. 4). This arc is measured at that instant in a prototypical beat when there is maximum curvature (a decision generally based upon subjective visual judgment). This distance can be normalized by the straight line distance between the sperm head-midpiece junction and the first flagellar inflection point, thus creating a dimensionless *curvature ratio* that is independent of sperm size.[51]

The kinematics of the sperm head are, in principle, far easier to measure than the flagellar kinematics, even though they reveal less about the details of the flagellar bending mechanism. With the advent of CASA (see below), data on sperm head kinematics have received increasing attention. FIGURE 5 illustrates the current set of parameters of sperm head motion that can be obtained from most CASA systems. These are all time-average parameters, *i.e.*, they are computed over a known time interval. The vigor of motion is measured by the three velocities: *curvilinear velocity* (VCL, the time-average velocity of the sperm head along its actual curvilinear trajectory), *straightline velocity* (VSL, the time average velocity of the sperm head as projected along the straight line between its first and final detected positions), and *average-path velocity* (VAP, the time average velocity of the sperm head as projected along its spatial average trajectory; this average path is computed via a mathematical smoothing of the actual curvilinear path, as described below). To some extent, sperm vigor is also described by the *beat cross frequency* (BCF, the time-average rate at which the curvilinear path crosses its average path). The pattern of motion is measured by the dimensionless ratios: *linearity* (LIN, the ratio of projected length to total length of the curvilinear trajectory), *wobble* (WOB, the degree of oscillation of the curvilinear path about its spatial average path), and *straightness* (STR, the effective linearity of the average path). The pattern of sperm head motion is also measured by the *amplitude of lateral head displacement* (ALH, the average or maximum amplitude of lateral distances of the actual sperm head trajectory about its spatial average path). Notably, there is no unique definition of ALH, even for a fixed definition of average path, and different CASA instruments measure it differently (see below).

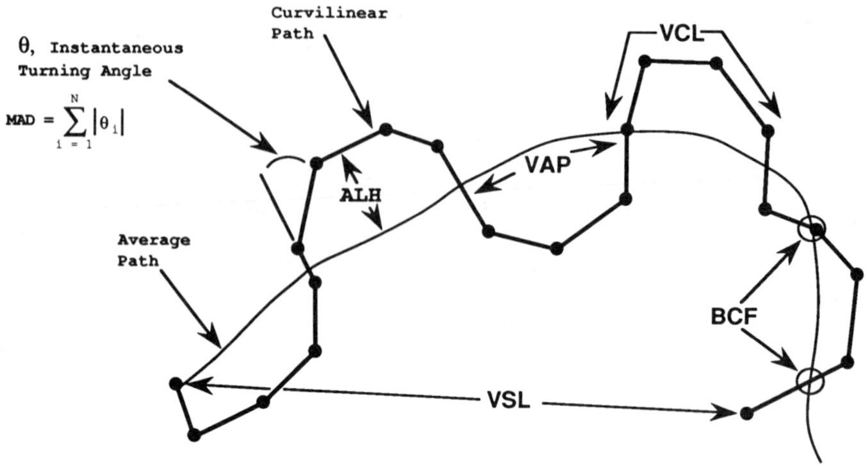

FIGURE 5. Definition of parameters of sperm head motion typically determined by CASA analysis.

There are several new experimental approaches to describing sperm kinematics that are worthy of mention. The instantaneous curvilinear velocity of the sperm is not constant, but varies in time, in a generally periodic fashion. Sperm periodic motion can be decomposed into a set of fundamental frequencies or harmonics, using techniques such as Fourier analysis.[43] This approach may provide a more accurate link between flagellar beat frequency and sperm head motions than does the BCF. The shape of the sperm head trajectory can be described by computing its *fractal dimension*, a measure of its space filling capacity.[52] Another recently applied concept in the characterization of sperm kinematics is that an entire set of parameters, not simply individual ones, is necessary to describe a single sperm. This has led to the implementation of multivariate statistical methods in which comparisons and prediction are made using a set of variables.[53-55] For example, individual sperm can be grouped and compared using cluster analysis techniques and multivariate analysis of variance. Prediction can be achieved using multiple regression methods, continuous or logistic. These multivariate approaches appear quite promising, and are likely to receive increasing implementation.

It is also worth noting that mechanical parameters, computed from sperm kinematics, also serve to characterize the biology of the cells. For example, when the sperm is abutted against the zona pellucida, the flagellar thrust and torque are more meaningful in understanding the process of zona penetration than flagellar beat characteristics alone.[36,56] The hydrodynamic power expended by a sperm is a basic component of the cell's energy budget. Analysis of the flagellar bending mechanism utilizes knowledge of the instantaneous bending moment distribution along the flagellum.[8,9] These derived biophysical quantities require sufficient experimental effort (flagellar analysis) and mathematical computation that their use is primarily restricted, at present, to basic biological studies of sperm function.

MEASUREMENT OF SPERM MOTILITY

Objective measurement of sperm motion can be performed using methods that are either direct or indirect. A direct method is one in which individual sperm cells are visualized and their motion recorded, for example using cine- or videomicrography. Indirect methods, such as spectrophotometry or laser-Doppler velocimetry,[57] estimate the mean swimming speed of sperm by measuring some optical property of the entire suspension. Such methods are fast and capable of automation. However, their calculations require assumptions about the randomness of sperm motion in the suspensions, which are frequently invalid, especially when large numbers of immotile cells are present. For these reasons, and the advent of automated direct techniques (CASA), the indirect methods are now seldom used.

At present, there are two principal indirect methods being used to study sperm motion: time-exposure micrography and videomicrography. Videomicrographic approaches have now almost completely superseded the earlier cinemicrographic ones: because of the immediate availability of the recorded images, and the ability to directly digitize the images. Time-exposure micrography is a method now over 40 years old.[58] In its simplest form, the shutter of a still frame camera is held open for one second, using constant illumination, generally with dark field microscopic optics.[59] The trajectories of swimming sperm can be identified as *tracks* on the developed film, and measured for various movement characteristics.[5] A variation on this approach is termed "multiple exposure photomicrography," in which the illumination is stroboscopic.[60] Here the sperm paths appear as *chains* of individual exposures. Analogous movement characteristics can be measured. Variations on this stroboscopic approach have been in use for many years by cell biologists interested in flagellar motion.[61] Here a sequence of instantaneous exposures is created with higher spatial resolution, to enable visualization and analysis of the flagellum throughout a beat cycle. Analysis of the sperm tracks and images created by the multiple exposure approaches can be facilitated by manual application of an electric digitizer to the images.

In the late 1970s, as the original reel-to-reel video recording methods were replaced by standardized video cassette systems, and as the optical resolution of the video cameras and recorders improved, practical use of videomicrography for sperm motion analysis became possible.[62] Originally, the video tapes were analyzed manually, using frame-by-frame projection. Simple determination of sperm straightline velocities could be performed using a transparent overlay containing concentric rings.[62] Soon, the manually controlled electronic digitizers were applied to frame-by-frame analysis.[41,45] The development of automatic video image digitization technology inevitably lead to its application in sperm motion analysis.[63,64] The CASA technology has been available commercially for over seven years, and is now utilized in many hundreds of laboratories, worldwide. At present, CASA technology is almost exclusively directed to measurement of the kinematics of the sperm head, although some progress has been made on the more challenging problem of flagellar analysis.[65] The principles of CASA were the subject of a recent review[5] and will not be re-reviewed here. However, some comments and caveats on the current state of the art/science are in order. The hardware and software for identifying and tracking individual sperm, and for computing particular movement characteristics, differ among the commercially available systems. We do not yet fully understand the accuracy of measurement of the systems, nor has it been optimized. Such systems have difficulty distinguishing spermatozoa from other cells, distinguishing motile from non-motile spermatozoa, and continuing to identify the paths of individual sperm when they are crossed by those of other sperm.[5] Such problems are paramount in human semen, which can have a relatively high sperm concentration (as compared to sperm capacitating *in vitro*), and large numbers of both non-motile sperm and other cells and debris. Such problems can be lessened, to some extent, by dilution of the semen.[66,67] However, the optimal conditions and procedures for such dilution have not yet been determined. Nonetheless, standardized operating procedures for CASA analysis of human semen are under development, and these will substantially improve the historic imprecision of such analysis. In some respects, CASA analysis of human sperm during capacitation *in vitro* poses fewer problems, since the concentration is much lower, the percent motility is higher, and there is little background particulate debris. The principal problem here is the rapidity and complexity of sperm motion, especially as hyperactivation develops. The typical CASA approach is to analyze sperm at a video sampling rate of 30 frames/sec for a time interval of no more than 0.5–0.67 sec. Such conditions of sampling cannot fully delineate the full geometric complexity of hyperactivated sperm paths, which would require higher framing rates and longer sampling intervals.[41,43,44] Nonetheless, there has been meaningful progress in the standardization of CASA analysis of human sperm hyperactivation, despite the limitations in its kinematic accuracy.[42,68] The present clinical goal is primarily to classify sperm as being hyperactivated, rather than to probe the kinematic nuances of such hyperactivation. This endpoint may be compatible with the understandably diminished measurement accuracy which currently exists. Indeed, an important challenge in the further development of CASA technology and methodology *per se*, is to understand and quantitate the degrees of accuracy and precision needed for any particular biomedical application, given the biological variability inherent in sperm motion for that application.

CONCLUSIONS

Sperm motility is a complex phenomenon, the understanding of which requires the integration of cell biology with reproductive physiology, biochemistry, biophysics and clinical andrology. Following insemination, mammalian spermatozoa exhibit a sequence of different types of motility, as the cells progress toward the egg. Such changes appear to be modulated by the female reproductive tract, to coordinate the union of both fertile sperm and eggs. However, mechanisms of such motility modulation are relatively poorly understood.

Measurement of sperm motility is entering a new era, in which objective, rapid methods are becoming accessible to a broad spectrum of laboratories, for which sophisticated engineering expertise is not required. This accessibility offers the prospect of significant increases in our understanding of the relationships between motility and sperm cell biology, transport through the female and fertilization, infertility, contraception and toxicology. Despite their obvious promise, and preliminary successes, the new CASA methods must remain the subject of careful scrutiny and analysis. At present, we do not yet know how accurate these methods are, nor how accurate they need to be to address successfully particular biomedical questions. Further technological developments will improve CASA accuracy, as well as precision. The challenge will be to apply these methods not just with thoroughness but, also, with biomedical wisdom.

REFERENCES

1. Drobnis, E. Z. & D. F. Katz. 1990. Videomicroscopy of mammalian fertilization. *In* Handbook On Mammalian Gamete Biology. P. Wassarman, Ed.: 269–300. CRC Press. New York.
2. Mortimer, D. 1978. Selectivity of sperm transport in the female genital tract. *In* Spermatozoa, Antibodies and Infertility. J. Cohen & W. F. Hendry, Eds.: 37–53. Blackwell, Oxford.
3. Overstreet, J. W. 1983. Transport of gametes in the reproductive tract of the female mammal. *In* Mechanism and Control of Animal Fertilization. J. F. Hartmann, Ed.: 499–543. Academic Press. New York.
4. Katz, D. F., E. Z. Drobnis & J. W. Overstreet. 1989. Factors regulating mammalian sperm migration through the female reproductive tract and oocyte vestments. Gamete Res. **22:** 443–469.
5. Boyers, S. P., R. O. Davis & D. F. Katz. 1989. Automated semen analysis. *In* Current Problems in Obstetrics and Gynecology and Fertility. R. L. Barbieri, Ed. **12:** 167–200. Year Book Medical Publishers, Inc. New York.
6. Katz, D. F. & E. Z. Drobnis. 1990. The analysis and interpretation of sperm forces. *In* Fertilization in Mammals. B. D. Bavister, J. Cummins & E. R. S. Roldan, Eds.: 125–137. Serono Symposia. Norwell, MA.
7. Fawcett, D. W. 1975. The mammalian spermatozoon. Dev. Biol. **44:** 394–436.
8. Blum, J. J. & M. Hines. 1979. Biophysics of flagellar motility. Q. Rev. Biophys. **12:** 103–108.
9. Brokaw, C. J. 1981. Introduction: Generation of the bending cycle in cilia and flagella. *In* Mechanism and Control of Ciliary Movement. C. J. Brokaw & P. Verdugo, Eds.: 137–141. Alan R. Liss. New York.
10. Tash, J. S. & A. R. Means. 1983. Cyclic adenosine 3′,5′ monophosphate, calcium and protein phosphorylation in flagellar motility. Biol. Reprod. **28:** 75–104.
11. Brokaw, C. J. 1965. Non-sinusoidal bending waves of sperm flagella. J. Exp. Biol. **43:** 155–169.
12. Gibbons, B. H. & I. R. Gibbons. 1972. Flagellar movement and adenosine triphosphatase activity in sea urchin sperm extracted with Triton X-100. J. Cell Biol. **54:** 74–97.
13. Rikmenspoel, R. 1984. Movements and active moments of bull sperm flagella as a function of temperature and viscosity. J. Exp. Biol. **108:** 205–230.
14. Suarez, S. S, D. F. Katz, D. H. Owen, J. B. Andrew & R. L. Powell. 1991. Evidence for the function of hyperactivated motility in sperm. Biol. Reprod. **44:** 375–381.
15. Morales, P., D. F. Katz, J. W. Overstreet, S. J. Samuels & R. J. Chang. 1988a. The relationship between the motility and morphology of spermatozoa in human semen. J. Androl. **9:** 241–247.
16. David, G., C. Serres & P. Jouannet. 1981. Kinematics of human spermatozoa. Gamete Res. **4:** 83–95.
17. Gibbons, R. A. & P. E. Mattner. 1971. The chemical and physical characteristics of the cervical secretion and its role in reproductive physiology. *In* Pathways to Conception. A. I. Sherman, Ed.: 143–155. Charles C Thomas. Springfield, IL.
18. Meyer, F. A. & A. Silberberg. 1980. The rheology and molecular organization of epithelial mucus. Biorheology **17:** 163–168.
19. Wolf, D. P., L. Blasco, M. Khan, *et al.* 1977. Human cervical mucus: I. Rheological characteristics. Fertil. Steril. **28:** 41–46.
20. Powell, R. L., G. R. Fulford & D. F. Katz. 1988. Analysis of sperm motion in a linear viscoelastic fluid (Abstract). The American Physical Society. Buffalo, NY.
21. Mattner, P. E. 1966. Formation and retention of the spermatozoan reservoir in the cervix of the ruminant. Nature **212:** 1479–1480.
22. Clegg, E. D. 1983. Mechanisms of mammalian sperm capacitation. *In* Mechanism and Control of Animal Fertilization. J. F. Hartmann, Ed.: 177–212. Academic Press. New York.
23. Cooper, G. W., J. W. Overstreet & D. F. Katz. 1979. Sperm transport in the reproductive tract of the female rabbit: Motility patterns and the flagellar activity of spermatozoa. Gamete Res. **2:** 35–42.
24. Olds-Clarke, P. 1986. Motility characteristics of sperm from the uterus and oviducts of female mice after mating to congenic males differing in sperm transport and fertility. Biol. Reprod. **34:** 453–467.
25. Behboodi, E., D. F. Katz, J. W. Overstreet & A. W. Hendrickx. 1989. The movement of cynomolgus and rhesus monkey spermatozoa collected from the lower female reproductive

tract. Gamete Res. **24:** 333–342.

26. OVERSTREET, J. W. & G. W. COOPER. 1975. Reduced sperm motility in the isthmus of the rabbit oviduct. Nature **258:** 718–719.
27. SUAREZ, S. S. 1987. Sperm transport and motility in the mouse oviduct: Observations in situ. Biol. Reprod. **36:** 203–210.
28. JOHNSON, L. L., D. F. KATZ & J. W. OVERSTREET. 1981. The movement characteristics of rabbit spermatozoa before and after activation. Gamete Res. **4:** 275–282.
29. SUAREZ, S. S. & R. A. OSMAN. 1987. Initiation of hyperactivated flagellar bending in mouse sperm within the female reproductive tract. Biol. Reprod. **36:** 1191–1198.
30. YANAGIMACHI, R. 1969. In vitro acrosome reaction and capacitation of golden hamster spermatozoa by bovine follicular fluid and its fractions. J. Exp. Zool. **170:** 269–280.
31. YANAGIMACHI, R. 1970. The movement of golden hamster spermatozoa before and after capacitation. J. Reprod. Fertil. **23:** 193–196.
32. GWATKIN, R. B. L. & O. F. ANDERSON. 1969. Capacitation of hamster spermatozoa by bovine follicular fluid. Nature **224:** 1111–1112.
33. PHILLIPS, D. M. 1972. Comparative analysis of mammalian sperm motility. J. Cell Biol. **53:** 561–573.
34. SUAREZ, S. S. 1988. Hamster sperm motility transformation during development of hyperactivation in vitro and epididymal maturation. Gamete Res. **19:** 51–65.
35. DROBNIS, E. Z., A. I. YUDIN, G. N. CHERR & D. F. KATZ. 1988a. The kinematics of hamster sperm during penetration of the cumulus cell matrix. Gamete Res. **21:** 367–383.
36. DROBNIS, E. Z., A. I. YUDIN, G. N. CHERR & D. F. KATZ. 1988b. Hamster sperm penetration of the zona pellucida: Kinematic analysis and mechanical implications. Dev. Biol. **130:** 311–323.
37. BURKMAN, L. J. 1984. Characterization of hyperactivated motility during capacitation: Comparison of fertile and oligospermic sperm populations. Arch. Androl. **13:** 153–165.
38. ROBERTSON, L., D. P. WOLF & J. S. TASH. 1988. Temporal changes in motility parameters related to acrosomal status: Identification and characterization of populations of hyperactivated human sperm. Biol. Reprod. **39:** 797–805.
39. MORTIMER, S. T. & D. MORTIMER. 1990. Kinematics of human spermatozoa incubated under capacitating conditions. J. Androl. **11:** 195–203.
40. MORALES, P., J. W. OVERSTREET & D. F. KATZ. 1988b. Changes in human sperm movement during capacitation in vitro. J. Reprod. Fertil. **83:** 119–128.
41. MORTIMER, D., E. F. CURTIS & A. RALSTON. 1988. Semi-automated analysis of manually reconstructed tracks of progressively motile human spermatozoa. Hum. Reprod. **3:** 303–309.
42. MACK, S. O., J. S. TASH & D. P. WOLF. 1989. Effect of measurement conditions on quantification of hyperactivated human sperm subpopulations by digital image analysis. Biol. Reprod. **40:** 1162.
43. DAVIS, R. O. & D. F. KATZ. 1988. Quantitative analysis of sperm motion kinematics from real-time video-edge images. Proc. Int. Soc. Optical Eng. **832:** 14–20.
44. KATZ, D. F., D. H. OWEN & R. L. POWELL. 1990. Interpretation of CASA measurement of sperm head motions: Hydrodynamic correlates with flagellar beat kinematics. Annual Meeting of the American Fertility Society, Washington, D.C.
45. NEILL, J. M. & P. OLDS-CLARKE. 1987. A computer-assisted assay for mouse sperm hyperactivation demonstrates that bicarbonate but not bovine serum albumin is required. Gamete Res. **18:** 121–140.
46. BROKAW, C. J. 1967. Adenosine triphosphate usage by flagella. Science **156:** 76–78.
47. DENEHY, M. A., D. HERBISON-EVANS & B. V. DENEHY. 1975. Rotational and oscillatory components of the tailwave in ram spermatozoa. Biol. Reprod. **13:** 289–297.
48. ISHIJIMA, S. & H. MOHRI. 1985. A quantitative description of flagellar movement in golden hamster spermatozoa. J. Exp. Biol. **114:** 463–475.
49. ISHIJIMA, S., S. OSHIO & H. MOHRI. 1986. Flagellar movement of human spermatozoa. Gamete Res. **13:** 185–191.
50. DRESDNER, R. D. & D. F. KATZ. 1981. Relationships of mammalian sperm motility and morphology to hydrodynamic aspects of cell function. Biol. Reprod. **25:** 920–930.
51. SUAREZ, S. S., D. F. KATZ & J. W. OVERSTREET. 1983. Movement characteristics and acrosomal status of rabbit spermatozoa recovered at the site and time of fertilization. Biol. Reprod. **29:** 1277–1287.
52. DAVIS, R. O. & D. F. KATZ. 1989. Fractal dimensions and the classification of sperm swimming trajectories (Abstract). Annual Meeting of the American Society of Andrology.

53. Davis, R. O., D. F. Katz & J. B. Andrew. 1988. Hi-speed harmonic analysis of human sperm motion: Characterization and discrimination of semen and in vitro capacitation (Abstract). 44th Annual American Fertility Society Meeting, Atlanta, GA.
54. Ginsburg, K. A., A. G. Sacco & K. S. Moghissi, 1988. Morphology data do not improve the predictive ability of movement analysis in sperm fertility assessment (Abstract). Annual Meeting of the American Fertility Society.
55. Vantman, D., S. M. Bands, G. Koukoulis, L. Dennison & R. J. Sherins. 1989. Assessment of sperm motion characteristics from fertile and infertile men using a fully automated computer assisted semen analyzer. Fertil. Steril. **51:** 156–161.
56. Baltz, J., D. F. Katz & R. Cone. 1988. The mechanics of sperm egg interaction at the zona pellucida. Biophys. J. **54:** 643–654.
57. Jouannet, P., B. Volochine, P. Deguent, *et al.* 1977. Light scattering determination of various characteristic parameters of spermatozoa motility in a series of human sperm. Andrologia **9:** 36–49.
58. Rothschild, V. 1949. Measurements of sperm activity before artificial insemination. Nature **163:** 358–359.
59. Overstreet, J. W., D. F. Katz, F. W. Hanson & J. Fonseca. 1979. A simple inexpensive method for objective assessment of human sperm movement characteristics. Fertil. Steril. **31:** 162–172.
60. Makler, A. 1978. A new multiple exposure photography method for objective human spermatozoal motility determination. Fertil. Steril. **30:** 192–199.
61. Cooper, T. G. & D. M. Woolley. 1982. Stroboscopic illumination for the assessment of hyperactivated motility of mouse spermatozoa. J. Exp. Zool. **223:** 291–294.
62. Katz, D. F. & J. W. Overstreet. 1981. Sperm motility assessment by videomicrography. Fertil. Steril. **35:** 188–193.
63. Liu, Y. T. & P. K. Warme. 1977. Computerized evaluation of sperm cell motility. Comp. Biomed. Res. **10:** 127–138.
64. Katz, D. F., R. O. Davis, B. A. Delandmeter & J. W. Overstreet. 1985. Real-time analysis of sperm motion using automatic video image digitization. Comput. Meth. Prog. Biomed. **21:** 173–182.
65. Stephens, D. T., S. Vijayaraghavan & S. S. Hoskins. 1988. Computerized flagellar analysis of the effects of the intracellular Ca^{2+} binding compounds fura 2, quin 2 and bapta on bovine sperm flagellar waveform (Abstract). Biol. Reprod. **38:** 89.
66. Vantman, D., G. Koukoulis, L. Dennison, M. Zinaman & R. J. Sherins. 1988. Computer-assisted semen analysis: Evaluation of method and assessment of the influence of sperm concentration on linear velocity determination. Fertil. Steril. **49:** 510–516.
67. Davis, R. O., M. F. Obasaju, J. B. Andrew & D. F. Katz. 1989. Effects of dilution with homologous seminal plasma (HSP) and phosphate-buffered saline (PBS) on computer-aided sperm analysis (CASA) measures of human seminal sperm motion. Annual meeting of the American Fertility Society, San Francisco, CA.
68. Burkman, L. J. 1991. Discrimination between nonhyperactivated and classical hyperactivated motility patterns in human spermatozoa using computerized analysis. Fertil. Steril. **55:** 363–371.

Clinical Use and Misuse of Automated Semen Analysis

RICHARD J. SHERINS

Division of Andrology
Genetics & IVF Institute
3020 Javier Road
Fairfax, Virginia 22031

INTRODUCTION

Unlike animal husbandry, where fertility potential of a male can be tested against multiple female partners, human male fertility prediction has historically relied upon semen analysis. The use of semen quality as an accurate predictive measure of a man's fertility potential has been hampered by a wide variety of problems (TABLE 1). These include variability in sample collection and methods of analysis, poor subject selection criteria, and inability to detect pregnancy reliably when there is early embryo loss. The sperm count has been the primary focus of interest and not the sperm functional ability. With newer objective measures of sperm analysis, such as computer-assisted sperm analysis (CASA), methods of analysis have still not been standardized and data not appropriately analyzed statistically.

Historically, clinicians have relied on sperm concentration as the principal semen parameter for fertility prediction. However, for serious students of the field, "oligospermia" is no more informative than "anemia" in providing insight into the mechanism of the problem. While the normal range for sperm concentration is 20–250 $\times$ 10^6/ml, in some studies as many as 20% of patients with less than 20 $\times$ 10^6/ml have been shown to be able to impregnate their spouse.[1] However, these data usually have not accounted for fecundability, *i.e.*, the rate by which pregnancy is achieved.

Recently, among men with isolated gonadotropin deficiency, pituitary hormone replacement has been shown to induce sperm production leading to a 95% fertility rate, with 6 months average time to conception, despite a low mean sperm concentration (FIG. 1) of only 16 $\times$ 10^6/ml.[2] Thus, sperm number *per se* may be misleading as a predictor of fertility potential. These data suggest that it is the functional capacity of sperm, rather than the actual sperm number, which is critical to whether or not a man can impregnate his partner. Functional abnormalities would include processes which 1) impair sperm motion and prevent sperm from reaching the egg, 2) interfere with ability of sperm to capacitate, 3) inhibit sperm binding to the zona pellucida, 4) inhibit the acrosome reaction and sperm penetration into the perivitelline space, and 5) alter sperm-egg fusion and penetration into the egg.

Motility disorders have long been recognized as an important component of male infertility. Traditional methods for assessing sperm motion are subjective and highly variable;[1] they include the fraction of motile sperm (% motility) and the quality of progressive movement (ranking 0 to 4). During the last decade there has been a rapid proliferation of long-awaited new methods to assess sperm motion parameters objec-

TABLE 1. Problem Areas in Fertility Assessment of the Male Which Hamper Physician Utilization of Semen Analysis Data to Accurately Predict Fertility Potential

- Semen analysis has previously been subjective
- Semen collection performed under non-standardized conditions
- Semen quality is inherently variable
- Insufficient number of data to provide reliable statistical analysis
- Poorly defined study groups
- Fertility status of wife ignored
- Insensitive methods for detection of conception with early embryo loss
- Deceptive non-spousal pregnancies have not been systematically excluded
- Direct correlations of sperm measures to actual fertilization of spouses eggs have been rarely employed
- Objective measures of sperm functions have not been standardized

tively.[3,4] These have now culminated in the evolution of "machine vision" technology or automated computer-assisted sperm analysis (CASA) to allow objective systematic assessment of sperm motion.[5] Computer algorithms characterize both the *pattern* and *vigor* of sperm motion. The CASA methodology increases accuracy and precision of the measurement and allows for standardization among laboratories. Even in its early state of development, CASA has provided new insights into the heterogeneity of sperm movement in semen as well as events which transpire during capacitation.

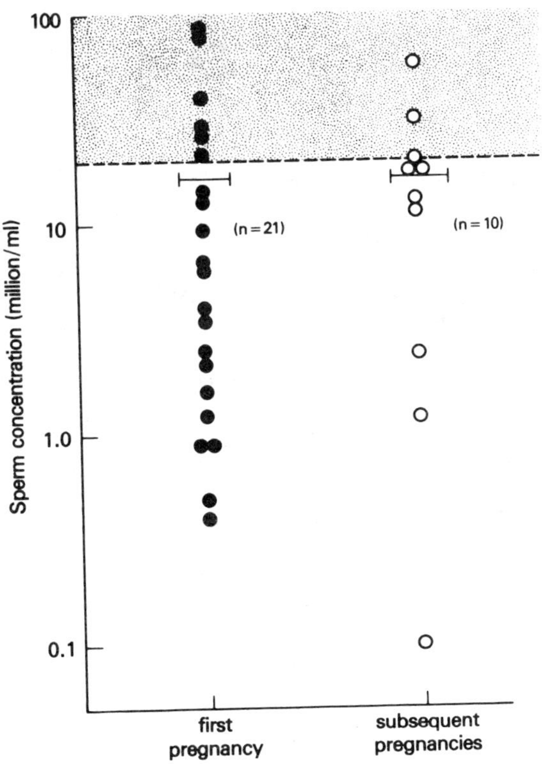

FIGURE 1. Mean sperm concentrations at the time of first conception (*closed circles*) and at the time of subsequent (second or third) conception (*open circles*) in men with isolated hypogonadotropic hypogonadism treated with gonadotropins. The number in parentheses represents the number of observations and the horizontal bars represent the mean of each group. The shaded area represents the conventional range of "normal."[2]

This chapter is written to provide insight into the clinical use and misuse of automated semen analysis. It emphasizes the critical importance of standardization, not only of semen collection and sample preparation for analysis, but also of parameter setting of equipment and operating procedures. As will be discussed, despite a variety of potential sources of error, CASA methodology can now provide long-awaited objectivity to sperm motion analysis. Potential sources of error can be minimized by use of disciplined technique in sample collection and analysis.

SEMEN COLLECTION

As ejaculation is an excretory function, semen quality has been shown to vary markedly even under conditions of strictly controlled abstinence.[1] With increasing intervals of abstinence sperm counts increase during seven to ten days while motility, viability, morphology, and fertilization potential frequently deteriorate.[6] Accordingly, any study of seminal characteristics requires strict abstinence control, not only to be able to assess sequential ejaculates within a subject but also to be able to make comparisons between subjects.[1] Traditionally, we prefer to obtain semen after 1 full day of sexual rest, that is 36 to 48 hours between ejaculations, with a background ejaculatory frequency of three times per week. This interval does not disrupt the sexual habits of the couple.

Considering within-subject variability of seminal characteristics, we have reported the need to assess approximately three semen specimens to establish a relatively stable baseline of values and to assess sperm parameters during more than one sperm cycle (74 days in the human) to recognize trends in semen quality.[1] We suggest that samples be collected by masturbation in appropriate, private collection rooms proximate to the laboratory; this facilitates prompt and standardized sperm processing.

Such measures reduce variability among samples collected from an individual, but still leave remarkable within-subject variations in sperm count, motility characteristics, and other semen parameters owing to the excretory nature of the product. Comparison of sperm measures analyzed in different laboratories is complicated by lack of standardization of semen collection procedures; most notably, abstinence intervals vary widely, semen may not be collected in a facility proximate to the laboratory, temperature and time to sample processing vary, and methods of semen collection other than masturbation, which alter semen quality, may be required for some individuals because of personal preference (condom, withdrawal, lubricants).

CASA TECHNOLOGY

CASA involves digitalization of sperm images from a microscopic field. The technical aspects of this process have been well summarized by Dr. Russell Davis in an extensive post graduate course review at the American Fertility Society.[5,7] Images are recorded by videocamera and projected onto a videomonitor for user convenience. Simultaneously, images of each sperm head are recorded electronically (digitalized) and also projected onto a videomonitor to form the equivalent of a multiple-exposure photomicrograph. Sperm heads appear as negative images, and contrast is adjusted (gray scale) so that the size of the real and digitalized images are equal. Individual picture elements in the field, called pixels, are illuminated to form the image of the sperm. Pixels are arranged as discrete dots on horizontal lines and are illuminated only when they correspond with a sperm's image. The central spatial location (centroid) of each sperm head is then computed and individual sperm trajectories are calculated by a computer program. In this way sperm parameters, such as concentration, percent motility and sperm motion characteristics can be measured automatically. A complete video picture, called a field, consists of two half-pictures, called frames. Each frame is formed by illuminating the relevant pixels on the odd set of video lines, then repeating this process for the even set of lines. Each set of odd or even video lines is illuminated every 1/60 second. This process of illuminating alternate sets of video lines is called interlacing. The speed with which interlacing is done is called the video framing rate. In standard video technology, each half-image, or video frame, is formed every 1/60 second, hence, the complete picture, or field, is formed only every 1/30 second. In this case, we would say that the video framing rate is 30 frames per second (Hz). Cells are counted as motile if movement occurs in two or more video frames and sperm velocity is calculated for cells that are tracked for 3 or more points of observation as set by the observer. The pixel scale (relative digitalized length/real image length) on the videomonitor is pre set at 0.688 and the velocity window set to record cells moving between 8 and 300 μm/sec.

Using current computer algorithms, CASA provides estimates of sperm concentration, percent motility, straight-line velocity (VSL), curvilinear velocity (VCL), velocity of the average path (VAP), linearity (L), amplitude of lateral head displacement (ALH) and beat cross frequency (BCF).

SOURCES OF VARIATION DURING CASA

CASA offers great potential in its ability to generate objectively large data sets of sperm characteristics. However, a number of problems can arise in obtaining accurate and precise results (TABLE 2). Errors can result from method of semen preparation, machine settings, choice of counting chamber, and sperm sampling bias.[8-12] Rigorous and disciplined quality assurance steps are required to provide optimal data. Training and monitoring of staff responsible for data acquisition is of the highest priority.

Threshold Setting

Adjusting the quality of the digitized image during CASA, threshold setting (gray scale), is a critical step which determines whether or not a sperm head is adequately

TABLE 2. Equipment Setting Factors and Sperm Processing Conditions Which Affect CASA Results

- Threshold setting of digitized image (gray scale)
- Video framing rate
- Number of tracking points
- Temperature
- Sperm concentration
- Choice of counting chamber
- Bias in selecting which cells are analyzed

defined to be included in computer computations.[10] Loss of data from the sample, variability of data within and between subjects, and differences in data between laboratories will result from inattention to the gray scale level. At the present time the threshold setting must be adjusted subjectively by the CASA user; generally, the digitized sperm head image is set to be slightly larger than the real image of the sperm.

Video Framing Rate

Sperm motion is complex, including rotatory motions, angular deviations of the head and varying vigor of its movement. Within semen there is increasing evidence for marked heterogeneity in sperm motion characteristics. The speed with which the digitized sperm images are collected (video framing rate) markedly influences the apparent sperm trajectory and how well it is characterized.[13] The video framing (digitization) rate influences significantly the apparent curvilinear velocity, lateral head amplitude, beat cross frequency and average path velocity, but seems to have no effect on straight-line velocity. Currently, most CASA equipment available has used a digitizing rate of 30 Hz (frames per second), which seems adequate for measurement of most semen parameters, but higher framing rates may be required to more accurately depict sperm motion characteristics under capacitating conditions and for measures of lateral head amplitude.

Tracking Points

The number of tracking points (frames analyzed) at a given video framing rate significantly affects calculated sperm motion characteristics (VCL, L and ALH).[10,12] At high sperm concentration (>20 million/ml), a progressive decline in apparent curvilinear velocity occurs when utilizing increasing numbers of tracking points.[12] At low sperm concentration, differences in tracking points primarily affect observed linearity (FIG. 2); at a reduced number of tracking points, most sperm appear to be moving in straight lines, while at higher tracking observations a full spectrum of linearities is recorded.[12] Accordingly, we utilize 20 tracking points for our CASA measurements, and most recent studies record with 15 to 20 fields of observations at a 30 Hz framing rate.

Temperature

Studies show that sperm motility varies significantly with ambient temperature.[14] Hence, some form of temperature regulation is recommended for CASA. Even for the relatively small differences between room temperature and 37°C, sperm velocity and linearity increase with rising temperature. Accordingly, we recommend keeping semen specimens at 37°C (incubator) from the time of collection through liquefaction and sperm processing, and utilize a stage warmer (37°C) during CASA.

Sperm Concentration

Using existing CASA methodology (CellSoft), high sperm concentration impacts significantly on estimation of curvilinear velocity.[12,14,15] Even with recent advances

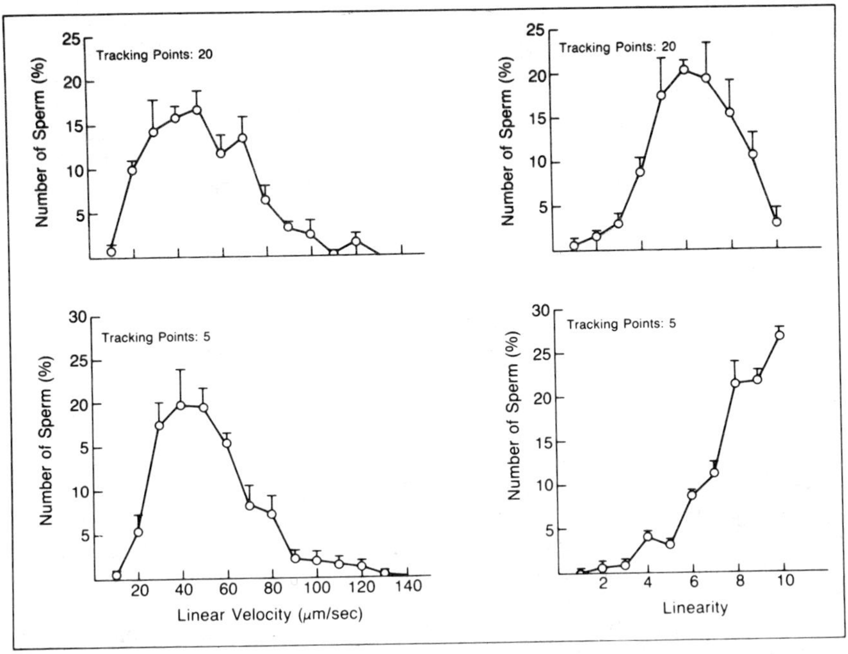

FIGURE 2. Curvilinear velocity (mean ± SE) and linearity distribution (percent) of sperm in seminal plasma tracked for either 5 or 20 points.[12]

in computer programming for newer instruments, assessing motion characteristics at high sperm concentration may still present problems and the user should consider these. At high sperm concentration (>20 million/ml), utilizing 20 tracking points, there is exclusion of sperm tracks interrupted by cell-cell collisions. This decreases significantly the number of data available for CASA calculations and excludes the faster moving sperm from estimates of VCL and L.[12] Since the heterogeneity of sperm motion in semen requires relatively long sperm tracking observations to provide accurate measures of VCL and L, dilution of semen to below 20 million/ml is recommended to avoid concentration-induced bias. Using the CellSoft program (Cryo Resources, Inc., New York), there is a higher fraction of utilizable data and higher curvilinear velocity estimates when measures are performed at concentrations <20 million/ml. VCL varies inversely, but not linearly, with sperm concentration. To avoid changing rheological properties and other aspects of the seminal milieu, semen should be diluted with an aliquot of the subject's own seminal plasma (10–100 μl aliquot centrifuged at 16,000 × *g* for 5 min to obtain cell-free seminal fluid).

Counting Chamber

The source and use of the sperm-counting chamber can contribute to systematic errors in CASA. The depth of the chamber is critical since, with moving sperm, cells frequently swim out of the field of focus when the distance is greater than 10 μm. In earlier studies, a precision Makler chamber (Sefi-Medical Instruments, Haifa, Israel) was utilized by most laboratories for viewing. Even so, care must be taken not to overfill the chamber, which leads to overestimation of both sperm concentration and percent motility.[14,16] This appears to be due to a technical artifact. More recently, disposable microcell chambers (Fertility Technologies, Inc., Natick, MA) have become available, which appear to provide more accurate and precise measures for moving cells.

Sampling Bias

Semen does not contain a homogeneous mix of sperm, and cell number and motility vary widely across multiple microscopic fields. Accordingly, the number of cells observed, the number of microscopic fields utilized and the randomness of sampling become critical issues if one is to obtain an accurate representation of values from a given sample.[8,12,14] At very low cell density (<10 million/ml) sampling bias is especially important. Most laboratories have shown appropriate accuracy and precision in CASA utilizing 100–200 cells from randomly selected viewing fields with coefficients of variation approximately 10% at 50 million/ml and 50% at 10 million/ml, in keeping with previous estimates of cell density by manual measurements. However, at severely oligospermic levels, sampling bias is especially noteworthy because it is effortful and time consuming to collect adequate numbers of cells to measure and every effort must be made to avoid focusing on only the highly motile sperm. Replicate measurements are essential for samples with low counts. Training, discipline and monitoring of staff is critical if one is to reduce sampling bias to a minimum.

CASA RESULTS FROM SEMEN

Sperm Concentration

Several studies have shown that CASA instruments are inaccurate in estimating sperm concentration in semen at values below 20 million/ml and above 100–150 million/ml. At low concentration, CellSoft overestimates sperm density by about 30%–50% relative to measurements made manually on fixed cells.[8,12,15,17] This seems to be due to counting of non-sperm particles. CellTrak and Hamilton-Thorn instruments appear to show a lesser error in this regard. At high cell density, cells may merge optically, at which point their data would be excluded from calculation because size criteria exceed those of normal sperm.

Depending on the laboratory, CASA estimates of sperm density may or may not be convenient or accurate. In evaluating samples primarily of normal men, *i.e.*, cryobank and/or routine semen screening, sperm concentrations generally fall in the convenient range for accurate CASA estimates; samples with concentrations exceeding 100 million/ml must be diluted. For andrology laboratories surveying semen primarily from infertile men, severely oligospermic samples (<10 million/ml) require manual counting measures for acceptable, accurate estimates. As described above, large errors in estimating low sperm concentration are in striking contrast to the improved accuracy in estimating motility characteristics at low sperm density.

Motion Characteristics

Vantman *et al.*[18] have assessed sperm motion characteristics from normal fertile donors and men with infertility using optimized CASA conditions as described above. Semen was collected after 36 to 48 hours abstinence among men also requested to have maintained prior ejaculatory frequency 2 to 3 times per week. Semen was analyzed soon after liquefaction under temperature-controlled conditions. If the initial analysis revealed a sperm concentration higher than 30 million/ml the sample was diluted with the patient's own seminal plasma to a density <20 million/ml. CASA was performed by CellSoft. Fifteen to twenty random microscopic fields were analyzed for each specimen, collecting data from approximately 100 cells. Data were analyzed utilizing 20 tracking points at a video framing rate of 30 Hz.

Among fertile donors, sperm VCL and L showed approximately symmetric and possibly gaussian distributions, whereas among infertile men VCL and L were *not* symmetric and thus not gaussian distributions (FIG. 3). Comparisons of means between groups is thus not appropriate mathematically. Inspection of individual frequency distributions of VCL and L shows significant heterogeneity. Two or more distinct subpopulations of motile sperm are evident in many semen specimens.

In view of the nongaussian distributions, cumulative distribution of the percent of cells measured at increasing intervals of VCL and L can be computed and a weighted average for fertile and infertile males constructed (FIG. 4). For VCL, 40 μm/sec is the point of maximum difference between infertile patients and fertile men (Vc_{40}), where only 38% of the cells of fertile men are at or below this cumulative velocity, while 60% of the sperm from infertile patients fall at or below this level. For linearity the greatest difference is observed at L_3 where 26% of cells from infertile men compared to 13% of cells from fertile donors fall at this level.

To further discriminate between fertile and infertile males, Vantman *et al.* applied

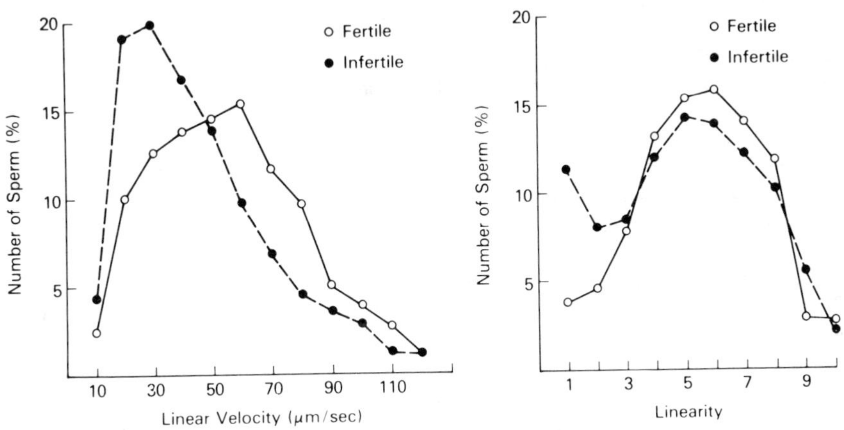

FIGURE 3. Mean frequency distributions of sperm curvilinear velocity and linearity in semen from fertile and infertile men. Data are shown as sperm number (percent) at increasing intervals of curvilinear velocity and linearity.[18]

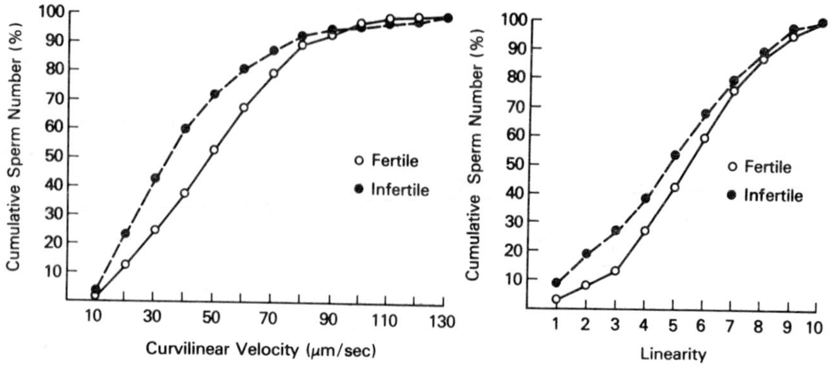

FIGURE 4. Weighted average of the cumulative percent distributions of sperm curvilinear velocity and linearity in semen from fertile and infertile men.[18]

co-variance analysis to these cumulative distributions of sperm motion characteristics. Vc_{40} and L_3 for each patient were plotted in reference to the weighted average of Vc_{40} and L_3 for fertile men (FIG. 5). For convenience, the mean Vc_{40} and L_3 for fertile men are reset to zero. Accordingly, by quadrant analysis, patient specimens with more cells at Vc_{40} than the mean value of fertile donors are slower (located to the left of the center line) and patient specimens with less cells at Vc_{40} than the mean value for fertile men are faster (located to the right of the center line). Using the same approach for linearity, samples with poor linearity have a higher percent of cells at L_3 than the mean for fertile men, and samples with better linearity have a lower percent of cells at L_3 than that observed for fertile men. Using this method, it was possible to distinguish four different subpopulations of infertile individuals: 1) those in whom sperm are slower and less linear (lower left quadrant); 2) those in whom sperm are faster and more linear (upper right quadrant); 3) those in whom sperm are faster but less linear (lower right quadrant); and 4) those in whom sperm are slower but more linear than those of fertile men (upper left quadrant).

By chi-square analysis, the data from fertile men are evenly distributed in the four quadrants and tightly clustered around the centroid (FIG. 5), whereas the data from patients fall predominantly in the lower left quadrant ($p < 0.001$). The lower left quadrant represents sperm cells that are both slower and less directional than those from average fertile males. However, not all of the cells from infertile males fall in this quadrant, as some patients have sperm that are similar to or faster and more directional than their fertile counterparts.

Using the above described quadrant analysis, a boundary line was computed, based on the distance of the individual patient data set at Vc_{40}, L_3 from the Vc_{40}, L_3 values of fertile men. This boundary separates 43 of 53 infertile men (81%), and 18 of 20 fertile men (90%), on the basis of the Vc_{40} and L_3 values.

Davis and associates, using a CellTrak-S instrument (Motion Analysis, Inc., Santa Rosa, CA) under optimal conditions, applied multivariate cluster analysis to straight-line velocity (VSL), curvilinear velocity (VCL), linearity (L) and mean angle of deviation (MAD) and could correctly classify semen belonging to fertile or infertile subjects.[19,20] Such multivariate analysis is certainly feasible with data derived by CASA

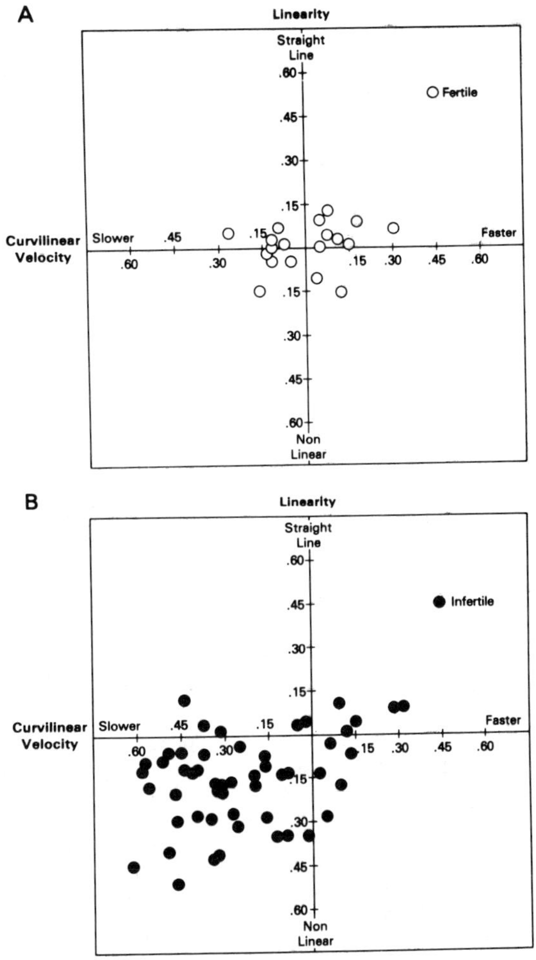

FIGURE 5. Distribution of curvilinear velocity and linearity values at Vc_{40} and L_3; individual values are compared to the weighted average values for normal men at that level. The top panel shows values from fertile men and the lower panel shows values for infertile men. The numbers placed along the vertical and horizontal axes represent the fraction of cells falling above or below the mean cumulative distribution value at Vc_{40}/L_3 for normal men.[18]

and may offer a more robust analysis of sperm motion to identify men more likely to be infertile.

SUMMARY

During the past six years, there has been an explosion of technology which allows automated machine-vision for sperm analysis.[21] CASA clearly provides an opportunity for objective, systematic assessment of sperm motion. But there are many caveats in using this type of equipment. CASA requires a disciplined and standardized approach to semen collection, specimen preparation, machine settings, calibration and avoidance of sampling bias. Potential sources of error can be minimized.

Unfortunately, the rapid commercialization of this technology preceded detailed statistical analysis of such data to allow equally rapid comparisons of data between different CASA machines and among different laboratories. Thus, it is now imperative that we standardize use of this technology and obtain more detailed biological insights into sperm motion parameters in semen and after capacitation before we empirically employ CASA for studies of fertility prediction.

In the basic science arena, CASA technology will likely evolve to provide new algorithms for accurate sperm motion analysis and give us an opportunity to address the biophysics of sperm movement. In the clinical arena, CASA instruments provide the opportunity to share and compare sperm motion data among laboratories by virtue of its objectivity, assuming standardized conditions of utilization. Identification of men with specific sperm motion disorders is certain, but the biological relevance of motility dysfunction to actual fertilization remains uncertain and surely the subject for further study.

REFERENCES

1. Sherins, R. J., D. Brightwell & P. M. Sternthal. 1977. Longitudinal analysis of semen of fertile and infertile men. *In* New Concepts of the Testis in Normal and Infertile Men: Morphology, Physiology and Pathology. P. Troen & H. Nankin. Eds.: 473–488. Raven Press. New York.
2. Burris, A. S., R. V. Clark, D. J. Vantman & R. J. Sherins. 1988. A low sperm concentration does not preclude fertility in men with isolated hypogonadotropic hypogonadism after gonadotropin therapy. Fertil. Steril. **50:** 343–347.
3. Katz, D. F. & J. W. Overstreet. 1981. Sperm motility assessment by videomicrography. Fertil. Steril. **35:** 188–193.
4. Overstreet, J. W., D. F. Katz, F. W. Hanson & J. R. Fonseca. 1979. A simple inexpensive method for objective assessment of human sperm movement characteristics. Fertil. Steril. **31:** 162–172.
5. Katz, D. F. & R. O. Davis. 1987. Automatic analysis of human sperm motion. J. Androl. **8:** 170–181.
6. Mortimer, D. 1985. The male factor in infertility. Part I: Semen analysis. *In* Current problems in Obstetrics, Gynecology and Fertility. J. M. Leventhal, Ed.: 3–87. Year Book Medical Publishers, Chicago.
7. Davis, R. O. 1990. The promise and pitfalls of computer aided sperm analysis. Post Graduate Course IV: Basic and Clinical Aspects of Male Infertility. American Fertility Society. Washington, D.C. November, pp. 108–154.
8. Ginsburg, K. A., K. S. Moghissi & E. L. Abel. 1988. Computer-assisted semen analysis: Sampling errors and reproducibility. J. Androl. **9:** 82–90.
9. Knuth, U. A., C. H. Yeung & E. Nieschlag. 1987. Computerized semen analysis: Objective measurement of semen characteristics is biased by subjective parameter setting. Fertil. Steril. **48:** 118–124.
10. Mack, S. O., D. P. Wolf & J. S. Tash. 1988. Quantitation of specific parameters of motility in large numbers of human sperm by digital image processing. Biol. Reprod. **38:** 270–281.
11. Mortimer, D. & S. T. Mortimer. 1988. Influence of system parameter settings on human sperm motility analysis using CellSoft. Human Reprod. **3:** 621–625.
12. Vantman, D., G. Koukoulis, L. Dennison, M. Zinaman & R. J. Sherins. 1988. Computer-assisted semen analysis: Evaluation of method and assessment of the influence of sperm concentration on linear velocity determination. Fertil. Steril. **49:** 510–515.
13. Mortimer, D., C. Serres, S. T. Mortimer & P. Jouannet. 1988. Influence of image sampling frequency on the perceived movement characteristics of progressively motile human spermatozoa. Gamete Res. **20:** 313–327.
14. Mack, S. O., J. S. Tash & D. P. Wolf. 1989. Effect of measurement conditions on quantification of hyperactivated human sperm subpopulations by digital image analysis. Biol. Reprod. **40:** 1162–1169.

15. Mortimer, D., N. Goel & M. A. Shu. 1988. Evaluation of the CellSoft automated semen analysis system in a routine laboratory setting. Fertil. Steril. **50:** 960–968.
16. Yanagida, K., K. Hoshi, A. Sato & L. Burkman. 1990. Automated semen analysis shows an increase in sperm concentration and motility with time in Makler chambers having excess sample volume. Human Reprod. **5:** 193–196.
17. Knuth, U. A. & E. Nieschlag. 1988. Comparison of computerized semen analysis with the conventional procedure in 322 patients. Fertil. Steril. **49:** 881–885.
18. Vantman, D., S. M. Banks, G. Koukoulis, L. Dennison & R. J. Sherins. 1989. Assessment of sperm motion characteristics from fertile and infertile men using a fully automated computer-assisted semen analyzer. Fertil. Steril. **51:** 156–161.
19. Davis, R. O. & J. W. Overstreet. 1990. A provisional standard for normal progression in semen assessed by CASA (computer aided sperm analysis). American Fertility Society. Washington, D. C. November, Abstract P88.
20. Davis, R. O., J. W. Overstreet, R. H. Asch & S. J. Silber. 1990. The use of CASA (computer aided sperm analysis) in predicting the clinical outcome of IVF when epididymal sperm are used for insemination. American Fertility Society. Washington, D. C. November, Abstract P5.
21. Boyers, S. P., R. O. Davis & D. F. Katz. 1989. Automated semen analysis. Curr. Prob. Ob/Gyn & Fertil. **5:** 167–200.

Reactive Oxygen Species and Human Spermatozoa[a]

CLAUDE GAGNON,[b,c] AKIRA IWASAKI,[d]
EVE DE LAMIRANDE,[b] AND NEIL KOVALSKI[b]

[b] *Urology Research Laboratory*
Royal Victoria Hospital
Faculty of Medicine, McGill University
Montréal, Québec, Canada H3A 1A1

[d] *Department of Urology*
Yokohama City University
Yokohama, 232 Japan

INTRODUCTION

Reactive oxygen species (ROS) such as hydrogen peroxide (H_2O_2), the superoxide anion ($^{\cdot}O_2^-$) and the hydroxyl radical ($^{\cdot}OH$), can be generated by living cells incubated under aerobic conditions.[1] To counteract the effect of ROS, cells possess systems that scavenge ROS to prevent internal cellular damage. Whereas there is little known on the sperm enzymatic systems involved in the generation of ROS, the presence of several enzymes involved in their neutralization, such as superoxide dismutase,[2-6] catalase,[7] and the glutathione peroxidase/reductase system, has been documented.[8-10] Thus, imbalance between the generation of ROS and their destruction can result in cellular damage.

It has been reported more than four decades ago that ROS can be toxic to spermatozoa and that catalase can confer protection.[11-13] Human spermatozoa are especially sensitive to lipid peroxidation induced by oxygen reactive species because of their high content of polyunsaturated fatty acids.[9,14,15] The lipoperoxidative lethal point, which corresponds to the level of peroxidation that will kill spermatozoa, has been calculated at 100 nmole of malonaldehyde formed per 10^8 cells.[9] The formation of malonaldehyde, a by-product of membrane lipoperoxidation, has been inversely correlated with the percentage of motile cells and positively correlated with mid-piece morphological defects in human spermatozoa.[16] The group of Aitken has reported that damaged or deficient spermatozoa form higher levels of ROS than normal motile spermatozoa.[17,18] It was suggested that ROS formation could be a cause for idiopathic infertility.[17,18]

In this chapter, we will first report on the incidence of ROS formation in the semen

[a] The authors acknowledge the financial support of the Medical Research Council of Canada.

[c] Address all correspondence to Dr. Claude Gagnon, Director, Urology Research Laboratory, Royal Victoria Hospital, Room H6.47, 687 Pine Ave. W., Montréal, Québec, Canada, H3A 1A1.

of a population of infertile patients. We will then address the possibility that leukocytes present in the male reproductive tract can cause damage to spermatozoa, and finally, we will discuss the mechanism by which ROS can cause sperm damage in conditions where viability is not affected.

INCIDENCE OF ROS FORMATION IN INFERTILE PATIENTS

To investigate whether ROS formation could be a significant factor in male infertility, the incidence of ROS formation was determined in the semen of an unselected population of patients consulting for infertility. Measurements of ROS formation were performed on whole semen rather then washed spermatozoa since several factors, both of cellular and secretory origins, could affect ROS formation and sperm function. For these experiments, ROS formation was determined 2–3 hours after semen collection by luminescence using luminol and a LKB computer-driven luminometer, at 27.7°C. Results indicated that 25% of the semen from 172 patients who were not azoospermic generated easily detectable amounts of ROS (>10 m V/s/10^9 spermatozoa). On the other hand, none of the six semen specimens from azoospermic patients and none of the 12 from fertile donors currently used in our laboratory produced ROS.[19,20]

In the group of patients, there was no difference in the incidence of ROS formation in semen samples in which the volume was smaller than 1.5 ml, higher than 2.5 ml or between these two values. However, there was a significant negative correlation ($r = 0.35$, $p < 0.05$) between the level of ROS formation and semen volume in these specimens.[20] Since the seminal vesicles contribute the majority of the semen volume, these results may suggest that secretions from these glands contain scavenging systems that decrease the detection of ROS measured by chemiluminescence.

The level of ROS formation was also inversely correlated with the percentage of motile cells ($r = 0.46$, $p < 0.05$), and the incidence of ROS formation was the lowest in sperm populations with more than 60% motile cells. Similarly to motility, linearity was inversely correlated with ROS formation ($r = 0.33$, $p < 0.05$).[19,20] These results suggest that damaged spermatozoa were mainly responsible for the generation of ROS.

Separation of cellular elements from semen, on a discontinuous Percoll gradient made of 20, 40, 65 and 95% Percoll layers, indicated that seminal plasma did not produce ROS, and that cells accumulating at the 40–65% and 65–95% interface (the 95% layer was combined with the latter interface) were responsible for the majority of ROS formed. The 40–65% interface contained few motile spermatozoa, occasional round cells, and a majority of immotile and morphologically abnormal spermatozoa. On the other hand, the 65–95% interface contained spermatozoa that were morphologically normal with an adequate intrinsic density. Whereas in gradients on which semen from fertile men were centrifuged, the latter Percoll interface contained 70–85% of the initial sperm population with a motility above 70–80%,[21] the same interface from gradients on which semen from patients were centrifuged may contain only 20–50% of the spermatozoa in semen, and be characterized by a motility ranging from 0 to 50%. Thus, spermatozoa that are morphologically normal under the light microscope, and have the right density, may be biochemically and functionally abnormal. We hypothesize that these spermatozoa are responsible for the ROS detected in the lower Percoll interface. The level of ROS generated in this Percoll layer was also inversely correlated with the percentage of motile spermatozoa and their linearity.[20]

EFFECT OF SPERM WASHING PROCEDURES ON ROS FORMATION

It has long been known that washing spermatozoa by repeated centrifugation-resuspension cycles results in a decrease in the quality of sperm motility. To investigate whether centrifugation damage could be linked to ROS formation, semen samples from patients were either centrifuged on Percoll gradient and the 65–95% interface analyzed or subjected to repeated (3×) centrifugation-resuspension cycles with fresh physiological buffer and the pellet analyzed. Analysis of the data revealed that washed spermatozoa in the 65–95% interface produced 4-fold more ROS than the whole semen. On the other hand, spermatozoa washed by repeated centrifugation-resuspension cycles generated 21-fold higher levels of ROS than the original semen when normalized for the number of spermatozoa. Adding back seminal plasma to spermatozoa washed by multiple centrifugations reduced ROS detected from 406 mV/s/10^9 spermatozoa to 61 mV/s/10^9 spermatozoa, a value similar to that obtained with spermatozoa subjected to 3 cycles of centrifugation-resuspension but without removal of seminal plasma (71 mV/s/10^9 spermatozoa). However, the latter two values were still 8-fold higher than the 8 mV/s/10^9 spermatozoa detected in the original semen.[20]

Thus, it would appear that morphologically abnormal and biochemically/functionally abnormal (but not dead) spermatozoa present in semen cause ROS formation. Centrifugation and removal of seminal plasma increase ROS detection.

NEUTROPHILS, INFECTION AND POSSIBLE DAMAGE TO SPERM FUNCTION

Concentrations of neutrophils above 1 million/ml are occasionally found in semen of patients consulting for infertility. The detection of these polymorphonuclear cells is currently based on the content of myeloperoxidase[22] or the presence of specific antigens. However, in the last case, antibodies that generally recognize all leukocytes are often used.[23] Since the presence of active neutrophils is a better reflection of an active acute infection than the whole leukocyte population, a test to determine active neutrophil concentration was developed. This new test, in contrast to the previous tests, such as the myeloperoxidase assay by histochemical techniques, determines the concentration of functionally active neutrophils. The new assay is based on the capacity of active neutrophils to generate ROS upon stimulation by invading microorganisms or by synthetic stimulants such as phorbol myristate acetate (PMA). The superoxide anion generated reduces nitroblue tetrazolium (pale yellow color) to formazan (blue color).[24] Although this test is less sensitive than the histochemical myeloperoxidase assay, the sensitivity obtained (0.5×10^6 polymorphonuclear leukocytes per ml of semen) is 2-fold below the level considered by the World Health Organization[25] as evidence of possible genital tract infection. The advantages of this assay include its simplicity, its low cost, and an objective assessment of functionally active polymorphonuclear leukocytes in semen.

To address the question whether active neutrophils could affect sperm function, PMA-stimulated neutrophils were incubated with spermatozoa. Although neutrophils only produced ROS in the first 30 min, the percentage of motile spermatozoa was affected 2–3 hours later for neutrophil concentrations above 2×10^6 cells/ml. However, at a later time (5 h), neutrophil concentrations as low as 0.6×10^6 cells/ml caused a decrease in motility of at least 30%. Addition of superoxide dismutase significantly reduced the amount of ROS detected by chemiluminescence and NBT, but without conferring any protection on sperm motility. On the other hand, catalase was able to prevent most of the damage done to sperm motility.[26] Whereas pools of human seminal plasma can prevent most of the damage caused by ROS produced by neutrophils, individual sperm samples seemed to confer a wide range of protection from full protection to none (unpublished data).

EFFECTS OF ROS ON MOTILITY AND VIABILITY OF HUMAN SPERMATOZOA

To further investigate the effects of ROS on sperm viability and motility, we have used xanthine (X) and xanthine oxidase (XO), which produces the superoxide anion (and subsequently H_2O_2 after dismutation), as a source of ROS. When X+XO at concentrations above 1 mM and 0.05 U/ml, respectively, were incubated with Percoll-washed motile spermatozoa from a fertile donor, sperm motility was arrested within 30–60 min. A drop of 30–50% in sperm viability was always associated with these experimental conditions. However, at lower ROS concentrations (0.3–0.6 mM X + 0.05 U XO/ml), viability was only marginally affected. Under these conditions, although ROS were present in solution for only one hour, the percentage of motile cells was only affected at 1.5 h after the addition of ROS. The drop in the percentage of motile cells occurred abruptly, in contrast to the flagellar beat frequency which was affected shortly but progressively after ROS addition. The decrease in beat frequency reached a value of 27% of control within the first hour after the addition of X+XO (TABLE 1).[27,28]

ROS have long been known to cause damage to cells by interfering with membrane function. To determine whether the effects on sperm motility could also be caused by modifications on the sperm axoneme, the motor responsible for sperm movement, demembranated sperm models were prepared as previously described.[29,30] These sperm models are prepared by demembranation of motile intact spermatozoa with Triton X-100; the motility of these immotile, demembranated spermatozoa is

TABLE 1. Effect of ROS on the Motility Parameters and ATP Level of Intact Spermatozoa

	Intact Spermatozoa		
Time (h)	Motility (% of control)	Beat Frequency (% of control)	ATP Level (% of control)
0	100	100	100
0.5	100	55	25
1	100	27	12
1.5	0	0	5
2.5	0	0	5
24	25	25	25

Percoll-washed spermatozoa from a fertile donor were incubated with xanthine (0.6 mM) and xanthine oxidase (0.05 U/ml). The percentage of motile spermatozoa and their flagellar beat frequency were measured at various time periods after addition of ROS. Sperm ATP levels were determined by the luciferine-luciferase assay. These results from one experiment are representative of 5 other experiments.

TABLE 2. Effect of ROS on the Motility Parameters of Demembranated Spermatozoa

Time (h)	Motility (% of control)	Beat Frequency (% of control)
0	100	100
0.5	100	100
1	50	100
1.5	25	100
2.5	0	0
24	25	100

Percoll-washed spermatozoa were treated as described in TABLE 1. At various time intervals after the initiation of ROS treatment, spermatozoa were demembranated with Triton X-100, and motility was reinitiated by the addition of 0.5 mM Mg ATP.[30] These results from the same experiment reported in TABLE 1 are representative of 5 other experiments.

then reactivated by the addition of a source of energy, ATP. Sperm models from ROS-treated intact spermatozoa could reactivate motility with a decreased percentage and duration of reactivation when compared to control untreated spermatozoa (TABLE 2). On the other hand, their flagellar beat frequency was not affected. It is worth mentioning that when intact spermatozoa were immobilized by ROS treatment, the reactivation of the sperm models was still possible, but for only an additional 30 min.[27,28]

The most surprising aspect of these experiments was that the motility of intact spermatozoa could spontaneously recover after several hours of arrest (TABLE 1). This was associated with the reappearance of motility in sperm models when challenged with ATP (TABLE 2).

IMPORTANCE OF ATP IN ROS DAMAGE TO SPERMATOZOA

Since ATP concentration determines the flagellar beat frequency of demembranated spermatozoa,[31] and ROS treatment caused a rapid decrease in flagellar beat frequency of intact spermatozoa, the level of ATP in control and ROS-treated cells was investigated. The level of ATP decreased rapidly following ROS treatment. The fall in ATP concentration was even steeper than that of the flagellar beat frequency. This discrepancy in the kinetics of these two parameters is not unexpected since the concentration of ATP within human spermatozoa is 4.5 mM,[32] a value much higher than the 0.3–0.4 mM ATP required for half maximal beat frequency in demembranated sperm models.[33] At the time when intact sperm motility ceased after ROS treatment, the level of ATP was 10- to 20-fold lower than that found in control spermatozoa.[34]

The importance of the drop in ATP concentration after ROS treatment was further emphasized by the following series of observations. The addition of lactate and pyruvate together with ROS to intact spermatozoa completely prevented the decrease in intracellular ATP concentration, the drop in flagellar beat frequency and the fall in sperm motility generally seen a few hours after ROS treatment. Furthermore, spermatozoa immobilized by ROS treatment, and supplemented with pyruvate + lactate reinitiated motility much earlier than their counterparts supplemented with buffer only (unpublished data).

TABLE 3. Effect of ROS Scavengers on the Motility of Spermatozoa Treated with X + XO

		Intact Spermatozoa			Demembranated Spermatozoa	
		Motility 2h				
Product	Concentration	%	Hz	Recovery 24h	Motility 2h (%)	Recovery 24h
None	–	0	0	No	0	No
Catalase	0.03 mg/ml	Total protection			Total protection	
	0.008 mg/ml	Total protection			Total protection	
	0.003 mg/ml	100	50	Total	100	Total
SOD	1.0 mg/ml	50	50	Total	Total protection	
	0.25 mg/ml	0	0	Partial	25	Partial
	0.10 mg/ml	0	0	Partial	0	Partial
DMSO	140 mM	0	0	Partial to total	0	Partial Partial
Dithiothreitol	1 mM	No protective effect against xanthine + xanthine oxidase				
Glutathione	1 mM					
Butylated hydroxytoluene	1 mM					
Sodium benzoate	100 mM					
Mannitol	100 mM					
Taurine	25 mM					
Hypotaurine	25 mM					

Spermatozoa were treated with XO (0.05 U/ml) + X (0.6 mM) in the absence or the presence of scavengers. Motility was evaluated 2 h and 24 h after the beginning of ROS treatment. Control (no treatment) spermatozoa had high motility ($\geq$75%, Hz: 4.5 $\pm$ 0.3 beat/sec) and their reactivation was above 75%. Results are expressed as percentage of control values.

EFFECTS OF ROS SCAVENGERS ON X + XO–TREATED SPERMATOZOA

To determine which of ROS produced by X + XO caused the damage to sperm motility, ROS-treated spermatozoa were incubated with various scavengers. Since X + XO can produce the superoxide anion which can be spontaneously or enzymically dismutated into H_2O_2 and O_2, and that $\cdot O_2^-$ and H_2O_2 can react together through the Haber Weiss reaction to produce the very toxic hydroxyl radical, superoxide dismutase, catalase and DMSO were used to scavenge $\cdot O_2^-$, H_2O_2 and $\cdot OH$, respectively. Of these scavengers only catalase at concentrations as low as 0.008 mg/ml conferred full protection on spermatozoa incubated with X and XO (TABLE 3). The addition of superoxide dismutase at a high concentration (1 mg/ml) conferred only partial protection, whereas 140 mM DMSO mainly helped the recovery of motility without affecting its fall. It would then appear from these results that H_2O_2 is the primary toxic ROS responsible for most damage done to spermatozoa. However, $\cdot O_2^-$ and $\cdot OH$ may, to some extent, also contribute to the toxicity of X + XO on human spermatozoa.

CONCLUSION

Normally, there is a fine balance between the amounts of ROS produced and scavenged by a cell. Cellular damage arises when this equilibrium is disturbed, especially when the increase in ROS produced cannot be eliminated by the reserve of scavenging systems. Such a disruption occurs in at least 25% of the semen of patients consulting for infertility. However, whether the disruption in ROS equilibrium is due to a decreased scavenging capacity or to an enhanced ROS production remains to be seen.

The clinical significance of leukocytes in male and female reproductive tracts remains controversial. However, the data summarized above indicate that stimulated leukocytes can produce an outburst of ROS that will decrease sperm motility over long periods of time, even at concentrations below 1×10^6 cells/ml. Whereas human seminal plasma has enormous scavenging capacity for the superoxide anion produced by activated leukocytes, the situation may be quite different in extracellular fluids surrounding spermatozoa in the male and female reproductive tracts.

The observation that exogenously added ROS affect sperm motility by decreasing the intracellular ATP level before affecting viability, raises the possibility that the poor sperm velocity frequently seen in the semen of infertile patients, which is a reflection of flagellar beat frequency, may be due to abnormally low levels of ATP. Whether this deficiency can be corrected by incubations with metabolic precursors known to increase cellular ATP levels remains to be investigated.

ACKNOWLEDGMENT

We are grateful to Mrs. Lina Ordonselli for her secretarial assistance.

REFERENCES

1. GRISHAM, M. B. & J. M. MCCORD. 1986. Chemistry and cytotoxicity of reactive oxygen metabolites. *In* Biology of Oxygen Radicals. A. E. Taylor *et al.*, Eds.: 1–18. American Physiological Society. Bethesda, MD.
2. ABU-ERREIZH, G., L. MAGNES & T. K. LI. 1978. Isolation and properties of superoxide dismutase from ram spermatozoa and erythrocytes. Biol. Reprod. **18:** 554–560.
3. MANELLA, M. R. F. & R. JONES. 1980. Properties of spermatozoa superoxide dismutase and lack of involvement of superoxides in metal-ion-catalysed lipid-peroxidation reactions in semen. Biochem. J. **191:** 289–296.
4. NISSEN, H. P. & H. W. KREYSEL. 1983. Superoxide dismutase in human semen. Klin. Wochenschr. **61:** 63–65.
5. ALVAREZ, J. G. & B. T. STOREY. 1983. Role of superoxide dismutase in protecting rabbit spermatozoa from oxygen toxicity due to lipid peroxidation. Biol. Reprod. **28:** 1129–1136.
6. ALVAREZ, J. G. & B. T. STOREY. 1984. Lipid peroxidation and the reactions of superoxide and hydrogen peroxide in mouse spermatozoa. Biol. Reprod. **30:** 833–841.
7. JEULIN, C., J. C. SOUFIR, P. WEBER, D. LAVAL-MARTIN & R. CALVAYRAC. 1989. Catalase activity in human spermatozoa and seminal plasma. Gamete Res. **24:** 185–196.
8. LI, T. K. 1975. The glutathione and thiol content of mammalian spermatozoa and seminal plasma. Biol. Reprod. **12:** 641–646.
9. ALVAREZ, J. G., J. C. TOUCHSTONE, L. BLASCO & B. T. STOREY. 1987. Spontaneous lipid peroxidation and production of hydrogen peroxide and superoxide in human spermatozoa—Superoxide dismutase as major enzyme protectant against oxygen toxicity. J. Androl. **8:** 338–348.
10. ALVAREZ, J. G. & B. T. STOREY. 1989. Role of glutathione peroxidase in protecting mammalian spermatozoa from loss of motility caused by spontaneous lipid peroxidation. Gamete Res. **23:** 77–88.
11. MCLEOD, J. 1943. The role of oxygen in the metabolism and motility of human spermatozoa. Am. J. Physiol. **138:** 512–518.
12. TOSIC, J. 1947. Mechanism of hydrogen peroxide formation by spermatozoa and the role of amino acids in sperm motility. Nature **159:** 544–545.
13. TOSIC, J. & A. WALTON. 1950. Metabolism of spermatozoa. Formation of hydrogen peroxide by spermatozoa and its effects on motility and survival. Biochem. J. **47:** 199–206.
14. JONES, R., T. MANN & R. SHERINS. 1979. Peroxidative breakdown of phospholipids in human spermatozoa, spermicidal properties of fatty acid peroxides and protective action of seminal plasma. Fertil. Steril. **31:** 531–537.
15. AITKEN, R. J. & J. S. CLARKSON. 1987. Cellular basis of defective sperm function and its association with the genesis of reactive oxygen species by human spermatozoa. J. Reprod. Fertil. **81:** 459–469.
16. RAO, B., J. C. SOUFIR, M. MARTIN & G. DAVID. 1989. Lipid peroxidation in human spermatozoa as related to midpiece abnormalities and motility. Gamete Res. **24:** 127–134.
17. AITKEN, J. R. & J. S. CLARKSON. 1988. Significance of reactive oxygen species and antioxidants in defining the efficacy of sperm preparation techniques. J. Androl. **9:** 367–376.
18. AITKEN, J. R., J. S. CLARKSON & S. FISHEL. 1989. Generation of reactive oxygen species, lipid peroxidation and human sperm function. Biol. Reprod. **40:** 183–197.
19. IWASAKI, A. & C. GAGNON. 1989. Free radical formation in human semen: Incidence and correlation with motility. 35th Annual Meeting of the Canadian Fertility and Andrology Society, Vancouver. Abstract 25.
20. IWASAKI, A. & C. GAGNON. 1991. Formation of reactive oxygen species in spermatozoa of infertile patients. Fertil. Steril. In press.
21. CHAPEAU, C. & C. GAGNON. 1987. Nitrocellulose and polyvinyl coatings prevent sperm adhesion to glass without affecting the motility of intact and demembranated human spermatozoa. J. Androl. **8:** 34–40.
22. BARRATT, C. L. R., A. ROBINSON, R. C. SPENCER, G. R. KINGHORN, A. WHITE, P. E. HARRISON, E. KESSOPOULON & I. D. COOKE. 1990. Seminal peroxidase positive cells are not an adequate indicator of asymptomatic urethral genital infection. Int. J. Androl. **13:** 361–370.

23. AITKEN, R. J. & K. M. WEST. 1990. Analysis of the relationship between reactive oxygen species production and leukocyte infiltration in fractions of human semen separated on Percoll gradients. Int. J. Androl. **13:** 433–451.
24. KOVALSKI, N., E. DE LAMIRANDE & C. GAGNON. 1991. Determination of neutrophil concentration in semen by measurement of superoxide radical formation. Fertil. Steril. In press.
25. WHO. 1987. Laboratory manual for the examination of human semen and semen-cervical mucus interaction. Cambridge University Press. Cambridge, UK.
26. KOVALSKI, N., E. DE LAMIRANDE & C. GAGNON. 1991. Dimethylsulfoxide and catalase protect against neutrophil induce loss of sperm motility. Canadian Fertility and Andrology Society, Québec. Abstract TP27.
27. DE LAMIRANDE, E., A. IWASAKI & C. GAGNON. 1992. Reactive oxygen species affect sperm axoneme. In press.
28. DE LAMIRANDE, E., A. IWASAKI & C. GAGNON. 1990. Free radicals also affect sperm axoneme. 36th Annual Meeting of the Canadian Fertility and Andrology Society, L'Esterel, Québec. Abstract 14.
29. MOHRI, H. & R. YAMAGIMACHI. 1980. Characteristics of motor apparatus in testicular epididymal and ejaculated spermatozoa. Exp. Cell Res. **127:** 191–196.
30. DE LAMIRANDE, E. & C. GAGNON. 1983. Aprotinin and a seminal plasma factor inhibit the motility of demembranated reactivated rabbit spermatozoa. Biol. Reprod. **28:** 788–796.
31. GIBBONS, B. H. & I. R. GIBBONS. 1972. Flagellar movement and adenosine triphosphatase activity in sea urchin extracted with Triton X-100. J. Cell Biol. **54:** 75–97.
32. FORD, W. C. C. & A. HARRISON. 1983. D-[1-^{14}C] mannitol and [U-^{14}C] sucrose as extracellular space markers for human spermatozoa and the rupture of 2-deoxyglucose. J. Reprod. Fertil. **69:** 479–487.
33. COSSON, M. P. & C. GAGNON. 1988. Protease inhibitor and substrates block motility and microtubule sliding of sea urchin and carp spermatozoa. Cell Motil. Cytoskeleton **10:** 518–527.
34. DE LAMIRANDE, E. & C. GAGNON. 1991. ATP depletion plays an important role in the inhibition of sperm motility observed after treatment with reactive oxygen species. 11th North American Testis Workshop, Montreal. Abstract 116.

The Effects of Moderate Heating of the Testes and Epididymides of Rams by Scrotal Insulation on Body Temperature, Respiratory Rate, Spermatozoa Output and Motility, and on Fertility and Embryonic Survival in Ewes Inseminated with Frozen Semen[a]

R. MIEUSSET,[b] P. I. QUINTANA CASARES, L. G. SANCHEZ-PARTIDA, S. F. SOWERBUTTS, J. L. ZUPP, AND B. P. SETCHELL

Department of Animal Sciences
Waite Agricultural Research Institute
University of Adelaide
Glen Osmond, South Australia 5064, Australia

INTRODUCTION

Elevation of testicular temperature above normal levels is well known to induce alterations in spermatogenesis in mammals with scrotal testes.[1] Depressed spermatogenesis was observed when ambient temperature was raised or a large increase in testicular temperature was induced for a short period or when the increased temperature was obtained through surgically induced cryptorchidism. Whatever the kind of elevation in temperature, fertility was reported to be depressed or even suppressed.[2] Such a depression in fertility of females mated to or inseminated with semen from heat stressed males could be due either to a failure of sperm transport in the female,[3] or to a failure in fertilization or an increase in embryonic loss or both.[4,5]

In humans, in whom experiments are obviously less easy to perform, some evidence seems to indicate that such a relation between testicular temperature and functions could exist. Spermatogenesis was depressed by a large increase induced in body temperature[6] or in scrotal temperature,[7] and by a slight and repeated increase in testicular temperature of fertile men.[8] An elevated scrotal temperature was observed in

[a] Financial support for this project was provided by CECOS Midi-Pyrénées and INSERM U168 (Toulouse, France) for R. Mieusset and by a small grant from the Australian Research Council.

[b] *Present address and address for all correspondence:* R. Mieusset, M.D., Centre de Stérilité Masculine, Hôpital La Grave, 31052, Toulouse Cedex, France.

about one third of infertile men.[9,10] Moreover, chronic treatment by cooling the scrotum was reported to improve semen characteristics[11] and to lead to pregnancy in the partners of 25% of the men with elevated scrotal temperatures.[12]

The aim of the present study was to assess the modifications in spermatogenesis of rams subjected to a moderate and repeated increase in scrotal temperature, *i.e.*, similar to the values observed in infertile men, for 8, 16, or 24 hours/day, as well as to assess the fertility of ewes inseminated with frozen semen from rams submitted to a 16 hours/day insulation regimen.

MATERIALS AND METHODS

Treatments

Fully fleeced mature Australian Merino rams, 3 to 5 years old and weighing 65 to 75 kg, were kept in individual pens under a 16 hour-light and 8 hour-dark regimen in 3 rooms (8 rams per room) in which ambient temperature ranged between 19 and 23°C. In each room, 4 rams were used as control and 4 rams submitted to an identical regimen of scrotal heating for either 8, 16, or 24 hours/day. The scrotum was heated by means of an insulating bag made up of one layer of aluminum foil sandwiched between two layers of cotton cloth, with a supplementary layer of water proof cotton cloth on the outside.[13] The bag was held around the scrotum by four tapes tied over the back of the rams. The starting of the heating period was on 18 December 1989 for the 8 h/day regimen, 15 January 1990 for 16 h/day, and 2 May 1990 for 24 h/day.

Before the main experiment, the effects of the scrotal insulation were evaluated in 10 other rams with 3 controls in conditions identical to the experimental ones. A thermistor probe (Yellow Spring, USA) was inserted between the tunica vaginalis and the scrotal skin under xylazine sedation (0.4 ml *i.v.*; Rompon, Bayer) on day 1. On day 2, temperatures and respiratory rates were recorded every five minutes for 200 min before an insulating bag was applied and for 220 min afterwards. Then the bag was left in place for 24 hours and the parameters recorded again on day 3, for 260 min with the bag on and during the 220 minutes following the removal of the bag.

Semen Analyses

Semen was collected twice a week for all rams by artificial vagina. Sperm count was assessed manually (Improved Neubauer Cell, Weber, England) and motility by a computerized image analyser (Hamilton Thorne Motility Analiser, Daintree Ind., Australia).

Fertility Assessment

Fertility was assessed for the group of 8 rams in which 4 rams were submitted to scrotal insulation for 16 hours per day.

Semen Freezing

Semen of the 8 rams was frozen on days 49 before and 4, 15 and 21 during the insulation period. Semen was diluted 5-fold with tris-glucose-egg yolk-glycerol at 32°C with pH controlled at 7 with citric acid and pellet-frozen on dry ice.[14] The pellets were kept in liquid nitrogen until insemination.

Insemination

The oestrus cycles of 636 mature Merino ewes were synchronized with progestagen sponges (Repromap, Upjohn, Australia) left *in situ* for 12 days and with 400 I.U. of PSMG (Folligon, Intervet, Australia) injected *i.m.* at the time of sponge removal. Insemination was performed through a laparoscope by deposition in all animals of 50 million spermatozoa in each uterine horn.

Pregnancy Diagnosis

Determinations of pregnancy were performed on each ewe 17 and 65 days after insemination. The first diagnosis was made by determining the plasma progesterone concentrations at day 17 with a R.I.A. assay[15] and a pregnancy recorded when the progesterone value was at least 2 ng/ml.[16] Ultrasonic examination was used to determine pregnancy at day 65, and a female was considered to have lost its embryo if pregnant on day 17 but not on day 65.

Statistical Analysis

Between-group comparisons of the semen characteristics and temperature values were done by unpaired Student's t-test, and within-group comparisons by paired Student's t-test. The numbers of pregnant females were compared by chi-square test.

RESULTS

Thermal and Respiratory Effects of Scrotal Insulation

Intrascrotal Temperatures

Intrascrotal temperature was significantly increased about 2°C by scrotal insulation: 33.69 $\pm$ 0.13°C (mean $\pm$ SEM) before versus 35.76 $\pm$ 0.10°C after bag on ($p < 0.001$) in the insulated group (FIG. 1). Such an increase was still observed after 24 hours with the bag on (FIG. 2): 36.35 $\pm$ 0.06°C in the insulated group versus 34.49 $\pm$ 0.11°C in the control group ($p < 0.001$). After the bag was taken off (FIG. 2), intrascrotal temperature of the insulated group returned to control values in about 20 minutes, and mean values during the subsequent 220 min did not differ between the two groups (34.26 ± 0.17°C in the insulated group vs. 34.32 ± 0.10°C in the control group).

Rectal Temperatures

A slight but significant decrease in rectal temperature (FIG. 1) was induced by scrotal insulation (38.90 ± 0.02°C before vs. 38.30 ± 0.05°C after the bag was on; $p < 0.01$), while no modifications occurred during the same periods in the control rams (38.70 ± 0.02°C before vs. 38.56 ± 0.02°C after). Such a decrease was still present after 24 hours with the bag on (FIG. 2): 38.38 ± 0.03°C in the control group vs. 38.12 ± 0.03°C in the insulated group ($p < 0.01$). Removal of the bag was followed by a slight but significant increase in rectal temperature value in the insulated group (38.12 ± 0.03°C when bag on vs. 38.52 ± 0.03°C when bag off; $p < 0.01$), while mean values were respectively 38.38 ± 0.03°C and 38.35 ± 0.03°C during the same periods in the control group.

Respiratory Rates

Respiratory rate was significantly higher during the insulated period than before (59.4 ± 2.5/min vs. 83.4 ± 3.5/min; $p < 0.01$), while no significant modifications occurred in the control group for the same periods (46.5 ± 2.2/min vs. 48.5 ± 2.1/min). Removal of the bag after 24 hours insulation was followed by a recovery to a normal respiratory rate (86.4 ± 3.4/min with bag on vs. 62.7 ± 2.7/min after bag off).

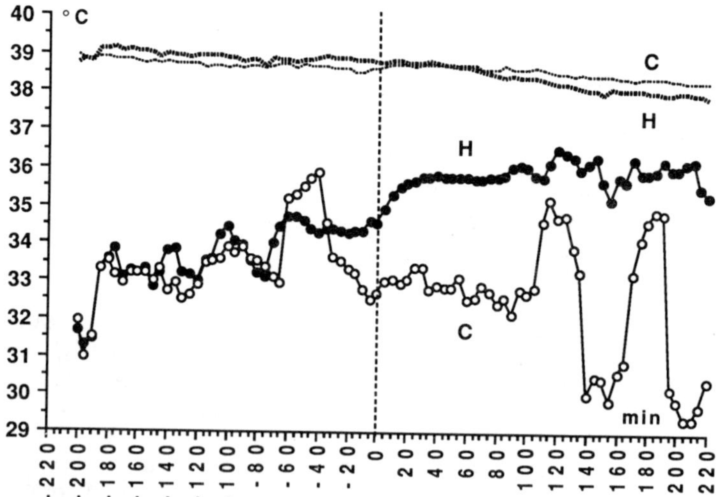

FIGURE 1. Temperatures and scrotal insulation. Mean rectal and intrascrotal temperatures in 3 control (C) and 10 insulated (H) rams during 220 minutes before and 220 minutes after the bag was on.

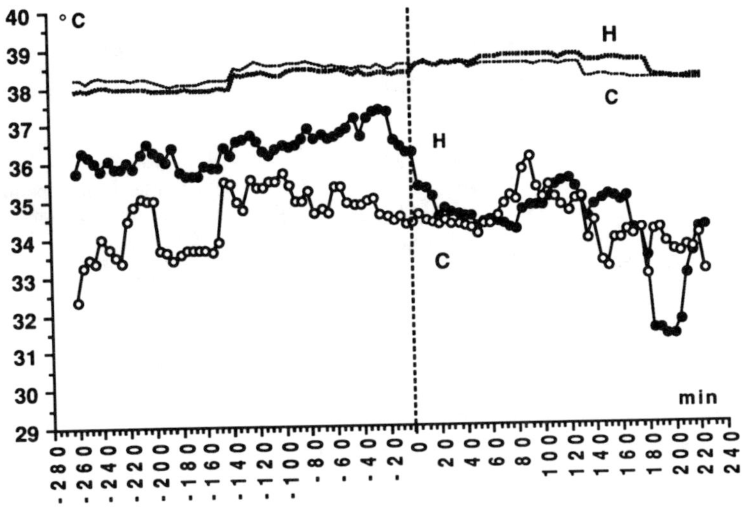

FIGURE 2. Temperature after one day of scrotal insulation. Mean rectal and intrascrotal temperatures in 3 control (C) and 10 insulated (H) rams during 260 minutes with the bag on for 24 hours and during the 230 minutes following the withdrawal of the bag.

Effects of a 2°C Elevated Intrascrotal Temperature on Spermatozoa Output and Motility

With scrotal insulation for 8 h/day, no significant effect on total sperm count (TSC) could be seen (FIG. 3) during the 162 consecutive days of insulation (2.72 $\pm$ 0.13 (mean $\pm$ SEM) vs. 3.34 $\pm$ 0.19 $\times$ 10^9 spermatozoa/ejaculate). On the other hand, the percentage of motile spermatozoa (motility) was irregularly depressed with 3 marked falls around days 60, 100, and 165 (FIG. 4). During the whole insulating period, the mean value of motility was significantly lower in the heated than in the control group: 57.6 $\pm$ 1.9 vs. 72.6 $\pm$ 1.2% ($p < 0.01$). Recovery to the control values did not occur until 30 days after insulation was stopped.

A slight depression of TSC was observed from day 100 when scrotal insulation was 16 h/day for 144 consecutive days (FIG. 5), and the mean TSC value was slightly but significantly lower in the heated than in the control group (3.21 $\pm$ 0.2 vs. 4.45 $\pm$ 0.3 $\times$ 10^9 spermatozoa/ejaculate; $p < 0.01$). Recovery to control values occurred 30 days after insulation was stopped. Depression in motility (FIG. 6) appeared earlier and continued longer than in the 8 h/day insulation, with a mean value during the 144 insulation days significantly lower in the insulated than in the control group: 41.2 $\pm$ 2.5 vs. 75.3 $\pm$ 2.7% ($p < 0.01$). Recovery to control values occurred within 40 days after the end of insulation.

When scrotal insulation was 24 h/day for 30 days, a fall in TSC started on day 12 and was marked from day 19 to 58, with recovery within 80 days after insulation was stopped (FIG. 7). Mean TSC was lower in the insulated than in the control group during the whole insulation period (2.03 $\pm$ 0.7 vs. 4.3 $\pm$ 0.4 $\times$ 10^9 spermatozoa/ejaculate; $p < 0.04$). Motility was depressed as early as day 9 until day 70 and fell

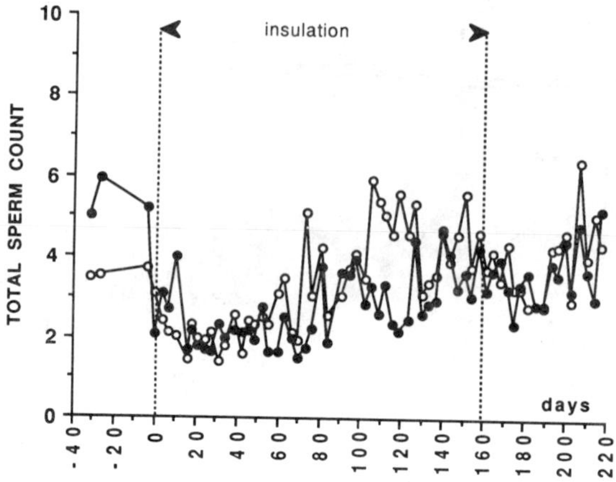

FIGURE 3. Effects of 8 h/day of scrotal insulation on spermatozoa output. Mean total sperm count (10^9 spermatozoa/ejaculate) in 4 control rams (*open circles*) and in 4 rams with scrotal insulation 8 h/day (*solid circles*) for 162 consecutive days.

to almost zero (FIG. 8) with a mean value lower than in the control 21.7 $\pm$ 8.9% vs. 77.9 $\pm$ 3.1% ($p < 0.001$).

Briefly, TSC was not affected by an 8 h/day increase of 2°C in scrotal temperature even after 162 consecutive days exposure, but was reduced from day 100 with a 16 h/day insulation, and drastically depressed within 20 days when scrotal insulation was continuous. On the contrary, motility was always affected by such an increase in scrotal temperature whatever the duration of the daily exposure, and this depression always preceded impairment in the TSC.

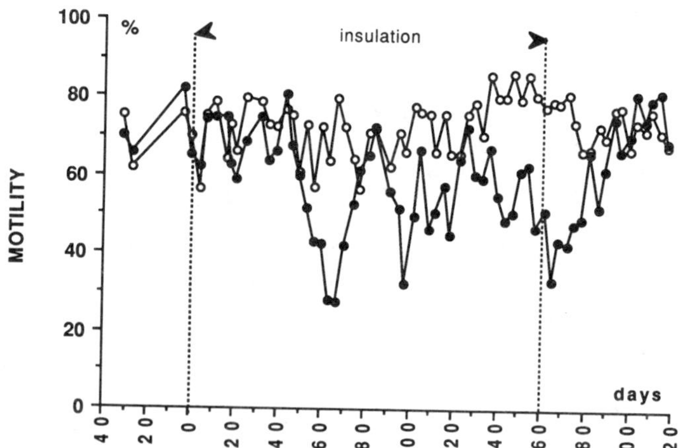

FIGURE 4. Effects of 8 h/day of scrotal insulation on motility percentage. Mean percentage of motile spermatozoa in 4 control rams (*open circles*) and in 4 rams with scrotal insulation 8 h/day (*solid circles*) for 162 consecutive days.

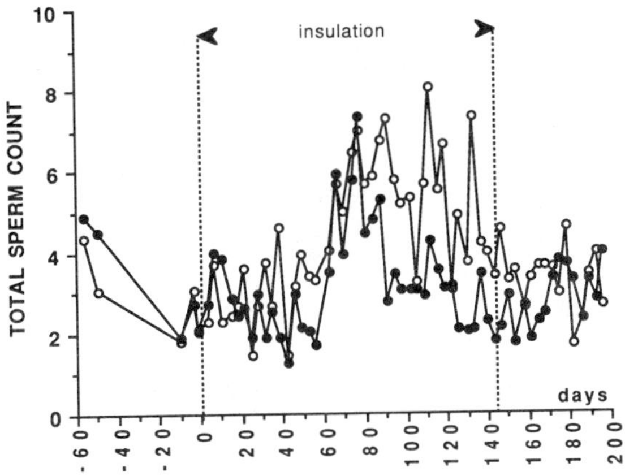

FIGURE 5. Effects of 16 h/day of scrotal insulation on spermatozoa output. Mean total sperm count (10^9 spermatozoa/ejaculate) in 4 control rams (*open circles*) and in 4 rams with scrotal insulation 16 h/day (*solid circles*) for 144 consecutive days.

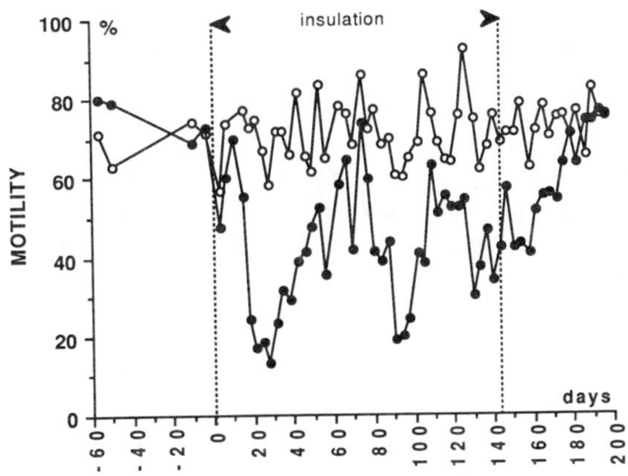

FIGURE 6. Effects of 16 h/day of scrotal insulation on motility percentage. Mean percentage of motile spermatozoa in 4 control rams (*open circles*) and in 4 rams with scrotal insulation 16 h/day (*solid circles*) for 144 consecutive days.

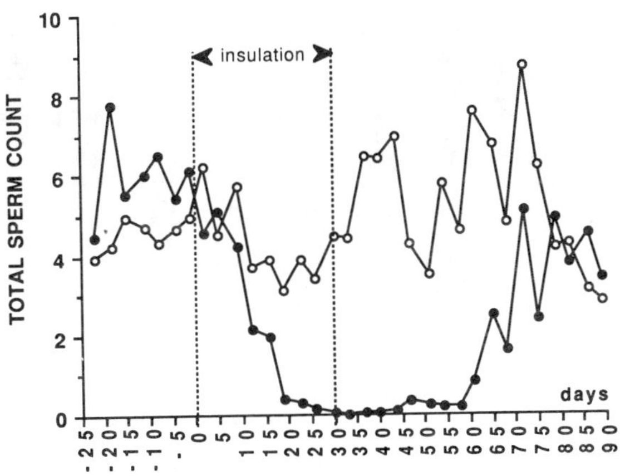

FIGURE 7. Effects of 16 h/day of scrotal insulation on spermatozoa output. Mean total sperm count (10^9 spermatozoa/ejaculate) in 4 control rams (*open circles*) and in 4 rams with scrotal insulation 24 h/day (*solid circles*) for 30 consecutive days.

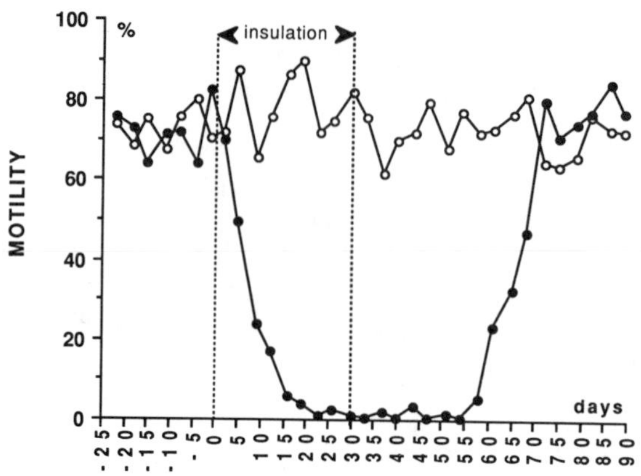

FIGURE 8. Effects of 24 h/day of scrotal insulation on motility percentage. Mean percentage of motile spermatozoa in 4 control rams (*open circles*) and in 4 rams with scrotal insulation 24 h/day (*solid circles*) for 30 consecutive days.

Effects on Fertility of a 2°C Increase in Scrotal Temperature for 16 h/day

Semen Characteristics of Samples Chosen for Freezing

No statistically significant differences were observed in TSC 49 days before heating or on day 4, 15, and 21 of scrotal insulation between heated and control groups (FIG. 9). Mean motility (FIG. 10) was not affected in the semen frozen before treatment or on days 4 and 15 of insulation, but was significantly lower in the sample frozen on day 21 from the insulated than from the control groups (16.8 ± 6.4% vs. 74.6 ± 0.9%;

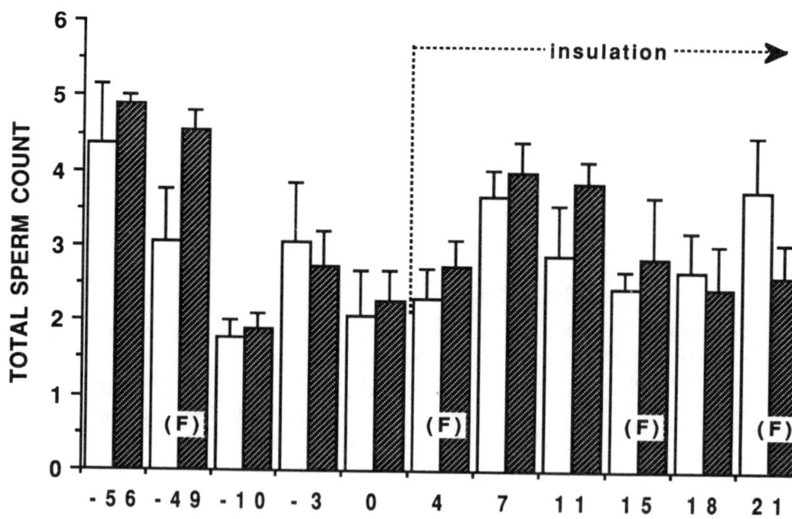

FIGURE 9. Spermatozoa output on days chosen for freezing semen. Total sperm count (mean ± SEM) in 4 control (*open bars*) and in 4 rams with 16 h/day of scrotal insulation (*hatched bars*) when freezing (F) the semen.

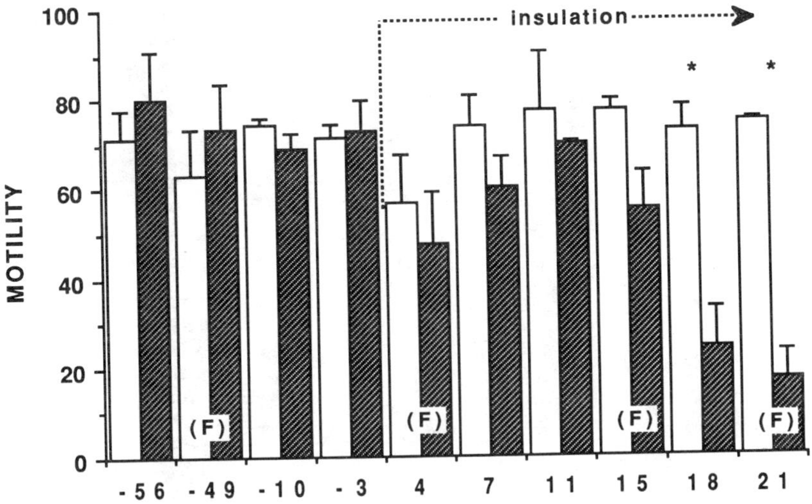

FIGURE 10. Sperm motility on days chosen for freezing semen. Percentage of motile spermatozoa (mean ± SEM) in 4 control (*open bars*) and in 4 rams with scrotal insulation for 16 h/day (*hatched bars*) when freezing (F) the semen. * = $p < 0.001$ with control group value on the same day.

$p < 0.001$). Such a difference was already apparent by day 18 of heating with 24.3 ± 8.5% motile vs. 72.6 ± 5.5%, respectively ($p < 0.003$).

Fertilization Rate

No statistically significant difference was observed in the pregnancy rate 17 days after insemination between the females inseminated with frozen semen from control rams and those inseminated with frozen semen from insulated rams collected before treatment (56% vs. 60.6%), at day 4 (65.2% vs. 71.8%) and at day 15 (66.7% vs. 63.6%) of insulation (FIG. 11). While a slightly lower pregnancy rate was obtained with semen from insulated rams at day 21 of insulation, this value was not significantly lower than with semen from control rams (48.2% vs. 60.3%).

Embryonic Survival

Pregnancy rate 65 days after insemination did not differ between ewes inseminated with semen collected before treatment from control (22.7%) and insulated (25.2%) rams (FIG. 11). However, pregnancy rate 65 days after insemination was significantly lower in the insulated than in the control rams with semen collected at day 4 (15.3 vs. 29.3%, $p < 0.03$), at day 15 (13.6 vs. 27.3%, $p < 0.04$), and at day 21 (3.5 vs. 20.6%, $p < 0.001$) of the insulation period.

Embryonic loss, calculated as the number of females no longer pregnant 65 days after insemination divided by the number of females pregnant 17 days after insemi-

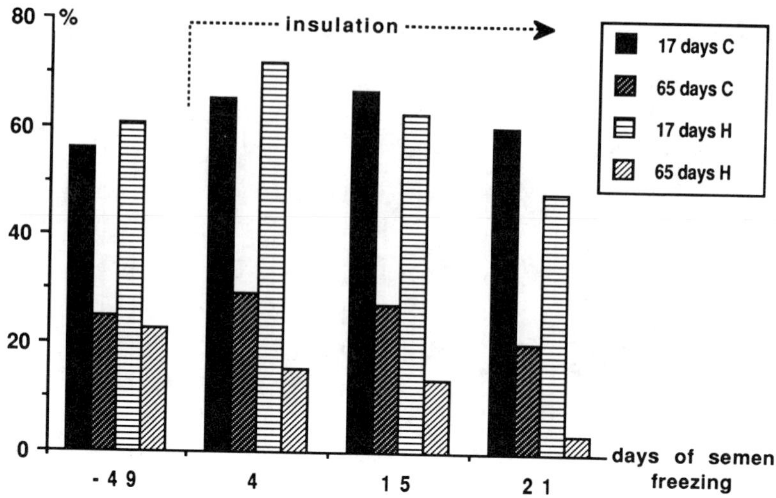

FIGURE 11. Pregnancy rate of ewes inseminated with frozen semen. Percentage of pregnant ewes (number of pregnant ewes/number of inseminated ewes) at 17 days and 65 days after insemination with frozen semen from control rams (C) and from scrotal-insulated rams for 16 h/day (H). Semen was frozen on days 49 before and 4, 15, and 21 during the scrotal insulation period.

nation, was similar in ewes inseminated with semen collected before treatment from control (28/51) and heated (25/40) rams. Embryonic loss was significantly higher in females inseminated with semen collected from insulated rams than from controls at day 4 (48/61 vs. 33/60, $p < 0.006$), at day 15 (44/56 vs. 26/44, $p < 0.04$), and at day 21 (38/41 vs. 25/36, $p < 0.003$) of the insulation period (FIG. 12).

DISCUSSION

An increase of 2°C in intrascrotal temperature of fully fleeced rams induced a decrease in body temperature. This decrease appeared later and was of less intensity

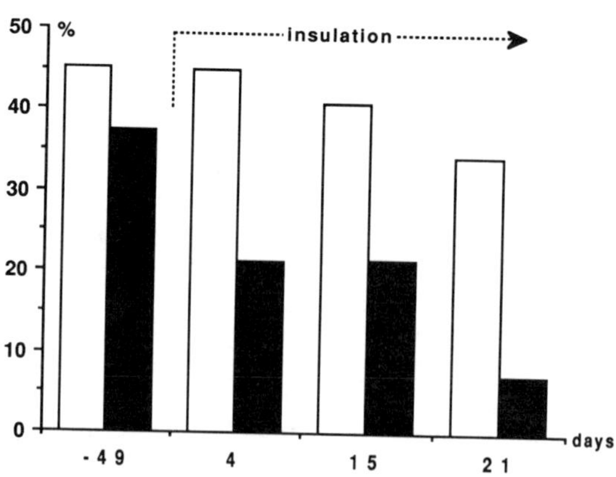

FIGURE 12. Embryonic survival and scrotal insulation. Percentage of embryonic survival (number of ewes still pregnant at 65 days/number of pregnant ewes at 17 days) in ewes inseminated with frozen semen from control rams (*open bars*) and from scrotal-insulated rams for 16 h/day (*solid bars*). Semen was frozen on days 49 before and 4, 15, and 21 during the scrotal insulation period.

than the one obtained during heating of the scrotum to 40 to 45°C in fully fleeced rams.[17] However, an adaptation to the increase in intrascrotal temperature occurred as shown by the constant value of the decrease in rectal temperature 2 hours and 24 hours after insulation. These results in rams differ from those in bulls in which the response to a 4°C increase in intrascrotal temperature did not involve a simultaneous decline in body temperature.[18] The moderate elevation in intrascrotal temperature induced an increase in the respiratory rate similar to that seen with a large increase in temperature,[17] but of less intensity. These results are in agreement with a previous statement that a full polypnea response developed only when the scrotum of rams was warmed to above 39°C.[17,19] The present results indicate that a moderate increase of 2°C in intrascrotal temperature does induce general modifications in the body such as a slight increase in respiratory rate and decrease in body temperature. These results support the view that the scrotum may act as an "early warning" system for general thermoregulatory mechanisms.[20]

An intrascrotal heating of about 4°C obtained through a 24 h/day insulation for 2 days was reported without any effect on spermatozoa output in bulls,[18] but induced a drastic depression in spermatozoa output when continued for 14 to 21 successive days in rams.[21] It has been assumed that depression in production of spermatozoa is linked to the length of exposure to a given increase in temperature;[22] but this does not seem to be true when intrascrotal elevation in temperature is as low as 2°C, since no effect could be seen on spermatozoa output even after 162 successive days of exposure to an 8 h/day insulation regimen.

Concerning motility of spermatozoa, comparisons with other experiments in which scrotal insulation was used are difficult as this parameter was not often studied. Changes in motility have been reported in semen from heat experiments using large increases in scrotal temperature for short times,[23,24] but in the present experiments a moderate elevation in intrascrotal temperature altered motility even with a daily exposure of 8 h/day. When a depression in spermatozoa output was induced, the latter was always preceded by a depression in motility. It seems reasonable to conclude that motility is more sensitive to a moderate increase in intrascrotal temperature than spermatozoa output.

No difference was observed in the fertilization rate of females inseminated with semen from control and insulated rams: a moderate increase of 2°C in intrascrotal temperature for 16 h/day does not seem to have impaired the fertilization capacity of spermatozoa even after 21 successive days of exposure. However, a reduced fertilization rate was reported in previous studies of heating in rams, boars and rats. Such a discrepancy in the effect of heat on the fertilization capacity of spermatozoa could be explained 1) by the use of a reduced number of males or females;[25–28] 2) by different effects on spermatogenesis when elevation in testicular temperature was large[5,26] or obtained through an increase in whole body temperature;[25,27–29] or 3) by fertility assessment when the semen was drastically altered by a long heat exposure.[4,30] In some other studies dealing with the effect on fertilization capacity of spermatozoa heated either directly as in rabbit[31] or through general or scrotal heating as in mice,[32,33] no modification in the fertilization rate was reported, but an increase in embryonic loss was observed. The technique used in the present study for the intra-uterine insemination does interfere with embryonic survival, as previously reported,[34] since the embryonic mortality rate was greater than 50% in the ewes inseminated with frozen semen from control rams. However, the embryonic loss was significantly greater in the females inseminated with frozen semen from rams subjected to a 2°C increase in intrascrotal temperature than in those inseminated from control rams.

As the passage of spermatozoa through the epididymis of the ram requires 11 to 14 days,[35] the increase in the embryonic loss observed as early as day 4 of scrotal insulation must indicate an effect of heat on the epididymal spermatozoa, even if no modifications could be detected in any of the semen characteristics studied. These facts are in disagreement with the current view that the epididymis and epididymal spermatozoa are resistant to heat. This opinion was based on the absence of any modification in the morphology or motility of spermatozoa before 14 days after general or large scrotal heating in rams[23,24] or before 14 days of general heating in boars.[4] However, the results of several other experiments seem to indicate that some functions of the epididymis could be temperature dependent: 1) temperature of the cauda epididymis was 4°C below rectal temperature in conscious rats[36] and 1.9°C in conscious boars;[37] 2) elevation of epididymal temperature in cryptepididymal rabbits was associated with an increased incidence of both dead and decapitated spermatozoa[38] and with a depressed secretory activity[39] and water and ion transport function[40] of the cauda epididymis epithelium; 3) the lower temperature of the scrotum was reported to be a major determinant of the sperm storage capacity of the rat cauda epididymis, and elevation of epididymal temperature induced an accelerated passage of spermatozoa through the epididymis in rat, rabbit and dog with most of the spermatozoa dying or losing their motility,[41,42] although in these experiments the effects of temperature were confounded with those of physical separation of the epididymis from the testis; 4) in induced cryptorchid rabbits, the onset of fertilization failure preceded any significant spermatozoa death or loss of motility in ejaculated semen;[43] 5) scrotal heating of the testes of rams induced a depression in the metabolic activity of ejaculated spermatozoa and the speed of the onset of this alteration suggested that the epididymis was a site of action;[44] and 6) in the rat, mouse and bull, the lower temperature of the cauda epididymis was shown to facilitate the storage of spermatozoa by enhancing oxygen availability.[45]

While different mechanisms can be evoked for the increase in embryonic loss when males were heat stressed,[5] the present results support the strong presumption that the fate of the embryo could be linked to some characteristics of the spermatozoa, but further studies are required to clearly define if the embryo loss occurred before or after implantation, and for which intensity of temperature elevation.

CONCLUSION

The results of the present experiment show that a moderate elevation of about 2°C in intrascrotal temperature by scrotal insulation of conscious rams induces: 1) general modifications such as a slight but significant increase in the respiratory rate (of about 30%) and decrease in body temperature (0.25 to 0.50°C); 2) no modification in spermatozoa output with an 8 h/day scrotal insulation, even when exposure was as long as 162 consecutive days; 3) a decrease in spermatozoa output with a 16 h/day scrotal insulation, the decrease happening sooner and being very severe for a 24 h/day scrotal insulation; 4) always a depression in the percentage of motile spermatozoa, even with 8 h/day of scrotal insulation, with the alteration in motility always preceding that in spermatozoa output; 5) no effect on the fertilization capacity of spermatozoa from rams subjected to a 16 h/day scrotal insulation for as long as 21 consecutive days; 6) an increase in the embryonic loss in females inseminated with frozen semen from rams subjected to 16 h/day scrotal insulation; and 7) a potential heat effect on epididymal spermatozoa as indicated by the increase in embryonic loss as early as day 4 in a 16 h/day scrotal insulation program, without any modification in the semen characteristics.

From these results and those already reported in the literature, we suggest that the sequence of the heat effects on spermatogenesis could be firstly a reduction in the capacity of the spermatozoa to produce a viable embryo, secondly an alteration in the motility of spermatozoa, thirdly a decrease in the capacity of spermatozoa to fertilize the ovum, and finally a decrease in the spermatozoa output.

REFERENCES

1. WAITES, G. M. H. & B. P. SETCHELL. 1990. Physiology of the mammalian testis. *In* Marshall's Physiology of Reproduction. Vol. 2. G. E. Lamming, Ed.: 1–105. Churchill Livingstone. London.
2. WAITES, G. M. H. 1968. Temperature and fertility in mammals. *In* Proceedings of the International Congress on Reproduction and Artificial Insemination, Paris. Vol. 1: 235–252.
3. ASDELL, S. A. & G. W. SALISBURY. 1941. The viability of spermatozoa in the abdominal epididymis and the failure of motile sperms to fertilize ova. Am. J. Physiol. **132:** 791–799.
4. WETTEMANN, R. P. & F. W. BAZER. 1985. Influence of environmental temperature on prolificacy of pigs. J. Reprod. Fertil. (Suppl.) **33:** 199–208.
5. SETCHELL, B. P., M. J. D'OCCHIO, M. J. HALL, M. S. LAURIE, M. J. TUCKER & J. L. ZUPP. 1988. Is embryonic mortality increased in normal female mated to subfertile males? J. Reprod. Fertil. **82:** 567–574.
6. MACLEOD, J. & R. S. HOTCHKISS. 1941. The effect of hyperpyrexia upon spermatozoa counts in men. Endocrinology **28:** 780–784.
7. WATANABE, A. 1959. The effect of heat on human spermatogenesis. Kyushu J. Med. Sci. **10:** 101–107.
8. MIEUSSET, R., L. BUJAN, A. MANSAT, F. PONTONNIER & H. GRANDJEAN. 1987. Hyperthermia and human spermatogenesis: Enhancement of the inhibitory effect obtained by artificial cryptorchidism. Int. J. Androl. **10:** 571–580.
9. MIEUSSET, R., L. BUJAN, C. MONDINAT, A. MANSAT, F. PONTONNIER & H. GRANDJEAN. 1987. Association of scrotal hyperthermia with impaired spermatogenesis in infertile men. Fertil. Steril. **48:** 1006–1011.
10. ZORGNIOTTI, A. W. & A. I. SEALFON. 1988. Measurement of intrascrotal temperature in normal and subfertile men. J. Reprod. Fertil. **82:** 563–567.
11. ROBINSON, D. & J. ROCK. 1968. Control of human spermatogenesis by induced changes of intrascrotal temperature. JAMA **204:** 80–87.
12. ZORGNIOTTI, A. W., M. S. COHEN & A. I. SEALFON. 1986. Chronic scrotal hypothermia: Results in 90 infertile couples. J. Urol. **135:** 703–708.
13. MALMGREM, L. & K. LARSON. 1989. Experimentally induced testicular alterations in boars: Histological and ultrastructural findings. J. Vet. Med. A **36:** 3–14.
14. EVANS, G. & W. M. C. MAXWELL. 1987. Use of frozen semen in sheep. *In* Salamon's Artificial Insemination of Sheep and Goats. G. Evans & W. M. C. Maxwell, Eds.: 122–124. Butterworths. Sydney.
15. D'OCCHIO, M. J., D. R. GIFFORD, R. M. HOSKINSON, T. WEATHERLY & B. P. SETCHELL. 1988. Gonadotrophin secretion and ovarian responses in prepubertal heifers actively immunized against androstenedions and oestradiol-17B. J. Reprod. Fertil. **83:** 159–168.
16. ROBERTSON, H. A. 1977. Reproduction in the ewe and the goat. *In* Reproduction in Domestic Animals, 3rd edition. H. H. Cole & P. T. Cupps, Eds.: 475–498. Academic Press. New York.
17. WAITES, G. M. H. 1962. The effect of heating the scrotum of the ram on respiration and body temperature. Q. J. Exp. Physiol. **47:** 314–323.
18. WILDEUS, S. & K. ENTWISTLE. 1983. Spermiogram and sperm reserves in hybrid *Bos indicus* × *Bos taurus* bulls after scrotal insulation. J. Reprod. Fertil. **69:** 711–716.
19. WAITES, G. M. H. & C. R. MOULE. 1961. The relation of vascular heat exchange to temperature regulation in the testis of the ram. J. Reprod. Fertil. **2:** 213–224.
20. SETCHELL, B. P. 1978. The scrotum and thermoregulation. *In* The Mammalian Testis. B. P. Setchell, Ed.: 90–108. Elek Book. London.

21. GLOVER, T. D. 1955. Some effects of scrotal insulation on the semen of rams. Proc. Soc. Study Fertil. **7:** 66–75.
22. FOWLER, D. G. 1969. Skin folds and Merino breeding. 7. The relations of heat applied to the testis and scrotal thermoregulation to fertility in Merino ram. Aust. J. Exp. Agric. Anim. Husband. **8:** 142–148.
23. MOULE, G. R. & G. M. H. WAITES. 1963. Seminal degeneration in the ram and its relation to the temperature of the scrotum. J. Reprod. Fertil. **5:** 433–436.
24. WAITES, G. M. H. & B. P. SETCHELL. 1964. Effect of local heating on blood flow and metabolism in the testis of conscious ram. J. Reprod. Fertil. **8:** 339–349.
25. FOWLER, D. G. & R. B. DUN. 1966. Skin folds and Merino breeding. 4. The susceptibility of rams selected for a high degree of skin wrinkle to heat induced infertility. Aust. J. Exp. Agric. Anim. Husband. **6:** 121–127.
26. BRADEN, A. W. H. & P. E. MATTNER. 1970. The effects of scrotal heating in the ram on semen characteristics, fecundity and embryonic mortality. Aust. J. Agric. Res. **12:** 509–518.
27. RATHORE, A. K. 1968. Effects of high temperature on sperm morphology and subsequent fertility in Merino sheep. Proc. Aust. Soc. Anim. Prod. **7:** 270–274.
28. RATHORE, A. K. 1970. Fertility of rams heated for 1, 2, 3 and 4 days mated to superovulated ewes. Aust. J. Agric. Res. **21:** 355–358.
29. HOWARTH, B. 1969. Fertility in the ram following exposure to elevated ambient temperature and humidity. J. Reprod. Fertil. **19:** 179–183.
30. DUTT, R. H. & E. C. SIMPSON. 1957. Environmental temperature and fertility of Southdown rams early in the breeding season. J. Anim. Sci. **16:** 136–143.
31. HOWARTH, B., C. W. ALLISTON & L. C. ULBERG. 1965. Importance of uterine environment on rabbit sperm prior to fertilization. J. Anim. Sci. **24:** 1027–1032.
32. BELLVÉ, A. R. 1972. Viability and survival of mouse embryos following parental exposure to high temperature. J. Reprod. Fertil. **30:** 71–81.
33. BURFENING, P. J., D. S. ELLIOT, E. J. EISEN & L. C. ULBERG. 1970. Survival of embryos resulting from spermatozoa produced by mice exposed to elevated ambient temperature. J. Anim. Sci. **30:** 578–582.
34. MAXWELL, W. M. C., G. L. BUTLER & H. R. WILSON. 1984. Intra-uterine insemination of ewes with frozen semen. J. Agric. Sci., Camb. **102:** 233–235.
35. ORTAVANT, R. 1954. Détermination de la vitesse de transfert des spermatozoïdes dans l'épididyme du bélier à l'aide du 32P. C. R. Soc. Biol. Paris **147:** 1152–1155.
36. BROOKS, D. E. 1973. Epididymal and testicular temperature in the unrestrained conscious rat. J. Reprod. Fertil. **35:** 157–160.
37. STONE, B. A. 1981. Thermal characteristics of the testis and epididymis of the boar. J. Reprod. Fertil. **63:** 551–557.
38. GLOVER, T. D. 1960. Spermatozoa from the isolated cauda epididymidis of rabbits and some effects of artificial cryptorchidism J. Reprod. Fertil. **1:** 121–129.
39. JONES, R. 1974. The effects of artificial cryptorchidism on the composition of epididymal plasma in the rabbit. Fertil. Steril. **25:** 432–438.
40. RASWEILER, J. J. & J. M. BEDFORD. 1982. Biology of the scrotum. III. Effects of abdominal temperature upon the epithelial cells of the rat cauda epididymidis. Biol. Reprod. **26:** 691–705.
41. BEDFORD, J. M. 1978. Influence of abdominal temperature on epididymal function in the rat and rabbit. Am. J. Anat. **152:** 509–522.
42. FOLDESY, R. G. & J. M. BEDFORD. 1982. Biology of the scrotum. I. Temperature and androgen as determinants of the sperm storage capacity of the rat cauda epididymidis. Biol. Reprod. **26:** 673–682.
43. CUMMINS, J. M. 1973. The effects of artificial cryptorchidism in the rabbit on the transport and survival of spermatozoa in the female reproductive tract. J. Reprod. Fertil. **33:** 469–479.
44. BROWN-WOODMANN, P. D. C., H. MOHRI, A. DARIN-BENNET, C. D. SHOREY & I. G. WHITE. 1976. Metabolic and ultrastructural changes in ejaculated spermatozoa induced by heating the testes of rams. J. Reprod. Fertil. **46:** 501–502.
45. DJAKIEW, D. & R. CARDULLO. 1986. Lower temperature of the cauda epididymidis facilitates the storage of sperm by enhancing oxygen availability. Gamete Res. **15:** 237–245.

Sperm Capacitation and the Acrosome Reaction

BAYARD T. STOREY

Division of Reproductive Biology
Department of Obstetrics & Gynecology
University of Pennsylvania Medical Center
Philadelphia, Pennsylvania 19104-6080

INTRODUCTION

For the mammalian spermatozoon, the process of maturation requires residence in both the male and female reproductive tract before the sperm is equipped to fertilize its conspecific egg when the two gametes meet in the oviduct. Sperm in the cauda epididymidis and the vas deferens have completed their basic education during transit through the epididymal lumen and are almost ready to fertilize the egg. Their finishing school *in vivo* is the female reproductive tract, in which they attain the capacitated state. Capacitation enables the sperm to undergo a specialized exocytotic reaction, the acrosome reaction, upon meeting the egg's extracellular matrix coat, the zona pellucida. The acrosome reaction is obligate for fertilization. It enables the sperm to penetrate the zona pellucida, enter the perivitelline space, and bind to the egg's plasma membrane. The plasma membrane at the equatorial segment of the acrosome-reacted sperm has become capable of fusing with the egg's plasma membrane. Once this fusion is complete, the sperm enters the egg, the male pronucleus is formed, and fertilization is underway. The links between the processes of capacitation and acrosome reaction in mammalian sperm are examined in this brief account, using the mouse as the primary model, with discussion of possible reaction mechanisms.

Capacitation of mammalian sperm was first identified by Austin[1] and Chang[2] as required for fertilization, based on the observation that rabbit sperm would not fertilize rabbit eggs *in vivo* if their residence time in the female reproductive tract prior to ovulation was less than 6 hours. Similar results were obtained with rat sperm;[3] the minimum residence time in this case was 4 hours. The term capacitation was introduced by Austin[4] and was taken to encompass the physiological changes undergone by the spermatozoon before it could penetrate the egg. *In vitro* capacitation of epididymal mouse sperm was achieved by Iwamatsu and Chang,[5,6] using heated bovine follicular fluid. A completely defined medium for fertilization of mouse eggs *in vitro* was provided by Toyoda *et al.*[7,8] The key components in this medium were bovine serum albumin (BSA) and energy substrates; the remaining components were those used to make Krebs-Ringer bicarbonate medium. The medium of Toyoda *et al.*[7] was shown to be able to capacitate sperm as well as to provide a medium supportive of the early processes of egg fertilization. This medium, along with the refinements suggested by Miyamoto and Chang[9] has proven to be the "workhorse" of mouse *in vitro* fertilization studies.

The definition of capacitation is still controversial. Should it include the acrosome reaction or should it refer only to those reactions leading up to the acrosome reaction? Austin[10] advocated separation of the two processes, while Chang and Hunter,[11] in the same year, grouped both processes as part of capacitation. The controversy has been summarized in a recent article by Chang.[12] Here, we take the view that capacitation is the process which readies the sperm to undergo the acrosome reaction; the acrosome reaction itself is considered a separate process. The experimental evidence for differentiating the two processes is first considered. The possible reactions leading to the acrosome reaction, their participants, and their mechanisms are discussed in the section following. The implications of these acrosome reaction mechanisms for those involved in capacitation are then briefly discussed.

DIFFERENTIATION OF THE ACROSOME REACTION AND CAPACITATION INTO SEPARATE PROCESSES

Differentiation between capacitation and the acrosome reaction is possible in mouse sperm, because independent assays for the two processes are available. Both utilize the fluorescent probe, chlortetracycline (CTC). The fluorescence assay for capacitation[13] was adapted from an earlier CTC fluorescence probe method developed to track the acrosome reaction in mouse sperm.[14] The fluorescence patterns observed using this assay are shown schematically in FIGURE 1. Under the precise set of conditions for capacitation of mouse sperm established by the extensive studies of Wolf and coworkers,[15-18] the "B" pattern, characteristic of capacitated sperm (FIG. 1), increases from less than 20% at the first observable time point of 10 min to over 80% at 60 minutes. During this period the "F1" and "F2" patterns (FIG. 1) decrease in synchrony with the B pattern increase. The B pattern percentage remains constant for the next 30 min and then declines as the acrosome reaction, assayed as increase in pattern "AR" (FIG. 1), occurs spontaneously at a slow rate. This is the same time course for capacitation, as assayed by fertilization, that had been determined in the studies by Wolf and coworkers cited above. The time course depends on the concentration of BSA in the medium.[19,20] The capacitation time of 60 to 90 min was found with 20 mg/ml of BSA; lower concentrations required longer times. No spontaneous acrosome reactions were observed in uncapacitated sperm:[13] capacitation of mouse sperm is required for the spontaneous acrosome reaction to occur.

A clearer differentiation between capacitation and the acrosome reaction is obtained in the case of the induction of acrosomal exocytosis in mouse sperm by the zona pellucida of the mouse egg. Mouse sperm bind to zonae pellucidae of eggs with plasma membrane intact[21] and, if capacitated, exhibit the B fluorescence pattern (FIG. 1) in the presence of CTC.[14] Once bound to the zona pellucida, the sperm undergo the acrosome reaction as shown by loss of the B pattern and eventual acquisition of the AR pattern (FIG. 1). This reaction is inhibited by the compound, 3-quinuclidinyl benzilate (QNB).[22,23] In the presence of QNB, the sperm remain attached to the zona pellucida; a high percentage of the cells exhibit the B fluorescence pattern with only a slow decline of this percentage over time, corresponding to the rate of the spontaneous acrosome reaction. The compound QNB does not inhibit the spontaneous reaction.[22] The acrosome reaction induced in sperm bound to the zona pellucida is presumed to be the physiological form of the acrosome reaction, since it occurs in the sperm best located to penetrate the zona pellucida as a result of this exocytotic process. This reaction occurs only in capacitated sperm displaying the B fluorescence pattern with

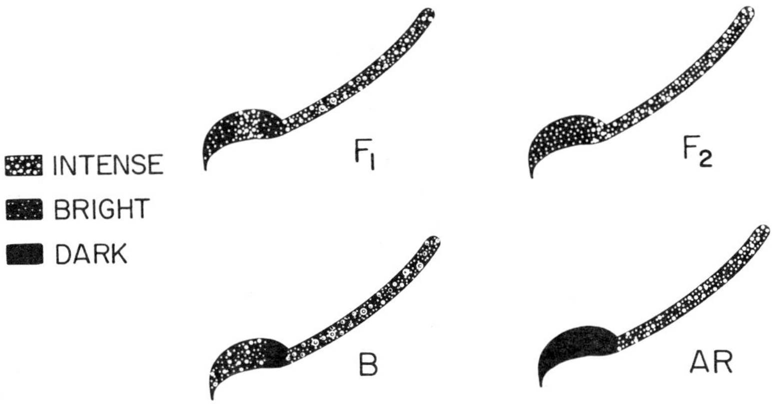

FIGURE 1. Schematic depiction of CTC fluorescence patterns observed on mouse spermatozoa during capacitation and the acrosome reaction. Sperm freshly isolated from the cauda epididymis, which are uncapacitated, show patterns F1 (upper left) and F2 (upper right). As sperm are incubated in medium in the presence of BSA to capacitate them, patterns F1 and F2 are lost and pattern B (lower left) appears. At 60–90 min incubation, about 85% of the sperm have acquired pattern B. Sperm incubated for long times in the presence of zonae pellucidae undergo the acrosome reaction and display pattern AR (lower right). (Adapted from Fig. 1 of Ward & Storey.[13])

CTC; uncapacitated sperm do not undergo the zona-induced acrosome reaction.[13,22] The requirement that the sperm be capacitated for the zona-induced reaction to occur provides a useful operational definition of capacitation. Mouse spermatozoa may be termed capacitated if they undergo the relatively rapid zona-induced acrosome reaction which is sensitive to inhibition by QNB.

The zona-induced acrosome reaction also occurs in capacitated bovine sperm.[24] Capacitation of bovine sperm *in vitro* requires that heparin, in addition to BSA, be in the medium. The processes of capacitation and the acrosome reaction can be differentiated in this species, since capacitation can be shown to be an absolute prerequisite for the zona-induced acrosome reaction to occur.[24,25] In a given sample of bovine sperm, only about half the cells actually become capacitated. These can be distinguished from their non-capacitated fellows by their ability to increase intracellular Ca^{2+} induced by added solubilized zonae. Only those cells that show this intracellular Ca^{2+} increase go on to complete the acrosome reaction.[26]

THE ACROSOME REACTION: PARTICIPANTS AND REACTIONS

As pointed out above, there are two forms of the acrosome reaction. One is the spontaneous acrosome reaction that occurs slowly in sperm in suspension in the absence of stimulatory agents.[22,27,28] The other is the acrosome reaction induced by the zona pellucida,[22,26,29] considered to be the one operative *in vivo*.[30] Both the spontaneous and the induced reactions produce acrosome-reacted sperm capable of fertilizing eggs.[18,31] It thus seems reasonable to postulate that both reactions go through the same pathway and involve the same intracellular components. The difference between the induced and the spontaneous acrosome reaction is that the zona increases the rates of the participating reactions such that the entire process occurs in a far shorter time. A rate difference is also observed between structurally intact, isolated zonae and solubilized zonae: the acrosome reaction occurs more rapidly with solubilized zonae and does not display the lag period of 30 min seen with the structurally intact zonae.[22,29] The zona-induced acrosome reaction in mouse sperm has received the most attention, and will be considered first in this discussion. The relation of the induced to the spontaneous reaction in this species will then be examined briefly.

The Zona-induced Acrosome Reaction: Participants

The specific agonist for induction of the mouse sperm acrosome reaction was shown by Bleil and Wassarman[29] to be the glycoprotein ZP3, one of the three glycoproteins making up the zona pellucida of the mouse egg.[32] ZP3 was also shown to be the zona glycoprotein mediating the binding of the sperm cell to the zona matrix structure,[33] designated here for convenience as the mechanical binding reaction to distinguish it from the acrosomal exocytosis induction reaction. The mechanical binding reaction appears to involve at least four components displaying cooperative interactions. Its complexities are beyond the scope of this review; the reader is referred to the detailed account of Storey and Kopf.[34] The induction reaction, with a specific agonist initiating a chain of reactions culminating in an exocytotic process, bears a strong resemblance to ligand-mediated exocytotic reactions in somatic cells proceeding through an intracellular signal transduction system.[35] One example is IgE-induced granule exocytosis in mast cells,[36-38] which involves aggregation of the IgE receptors.[37] Leyton and Saling[39] demonstrated that aggregation of ZP3 glycopeptides by crosslinking induced the acrosome reaction while the glycopeptides alone were ineffective under the same conditions.

The first place to look for sperm participants in the zona-induced acrosome reaction would be among those sperm plasma membrane proteins binding ZP3. Unfortunately, candidate proteins are few in number. Only two have been found to date that bind ZP3 in their purified form. One is a 95 kDa protein, p95, reported by Leyton and Saling;[40] p95 not only binds ZP3, it shows tyrosine kinase (TK) activity that is markedly stimulated on binding ZP3.[41,42] This protein is at present the prime candidate for the sperm plasma membrane receptor for a ZP3 ligand acting as agonist for the induced acrosome reaction. The other sperm plasma membrane with ZP3 binding activity is a 56 kDa protein, p56, described by Bleil and Wassarman.[43] This protein binds ZP3 with high affinity under non-denaturing conditions, and a crosslinked complex between the two proteins can be obtained. The binding is specific, in that ZP2, the partner of ZP3 in forming the structural filaments of the intact zona pellucida,[44] does not bind to p56. The p56 protein has no known function at present.

One protein that must be a participant in the zona-induced acrosome reaction appears as a doublet on gel electrophoresis with M_r = 200/220 kDa, designated p200/220, and is the antigen recognized by the monoclonal antibody M42.[45] This antibody blocks fertilization by inhibiting the zona-induced acrosome reaction at its initiation.[46] Use of the fluorescent probe CTC revealed that the sperm under conditions of M42 inhibition retained the B pattern of fluorescence.[47] The antibody therefore has the same functional effect on the zona-induced acrosome reaction as QNB. When purified by gel electrophoresis, p200/220 does not bind ZP3, but this is most probably due to denaturation of the protein on the SDS gel.

Another class of proteins shown to participate in the zona-induced acrosome reaction are the GTP-binding regulatory proteins, or G proteins. This group of proteins includes G_s, G_i, G_o, G_z, and transducin, any one of which may play a critical role as a signal transducing element in coupling agonist ligand-receptor activation to the targeted effects in a given cell through the series of intracellular reactions involved in cell signaling.[48,49] Kopf *et al.*[50] have demonstrated the presence of G proteins of the G_i class in mammalian sperm, with the α subunit of the heterotrimeric protein appearing with M_r = 41 kDa on gel electrophoresis. A distinguishing characteristic of this class of G protein is inactivation by the bacterial toxin, pertussis toxin, due to ADP-ribosylation of the α subunit. Endo *et al.*[51,52] were able to block the zona-induced acrosome reaction at the initiation stage by treatment of the mouse sperm with pertussis toxin. This is the same stage at which QNB and M42 also act as inhibitors. Further evidence that the G_i protein was participating in the induced reaction was specific protection from pertussis toxin inactivation by the GTP analog, GTPγS.[51] Inhibition by pertussis toxin of the zona-induced acrosome reaction in bovine sperm was also demonstrated,[26] strongly implying that cell signaling involving these components is a feature common to this reaction in mammalian sperm.

The proteins described above as participants in the zona-induced acrosome reaction have been separated and characterized with regard to M_r by gel electrophoresis. Three other components have been shown functionally to be actual or likely participants, but no individual proteins have been identified that correspond to these functional activities. One of these components is the putative protein that binds QNB with resulting inhibition of the acrosome reaction. Scatchard analysis of ^{3}H-QNB binding to sperm cells yielded values of K_D = 5 nM with B = 6000 sites per cell.[23] The Scatchard plot was linear and the Hill coefficient was unity, indicating a single group of homogeneous receptors acting independently without cooperativity. The property of QNB binding suggests that this protein may resemble a muscarinic receptor, but pharmacological characterization also indicates definite differences.[23] The possibility that the QNB protein, designated for convenience SQBP for Sperm QNB Binding Protein, may act as an activatable Ca^{2+} channel is discussed in a later section of this review.

The second component is protein kinase C (PK-C). Evidence for its participation in the zona-induced acrosome reaction was provided by the effects of biologically active phorbol esters reported by Lee *et al.*[53] The ester 12-O-tetradecanoyl, 13-O-phorbol acetate (TPA) changed the time course of the zona-induced acrosome reaction by accelerating the early stage and slowing down the later stage. These esters are known potent activators of PK-C;[54] they profoundly affect the zona-induced acrosome reaction, thereby implicating PK-C as a participant.

The third component is phospholipase C (PL-C), specific for hydrolysis of phosphotidyl inositol 4,5-diphosphate to diacylglycerol (DAG) and 1,4,5-inositol triphosphate. Roldan and Harrison[55-57] have shown that this activity is present in mammalian sperm from five species, including mouse and human. It is of interest that PK-C activity could not be demonstrated in ram sperm, while PL-C could be.[55] The experiments with ram sperm were carried out with the divalent cation ionophore, A23187, as activator of the acrosome reaction. No experiments to date have been reported which speak to the activation of this enzymatic activity by the zona pellucida.

The Zona-induced Acrosome Reaction: Reactions

The list of identified and putative participants in the zona-induced acrosome reaction includes enzymatic activities that have been shown to drive intracellular signal transduction in somatic cells.[35,48,49,54,58] The problem is to discern the sequence in which these reactions function to provide a signal transduction chain. In this section, studies of the time courses of distinguishable stages of the zona-induced acrosome reaction in mouse sperm will be considered, in order to suggest a model for the mouse sperm signal transduction chain set into operation by ZP3.

The use of the fluorescent probe CTC provided an assay for the acrosomal status of mouse sperm interacting with the mouse zona pellucida as a function of time, with a time resolution of 5 minutes.[13] Application of this assay at 15–30 min intervals to track the progress of zona-induced acrosome reactions in sperm bound to structurally intact, isolated zonae showed that three fluorescent patterns appeared sequentially in time.[59] The first pattern observed at early incubation times was pattern B, described above (FIGS. 1 and 2), corresponding to capacitated, acrosome intact cells. As loss of pattern B occurred, it was replaced by an intermediate pattern "S" (FIG. 2). The pattern seen at late times was pattern AR, corresponding to completely reacted sperm (FIGS. 1 and 2). The studies with CTC were supplemented with fluorescent 9-aminoacridine derivatives,[59,60] which act as pH probes.[61] These probes localize to intracellular compartments with lumen pH lower than that of the suspending medium, with enhancement of fluorescence.[62] The preferred probe was *N*-(*n*-dodecyl)-9-aminoacridine (NDAA), which localizes to the acrosomal region as shown by bright fluorescence over the anterior portion of the head (FIG. 2); this is designated pattern N. This fluorescence is lost in acrosome-reacted sperm.[60] The time course of the disappearance of pattern N followed the loss of CTC pattern B and onset of CTC pattern S. These four fluorescence patterns and the sequence of their appearance and disappearance are shown in FIGURE 2.

Loss of pattern N is due to equilibration of the acidic acrosomal compartment and the outside medium with resulting loss of the pH gradient between them. The observation that loss of pattern N followed loss of pattern B and appearance of pattern S indicated that pattern N loss marked a boundary between two stages of the zona-induced acrosome reaction. The time course measurements described above were, by design of the experiment, carried out by assessing the fluorescence patterns on a large number of sperm bound to structurally intact zonae and so determining the percentage of a given pattern in the population of cells at the selected time points. This mode of kinetic measurement was designated "population kinetics." An alternative mode of kinetic measurement was direct determination of the rate of loss of fluorescence pattern N in individual cells, designated "single cell kinetics." The population kinetics showed a characteristic lag time of 30 min, after the sperm had bound to the zonae, before onset of loss of pattern B could be observed. The half time for loss of pattern B was 50 min, with the loss being complete in 180 minutes. Pattern N loss lagged behind pattern B loss, being complete in 210 min with a half time of 60 minutes. Pattern S was maximal at 150 min and had disappeared at 210 min, at which time pattern AR had become maximal. The single cell kinetics showed that loss of pattern N from the individual cell was rapid and constant, with a half time of 2.1 minutes. The population kinetics derive from the differing lag times to loss of pattern N fluorescence, which varied from 30 min to 150 min for 50 samples ob-

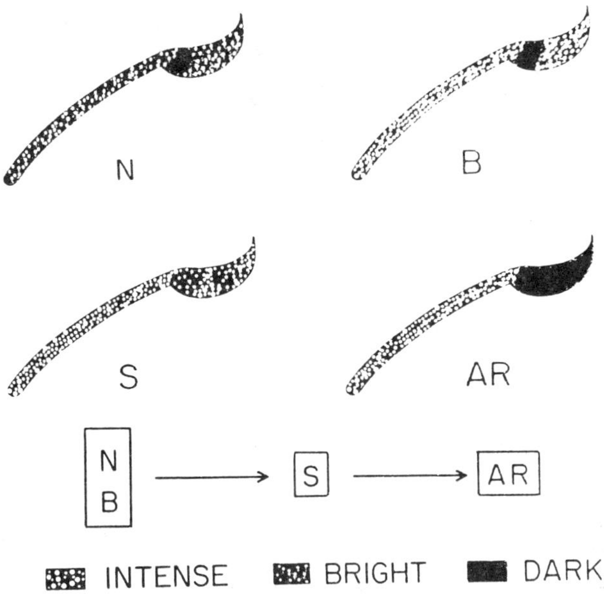

FIGURE 2. Schematic depiction of CTC and NDAA fluorescence patterns observed on capacitated mouse spermatozoa bound to isolated, structurally intact zonae pellucidae under conditions of incubation favoring zona-induction of the acrosome reaction. NDAA pattern N (upper left) resembles CTC pattern B (upper right). Both patterns are seen at early times in capacitated sperm bound to zonae. As the incubation time increases, pattern B is lost and is replaced by pattern S (lower left), which appears transiently, and is then in turn replaced by pattern AR (lower right). Pattern N loss follows pattern B loss with a short lag (see text). The temporal sequence of the appearance of the different fluorescent patterns is shown diagrammatically at the bottom of the FIGURE. (Adapted from Fig. 2 of Lee & Storey[59] and Fig. 1 of Lee & Storey.[60])

served. These results show that loss of pattern N is the reaction marking the transition between two stages of the acrosome reaction, which may be formulated functionally at this stage of the discussion in terms of the CTC fluorescence pattern changes as the B-to-S and S-to-AR transitions, the former being the first stage and the latter being the second stage.

Independent regulation of these two stages of the induced acrosome reaction is inferred from two separate lines of evidence. One line is the observation that biologically active phorbol esters such as TPA accelerate the B-to-S transition, but retard the S-to-AR transition, in sperm bound to isolated zonae, compared to the rates for these transitions seen in the absence of phorbol esters.[53] This effect is seen with 60 nM TPA in sperm bound to zonae, but the spontaneous acrosome reaction in sperm in suspension in the absence of zonae is unaffected by TPA up to the solubility limit of 10 μM. The second line of evidence comes from experiments with sperm bound to zonae from eggs treated with TPA. This treatment causes an egg-induced modification of ZP3 such that mechanical sperm binding and the induction of the B-to-S transition in the zonae-bound sperm are both unaffected, but the S-to-AR transition no longer takes place.[63,64] The sperm remain stalled in the S pattern. This made it possible to characterize the otherwise experimentally inaccessible transient S state.[65] It was found that sperm in this stalled S state retained their fluorescent N pattern, which indicates that the plasma membrane permeability barriers have remained intact. The sperm are not in an inhibited state, because addition of solubilized zonae from untreated eggs or the divalent cation ionophore A23187 induces the S-to-AR transition at the expected rate. This result confirms the supposition that the TPA treatment of the eggs partially debilitates ZP3, possibly by loss or modification of a ligand, such that ZP3 cannot initiate the second stage of the reaction. The sperm are induced to a poised or metastable state, however, as addition of the monovalent cation/H^+ exchange ionophore nigericin[66] also induces the S-to-AR transition. This ionophore has no effect on sperm in the B pattern state bound to zonae. The implication is that this stalled S state is the immediate precursor state to the rapid reaction causing loss of pattern N, and so it has been designated the S1 state.[65]

Another aspect of the reactions leading to the zona-induced mouse sperm acrosome reaction has been revealed by use of the Ca^{2+} fluorescent indicator, fura-2.[67] Mouse sperm treated with the tetra-acetoxymethyl ester of fura-2, which is permeant to membranes, load the probe onto the surface of the plasma membrane and into the acrosomal compartment.[60] The external probe on the plasma membrane can be quenched by addition of Mn^{2+}. This quenching leaves a bright arc of fluorescence overlying the anterior sperm head, which is emitted by fura–2 tetracarboxylate trapped in the acrosomal lumen and hence inaccessible to the exogenous Mn^{2+}. This fluorescence pattern is designated "F." Pattern F is lost from sperm bound to zonae with the same time course as assayed by population kinetics as pattern N. This result implies that the same process is causing loss of both patterns: a loss of membrane cation permeability barriers, allowing H^+ equilibration and quenching of fura-2 now made accessible to exogenous Mn^{2+}. The most plausible mechanism for the loss of these barriers is punctate apposition of the plasma and outer acrosomal membranes, followed by membrane fusion and pore formation at the points of apposition. This is the mechanism for the initiation of the membrane processes leading to the eventual vesiculation that completes the acrosome reaction, as envisioned by Bedford and Cooper.[28] It is also the mechanism for pore formation postulated as the first stage in granule exocytosis from mast cells.[36]

Other experimental observations that bear on the reactions driving zona-induced acrosomal exocytosis in mouse sperm are the following. 1) Extracellular Ca^{2+} is required for the reaction. In the absence of Ca^{2+}, the zona-induced acrosome reaction does not occur. Addition of ionophore A23187 accelerates the reaction in sperm bound to structurally intact zonae to such an extent that it is too rapid to follow by the CTC fluorescence pattern assay.[59] This effect is partially inhibited by QNB at concentrations that totally block the induced reaction in the absence of A23187. These results imply that a rise in intracellular Ca^{2+} is essential for the exocytotic reaction to proceed, and that the Ca^{2+} source is the extracellular medium. It further implies that the action of QNB is closely associated with the mechanism of rise in intracellular Ca^{2+}. While antibody M42 blocks the reaction at the B-to-S transition, it has no effect on the S-to-AR transition.[47] Earlier experiments reported by Florman *et al.*[68] indicate that the same is true for QNB. 3) Tyrphostin RG50864, a specific inhibitor of TK activity,[69] blocks the B-to-S transition and also markedly inhibits zona-induced autophosphorylation of p95.[42]

The Zona-induced Acrosome Reaction: A Model

A model for the zona-induced acrosome reaction in mouse sperm has been developed[34,70] from the experimental observations described above and based on the viewpoint that the acrosome resembles an overgrown exocytotic granule, rather than an overgrown lysosome. This viewpoint has illuminated the parallels between mast cell granule exocytosis in response to IgE and the sperm acrosome reaction in response to the zona pellucida, and so has led us to formulate the latter in terms of five stages, analogous to the five stages for the former proposed by Zimmerberg.[36] The five stages are shown in FIGURE 3, along with the assignments of CTC, NDAA, and fura-2 fluorescent patterns to each stage. In the **intact** stage, the outer acrosomal membrane (OAM) and the plasma membrane (PM) are separated by a narrow but finite cytosolic space. The sperm are capacitated, display the CTC fluorescent pattern B, and are prepared for the transition to the next stage upon activation by the zona pellucida. The next stage is the **poised** stage, in which the outer acrosomal membrane is apposed to the plasma membrane at many point junctions; but the two membranes, while adherent at these points, retain their separate integrities. The next stage is the **punctate** stage, in which the two membranes fuse at the point junctions to form pores just wide enough to allow passage of small ions and molecules, while the acrosomal matrix (AMX) remains intact. At the punctate stage, the membrane permeability barriers are lost, and the transition to the next stage, the **fenestrate** stage is driven primarily by osmotic effects.[71] The acrosomal matrix swells and begins to disperse. Macromolecules can pass in and out of the expanding pores. In the final, or **reacted** stage, the pores widen to the point that vesicles form, the matrix dispersion is completed, and all the membranes at the equatorial segment (EQ) fuse in a directed manner to seal in the remaining sperm cytosol. The inner acrosomal membrane (IAM) becomes the limiting membrane over the anterior portion of the sperm head. The sperm is now ready to penetrate the zona pellucida by binding to successive ZP2 molecules in its traverse through the matrix,[72] while acrosin and possibly other proteases cleave the ZP2/ZP3 filaments[44] in its path.

In this model, it is the transition from intact-to-poised and from poised-to-punctate that are mediated by the reactions of intracellular signal transduction. These two transitions are the ones whose independent regulation was discussed above. In terms of the fluorescence patterns, the intact-to-poised transition corresponds to the B-to-S1 transition for CTC, in which both NDAA and fura-2 fluorescence are retained over the acrosomal region of the head. Retention of these two fluorescence patterns are designated N+ and F+, respectively (FIG. 3). The poised-to-punctate transition corresponds to the loss of the NDAA and fura-2 head fluorescence patterns, which are for convenience designated the N+-to-N− and F+-to-F− transitions. The CTC patterns S2 and S3 are different degrees of spotty fluorescence that reflect the pore widening and onset of vesiculation. These, along with S1, were all subsumed under the S pattern classification in earlier studies.[47,51,59,60] The reacted state, in which the hybrid PM/OAM vesicles are lost, corresponds to the CTC fluorescence pattern AR. Based on this model, the first independently regulated transition accelerated by phorbol esters[53] is now reformulated as the B-to-S1 transition, while the second independently regulated transition retarded by phorbol esters is now reformulated as the N+-to-N− transition, rather than as the S-to-AR transition as was done above. The poised-to-punctate, or N+-to-N−, transition takes the acrosome reaction to the point of irre-

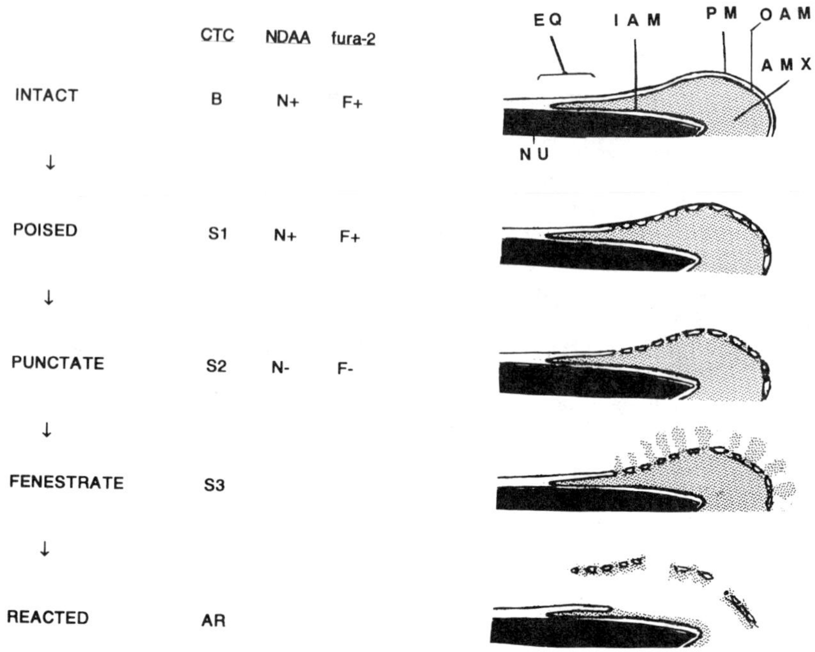

FIGURE 3. The five stages of the mouse sperm acrosome reaction shown in sequence. The first stage is the **intact** stage, shown at the top of the figure. The sperm cell has a fully intact plasma membrane (PM) overlying the outer acrosomal membrane (OAM), the equatorial segment (EQ), and the nucleus (NU), itself enclosed in its own nuclear membrane (not shown). The acrosomal matrix (AMX) is completely contained within the OAM and the inner acrosomal membrane (IAM). The second stage is the **poised** stage, in which the OAM and the PM have made point appositions, but both membranes have retained their integrity. The third stage is the **punctate** stage, in which the OAM and PM have fused at the point appositions to form pores. The AMX remains intact. The fourth stage is the **fenestrate** stage, in which the pores have widened and the AMX has begun to swell and disperse. The fifth stage is the **reacted** stage, shown at the bottom of the figure, in which the pores have widened to the point where hybrid vesicles of the OAM and PM have formed and have separated from the sperm head. Multiple membrane fusion has occurred at the EQ and the IAM is now the limiting membrane over the sperm head. The corresponding CTC fluorescent patterns are shown in the left column. The NDAA and fura-2 patterns are shown in the center and right columns. N+ and F+ indicate that the sperm display the N and F patterns; N− and F− indicate that these patterns have been lost.

versibility, after which it proceeds unregulated in response to osmotic forces.[71] Once the pores have formed, extracellular Ca^{2+} and H^{+} have free access to the acrosomal matrix, which then swells, thereby enlarging the pores to the point of vesiculation, and so driving the reaction to completion.

Mast cell granule exocytosis appears to share with the sperm acrosome reaction two sequential, independently regulated stages.[38] The first stage, in which granule apposition to the plasma membrane occurs, involves intracellular protein phosphorylation, while the second stage, in which membrane fusion and pore formation occurs, involves intracellular protein dephosphorylation. By analogy, we postulate that the intact-to-poised transition involves intracellular protein phosphorylation mediated by PK-C, with activation of PK-C by diacylglycerol (DAG). The intracellular DAG,

$[DAG]_i$, is released by activation of PL-C, which in turn is mediated by ZP3 activation of p95(TK) with increase in protein tyrosine phosphate (Tyr~P), both on p95 itself and presumably on other proteins. The latter protein, the only sperm plasma membrane protein to bind and respond to ZP3,[40–42] has the properties of a TK receptor of the type reported to activate PL-C directly or through the agency of a G protein.[73] This places p95(TK) as the primary receptor for the ZP3 ligand that initiates the zona-induced acrosome reaction. Activation of PK-C also requires Ca^{2+}, and increase of intracellular Ca^{2+}, $[Ca^{2+}]_i$, by influx from the extracellular medium is also postulated. It is suggested that this influx is mediated by SQNB, the QNB protein discussed above, in concert with a G_i protein. Induction of the first stage of the zona-induced acrosome reaction, the B-to-S1 transition, may be summarized in the set of hypothetical reactions listed below.

$$\text{ZP3} \Rightarrow \text{p95(TK)}\ \{A\}\ [\text{Tyr}{\sim}\text{P}]_i\uparrow\ \Rightarrow \text{PL-C}\ \{A\} \rightarrow [\text{DAG}]_i\uparrow \quad (1)$$
$$\Downarrow ?$$
$$\text{ZP3} \Rightarrow ?\ \text{SQPB-G}_i\ \{A\} \rightarrow [\text{Ca}^{2+}]_i\uparrow \quad (2)$$

$$[\text{Ca}^{2+}]_i\uparrow + [\text{DAG}]_i\uparrow\ \Rightarrow \text{PK-C}\ \{A\} \rightarrow [\text{pOAM}{\sim}\text{P}]_i\uparrow + [\text{pPM}{\sim}\text{P}]_i\uparrow \quad (3)$$

The symbol "{A}" in reactions **(1)–(3)** indicates activation of the enzyme or regulatory protein so marked. The symbol "↑" indicates an increase in the intracellular component. The final products of this set of three reactions are phosphorylated outer membrane proteins, $[pOAM{\sim}P]_i$, and phosphorylated plasma membrane proteins, $[pPM{\sim}P]_i$, where the subscript "i" here indicates that the phosphate ester groups, ~P, are in the cytosolic space, on the outer surface of the OAM and on the inner surface of the PM. It is these phosphorylated proteins that make the point apposition of the two membranes. Completion of reaction (3) marks the end of the intact-to-poised, or B-to-S1, transition. The two "?" indicate that the SQBP-G_i combination may be activated either by p95 or directly by ZP3. An important aspect of this model is that **both** the pathways leading to rise in $[Ca^{2+}]_i$ and $[DAG]_i$ must function. If the two are independently initiated by ZP3 ligands, the mechanism of initiation becomes comparable to the opening of a safe deposit box, for which two keys in concert are required.

The experimental support for this part of the model comes from the observations that: 1) phorbol esters that activate PK-C accelerate the B-to-S1 transition;[53] 2) extracellular Ca^{2+} is required for the acrosome reaction;[59,74] 3) the B-to-S1 transition is blocked by QNB,[59] by pertussis toxin which inactivates G_i proteins,[51,52] and by tyrphostin RG50864,[42] which is a specific and potent inhibitor of TK activity;[69] and that 4) ionophore A23187 overcomes the block to this transition by QNB and pertussis toxin.[52,59]

Induction of the second stage of the acrosome reaction is postulated to occur through the following reactions, which set in motion the protein dephosphorylations leading to pore formation by deactivation of PK-C and activation of protein phosphatases.

$$\text{ZP3} \Rightarrow ?\ \text{PTPase} \Rightarrow \text{p95(TK)}\ \{DA\}\ [\text{Tyr}{\sim}\text{P}]_i\downarrow\ \Rightarrow \text{PL-C}\ \{DA\} \rightarrow [\text{DAG}]_i\downarrow \quad (4)$$
$$\Uparrow ?$$
$$[\text{Ca}^{2+}]_i\uparrow\ \Rightarrow \text{DAG-K}\ \{A\} \rightarrow [\text{DAG}]_i\downarrow\ \Rightarrow \text{PK-C}\ \{DA\} \quad (5)$$

$$[\text{Ca}^{2+}]_i\uparrow\ \Rightarrow \text{CMDase}\ \{A\} \rightarrow [\text{SPB}]_i\uparrow\ \Rightarrow \text{PK-C}\ \{I\} \quad (6)$$
$$\Downarrow ?$$
$$\text{ZP3} \Rightarrow ?\ (\text{G}_E)\ \text{pPase} \Rightarrow [\text{pOAM}{\sim}\text{P}]_i\downarrow + [\text{pPM}{\sim}\text{P}]_i\downarrow\ \Rightarrow \text{Pore Form.} \quad (7)$$

The symbols "{A}" and "↑" stand for enzyme activation and intracellular component increase, respectively, as in reactions **(1)–(3)** above. In reactions **(4)–(7)**, the symbols "{DA}", "{I}", and "↓" stand for enzyme deactivation, enzyme inhibition, and intracellular component decrease, respectively. DAG kinase (DAG-K) removes DAG by phosphorylation, and so deactivates PK-C.[57] Ceramidase (CMDase) hydrolyzes ceramide to produce sphingosine base, $[SPB]_i$, an inhibitor of PK-C,[75] in the last step of the enzymatic pathway leading from the sperm's ample supply of sphingomyelin,[76] a pathway now recognized as active in intracellular regulation.[77] The postulated activation of phosphotyrosine phosphatase (PTPase) by ZP3 deactivates p95(TK) in this scheme, which leads to deactivation of PL-C, and so indirectly to further deactivation of PK-C through decreased production of $[DAG]_i$. This combined assault on PK-C activity allows dephosphorylation of $[pOAM{\sim}P]_i$ and $[pPM{\sim}P]_i$ by a postulated protein phosphatase (pPase) to dominate, thus leading to pore formation. The activation of pPase by ZP3 and involvement of a G protein, designated G_E, is suggested by analogy to the scheme proposed for the equivalent late-acting phosphatase by the Gomperts group.[78]

Experimental support for this formulation of the second stage comes from the observation that phorbol esters retard the Sl-to-AR transition,[53] presumably by maintaining activation of PK-C. The need for activation of this stage by ZP3 is suggested by the experiments with zonae from eggs treated with TPA, whose ZP3 appears to have lost the ability to activate the second stage while retaining full ability to activate the first stage of the induced acrosome reaction.[64,65] The possibility of an active PTPase is suggested by the participation of p200/220 in the reaction. This component has the M_r expected for the CD45 group of plasma membrane phosphotyrosine phosphatases.[79] The inhibitory action of Mab M42 could be explained by activation of p200/220 to dephosphorylate p95(TK), thus preventing activation of the first stage of the acrosome reaction as formulated in reactions **(1)–(3)** above. Experimental evidence for this action of Mab M42 comes from the observation of Leyton and Saling[40] that the degree of tyrosine phosphorylation on p95 is decreased relative to that seen in capacitated sperm by treatment of these sperm with the antibody. The sequence of stages is postulated to occur by the increase in $[Ca^{2+}]_i$ in the first stage, which then allows activation of the enzymes active in the second stage. While plausible, this aspect of the model is admittedly a bit speculative, and this has been noted by the "?" next to the postulated $[Ca^{2+}]_i$ activation pathways in reactions **(4)–(7)**. This model is accessible to experimental test, as it makes specific predictions about the increase and decrease of $[Ca^{2+}]_i$, $[DAG]_i$, and $[SPB]_i$, the p95(TK) phosphorylation state, and the phosphorylation state of proteins of the OAM and PM overlying the acrosomal region. A membrane preparation highly enriched in p95(TK) comprising membranes from this region of the mouse sperm head has recently been reported,[80] making the experimental determination of these protein phosphorylation states feasible.

The Spontaneous Acrosome Reaction

The spontaneous acrosome reaction in mouse sperm occurs much less rapidly than the zona-induced one, and the inhibitors of the zona-induced reaction have no effect on the spontaneous one.[22,51–53] It is proposed that the reaction sequence proposed in reactions **(1)–(7)** above can proceed, even in the absence of zona activation. A slow influx of Ca^{2+} could occur if the "leak" of this cation down its steep electrochemical gradient into the cell were to outpace the ion pump extruding it. Aggregation of p95(TK) could also occur at a finite rate resulting in its activation. The result would be eventual acrosomal exocytosis in the population of sperm cells independent of zona activation. Since the inhibitors of the zona-induced acrosome reaction work on the zona-dependent pathways, they would be expected to be without effect on the spontaneous reaction. This model leads to some ideas concerning the nature of the capacitation process, without which neither the spontaneous nor the zona-induced acrosome reaction in mouse sperm can occur.[13]

CAPACITATION AND THE ACROSOME REACTION

It is beyond the scope of this account to provide a review of the process of capacitation in mammalian sperm; the reader is referred to the excellent review by Saling[81] for this. The following comments are offered, based on the model of the acrosome reaction in mouse sperm described above. Go and Wolf[20] documented the efflux of cholesterol from mouse sperm during capacitation, and showed that BSA was essential to this process. This result was in full agreement with earlier observations of Davis[82,83] that the time required for capacitation in sperm from a number of mammalian species correlated with the time required for the loss of cholesterol to proceed to a level characteristic of the species. This loss of cholesterol has been postulated to increase fluidity of the sperm plasma membrane.[84] Were the plasma membrane too rigid, then the aggregation of p95(TK) required for its activation would be inhibited. Support for this concept comes from the observation of Leyton and Saling[40] that tyrosine phosphorylation on p95 is much less pronounced in uncapacitated than in capacitated mouse sperm. Loss of surface protein from the plasma membrane has also been shown to occur during capacitation.[81] This suggests that protein removal may in part promote the influx of Ca^{2+} into the cell. If neither p95(TK) activation nor Ca^{2+} influx can occur, then both the spontaneous and zona-induced acrosome reactions would be blocked. This hypothesis is experimentally accessible through studies of Ca^{2+} influx along with p95 activation in capacitated and uncapacitated mouse sperm.

CONCLUSIONS

The link between capacitation in mouse sperm and the acrosome reaction, whether spontaneous or zona-induced, is postulated to be the removal of the blocks to two reactions, the activation of p95(TK) through its aggregation and subsequent autophosphorylation[40,42] and the influx of Ca^{2+}. The details of the reactions mediating the removal of these blocks remain to be elucidated. While there are clear differences between murine and bovine sperm in this regard,[24,25] it is evident that similarities exist with regard to Ca^{2+} influx, since only those bovine sperm that show this influx in response to the acrosome reaction are capable of undergoing the zona-induced acrosome reaction.[26] It is hoped that the studies outlined and the reaction models presented in this discussion will be directly applicable to the question of capacitation and the physiologically relevant acrosome reaction in human sperm.

REFERENCES

1. AUSTIN, C. R. 1951. Australian J. Sci. Res. Ser. B. **4:** 581–596.
2. CHANG, M. C. 1951. Nature **168:** 697–698.
3. AUSTIN, C. R. 1985. *In* Biology of Fertilization. C. B. Metz & A. Monroy, Eds.: 121–155. Academic Press. New York.
4. AUSTIN, C. R. 1952. Nature **170:** 326.
5. IWAMATSU, H. & M. C. CHANG. 1969. Nature **224:** 919–920.
6. IWAMATSU, H. & M. C. CHANG. 1970. J. Exp. Zool. **175:** 271–282.
7. TOYODA, Y., M. YOKOYAMA & T. HOSI. 1971. Jap. J. Anim. Reprod. **16:** 147–151.
8. TOYODA, Y., M. YOKOYAMA & T. HOSI. 1971. Jap. J. Anim. Reprod. **16:** 152–157.
9. MIYAMOTO, H. & M. C. CHANG. 1973. J. Reprod. Fertil. **32:** 193–205.
10. AUSTIN, C. R. 1975. J. Reprod. Fertil. **44:** 155–166.
11. CHANG, M. C. & R. F. H. HUNTER. 1975. *In* Handbook of Physiology, Section 7: Endocrinology. Vol. V, Male Reproductive System. D. W. Hamilton & R. O. Greep, Eds.: 339–351. American Physiological Society. Washington, DC.
12. CHANG, M. C. 1984. J. Androl. **5:** 45–50.
13. WARD, C. R. & B. T. STOREY. 1984. Dev. Biol. **104:** 287–296.
14. SALING, P. M. & B. T. STOREY. 1979. J. Cell Biol. **83:** 544–555.
15. INOUE, M. & D. P. WOLF. 1974. Biol. Reprod. **11:** 558–565.
16. INOUE, M. & D. P. WOLF. 1975. Biol. Reprod. **13:** 340–348.
17. WOLF, D. P. & M. INOUE. 1976. J. Exp. Zool. **196:** 27–38.
18. WOLF, D. P., M. INOUE & R. A. STARK. 1976. Biol. Reprod. **15:** 213–221.
19. WOLF, D. P. 1979. *In* The Biology of the Fluids of the Female Genital Tract. F. K. Beller & G. F. B. Schumacher, Eds.: 407–414. Elsevier North Holland. Amsterdam
20. GO, K. J. & D. P. WOLF. 1985. Biol. Reprod. **32:** 145–153.
21. SALING, P. M., J. SOWINSKI & B. T. STOREY. 1979. J. Exp. Zool. **209:** 229–238.
22. FLORMAN, H. M. & B. T. STOREY. 1982. Dev. Biol. **91:** 121–130.
23. FLORMAN, H. M. & B. T. STOREY. 1982. J. Androl. **3:** 157–164.
24. FLORMAN, H. M. & N. L. FIRST. 1988. Dev. Biol. **128:** 453–463.
25. FLORMAN, H. M. & N. L. FIRST. 1988. Dev. Biol. **128:** 464–473.
26. FLORMAN, H. M., R. M. TOMBES, N. L. FIRST & D. F. BABCOCK. 1989. Dev. Biol. **135:** 133–146.
27. MCRORIE, R. A. & W. L. WILLIAMS. 1974. Annu. Rev. Biochem. **43:** 777–803.
28. BEDFORD, J. M. & G. W. COOPER. 1978. *In* Cell Surface Reviews. G. Poste & G. L. Nicholson, Eds. Vol. **5:** 65–125. Elsevier North Holland. Amsterdam.
29. BLEIL, J. D. & P. M. WASSARMAN. 1983. Dev. Biol. **95:** 317–324.
30. KOPF, G. S. & G. L. GERTON. 1990. *In* The Biology and Chemistry of Mammalian Fertilization. P. M. Wassarman, Ed. Vol. **1:** 153–203. CRC Press. Boca Raton, FL.
31. FLORMAN, H. M. & B. T. STOREY. 1981. J. Exp. Zool. **216:** 159–167.
32. BLEIL, J. D. & P. M. WASSARMAN. 1980. Dev. Biol. **76:** 185–202.
33. BLEIL, J. D. & P. M. WASSARMAN. 1980. Cell **20:** 873–882.
34. STOREY, B. T. & G. S. KOPF. 1991. *In* A Comparative Overview of Mammalian Fertilization. B. S. Dunbar & M. G. O'Rand, Eds.: 167–216. Plenum Publishing Corp. New York.
35. BERRIDGE, M. J. 1986. J. Cell Sci. (Suppl) **4:** 137–153.
36. ZIMMERBERG, J. 1987. Biosci. Reports **7:** 251–268.
37. METZGER, H. 1988. Adv. Immunol. **43:** 277–312.
38. GOMPERTS, B. D. 1990. Int. J. Exp. Pathol. **71:** 423–431.
39. LEYTON, L. & P. SALING. 1989. J. Cell Biol. **108:** 2163–2168.
40. LEYTON, L. & P. SALING. 1989. Cell **57:** 123–150.
41. SALING, P. M., D. O. BUNCH, P. LE GUEN & L. LEYTON. 1991. *In* Mammalian Fertilization. B. D. Bavister, J. Cummins & E. R. S. Roldan, Eds.: 239–252, Serono Symposia USA, Norwell.
42. LEYTON, L., D. O. BUNCH, P. LEGUEN, M. SELUB & P. M. SALING. 1990. *In* Gamete Interaction. N. Alexander, D. Griffin, J. Speiler & G. M. H. Waites, Eds.: 225–239. Wiley-Liss. New York.
43. BLEIL, J. D. & P. M. WASSARMAN. 1990. Proc. Natl. Acad. Sci. USA **87:** 5563–5567.
44. GREVE, J. M. & P. M. WASSARMAN. 1985. J. Mol. Biol. **181:** 253–264.
45. SALING, P. M. & K. A. LAKOSKI. 1985. Biol. Reprod. **33:** 527–536.
46. SALING, P. M. 1986. Dev. Biol. **177:** 511–519.

47. LEYTON, L., A. ROBINSON & P. M. SALING. 1989. Dev. Biol. **132:** 174–178.
48. ROSS, E. M. 1989. Neuron **3:** 141–152.
49. FREISSMUTH, M., P. J. CASEY & A. G. GILMAN. 1989. FASEB J. **3:** 2125–2131.
50. KOPF, G. S., M. J. WOOLKALIS & G. L. GERTON. 1986. J. Biol. Chem. **261:** 7327–7331.
51. ENDO, Y., M. A. LEE & G. S. KOPF. 1987. Dev. Biol. **119:** 210–216.
52. ENDO, Y., M. A. LEE & G. S. KOPF. 1988. Dev. Biol. **129:** 12–24.
53. LEE, M. A., G. S. KOPF & B. T. STOREY. 1987. Biol. Reprod. **36:** 617–627.
54. NISHIZUKA, Y. 1984. Nature **308:** 693–698.
55. ROLDAN, E. S. R. & R. A. P. HARRISON. 1988. Biochem. Biophys. Res. Commun. **155:** 901–906.
56. ROLDAN, E. S. R. & R. A. P. HARRISON. 1989. Biochem. J. **259:** 397–406.
57. ROLDAN, E. S. R. & R. A. P. HARRISON. 1990. Biochem. Biophys. Res. Commun. **172:** 8–15.
58. BIRNBAUMER, L., A. ABRAMOWITZ, Y. YATANI, K. OKABE, R. MATTERA, R. GRAF, J. SANFORD, J. CODINA & A. M. BROWN. 1990. Crit. Rev. Biochem. Mol. Biol. **25:** 225–244.
59. LEE, M. A. & B. T. STOREY. 1985. Biol. Reprod. **33:** 235–246.
60. Lee, M. A. & B. T. STOREY. 1989. Gamete Res. **24:** 303–326.
61. HUANG, C. S., S. J. KOPACZ & C. P. LEE. 1983. Biochim. Biophys. Acta **722:** 107–115.
62. JOHNSON, R. G., S. E. CARTY, B. J. FINGERHOOD & A. SCARPA. 1980. FEBS Lett. **120:** 75–79.
63. ENDO, Y., R. M. SCHULTZ & G. S. KOPF. 1987. Dev. Biol. **119:** 199–209.
64. ENDO, Y., P. MATTEI, G. S. KOPF & R. M. SCHULTZ. 1987. Dev. Biol. **123:** 574–577.
65. KLIGMAN, I., M. GLASSNER, B. T. STOREY & G. S. KOPF. 1991. Dev. Biol. **145:** 344–355.
66. PRESSMAN, B. C. 1976. Ann. Rev. Biochem. **45:** 501–530.
67. GRYNKIEWICZ, G., M. POENIE & R. Y. TSIEN. 1985. J. Biol. Chem. **260:** 3440–3450.
68. FLORMAN, H. M., P. M. SALING & B. T. STOREY. 1982. J. Androl. **3:** 373–381.
69. LYALL, R. M., A. ZILBERSTEIN, G. GAZIT, C. GILON, A. LEVITZKI & J. SCHLESSINGER. 1989. J. Biol. Chem. **264:** 14503–14509.
70. STOREY, B. T. 1992. *In* Comparative Spermatology 20 Years After. B. Baccetti, Ed. Raven Press. New York. In press.
71. CHANDLER, D. E., M. WHITAKER & J. ZIMMERBERG. 1989. J. Cell Biol. **109:** 1269–1278.
72. BLEIL, J. D. & P. M. WASSARMAN. 1986. J. Cell Biol. **102:** 1363–1371.
73. ULLRICH, A. & J. SCHLESSINGER. 1990. Cell **61:** 203–212.
74. YANAGIMACHI, R. 1975. Biol. Reprod. **13:** 519–526.
75. MERRILL, A. H., A. M. SERENI, V. L. STEVENS, Y. A. HANNUN, R. M. BELL & J. M. KINKADE. 1986. J. Biol. Chem. **261:** 12610–12615.
76. ALVAREZ, J. G., I. LOPEZ, J. C. TOUCHSTONE & B. T. STOREY. 1987. J. Liquid Chromatog. **10:** 3557–3573.
77. MERRILL, A. H. & V. L. STEVENS. 1989. Biochim. Biophys. Acta **1010:** 131–139.
78. CHURCHER, Y., I. M. KRAMER & B. D. GOMPERTS. 1990. Cell Reg. **1:** 523–530.
79. CHARBONNEAU, H., N. K. TONKS, K. A. WALSH & E. H. FISCHER. 1988. Proc. Natl. Acad. Sci. USA **85:** 7183–7186.
80. BUNCH, D. O. & P. M. SALING. 1991. Biol. Reprod. **44:** 672–680.
81. SALING, P. M. 1989. Oxford Rev. Reprod. Biol. **11:** 339–388.
82. DAVIS, B. K. 1980. Arch. Androl. **5:** 249–254.
83. DAVIS, B. K. 1981. Proc. Natl. Acad. Sci. USA **78:** 7560–7564.
84. LANGLAIS, J. & K. D. ROBERTS. 1985. Gamete Res. **12:** 183–224.

The Genetics of Sperm Function in Fertilization[a]

PATRICIA OLDS-CLARKE

Department of Anatomy and Cell Biology
Temple University School of Medicine
3400 N. Broad Street
Philadelphia, Pennsylvania 19140

MUTATIONS CAN BE USEFUL TOOLS IN THE STUDY OF FERTILIZATION

Mammalian fertilization is such a complex process that it has been difficult to identify and characterize all of the structural and regulatory components involved in gamete interaction. The study of mutations, in concert with other approaches, has been instrumental in elucidating the molecular basis of organelle function in other cell types. For example, analysis of mutations causing flagellar paralysis in *Chlamydomonas* has identified over 85 genes necessary for the assembly and function of this organelle.[1] This review will describe mutations which impair mammalian sperm function, with emphasis on studies published since a previous review of this topic.[2]

Although inherited alterations in human[3] and bull[4] sperm function are known, mutational analysis in large mammalian species is often difficult for ethical or economic reasons. The mouse, on the other hand, has been extensively used in genetic studies—it is the mammalian fruit fly. Because of this, the mouse offers a number of tools to aid the reproductive biologist in a genetic analysis. First, there is a long list of mutations which affect male fertility.[5,6] Second, assignment of mutations to a specific locus on a particular chromosome (mapping) is facilitated by the large numbers of mutations already mapped[7] and through the use of hybrids between *Mus musculus* (the laboratory mouse) and a closely related species, *Mus spretus*.[8] Finally, molecular probes for many parts of the genome[9] and testis-specific cDNA libraries are available.[10]

The power of these tools can be seen in the unraveling of the mechanisms by which two mutations, *Steel* (*Sl*) and *White-spotting* (*W*), cause sterility. These mutations, found on different chromosomes, cause the same triad of symptoms: a severe deficiency of hemopoietic tissue, hair pigmentation, and germ cells. Recently it was shown that the *W* locus includes the proto-oncogene *c-kit*, which codes for a transmembrane tyrosine kinase receptor, while the product of the *Sl* locus is the ligand for this receptor.[11] This implicates *c-kit* in the proliferation of primary germ cells.

Another reason for using the mouse for mutational analysis is the existence of congenic strains, which are genetically identical except in the region of the mutation. Sperm characteristics are the end result of interactions of alleles at many different

[a] The research for this paper was supported by NICHD Grant 15045.

loci. Therefore if sperm from a mutant are compared to sperm from a genetically unrelated wild-type male, differences between mutant and wild-type sperm could be due to the expression of alleles at other loci. When congenic strains are not available, siblings must be used. Differences in fertility or in sperm characteristics can definitively be ascribed to the mutation only if the mutant and the wild-type controls share a significant portion of their genomes.

This review will focus on four genetic mouse models of sperm dysfunction: abnormal spermatozoon head (*azh*), *bouncy* (*bc*), a mutation produced by insertional mutagenesis which may be within the *hotfoot* locus (*ho*), and the *t* complex. Because the *t* complex has such paradoxical effects on fertility, this system will be discussed last and in greater detail.

AZH ALTERS SPERM HEAD MORPHOLOGY

The mutation *azh* causes all sperm heads to have grossly abnormal shapes, presumably the result of abnormalities in the manchette and nuclear ring, structures important in shaping the sperm head during spermiogenesis.[12] Some *azh* male homozygotes were subfertile[13] and capacitated mutant sperm bound to the zona pellucida at a reduced level, relative to sperm from several noncongenic strains of normal mice.[14] That some mutant sperm can fertilize, in spite of their abnormal head shape, suggests that such abnormalities do not in themselves preclude successful sperm-egg interactions.

Sperm populations from *azh/azh* mice contain some motile flagella unattached to a head. We took advantage of this to determine whether the lack of a head affected flagellar movement. Motile flagella with and without heads were analyzed for speed and path shape using the Image–80 sperm motion analysis system as previously described.[15] As each sperm appeared on the videotape, it was classified as headless or headed, then traced for 1.0 sec at 30 frames/second. There were no significant differences in sperm swimming speed or straightness of path between headed and headless mutant sperm (TABLE 1). Because the sample size was small, subtle differences in motility could have been overlooked; nevertheless, motility was not appreciably affected even by such a gross abnormality as the absence of a head. This suggests that flagellar movement is not altered by dramatic differences in head size.

TABLE 1. Abnormal Head Shape and Motility of Sperm from *azh/azh* Mice

Minutes of Incubation	Sperm Head Type	No. Sperm Examined/Male[a]	Curvilinear Velocity (μ/sec)[a]	Linearity[a]
30	Abnormal[b]	36 ± 0.5	144 ± 12	46 ± 7
	None[b]	8 –	160 ± 6	40 ± 5
90	Abnormal	37 ± 4	161 ± 16	34 ± 4
	None	8 ± 4	181 ± 41	32 ± 4

[a] Mean of mean/male, ± Standard Deviation.

[b] Sperm from 4 *azh/azh* mice, back-crossed to C57BL/6J mice for seven generations (mice generously contributed by Dr. Marvin Meistrich, M.D. Anderson Hospital and Cancer Institute, Houston, TX).

BOUNCY MAY CAUSE DEFECTS IN SPERM-EGG INTERACTION

In a survey of mutations affecting post-testicular sperm function, sperm from *bouncy* homozygotes were unable to fertilize eggs *in vivo* despite normal epididymal sperm numbers.[16] *In vitro*, *bouncy* sperm fertilized fewer eggs than sperm from congenic wild-type males. When minimal sperm concentrations were used, fewer mutant sperm penetrated zona-free hamster eggs, suggesting that *bouncy* may alter sperm-egg binding or fusion. The caput epididymis of *bouncy* mice appeared to lack a secreted protein of M_r 18,000, suggesting that this protein could be important in sperm-egg interactions. If so, this mutant could be a promising model system in which to study how epididymis-sperm interactions affect sperm function.

INSERTIONAL MUTAGENESIS IN A TRANSGENIC MOUSE CAUSES FERTILIZATION DEFECTS

Production of transgenic mice occasionally causes sterility by insertional mutagenesis. Insertion of an altered dihydrofolate reductase gene at or near the *hotfoot* (*ho*) locus produced a transgenic line of mice that were male-sterile (females were subfertile).[17] Sperm from mice with the insertional mutation, ho^{Jwg}, could fertilize zona-drilled oocytes but were much less successful with zona-intact oocytes. Although no formal motility analysis was carried out, sperm appeared to move with decreased forward progression. Therefore ho^{Jwg} could affect either zona binding or zona penetration. Because the wild-type control mice were genetically unrelated to mice carrying ho^{Jwg}, it is unclear whether these effects on sperm function are due solely to the inserted DNA sequence.

THE *t* COMPLEX CONTAINS GENES AFFECTING SPERM FERTILIZING ABILITY

The *t* complex is a group of linked genes on chromosome 17. This complex is large, encompassing about 1% of the total genome[18] and containing at least four inversions.[19] These inversions prevent recombination between the *t* complex and the wild-type homologue, thus causing the *t* complex to be transmitted as though it were a single genetic unit. The *t* complex is transmitted by *t*/+ females to 50% of their offspring, but *t*/+ males transmit it to 90–99% of their offspring. All evidence suggests that in *t*/+ males, sperm carrying the complex (*t* sperm) have an advantage over wild-type sperm (+ sperm), such that very few + sperm ever fertilize eggs *in vivo.*[2] We showed by direct sperm competition tests between *t* sperm and + sperm from congenic +/+ males that *t* sperm had no advantage in fertilization *in vivo.*[20] Since *t* sperm have no advantage in fertilization over normal sperm, + sperm produced by *t*/+ males must be dysfunctional (FIG. 1).

Most *t* complexes include a lethal factor, precluding true homozygotes. The lethal factors are non-allelic, however, so that mice can be constructed carrying complementing lethals. These mice will be referred to as t^x/t^y mice, where x and y indicate different lethal factors, and t^x and t^y are referred to as different *t* "haplotypes." Female t^x/t^y mice are fertile while males are sterile[2] (FIG. 1).

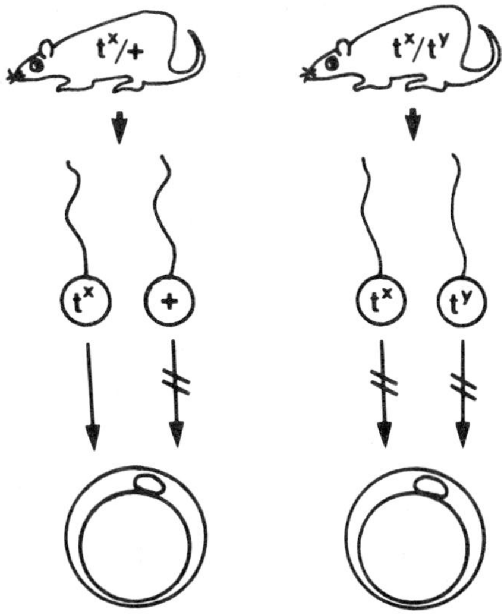

FIGURE 1. Fertilizing ability of sperm from males carrying one or two *t* haplotypes. In $t^x/+$ males, + sperm are dysfunctional relative to t^x sperm. In t^x/t^y males, all sperm are nonfunctional.

INTERACTION OF GENES IN THE *t* COMPLEX ALTERS FERTILIZING ABILITY

These effects on sperm function are due to the interaction of several genes within the *t* complex.[21] Although the nature of this interaction is not known, we have proposed the following hypothesis.[2] Genes located in various regions of the *t* complex, named *Tcd-1*, *Tcd-2*, *etc.*, are necessary for normal sperm function. All *t* haplotypes have defective alleles at these loci, resulting in sperm dysfunction even in heterozygotes.[22] Every *t* haplotype also includes another gene, *Tcr* (FIG. 2), which somehow compensates for the depleted levels of the products of Tcd^+ alleles, restoring sperm function. If *Tcr* is expressed only in haploid cells and its product is confined to *t* spermatids, then only *t* sperm will be "rescued" from the detrimental effects of the Tcd^t genes and thus be able to fertilize eggs. In genetic terms, *Tcr* acts as a second-site suppressor mutation for the effects of the Tcd^t products.[23] Mice with two *t* complexes have no normal alleles at the *Tcd* loci, and therefore their sperm are not helped by the presence of *Tcr*.

THE *t* COMPLEX CONTAINS MANY TESTIS-EXPRESSED GENES

The segment of DNA containing *Tcr* has been cloned; it contains a gene, *Tcp-10b*, which is part of a family of genes that encode testis-specific transcripts.[24,25] Members of this gene family, including *Tcp-10b*, are expressed in pachytene spermatocytes and round spermatids from both +/+ and *t*/+ mice. In round spermatids of *t*/+ mice a second transcript is also made, apparently from an alternative splicing event.[26] The *Tcp-10b* transcript which is unique to haploid cells from *t*/+ mice could encode a variant protein responsible for the *Tcr* phenotype.

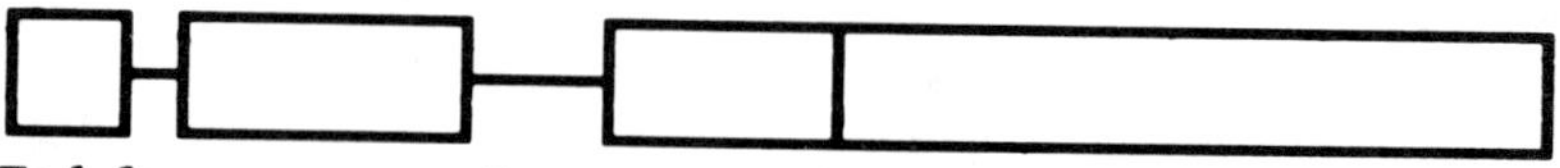

FIGURE 2. Map of the *t* complex region of chromosome 17, showing the approximate location of factors affecting male fertility (there may be more than three *Tcd* factors). The centromere is to the left. Positions of inversions relative to these factors are indicated by the boxes.

None of the *Tcd* genes have been identified, but testis-specific transcripts of clones located within the *t* complex have been reported,[27-30] and a number of *t*-specific proteins synthesized in testicular cells have been identified.[31] The gene for one of these proteins, *Tcp-1*, has some sequence homology to the chaperonin family;[32] since homologous sequences have been found in human beings, fruit flies, and yeast,[33] this locus may be important for a cell function common to all eukaryotes. In summary, there is as yet no evidence that any of these potential candidates for *Tcd* genes affect sperm function.

THE PHYSIOLOGICAL DIFFERENCE BETWEEN *t* AND + SPERM IN POPULATIONS FROM *t*/+ MALES IS UNKNOWN

Another approach to determining the nature of the *Tcd* genes is to identify abnormalities in the mutant cells and from them determine the underlying molecular mechanisms. Genes for these components can then be mapped to specific sites within the *t* complex. In searching for abnormalities among sperm from *t*/+ males, however, it cannot be assumed that all abnormalities are unique to + sperm. Some sperm abnormalities will be confined to + sperm, but others may be characteristic of all sperm in the population. Although it is now possible to genotype individual sperm using the polymerase chain reaction,[34] this approach has yet to be used with the *t* complex. Because there is currently no evidence that any of the sperm defects identified thus far are unique to + or *t* sperm, all sperm from *t*/+ males will hereafter be considered a single physiological type, "*t*/+ sperm."

THE *t* COMPLEX AFFECTS SPERM TRANSPORT TO THE SITE OF FERTILIZATION AND SPERM-EGG INTERACTION

The *t* complex has no obvious effects on male genital tract functions[16,20] or on the number of motile sperm reaching the uterus.[35] Sperm transport to the oviduct is affected, however. Virtually no sperm can be recovered from the oviduct after matings with t^x/t^y males, regardless of their genetic background,[36] and females mated to *t*/+ males had significantly fewer oviductal sperm than females mated to congenic +/+ males.[37]

The *t* complex also alters sperm-egg interaction. When sperm from t^x/t^y males were artificially inseminated into the ovarian bursa, so that sperm would be swept down into the oviduct with the eggs, the sperm were unable to fertilize.[38] *In vitro*, even drilling or removal of the zona pellucida did not allow sperm from t^x/t^y males

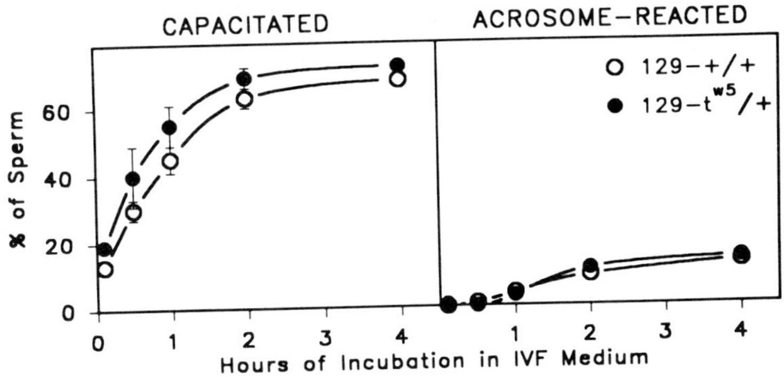

FIGURE 3 The mean ± SEM percent of capacitated and spontaneously acrosome-reacted sperm from four +/+ and $t^{w5}/+$ males of the 129 strain. Capacitation and the acrosome reaction were determined by the chlortetracycline assay (Ward & Storey, 1984, Dev. Biol. **104:** 287–296). Error bars not shown are smaller than the symbols.

to penetrate oocytes.[39,40] Evidence for defective *t*/+ sperm fertilizing ability *in vitro* is contradictory,[40-42] probably because alleles at loci outside the *t* complex can mitigate the effects of genes within the *t* complex.[43] Thus sperm from t^x/t^y males are incapable of sperm-egg fusion, but it is not clear what step or steps in fertilization are defective in *t*/+ sperm.

THE *t* COMPLEX ALTERS QUALITATIVE ASPECTS OF SPERM MOTILITY

The *t* complex causes no unique sperm ultrastructural abnormalities, and no differences could be found on silver-stained 2-dimensional gels of sperm proteins of congenic *t*/+, t^x/t^y, or +/+ males.[2] This suggests that the *t* complex regulates more subtle aspects of sperm function, *e.g.*, regulatory proteins.

Surface galactosyltransferase (GT) activity levels in *t*/+ sperm populations are twice those of congenic +/+ sperm populations, and levels in t^x/t^y sperm populations are fourfold higher.[44] GT has been implicated as one of the factors needed for sperm-zona binding,[45] suggesting it has an important function in fertilization. However, since *t*/+ sperm do not differ from congenic +/+ sperm in zona-binding ability[46] and since sperm of the BALB/c and 129 strains of mice with normal fertility have GT activity levels similar to sperm of t^x/t^y males,[47,48] elevated GT activity does not appear to affect fertilizing ability.

A premature acrosome reaction has been reported to be characteristic of sperm from mice carrying the t^{w5} haplotype when they are capacitated in medium supplemented with amino acids and glutathione.[49] We have repeated these experiments, capacitating sperm in a modified Krebs-Ringer-bicarbonate medium which will support fertilization *in vitro.* We found no differences in the levels of capacitation or spontaneous acrosome reactions between $t^{w5}/+$ sperm and congenic +/+ sperm (FIG. 3). In addition, sperm from mice carrying the t^{w32} haplotype were not different from congenic wild-type sperm in their rate of capacitation or acrosome reaction.[46,50] There-

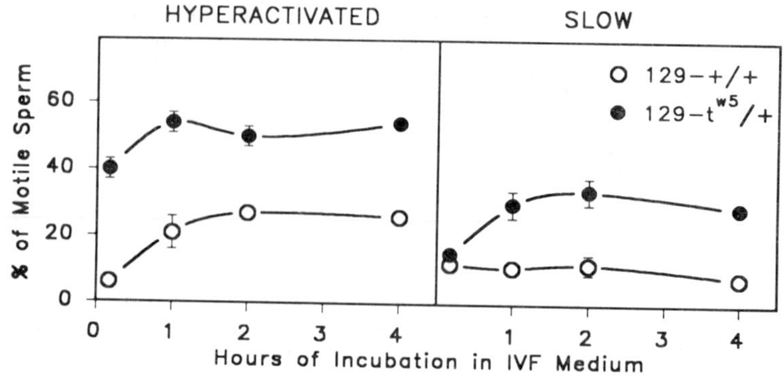

FIGURE 4. The mean ± SEM percent of hyperactivated and slow sperm from +/+ and $t^{w5}/+$ males of the 129 strain. Curvilinear velocity at 30 frames/sec (VCL) and linearity (LIN) were determined by the Hamilton-Thorn Motility Analyser. Hyperactivated sperm were defined as those with VCL >115 μm/sec and LIN < 42; slow sperm were defined as those with VCL between 20 and 115 μm/sec. Error bars not shown are smaller than the symbol.

fore an elevated level of spontaneous acrosome reactions is not a general characteristic of *t* haplotypes.

A decrease in progressiveness of motile sperm is characteristic of all *t* haplotypes thus far examined. We found that the progressive or straight-line velocity of *t*/+ sperm was significantly lower than that of congenic wild-type sperm, and that of t^x/t^y sperm was hardly measurable.[51] This was also true for sperm recovered from the uterus (TABLE 2). Recently we showed that nonprogressive $t^{w32}/+$ sperm from the male tract are of two types: some are prematurely hyperactivated, while others have abnormally low curvilinear velocities.[50] We have now repeated these experiments with $t^{w5}/+$ sperm, using the Hamilton-Thorn Motility Analyser (Hamilton-Thorn Research, Inc., Danvers, MA). As with $t^{w32}/+$ sperm, the large majority of $t^{w5}/+$ sperm are either prematurely hyperactivated, or slow (FIG. 4). Thus several types of nonprogressive motility may be characteristic of sperm populations from mice carrying one *t* haplotype, while all t^x/t^y sperm are slow.

TABLE 2. Effect of the *t* Complex on Uterine Sperm Motility

Male Genotype	No. of Sperm ($\times 10^6$)[a]	% Motile	% Slow[b]	% Progressive[b]
F1-+/+[c]	4.8 ± 0.9	76 ± 7	9 ± 3	91 ± 3
F1-$t^{w32}/+$	4.6 ± 0.3	78 ± 6	44 ± 9[d]	56 ± 9[d]
F1-t^{w32}/t^0	1.8 ± 1.0[e]	51 ± 7[e]	100 —[e]	0 —[e]

[a] Recovered one hour post-coitus.

[b] Motile sperm with a curvilinear velocity (VCL) <170 μm/sec were considered slow; progressive sperm were defined as those motile sperm with a VCL >170 μm/sec and a linearity >34 (data reanalyzed from Olds-Clarke, Biol. Reprod. **34:** 453, 1986; mean VCL of +/+ uterine sperm = 223 μm/sec).

[c] Five males of each genotype were tested, all of the (C3HXC57BL/6)F1 hybrid strain.

[d] Significantly different from F1-+/+ (Wilcoxon test, $p < 0.05$).

[e] Significantly different from F1-+/+ and F1-$t^{w32}/+$ (Wilcoxon test, $p < 0.05$).

The slow motility of some $t/+$ and all t^x/t^y sperm could explain their defective function in fertilization *in vivo*. Progressive motility is thought to be important in sperm transport through the female genital tract.[52] When sperm were recovered from the uteri of females mated to congenic $+/+$, $t/+$ or t^x/t^y males, at one hour post-coitus few sperm were hyperactivated. Therefore virtually all motile $+/+$ sperm were progressive, while only half the motile $t/+$ sperm and none of the t^x/t^y sperm were progressive (TABLE 2). This correlates well with the numbers of sperm reaching the oviduct (reduced for $t/+$ sperm and virtually nil for t^x/t^y sperm) and suggests that the slow motility of these sperm could keep them from reaching the oviduct, thus preventing them from participating in fertilization *in vivo*.

It is not known whether either premature hyperactivation or slow swimming speeds alters $t/+$ sperm transport through the egg investments. Motility cannot be the only sperm function affected by the *t* complex, however. As mentioned previously, t^x/t^y sperm are unable to penetrate zona-free oocytes. Since this function is not dependent on motility,[53] it seems likely that the *t* complex also contains factors affecting sperm-egg fusion.

THE *t* COMPLEX CAUSES INCREASED FLAGELLAR SENSITIVITY TO CALCIUM

The premature hyperactivation of $t/+$ sperm may be dependent on a specific flagellar curvature resembling a fishhook. This severe curvature within the midpiece is apparent during part of the beat cycle of hyperactivated rodent sperm, *e.g.*, hamster sperm at the zona surface[52] and mouse sperm recovered from the oviduct,[54] suggesting that it may be one component of hyperactivation. The fishhook was much more prevalent among motile $t^{w32}/+$ sperm, which hyperactivate prematurely, than in congenic wild-type sperm.[55]

The fishhook in both wild-type and mutant sperm is controlled by the action of calcium ions (Ca^{2+}) on some flagellar component. Concentrations of Ca^{2+} above 10^{-5} M induce the fishhook in the flagella of Triton X-100-extracted, ATP-reactivated rat and mouse sperm.[55,56] Reactivated $t^{w32}/+$ sperm, however, assumed the extreme flagellar curvature at a 10-fold lower Ca^{2+} concentration than congenic wild-type sperm.[55] Intact sperm also exhibit abnormal flagellar curvature. After prolonged incubation in Ca^{2+}, the entire flagellum of some motile $t/+$ sperm curl up; a similar "curlique" is assumed by motile t^x/t^y sperm immediately after release from the male tract (FIG. 5).

These observations suggest that the *t* complex alters some flagellar component that interacts with Ca^{2+}. The altered interaction results in an abnormal flagellar conformation which in turn could be the cause of the premature hyperactivation. Ca^{2+} can affect flagellar movement by its interaction with calmodulin,[57] by activating enzymes controlling cAMP levels,[58] or through both of these pathways.[59] It remains to be determined how the *t* complex alters Ca^{2+} control of flagellar movement.

SUMMARY OF THE *t* COMPLEX

Our working hypothesis is that in $t/+$ males, *Tcd* mutations cause potential defects in sperm motility and ability to penetrate oocytes. The *Tcr* product, synthesized in

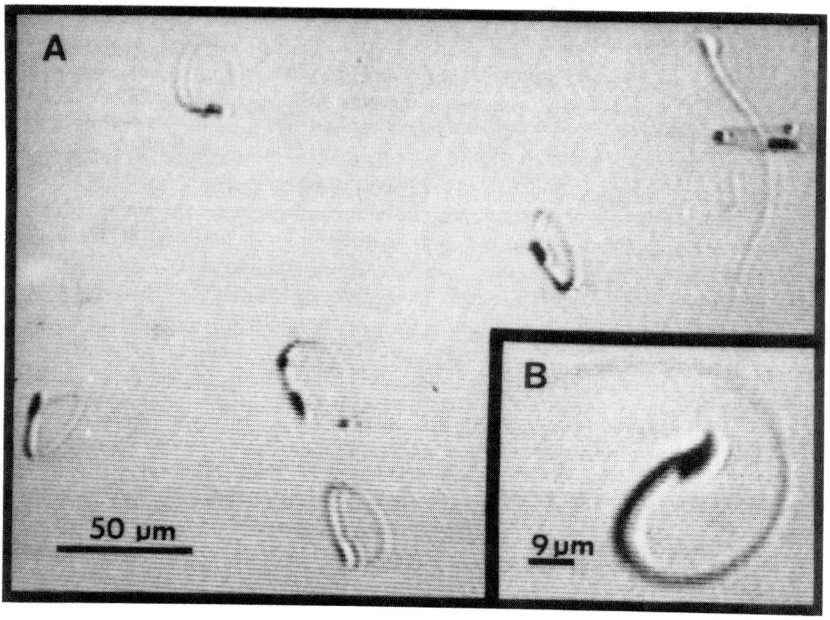

FIGURE 5. Mutant sperm flagellar curvature. A: Frame from videotape of sperm from a t^{w32}/t^{w5} male, immediately after isolation in medium with 1.7 mM calcium. Flagella of motile cells are curled, while the nonmotile flagellum remains straight. B: Frame from videotape of sperm from a $t^{w5}/+$ male incubated 4 hours in 1.7 mM calcium, showing a flagellar curvature similar to that seen in A.

t spermatids, somehow mitigates these defects; therefore only + sperm have difficulties in reaching and penetrating the egg. Sperm produced by t^x/t^y males have no normal alleles at *Tcd* loci, and thus show such severe defects in motility and egg-penetrating ability that even *Tcr* is unable to "rescue" these sperm. While it is likely that *Tcp-10* is the gene representing *Tcr*, *Tcd* genes and their functions are as yet unknown. The gene (or genes) altering motility is a candidate for the distal *Tcd* factor, since the non-progressive motility maps to this region of the *t* complex.[51] The major challenge for future studies is to identify the *Tcd* factors and fill the gap between results obtained with the traditional genetic approach and those obtained by "reverse genetics."

While the inversions which link these genes are unique to mice, it is likely that genes homologous to *Tcr* and *Tcd* are found in other mammalian species. A sequence homologous to *Tcp-10* exists in the human genome.[26] *Tcp-1* and four other genes located within the wild-type homologue of the *t* complex region have equivalents on human chromosome 6,[60] suggesting that many homologous genes in the *t* complex region have been retained during the evolution of mammals. Thus an understanding of the *t* complex could increase our knowledge of the genes needed for human sperm function.

MOUSE MUTATIONS PROVIDE INSIGHT INTO NORMAL SPERM FUNCTION IN FERTILIZATION

The mouse is an excellent model system for identifying and characterizing genes controlling sperm function in mammals, because of the extensive knowledge of the genetics of this species and because the gametes are easily manipulated *in vivo* and *in vitro*. Mutations altering sperm function in fertilization and cloned genes expressed during spermiogenesis have been identified. We must now seek to determine the molecular defects underlying the mutations and to understand how the products of the cloned genes affect sperm function. Advances in molecular gene technology combined with classic genetic analysis and tests of sperm function in mutant and transgenic mice can provide novel insight into systems regulating sperm function in fertilization.

ACKNOWLEDGMENTS

The author is grateful to Robin Sego and Roger Montemayor for their expert technical assistance, and to Dr. Lee Silver for mating pairs of 129-t^{w5}/+ mice.

REFERENCES

1. HUANG, B. P. 1986. *Chlamydomonas reinhardtii*: A model system for the genetic analysis of flagellar structure and motility. Int. Rev. Cytol. **99:** 181–216.
2. OLDS-CLARKE, P. 1988. Genetic analysis of sperm function in fertilization. Gam. Res. **20:** 241–264.
3. OLDS-CLARKE, P. 1990. Genetic analysis of sperm motility. *In* Controls of Sperm Motility: Biological and Clinical Aspects. G. Gagnon, Ed.: 43–52. CRC Press. Boca Raton, FL.
4. KOEFOED-JOHNSEN, H. H., J. B. ANDERSEN, E. ANDRESEN, E. BLOM & H. PHILIPSEN. 1980. The Dag defect of the tail of the bull sperm. Theriogenology **14:** 471–476.
5. HANDEL, M. A. 1987. Genetic control of spermatogenesis in mice. *In* Results and Problems in Cell Differentiation, W. Hennig, Ed. Vol. **15:** 1–62. Springer-Verlag. Berlin.
6. CHUBB, C. 1989. Genetically defined mouse models of male infertility. J. Androl. **10:** 77–88.
7. DOOLITTLE, D. P., M. T. DAVISSON, T. H. RODERICK & A. L. HILLYARD. 1990. The locus map of the mouse. Mouse Genome **87:** 14–27.
8. AVNER, P., L. AMAR, L. DANDOLO & J. L. GUENET. 1988. Genetic analysis of the mouse using interspecific crosses. Trends Genet. **4:** 18–23.
9. COMMITTEE FOR MOUSE CHROMOSOME 17. 1991. Maps of mouse chromosome 17: First report. Mamm. Genome **1:** 5–29.
10. HECHT, N. B. 1990. Regulation of 'haploid expressed genes' in male germ cells. J. Reprod. Fertil. **88:** 679–693.
11. WITTE, O. N. 1990. *Steel* locus defines new multipotent growth factor. Cell **63:** 5–6.
12. COLE, A., M. L. MEISTRICH, L. M. CHERRY & P. K. TROSTLE-WEIGE. 1988. Nuclear and manchette development in spermatids of normal and *azh/azh* mutant mice. Biol. Reprod. **38:** 385–401.
13. HUGENHOLTZ, A. P. 1984. Mouse News Lett. **71:** 34–35.
14. KOT, M. C. & M. A. HANDEL. 1987. Binding of morphologically abnormal sperm to mouse egg zonae pellucidae in vitro. Gamete Res. **18:** 57–66.
15. OLDS-CLARKE, P., H. M. BAER & W. L. GERBER. 1990. Human sperm motion analysis by automatic (Hamilton-Thorn Motility Analyser) and manual (Image–80) digitization systems. J. Androl. **11:** 52–58.
16. HOLLAND, M. K. & M.-C. ORGEBIN-CRIST. 1988. Epididymal protein synthesis and secretion in strains of mice bearing single gene mutations which affect fertility. Biol. Reprod. **38:** 497–510.
17. GORDON, J. W., J. UEHLINGER, N. DAYANI, B. E. TALANSKY, M. GORDON, G. S. RUDOMEN

& P. E. NEUMANN. 1990. Analysis of the *hotfoot* (*ho*) locus by creation of an insertional mutation in a transgenic mouse. Dev. Biol. **137:** 349–358.
18. SILVER, L. 1987. Mouse *t* haplotypes: A tale of tails and a misunderstood selfish chromosome. Curr. Top. Microbiol. Immunol. **137:** 64–69.
19. HAMMER, M. F., J. SCHIMENTI & L. M. SILVER. 1989. Evolution of mouse chromosome 17 and the origin of inversions associated with *t* haplotypes. Proc. Natl. Acad. Sci. USA **86:** 3261–3265.
20. OLDS-CLARKE, P. & B. PEITZ. 1985. Fertility of sperm from *t*/+ mice: Evidence that +-bearing sperm are dysfunctional. Genet. Res. **47:** 49–52.
21. LYON, M. F. 1986. Male sterility of the mouse *t*-complex is due to homozygosity of the distorter genes. Cell **44:** 357–363.
22. LYON, M. F. 1987. Distorter genes of the mouse *t*-complex impair male fertility when heterozygous. Genet. Res. **49:** 57–60.
23. DUTCHER, S. K. & F. G. LUX. 1989. Genetic interactions of mutations affecting flagella and basal bodies in *Chlamydomonas.* Cell Motil. Cytoskel. **14:** 104–117.
24. SCHIMENTI, J., J. A. CEBRA-THOMAS, C. L. DECKER, S. D. ISLAM, S. H. PILDER & L. M. SILVER. 1988. A candidate gene family for the mouse *t complex responder* (*Tcr*) locus responsible for haploid effects on sperm function. Cell **55:** 71–78.
25. ROSEN, L. L., D. C. BULLARD, L. M. SILVER & J. C. SCHIMENTI. 1990. Molecular cloning of the *t complex responder* genetic locus. Genomics **8:** 134–140.
26. CEBRA-THOMAS, J. A., C. L. DECKER, L. C. SNYDER, S. H. PILDER & L. M. SILVER. 1991. An allele- and haploid-specific product generated by alternative splicing from a mouse *t complex responder* locus candidate. Nature **349:** 239–241.
27. RAPPOLD, G. A., L. STUBBS, S. LABEIT, R. B. CRKVENJAKOV & H. LEHRACH. 1987. Identification of a testis-specific gene from the mouse *t*-complex next to a CpG-rich island. EMBO J. **6:** 1975–1980.
28. SORRENTINO, V., M. D. MCKINNEY, M. GIORGI, R. GEREMIA & E. FLEISSNER. 1988. Expression of cellular proto-oncogenes in the mouse male germ line: A distinctive 2.4-kilobase *pim-1* transcript is expressed in haploid postmeiotic cells. Proc. Natl. Acad. Sci. USA **85:** 2191–2195.
29. LADER, E., H.-S. HA, M. O'NEIL, K. ARTZT & D. BENNETT. 1989. *tctex-1*: A candidate gene family for a mouse *t* complex sterility locus. Cell **58:** 969–979.
30. MAZARAKIS, N. D., D. NELKI, M. F. LYON, S. RUDDY, E. P. EVANS, P. FREEMONT & K. DUDLEY. 1991. Isolation and characterization of a testis-expressed developmentally regulated gene from the distal inversion of the mouse *t*-complex. Development **111:** 561–571.
31. SILVER, L. M., K. C. KLEENE, R. J. DISTEL & N. B. HECHT. 1987. Synthesis of mouse *t* complex proteins during haploid stages of spermatogenesis. Dev. Biol. **119:** 605–608.
32. GUPTA, R. S. 1990. Sequence and structural homology between a mouse *t* complex protein TCP-1 and the 'chaperonin' family of bacterial (GroEL, 60–65 kDa heat shock antigen) and eukaryotic proteins. Biochem. Int. **20:** 833–841.
33. URSIC, D. & B. GANETZKY. 1988. A *Drosophila melanogaster* gene encodes a protein homologous to the mouse *t* complex polypeptide 1. Gene **68:** 267–274.
34. LI, H., U. B. GYLLENSTEN, X. CUI, R. K. SAIKI, H. A. ERLICH & N. ARNHEIM. 1988. Amplification and analysis of DNA sequences in single human sperm and diploid cells. Nature **335:** 414–417.
35. OLDS-CLARKE, P. 1986. Motility characteristics of sperm from the uterus and oviducts of female mice after mating to congenic males differing in sperm transport and fertility. Biol. Reprod. **34:** 453–467.
36. OLDS, P. 1970. Effect of the T locus on sperm distribution in the house mouse. Biol. Reprod. **2:** 91–97.
37. TESSLER, S. & P. OLDS-CLARKE. 1981. Male genotype influences sperm transport in female mice. Biol. Reprod. **24:** 806–813.
38. OLDS, P. 1971. Effect of the T locus on fertilization in the house mouse. J. Exp. Zool. **177:** 417–434.
39. MCGRATH, J. & N. HILLMAN. 1980. Sterility in mutant (t^{Lx}/t^{Ly}) male mice. III. In vitro fertilization. J. Embryol. Exp. Morphol. **59:** 49–58.
40. AHMAD, T., J. C. CONOVER, M. N. QUIGLEY, R. L. COLLINS, A. J. THOMAS, JR. & R. B. L. GWATKIN. 1989. Failure of spermatozoa from T/t mice to fertilize in vitro is overcome by zona drilling. Gamete Res. **22:** 369–373.

41. McGrath, J. & H. Hillman. 1980. The *in vitro* transmission frequency of the t^{12} mutation in the mouse. J. Embryol. Exp. Morphol. **60:** 141–151.
42. Garside, W. & N. Hillman. 1989. The *in vivo* and *in vitro* transmission frequencies of the t^{w5}-haplotype in mice. Genet. Res. **53:** 21–24.
43. Olds-Clarke, P. & S. McCabe. 1981. Genetic background affects expression of *t* haplotype in mouse sperm. Genet. Res. **40:** 249–254.
44. Macek, M. B. & B. D. Shur. 1988. Protein-carbohydrate complementarity in mammalian gamete recognition. Gamete Res. **20:** 93–109.
45. Benau, D. A. & B. T. Storey. 1988. Relationship between two types of mouse sperm surface sites that mediate binding of sperm to the zona pellucida. Biol. Reprod. **39:** 235–244.
46. Olds-Clarke, P. 1990. Variation in the quality of sperm motility and its relationship to capacitation. *In* Fertilization in Mammals. B. Bavister, J. Cummins & E. Roldan, Eds. Serono Symposium USA. Norwell, MA.
47. Shur, B. D. & D. Bennett. 1979. A specific defect in galactosyltransferase regulation on sperm bearing mutant alleles of the T/t locus. Dev. Biol. **71:** 243–259.
48. Shur, B. D. 1990. Galactosyltransferase activities on mouse sperm bearing multiple t^{lethal} and t^{viable} haplotypes of the T/t-complex. Genet. Res. **38:** 225–236.
49. Brown, J., J. A. Cebra-Thomas, J. D. Bleil, P. M. Wassarman & L. M. Silver. 1989. A premature acrosome reaction is programmed by mouse *t* haplotypes during sperm differentiation and could play a role in transmission ratio distortion. Development **106:** 769–773.
50. Olds-Clarke, P. 1989. Sperm from $t^{w32}/+$ mice: capacitation is normal, but hyperactivation is premature and nonhyperactivated sperm are slow. Dev. Biol. **131:** 475–482.
51. Olds-Clarke, P. 1983. Nonprogressive sperm motility is characteristic of most complete *t* haplotypes in the mouse. Genet. Res. **42:** 151–157.
52. Katz, D. F., E. Z. Drobnis & J. W. Overstreet. 1989. Factors regulating mammalian sperm migration through the female reproductive tract and oocyte investments. Gamete Res. **22:** 443–469.
53. Aitken, R. J., A. Ross & M. M. Lees. 1983. Analysis of sperm function in Kartagener's syndrome. Fertil. Steril. **40:** 696–698.
54. Phillips, D. M. 1972. Comparative analysis of mammalian sperm motility. J. Cell Biol. **53:** 561–573.
55. Lindemann, C. B., J. S. Goltz, K. S. Kanous, T. K. Gardner & P. Olds-Clarke. 1990. Evidence for an increased sensitivity to Ca^{2+} in the flagella of sperm from $t^{w32}/+$ mice. Mol. Reprod. Dev. **26:** 69–77.
56. Lindemann, C. B. & J. S. Goltz. 1988. Calcium regulation of flagellar curvature and swimming pattern in Triton X-100 extracted rat sperm. Cell Motil. Cytoskel. **10:** 420–431.
57. Otter, T. 1989. Calmodulin and the control of flagellar movement. *In* Cell Movement. F. D. Warner & J. R. McIntosh, Eds. Vol. **1:** 91–109. Alan R. Liss, Inc. New York.
58. Brokaw, C. J. 1987. Regulation of sperm flagellar motility by calcium and cAMP-dependent phosphorylation. J. Cell Biochem. **35:** 175–184.
59. Lindemann, C. B. & K. S. Kanous. 1989. Regulation of mammalian sperm motility. Arch. Androl. **23:** 1–22.
60. Nadeau, J., P. Grant & M. Kosowsky. 1990. Man on mouse homology map. Mouse Genome **87:** 59.

Sperm Proteins That Serve as Receptors for the Zona Pellucida and Their Post-Testicular Modification[a]

DIANA G. MYLES[b] AND PAUL PRIMAKOFF[b]

Department of Physiology
University of Connecticut Health Center
Farmington, Connecticut 06030

INTRODUCTION

Cell adhesion occurs at many developmental stages of a multicellular organism and may take the form of cell-cell adhesion or adhesion between cells and the extracellular matrix. Some cell adhesions are stable and act to form tissues, while others are transitory such as those that occur during activation of the immune system. An early step in mammalian fertilization is an adhesion step between the sperm surface and an extracellular coat, the zona pellucida, that surrounds the oocyte. Sperm binding must be transient, allowing the sperm to unbind and pass through the zona pellucida so the gamete membranes can come into contact with each other and fuse. How the unbinding is accomplished is not known.

In *in vitro* assays, sperm bind to the zona pellucida both before and after they acrosome react. The sperm of many species tested, including chinese hamster,[1] rabbit,[2] guinea pig,[3] and human,[4] can initiate binding to the zona whether they are acrosome-intact or acrosome-reacted. In mouse, however, it appears that only acrosome-intact sperm are able to initiate binding (see refs. 5 & 6 for review) and that acrosome-reacted sperm only bind after the sperm acrosome react on the zona pellucida.[7,8] This may reflect a required processing step for either the receptor on acrosome-reacted sperm or for the zona ligand that occurs when mouse sperm are bound to the zona during the acrosome reaction. Evidence indicates that the ligands and receptors may be different for acrosome-intact and acrosome-reacted sperm.[3,4,9]

It has been shown that the binding of acrosome-intact sperm to the zona pellucida can result in the induction of the sperm acrosome reaction.[5,10] The ligand-receptor interaction that initiates sperm exocytosis could be the same as or different from the interaction that is responsible for the binding of acrosome-intact sperm to the zona.[11]

[a] Research discussed from this laboratory, including unpublished data, was supported by National Institutes of Health Grants HD16580 and HD21989.

[b] Tel. (203) 679-2846; FAX (203) 679-1269.

IDENTIFICATION OF SPERM RECEPTORS FOR THE ZONA PELLUCIDA

A major focus in understanding the molecular bases of these phenomena is identification of the sperm surface molecules that are involved in sperm-zona adhesion. TABLE 1 lists approaches that could be used to identify the sperm receptors for zona proteins. Many of these approaches have been taken and a variety of sperm surface molecules have been identified that are implicated in sperm-zona binding (for recent reviews see refs. 5, 6, 11 & 12). These molecules may either be cell adhesion molecules that bind directly to the zona glycoproteins or they could be accessory molecules that are required for cell adhesion, but do not directly interact with the zona.

Because many different candidate sperm proteins have been identified by a variety of techniques, in several different species, certain questions are raised about these proteins. Are there multiple adhesion molecules on a sperm surface that bind to the zona? Are the cell adhesion molecules shared by sperm of many species or do the sperm of each mammalian species have different sperm adhesion molecules for the zona? In many cases sperm-zona adhesion is species specific, but adhesion of sperm to the zona of heterologous species can occur.[1,3,13]

It is also possible that not all of the candidate sperm proteins will prove to be cell adhesion molecules. The criteria applied so far to show that any individual sperm protein has a role in zona binding vary among the different studies. One of the most thoroughly investigated sperm surface receptors is the mouse surface protein, galactosyltransferase (GalTase). GalTase has been demonstrated to be a sperm cell adhesion molecule by a variety of experiments. The enzymatic activity of this adhesion protein has been taken advantage of to do experiments in which sperm-egg binding was inhibited by blocking or altering the transferase activity on the sperm or blocking or removing GalTase binding sites on the zona pellucida (reviewed in refs. 12 & 14). In addition, purified sperm surface GalTase, when pre-incubated with eggs, inhibits sperm binding.[15] As with GalTase, the strongest evidence that a protein is actually a cell adhesion molecule will be gained by using a combination of experiments. For cell adhesion molecules that do not have enzymatic activity a different set of experiments must be used. In other systems, cell adhesion molecules have been commonly identified and positively confirmed as cell adhesion molecules by a combination of the following criteria (for examples, see ref. 16). 1) Monoclonal antibodies (mAbs)

TABLE 1. Approaches to the Identification of Sperm Receptor Molecules for the Zona Pellucida

A. Inhibition studies
   1. Antibody inhibition
   2. Inhibition of molecular activity (*e.g.*, enzyme activity)
   3. Competition with purified ligand or receptor

B. Molecular alteration
   1. Chemical alteration of ligand or receptor
   2. Molecular "knock out" experiments to eliminate functional molecules

C. Demonstration of interactions
   1. With intact gametes (*e.g.*, crosslinking)
   2. *In vitro* interactions of purified components

or polyclonal antibodies to the protein are able to inhibit cell adhesion. 2) Purified protein will bind to the surface of target cells and prevent cell adhesion. The binding of the purified protein can be inhibited by the same antibodies that block cell-cell adhesion. 3) Heterologous cells, transfected with the appropriate cDNA and expressing the candidate protein, will bind to the target cell and antibody to the protein will inhibit this binding. Such a combination of criteria has so far not been applied to putative sperm cell adhesion molecules, but the use of such criteria would provide a clear demonstration of the function of a cell adhesion molecule in zona binding.

PH-20 AS A PROTEIN REQUIRED FOR BINDING OF ACROSOME-REACTED GUINEA PIG SPERM TO THE ZONA PELLUCIDA

The sperm surface protein, PH-20, has been demonstrated to have a required role in binding of acrosome-reacted guinea pig sperm to the zona pellucida[17] and homologues of the PH-20 gene are present in other mammalian species (mouse, rat, hamster, rabbit, bovine, monkey and human).[18] Initial identification of PH-20 as a protein required for guinea pig sperm-zona binding came from inhibition studies using monoclonal antibodies.[17] Three different mAbs were used; all three recognize the PH-20 protein, bind to the surface of sperm at the same level, and are of the same antibody class (IgG_1). The PH-22 mAb had no effect on zona binding (even at concentrations of 50 μg/ml of purified antibody), but the PH-20 mAb inhibited acrosome-reacted sperm binding up to 90% in a dose-dependent manner, with half maximal inhibition occurring at 2 μg/ml of purified antibody. (The third mAb, PH-21, gave an intermediate level of inhibition.) Several different polyclonal antibodies, and their Fab fragments, directed against affinity-purified PH-20 protein, also show high levels of inhibition of zona binding *in vitro* (ref. 20 and our unpublished results). In *in vivo* experiments, female guinea pigs, injected with purified PH-20 protein, became completely infertile during the period when antibody titers remained high.[19] Because the PH-20 protein is anchored in the membrane via glycosylphosphatidylinositol (GPI), it has been possible to release a major fraction of the protein from acrosome-reacted sperm using the phosphatidylinositol specific phospholipase C.[20] Acrosome-reacted sperm, treated with the enzyme, remain normally motile, but are inhibited from binding to the zona (our unpublished results).

A cDNA for PH-20 has been cloned and sequenced.[18] The mature protein is a single polypeptide of 468 amino acids and has six potential N-linked glycosylation sites, and twelve cysteine residues. It is endoproteolytically cleaved, at or near amino acid 290, into two polypeptides that are held together by at least one disulfide bond. PH-20 is a novel protein and does not have significant homology with known sequences. Current studies are aimed at testing its putative function as a sperm cell adhesion molecule or if it has some other activity in zona binding.

ALTERATION OF ZONA PROTEIN RECEPTORS IN PREPARATION FOR BINDING ACTIVITY

Apparently sperm do not exit the testis with an innate ability to bind to the zona pellucida and to fertilize eggs.[21] Besides changes in sperm motility, changes in the sperm surface are generally thought to be required (for review see refs. 22 & 23). These modifications may occur in both the male reproductive tract (during epididymal maturation) and in the female reproductive tract (during capacitation). Further modifications may be required for binding of acrosome-reacted sperm that might accompany the acrosome reaction itself.

Required surface modifications could fall into several different categories. Fertilization may require the addition of zona receptors to the sperm cell. Alternatively, the receptors may be present on immature sperm, but require either the removal of inhibitors or activation. After washing, mouse caput sperm are able to bind to the zona pellucida at 80% of the level of immobilized cauda sperm. This result is consistent with the finding that the GalTase is present on caput sperm and that washing removes inhibitors to GalTase activity.[24] It is also possible that existing receptor molecules must be processed or modified in some way on the surface before they become (fully) functional.[23] Modifications that occur to the guinea pig sperm surface protein, PH-20, have been studied in detail and will be discussed here as a model system in studying posttesticular changes that modify a protein that functions in zona binding.

Although PH-20 protein is associated with the guinea pig sperm surface when it leaves the testis, it undergoes a series of modifications, both during epididymal maturation and the acrosome reaction that may result in its activation (TABLE 2). Changes in the pattern of localization and in the level of surface expression occur both during epididymal maturation and following the acrosome reaction and result in increased surface density in particular regions of the surface. In other cell adhesion systems it has been shown that adhesion can be regulated by receptor density (for examples see refs. 16 & 25). During epididymal maturation, PH-20 protein loses its whole cell distribution, and becomes limited to just the posterior head surface.[26] At least part of this change in localization can be accounted for by the migration of PH-20 protein out of other region(s) into the posterior head domain resulting in a twofold increase in site density in the posterior head region.[27] An increase in site density also occurs for the GalTase receptor during epididymal passage. The fact that GalTase is only at 60% of its final density on caput sperm[28] has been suggested as an explanation for the lower binding of caput sperm (80%) compared to immobilized cauda sperm even after washing of the sperm.[24]

TABLE 2. Post-Testicular Changes in PH-20 Protein before Fertilization

	Epididymal Maturation	Acrosome Reaction	References
Localization	Whole cell becomes posterior head	Posterior head to inner acrosomal membrane	26, 29
Level of expression	Increase to 200% of testicular in the posterior head	Increase to 250% of surface expression on acrosome-intact	27, 30
Diffusion coefficient	10-fold increase from testicular	10-fold increase (100-fold from testicular)	20, 33
Post-translational processing	2 kD decrease in M_r	Endoproteolytic cleavage into two fragments	27, 36

A second migration and concentration of PH-20 protein occurs after the acrosome reaction, when PH-20 moves out of the posterior head domain into the inner acrosomal membrane (IAM) after these membrane domains become contiguous during the acrosome reaction.[29] There the migrating population of PH-20 protein joins a second population of PH-20 that is associated with the inner acrosomal membrane and therefore is revealed by the acrosome reaction. This increases the level of surface expression by about 2.5-fold what it was prior to the acrosome reaction, and increases the IAM population by about 163% of what it would be if no migration from the posterior head occurred.[30]

The migration of PH-20 not only changes the surface density, but also puts PH-20 in a new position on the surface at a time when it functions in the binding of acrosome-reacted sperm. Two other proteins, implicated in sperm-zona binding, change their pattern of surface localization during capacitation (2B1[31]) or after the acrosome reaction (GalTase[32]). The relocalization of the PH-20 protein brings it into a surface domain (IAM) where it is in the appropriate position to function in the binding of acrosome-reacted sperm. The migration of 2B1 during capacitation from the tail to the anterior head also brings it into the correct position to participate in the binding of acrosome-intact sperm to the zona. GalTase, that participates in the binding of acrosome-intact sperm to the zona, migrates after the acrosome reaction from the anterior head to the equatorial region and by its migration could actually act to give the sperm a push forward to begin penetration of the zona.

There is also an increase in the diffusion coefficient (the rate at which a protein diffuses) of the PH-20 protein at two stages in sperm maturation. During epididymal maturation the surface population, measured in the head plasma membrane, increased from $D = (1.9 \pm 0.31) \times 10^{-11}$ cm^2/sec to $D = (1.8 \pm 0.5) \times 10^{-10}$ cm^2/sec, an approximate 10-fold increase.[20,33] After the acrosome reaction, the total surface population of PH-20 (composed of the pre-existing IAM population and the migrated posterior head population) has a $D = (1.7 \pm 0.5) \times 10^{-9}$ cm^2/sec, approximately an additional 10-fold increase.[33] The total increase, therefore, in diffusion rate of surface PH-20 from testicular to acrosome-reacted sperm is about 100-fold. The free diffusion measured for PH-20 on acrosome-reacted sperm is consistent with the fact that it is anchored in the membrane with a lipid (GPI) anchor.[20] This increase in mobility of the PH-20 protein during sperm maturation and after the acrosome reaction is consistent with the idea of an increase in PH-20 protein activity in cell adhesion. Increased diffusion of cell adhesion molecules can promote cell adhesion by shortening the "catch" time between the initial binding of receptor and ligand and the time required for the formation of additional bonds through the redistribution of receptors into the contact region.[34,35]

PH-20 protein undergoes posttranslational modifications during both epididymal maturation and the acrosome reaction. PH-20 is made as a glycosylated single polypeptide chain and when immunoprecipitated from surface-labeled testicular sperm runs on reducing SDS-PAGE at 66 kD. It undergoes at least two processing steps. First during epididymal passage it is reduced to a size of 64 kD.[27] The second processing step is an endoproteolytic cleavage that generates two protein fragments held together by disulfide bond(s), so that when the protein is run on reducing SDS-PAGE it separates into two bands at 41–48 kD and 27 kD.[36] Although this second processing step may begin during epididymal passage, the bulk of this endoproteolytic cleavage occurs at the time of the acrosome reaction.[27,36] Post-translational modification is another possible way in which PH-20 protein function could be controlled. Proteolytic processing may activate an inactive form of the protein and in fact, proteolytic processing is a common means of regulation of protein function (for a review see ref. 37), including the proteolytic processing of cell adhesion molecules (for example see ref. 38).

SUMMARY AND CONCLUSIONS

The search for molecules on the surface of mammalian sperm that are responsible for the binding of sperm to the zona pellucida has led to the identification of a number of different surface proteins. Different experimental approaches have been used to identify these proteins and the strength of the evidence for their putative role in zona binding is therefore quite variable. In this paper we have discussed some of the approaches that are used to identify cell adhesion molecules and criteria that might be applied in future research. Further research will be required to answer questions as to whether multiple surface antigens are involved in zona binding and if the sperm receptors for the zona are conserved among species. Both of these results would be expected based on what is known about cell adhesion in other systems. We have also discussed the modifications that occur to surface proteins after the sperm leave the testis and how these modifications can potentially activate or increase the efficiency of the function of a protein in zona binding.

REFERENCES

1. Yanagimachi, R. 1981. Mechanisms of fertilization in mammals. *In* Fertilization and Embryonic Development *In Vitro.* L. Mastroianni, Jr. & J. D. Biggers, Eds.: 81–182. Plenum Publishing Corp. New York.
2. Kuzan, F. B., A. D. Fleming & G. E. Seidel, Jr. 1984. Successful fertilization *in vitro* of fresh intact oocytes by perivitelline (acrosome-reacted) spermatozoa of the rabbit. Fertil. Steril. **41:** 766–770.
3. Myles, D. G., H. Hyatt & P. Primakoff. 1987. Binding of both acrosome-intact and acrosome-reacted guinea pig sperm to the zona pellucida during in vitro fertilization. Dev. Biol. **121:** 559–567.
4. Morales, P., N. L. Cross, J. W. Overstreet & F. W. Hanson. 1989. Acrosome intact and acrosome-reacted human sperm can initiate binding to the zona pellucida. Dev. Biol. **133:** 385–392.
5. Saling, P. M. 1989. Mammalian sperm interaction with extracellular matrices of the egg. *In* Oxford Reviews of Reproductive Biology. S. R. Milligan, Ed. Vol. **11:** 339–388. Oxford University Press. Oxford.
6. Jones, R. 1990. Identification and functions of mammalian sperm-egg recognition molecules during fertilization. J. Reprod. Fertil. Suppl. **42:** 89–105.
7. Saling, P. M. & B. T. Storey. 1979. Mouse gamete interactions during fertilization in vitro. J. Cell Biol. **83:** 544–555.
8. Bleil, J. D., J. M. Greve & P. M. Wassarman. 1988. Identification of a secondary sperm receptor in the mouse egg zona pellucida: Role in maintenance of binding of acrosome-reacted sperm to eggs. Dev. Biol. **128:** 376–385.
9. Bleil, J. D. & P. W. Wassarman. 1990. Identification of a ZP3-binding protein on acrosome-intact mouse sperm by photoaffinity crosslinking. Proc. Natl. Acad. Sci. USA **87:** 5563–5567.
10. Bleil, J. C. & P. M. Wassarman. 1983. Sperm-egg interactions in the mouse: Sequence of events and induction of the acrosome reaction by a zona pellucida glycoprotein. Dev. Biol. **95:** 317–324.
11. Snell, W. J. 1990. Adhesion and signalling during fertilization in multicellular and unicellular organisms. Curr. Opin. Cell Biol. **2:** 821–832.

12. SHUR, B. D. 1989. Glycoconjugates as mediators of cellular interactions during development. Curr. Opin. Cell Biol. **1:** 905–912.
13. HARTMANN, J. F. 1983. Mammalian fertilization: Gamete surface interactions *in vitro. In* Mechanism and Control of Animal Fertilization. J. F. Hartmann, Ed.: 325–364. Academic Press. New York.
14. SHUR, B. D. 1989. Galactosyltransferase as a recognition molecule during fertilization and development. *In* The Molecular Biology of Fertilization. H. Schatten & G. Schatten, Eds.: 37–71. Academic Press. New York.
15. SHUR, B. D. & C. A. NEELY. 1988. Plasma membrane association, purification, and partial characterization of mouse sperm β1,4-galactosyltransferase. J. Biol. Chem. **263:** 17706–17714.
16. SPRINGER, T. A. 1990. The sensation and regulation of interactions with the extracellular environment: The cell biology of lymphocyte adhesion receptors. Ann. Rev. Cell Biol. **6:** 359–402.
17. PRIMAKOFF, P., H. HYATT & D. G. MYLES. 1985. A role for the migrating sperm surface antigen PH-20 in guinea pig sperm binding to the egg zona pellucida. J. Cell Biol. **101:** 2239–2244.
18. LATHROP, W. F., E. P. CARMICHAEL, D. G. MYLES & P. PRIMAKOFF. 1990. cDNA cloning reveals the molecular structure of a sperm surface protein, PH-20, involved in sperm-egg adhesion and the wide distribution of its gene among mammals. J. Cell Biol. **111:** 2939–2949.
19. PRIMAKOFF, P., W. LATHROP, L. WOOLMAN, A. COWAN & D. MYLES. 1988. Fully effective contraception in male and female guinea pigs immunized with sperm protein PH-20. Nature **335:** 543–546.
20. PHELPS, B. M., P. PRIMAKOFF, D. E. KOPPEL, M. G. LOW & D. G. MYLES. 1988. Restricted lateral diffusion of PH-20, a PI-anchored sperm membrane protein. Science **240:** 1780–1782.
21. YANAGIMACHI, R. 1988. Mammalian fertilization. *In* Physiology of Reproduction. E. Knobil & J. Neill, *et al.*, Eds.: 135–185. Raven Press, Ltd. New York.
22. EDDY, E. M., R. B. VERNON, C. H. MULLER, A. C. HAHNEL & B. A. FENDERSON. 1985. Immunodissection of sperm surface modifications during epididymal maturation. Am. J. Anat. **174:** 225–237.
23. MYLES, D. G. 1991. Sperm surface proteins of testicular origin: Expression and localization in the testis and beyond. *In* Cell and Molecular Biology of the Testis. C. Desjardins & L. L. Ewing, Eds. Oxford University Press. Oxford. In press.
24. MCLAUGHLIN, J. D. & B. D. SHUR. 1987. Binding of caput epididymal mouse sperm to the zona pellucida. Dev. Biol. **124:** 557–561.
25. DOHERTY, P., M. FRUNS, P. SEATON, G. DICKSON, C. H. BARTON, T. A. SEARS & F. S. WALSH. 1990. A threshold effect of the major isoforms of NCAM on neurite outgrowth. Nature **343:** 464–466.
26. PHELPS, B. & D. G. MYLES. 1987. The guinea pig sperm plasma membrane protein, PH-20, reaches the surface via two transport pathways and becomes localized to a domain after an initial uniform insertion. Dev. Biol. **123:** 63–72.
27. PHELPS, B. M., D. E. KOPPEL, P. PRIMAKOFF & D. G. MYLES. 1990. Evidence that proteolysis of the surface is an initial step in the mechanism of formation of sperm cell surface domains. J. Cell Biol. **111:** 1839–1847.
28. SCULLY, N. F., J. H. SHAPER & B. D. SHUR. 1987. Spatial and temporal expression of cell surface galactosyltransferase during mouse spermatogenesis and epididymal maturation. Dev. Biol. **124:** 111–124.
29. MYLES, D. G. & P. PRIMAKOFF. 1984. Localized surface antigens of guinea pig sperm migrate to new regions prior to fertilization. J. Cell Biol. **99:** 1634–1641.
30. COWAN, A. E., P. PRIMAKOFF & D. G. MYLES. 1986. Sperm exocytosis increases the amount of PH-20 antigen on the surface of guinea pig sperm. J. Cell Biol. **103:** 1289–1297.
31. JONES, R., R. SHALGI, J. HOYLAND & D. M. PHILLIPS. 1990. Topographical rearrangement of a plasma membrane antigen during capacitation of rat spermatozoa in vitro. Dev. Biol. **139:** 349–362.
32. LOPEZ, L. C. & B. D. SHUR. 1987. Redistribution of mouse sperm surface galactosyltransferase after the acrosome reaction. J. Cell Biol. **105:** 1663–1670.
33. COWAN, A. E., D. G. MYLES & D. E. KOPPEL. 1987. Lateral diffusion of the PH-20 protein on guinea pig sperm: Evidence that barriers to diffusion maintain plasma membrane domains in mammalian sperm. J. Cell Biol. **104:** 917–923.

34. BELL, G. I., M. DEMBO & P. BONGRAND. 1984. Cell adhesion. Competition between nonspecific repulsion and specific bonding. Biophys. J. **45:** 1051–1064.
35. EDIDIN, M. 1987. Rotational and lateral diffusion of membrane proteins and lipids: Phenomena and function. Curr. Top. Membr. Transp. **29:** 91–127.
36. PRIMAKOFF, P., A. E. COWAN, H. HYATT, J. TREDICK-KLINE & D. G. MYLES. 1988. Purification of the guinea pig sperm preparations that cleaves PH-20 into two disulfide-linked fragments. Biol. Reprod. **38:** 921–934.
37. NEURATH, H. 1989. Proteolytic processing and physiological regulation. Trends Biochem. Sci. **14:** 268–271.
38. OZAWA, M. & R. KEMLER. 1990. Correct proteolytic cleavage is required for the cell adhesive function of uvomorulin. J. Cell Biol. **111:** 1645–1650.

Index of Contributors

Subject Index